MEDICAL INVESTIGATION

has proved that every organ in the human body has the capacity to function satisfactorily for a minimum of one hundred years. Dr. Rothenberg tells how you can slow the aging process, increase your life span, and add zest to your later years, with a full coverage of the new discoveries in modern medicine and a definite health program for people over forty.

"Dr. Rothenberg covers virtually the entire field of health in his book, from abscesses to zinc antidotes. The information is given in simple question-and-answer form, and is couched in language anyone can grasp. . . . This strikes me as the most useful and comprehensive guide of its kind currently available."
  —John Barkham, *Saturday Review Syndicate*

"Dr. Rothenberg's explanations, written in a clear, concise manner, bring much-needed and easily understood medical advice to the older person and his family. Altogether this is another worthy and notable achievement by a distinguished colleague."
  —*MD Magazine*

ROBERT E. ROTHENBERG, M.D., is a Diplomate of the American Board of Surgery; a Fellow of the American College of Surgeons; Attending Surgeon at the French and Polyclinic Medical School and Health Center, New York; Attending Surgeon at the Jewish Hospital and Medical Center of Brooklyn; Former Civilian Surgical Consultant to the United States Army Hospital, Fort Jay, New York; and former Member of the Board of Directors of the Health Insurance Plan of Greater New York.

SIGNET Titles of Special Interest

HEALTH IN THE LATER YEARS

REVISED AND UPDATED

including
The Latest Information on
the MEDICARE PROGRAM *and*
SOCIAL SECURITY BENEFITS

ROBERT E. ROTHENBERG,
M.D., F.A.C.S.

Illustrated by
Sylvia and Lester V. Bergman

A SIGNET BOOK from
NEW AMERICAN LIBRARY
TIMES MIRROR

SIGNET TRADEMARK REG. U.S. PAT. OFF. AND FOREIGN COUNTRIES
REGISTERED TRADEMARK—MARCA REGISTRADA
HECHO EN CHICAGO, U.S.A.

SIGNET, SIGNET CLASSICS, SIGNETTE, MENTOR AND PLUME BOOKS
are published by The New American Library, Inc.,
1301 Avenue of the Americas, New York, New York 10019

FIRST PRINTING, APRIL, 1966

PRINTED IN THE UNITED STATES OF AMERICA

TO THE MEMORY OF MY
WONDERFUL FATHER, SIMON,
who remained young throughout
all of his seventy-eight years.

ACKNOWLEDGMENTS

For a manuscript of this scope, one must draw much of his material from the various textbooks on medicine, surgery, and geriatrics. To the authors of these texts, I wish to express my gratitude and my regret that the list of books is so long that it precludes individual mention.

A good deal of credit for the idea of this work goes to Milton S. Fox, the brilliant editor in chief of the art-book publisher Harry N. Abrams, Inc. His repeated urging played a conspicuous part in the author's ultimate decision to write the book.

I am greatly indebted to my secretary, Eileen F. Kessler, who labored long and conscientiously in assembling material, looking up references, and typing near-illegible script. Without her extraordinary devotion to duty, this book might never have been completed.

To Susan Ellis, medical writer and indexer, I shall always be grateful for the manner in which she helped to transpose spoken words into written manuscript.

I wish to record special appreciation to my dear friend James S. Hays, past president of the Home for Aged and Infirm Hebrews of New York, for his help in writing the chapter on institutional care, and to Jean Rothenberg, of Cincinnati, for her excellent suggestions concerning the chapter on hearing and deafness.

To Abradale Press, publishers of *The New Illustrated Medical Encyclopedia for Home Use,* to the American Cancer Society, to the Metropolitan Life Insurance Company, to the Sonotone Corporation, and to the U.S. Department of Health, Education and Welfare, I wish to extend my thanks for permission to use illustrations, charts, diagrams, and statistical data.

R. E. R.

HOW TO USE THIS BOOK

Illnesses and upsets in body function are not always limited to one system or to one organ. Thus, a kidney affliction may arise from, and be part of, a blood vessel or heart condition. Similarly, a stomach ailment may have its origin in a vitamin deficiency or in an emotional upheaval. For this reason, the reader may discover a topic classified under several different headings and discussed in several places in the book.

Certain topics have been removed from their logical medical classification and have been discussed as separate entities mainly because the lay public thinks of them in that way. For example, *Cataracts* is listed as a separate topic, although it might have been included in the discussion on *Eyes; Pneumonia* is discussed under that title, although it might have been dealt with under *Lungs*.

In order to find topics easily, the following procedure is recommended:

First scan the Alphabetical List of Subjects in the front of the book. On turning to a particular subject, one will find *related topics* listed directly beneath the heading. Under "Allergy," for example, are listed the related topics "Asthma; Drugs and Medicines; Skin." These related topics also appear in the Alphabetical List of Subjects. If the topic still cannot be found, turn to the Index, which begins on page 753.

CONTENTS

ALPHABETICAL LIST OF SUBJECTS

Contents

INTRODUCTORY REMARKS ON AGING

Since the very beginning, man has been aware of the ebb and flow of time. The constancy of the sun's appearance and disappearance afforded him a ready unit by which to calculate time's passage. He learned there was a time to work and a time to sleep, a time to hunt and a time to store away, a time to plant and a time to harvest. Later in his development, man discovered that the moon and the stars followed a regular pattern of behavior, and he was able to gauge the time of the month, the seasons, and the years by plotting and recording their movements. The knowledge of *time* was as important to him as the knowledge of space.

Throughout the ages, man has displayed a profound absorption in recording dates, in devising calendars, and in constructing devices to tell the time of day. A visit to almost any large museum containing relics of early civilizations will reveal the extraordinary precocity man has shown in making sure that time was recorded precisely and accurately. Ingenious sundials, elaborate calendars, and complicated timepieces were invented by primitive peoples who were centuries behind in the construction of many simpler but more important items necessary for survival. During the Middle Ages man expended a good deal of thought and energy on inventing many varieties of timepieces and clocks. If he had used a small portion of this effort for developing agricultural machinery instead, it is safe to conjecture that the cotton gin and the harvester might have been invented much earlier.

Ancient records show this same extraordinary concern for the recording of time and its passage. As a result, we are the legatees of huge quantities of chronological information chiseled into stones and tablets or scratched onto the surface of parchments. From these records historians can often determine the very day, thousands of years ago, on which a specific event took place.

Why this intense preoccupation with *time?* Although many factors were probably involved, much of man's concern with time originated in the awareness that a *limit* had been placed upon the amount of it he could spend on earth. This fact must have been painful to our ancestors, for they spent much of their lives propitiating the gods to permit them to stay alive and they devoted themselves passionately to the development of cults, beliefs, and religions that revolved around reincarnation and an afterlife. Life was so short thousands of years ago that man was unable to accept its physical termination as its true end.

In a sense, it is fortunate that these concepts, which projected man forward into a timeless future, were developed. Perhaps no single thought has afforded man more solace and comfort or has stimulated him to more good than the belief that there is a *hereafter* in which he may dwell happily forever!

Modern man, too, is intensely preoccupied with thoughts of time and age. He acknowledges with great reluctance the limitations placed on his span of life. So important is the concept of *age* that, from earliest infancy, a child is indoctrinated with endless admonitions about his age and the expected behavior for one who has lived his particular number of years. He is told from the very first that he is *older* or *younger* than his brother or sister. This immediately places upon him a responsibility for a certain type of behavior. He is asked innumerable questions concerning what he wants to be when he grows *older*. As an adolescent, he is scolded time and again not to act like a child but to be more *grown up*. It is only natural that by the time a child does reach maturity, he begins forthwith to worry about *growing old*. And so we see boys in their twenties worrying about the loss of a few hairs or the onset of fatigue after a strenuous day's work. Young women become alarmed upon discovering a gray hair or a slight wrinkle in the neck. One hears that an athlete is *an old man* when he reaches thirty or that a woman has lost her appeal when she passes twenty-five. A man of fifty is told to *act his age* when he is flirtatious or demonstrates interest in activities usually indulged in by younger men.

It should be pointed out that the anxiety created by the fear of aging has produced many beneficial side effects. It has spurred man to a never-ending search for greater knowledge and better tools to overcome things in his environment that might shorten his life-span. Modern man has been amazingly successful in this effort to prolong his life, but now he often finds himself perplexed by factors arising out of his achievements.

The recent dramatic increase in the number of people who are living into the seventh and eighth decades may be ascribed to many factors, including vastly improved hygiene and living conditions, mass vaccinations and immunizations, the eradication of many of the serious diseases of childhood and early adult life, the tremendous advances in surgery, the discovery of the antibiotic wonder drugs, and many other great accomplishments in the field of medicine. Although the world rejoices at this extension of the life-span, it finds itself overwhelmed by the enormous number of new problems that have been created. To cite just a few examples in the field of physical care: nursing homes for the aged are inadequate; homes for the aged are too few in number, and those in existence have long waiting lists for admission; hospitals for the care of the chronically ill are woefully lacking, and those in existence are understaffed; communities throughout the country lack sufficient apartments and hotels especially designed to meet the needs of elder citizens; recreational facilities for the aged have been established in only a few communities throughout the nation. The list could go on and on.

Although society has long since prescribed codes and rules of conduct for its children and young adults, it has not yet begun to crystallize its thinking about or to evolve standards for that large segment of its population that now lives into the seventies, eighties, and nineties. Furthermore, medical science has not yet fully developed specific methods and techniques for handling the many special problems of this older age group. One of the main purposes of this book is to explore some of the particular medical and social situations that have been created by the recent prolongation of the life-span.

It is obvious that the changes brought about by scientific advancement demand a reevaluation of present-day thinking on *age* and *aging*. Perhaps a great deal of our present and past thinking will have to be discarded, for the truths of one hundred years ago are not necessarily true today, and today's truths may not be valid one hundred years from now. In biblical times a man of thirty was old; he was old at forty two hundred years ago; today, he is often young in his sixties or seventies. This latter statement requires little to substantiate it. All one has to do is to look about him and note the virility and vigor of many of our contemporary world figures who are, or recently were, in their seventies or eighties. Although Michelangelo was a rarity in his time, the twentieth century can point to a host of people who have performed at peak efficiency after the proverbial three score and ten years: Eleanor Roosevelt, David Ben Gurion, Douglas MacArthur, Bernard Baruch, Oliver Wendell Holmes, Grandma Moses, Picasso, Toscanini, Konrad Adenauer, Harry Truman, Robert Frost, Pope John, and many others.

We should ask ourselves whether there still remains a basis for defining age merely in terms of the number of years that have elapsed since birth. It would seem more logical to carefully evaluate the present health of an individual and attempt to estimate the number of years that are left to him! If this were the practice, then the man of sixty with twenty years of life still to live could be described as ten years younger than the man of sixty with only ten years remaining. Further, a man of forty with but ten years left to him is a great deal older than a man of sixty with twenty years still to live!

Such a new system of defining age has real merit from a medical point of view, for people can truly be old in their twenties or thirties if they suffer from diseased kidneys, a damaged liver, or sclerotic blood vessels. Conversely, people can remain relatively young in their seventies if their vital organs have not undergone major degenerative changes.

It is estimated that by 1980 almost one out of every five persons in America and Europe will be sixty years of age or older. And it is fair to predict that if scientific progress continues at the same pace as it has during the last one hundred years, the average healthy man or woman of sixty may, by the turn of the next century, confidently expect to live an additional twenty to twenty-five more years. It is more difficult to predict what society's attitude toward this older age group will be, or how the problems created by their extended lifespan will be solved. If we can go by past experience, it can be assumed that these people will not want to waste the last quarter of their lives in secluded idleness, nor will they want to retire unnecessarily from social and physical activity. What provisions will be made to permit them to express themselves fully and to lead the active lives they will want?

The older person of the twenty-first century will, in all probability, consider enforced retirement at sixty or sixty-five years a great infringement of his right to be a full-fledged contributing member of society. And to make matters more complicated, this reluctance to retire may coincide with a period in our economic life when jobs will be fewer because of the wider utilization of automation techniques! The 20 percent of the population who will be over sixty can be just as capable as younger workers of manipulating the buttons that will run the machinery of the future! Moreover, in many instances, the greater wisdom and reliability that accompany maturity may make this group more attractive to employers than younger workers who change jobs frequently in the hope of earning more money or of being advanced more quickly to positions of greater importance. If this happens, how will the society of the next century react to it?

There is little doubt that new arrangements will have to be made for later retirement. Also, compulsory-retirement systems will have to be completely overhauled or discarded. By the same token, communities will have to embark upon new social planning that will take into account larger numbers of citizens in the sixty- to eighty-year age group. Accident and health insurance contracts will require changes to permit policies to remain in force during these later years. Pension systems will require radical revision to conform to new actuarial statistics and conditions. Medical care insurance, whether commercial, voluntary, or state subsidized, will have to be altered and liberalized to permit full coverage of the older segment of our population. And finally, there will have to be much new social legislation to provide for this ever-growing segment of the population.

Before proceeding further with the problems of life after sixty, it would perhaps be best to inquire into and inspect some of the medical aspects of the aging process.

When does one start to grow old?

Does the first gray hair or the first wrinkle really herald the beginning of the aging process?

Certainly they do not, for the process of aging begins even before one is born! Certain structures are functional only during the life of the embryo. As the time for birth approaches these structures show all the characteristic signs of aging and become functionless by the time the child is ready to be born. One can actually see some of these changes under a microscope. Microscopic examination of the blood vessels of the umbilical cord or the walls of the ductus arteriosus (an artery in the embryo's chest that shunts blood away from the lungs to the aorta) reveals the same typical thickening of the lining of the vessel walls, loss of elastic fibers, and narrowing or obliteration of their passageway that may be found in the arteriosclerosis of old age.

If the aging process does actually begin before birth, one might reasonably ask how long human life, under ideal conditions, can really last? What is a full life-span? Medical investigators have estimated that under ideal circumstances almost every organ in the body has the physical capability of functioning satisfactorily for a minimum of one hundred years. Post-mortem microscopic examinations of healthy organs of centenarians often reveal minimal evidences of deterioration. Of course, a span of one hundred years can be achieved only if *all* of the vital structures remain free from major degenerative changes. Although the "one-hundred year goal" has not yet been reached by medical science, it is one that we can confidently expect to attain sometime within the next two centuries.*

Throughout life, from earliest infancy, the body replaces worn-out cells. Most cells become old and die while the total body mechanism continues to grow and flourish. For instance, by the time an individual reaches maturity, he has none of the skin cells that he had at the time of birth. These cells are replaced thousands of times during life. Similarly, not a single red blood cell lives more than sixty to ninety days before being replaced by a new cell. Interestingly enough, there are exceptions to this replacement process. For example, brain cells, nerve cells, and muscle cells will not regenerate if they are destroyed. In one sense, we should be grateful to Nature for this because the continuous life and functioning of the same brain cells permits us to store and remember most of our past experiences. If there were brain-cell replacement, we would be forced to learn things over and over again. Furthermore, we would be unable to profit from the experience of our past. In another sense, it is unfortunate that nerve and muscle cells do not have the power to regenerate, for if they did, many of those paralyzed by a stroke, polio, or other diseases could grow new tissues that would permit the paralyzed structures to regain normal function.

As aging progresses more and more of the functioning cells of an organ are replaced by nonfunctioning cells. Thus, the elastic cells in the walls of arteries are replaced by fibrous tissues that do not have the faculty of expanding and contracting. In such organs as the heart, the liver, and the kidneys, functioning cells may be so completely replaced by inert fibrous tissue that normal function can no longer be maintained. The cartilages lining the bony joints may become so thinned out as one ages, and fibrous tissue and calcium deposits may become so widespread, that crippling arthritis may result.

It is important to note that the rate of aging varies greatly from organ to organ within the same body. For example, one notes that many people in their seventies or eighties retain

*At present there are ten thousand Americans who are one hundred years old or older.

good vision and hearing although they are losing their teeth or have suffered severe heart damage. Others who have excellent heart function may be totally blind or deaf.

Why do certain organs undergo early aging whereas others remain relatively healthy and young far into the later decades? Some of the reasons for this disparity are as follows:

1. If an organ has been attacked by serious disease in youth or during the middle years, it may deteriorate earlier. Thus, a kidney that was affected by nephritis during childhood is more likely to have its function impaired at an early adult age.

2. Heredity may play an important part in the rate at which organs show signs of aging. For instance, someone whose parents and grandparents were free from arteriosclerosis until very late in life has a good chance of inheriting blood vessels that will be able to resist arteriosclerotic changes. This is one of the reasons why longevity appears to be the rule in some families. Of course, it must be realized that such environmental factors as infections, accidents, tumor growths, and self-abuse can modify or nullify a fine heredity.

3. The environment in which a person lives frequently influences the rate at which the organs age. An obvious example is the skin. Sailors, farmers, and others who spend a great part of their lives in the open will develop old, weather-beaten, wrinkled skin at an earlier age than those who have been sheltered from the elements. As we all know, actors and actresses who, throughout most of their lives, have made it a practice to avoid overexposure to sun, cold, and wind often retain their youthful appearance well into their sixties.

4. The manner in which an organ has been used and cared for is very important in determining its ability to withstand aging. If one abuses or overuses a structure, it will degenerate more rapidly. It is well known that people who drink to excess or who permit themselves to grow too fat are much more likely to develop cirrhosis of the liver, high blood pressure, or diabetes while they are still young.

5. The functional adequacy of the arteries and nerves that supply an organ are essential in determining the rate at which that organ will show signs of deterioration. Although a kidney may be structurally sound, if the arteries

that supply it are sclerotic and narrowed, early degeneration and loss of kidney function will set in. By the same token, if the nerves that go to a group of muscles degenerate, those muscles will wither and lose their ability to function properly.

6. The endocrine glands (the pituitary, the thyroid, the parathyroids, the adrenals, the ovaries, and the testicles) play an important role in determining the rate at which various structures will show signs of aging. Serious disease involving one or more of these glands may lead to premature aging of an organ that is dependent upon its secretions.

7. Emotional factors influence the body to a tremendous degree. The exact nature of these influences cannot always be pinpointed, but it is generally recognized that the unstable, overemotional, neurotic individual is an exceptionally likely candidate for early development of heart disease, arteriosclerosis, and other degenerative disorders involving essential body structures.

Despite the inevitability of changes with age, much can be done to slow down the course of the aging process. Just as a fine piece of machinery can be made to last years longer than its usual span, so can the human body and mind—by careful maintenance throughout the early and middle years—be preserved to serve many additional productive years. One of the main purposes of this book is to outline methods and to suggest rules for the maintenance of better health in the later years. Scattered throughout the text are hints on how to prevent premature aging and programs for delaying the onset of many of the infirmities of old age.

Although this book is a compilation of medically accepted information concerning the diseases of the later years, it does *not* contain prescriptions for self-treatment; nor should it be used as a substitute for a physician's care.

The material recorded here will, it is hoped, be of interest and assistance not only to people past sixty but also to those in their forties and fifties who are just beginning to think of themselves in other than youthful terms. They, especially, may benefit from medical advice on how to delay the aging process and how to escape many of the avoidable illnesses of later life. In writing this book the author has made a conscious effort to direct much of the material to the children of aging parents. Since the life-span has been extended so greatly, more and more children are being charged with responsibility for the care of their aged parents. In like manner, nurses, companions, attendants, and social workers will find this work so organized that they can readily locate advice for the handling of the many special problems they will encounter in dealing with the aging and the aged.

Wherever possible in the text, complicated medical terms have been omitted and readily understood words have been substituted. In order to facilitate use of the book, subjects have been arranged alphabetically rather than according to body systems. A full index with cross references may be found at the end of the book.

The question-and-answer technique has been employed in this book because that is the way most medical problems come to the physician's attention. The questions contained here are those most often asked by older people and their families. The answers are those most often given by today's physicians. It should be remembered, however, that considerable variation exists in the interpretation of disease and in the advice that different physicians will give to their patients on the same subject. The medical information has been gathered from standard textbooks on geriatrics, from surgical and medical texts and journals, from personal communications with physicians who specialize in particular fields of geriatric care, and from the experience of the author during approximately thirty years of practice. It should also be emphasized that this book deals mainly with health and medical care *in the later years* and makes no claim to being a complete textbook on medicine for all people.

Finally, no attempt has been made to embellish the later years of life with attributes they do not possess. One cannot ignore the incontrovertible fact that it is far more pleasant to be thirty years old than to be seventy. On the other hand, a sincere effort has been made in writing this book to show that the later years can be good years if mental and physical health are maintained. Fortunately, older people are so endowed that, given a state of good health, they can derive almost as much pleasure and gratification from the later years as younger people derive from the earlier years.

ADRENAL GLANDS

See ENDOCRINE GLANDS AND HORMONES; FUNCTIONAL CHANGES WITH AGING; LONGEVITY; PREMATURE AGING; SEX HORMONES.

Where are the adrenal glands located and what is their appearance?

There is one on each side of the body, located just above and adjacent to the kidneys in the upper, back portion of the abdomen. They are small in size, measuring approximately one by two inches in diameter, yellowish in color, and triangular in shape.

What is the structure and function of the adrenal glands?

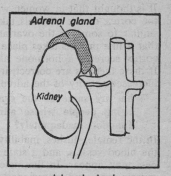

Adrenal gland

The adrenals are essential to normal body function in that they produce and secrete hormones that are necessary for the maintenance of life. Until the discovery of cortisone, patients suffering severe adrenal-gland failure would invariably die.

Each gland is divided into a cortex and a medulla.

The cortex produces hormones that influence the following body functions:

1. The maintenance of water and mineral balance.
2. The secretion of certain female and male sex hormones.
3. The storage, utilization, and maintenance of body proteins, sugars, and fats.
4. The production of chemicals vitally connected with the body's response to stress, strain, and injury.

The medulla of the adrenal gland produces and secretes adrenalin and noradrenalin (also known as epinephrine and norepinephrine). These hormones, after secretion into the bloodstream, have the following effects:

1. They increase the rate of blood coagulation (clotting).
2. They reduce muscle fatigue, thereby permitting sustained physical exertion.
3. They stimulate the heart by increasing the force of its contractions.

4. They increase the concentration of sugar in the blood, thereby making more sugar available to the body tissues.

Is adrenal function usually maintained at normal levels in aging individuals?

Yes, to a degree. There are, however, some investigators who believe that the aging process itself is accelerated or brought on by a decrease in adrenal function, particularly in the cortex. This contention has not been proved, although there is great similarity between the generalized weakness and slowing of metabolism that is seen in some older people and that seen in young people afflicted with disease of the adrenal glands.

Do the adrenal glands ever become overactive in older people?

It is thought that in women who have passed the menopause, the cortex of the adrenals takes over and secretes hormones similar to some of the ovarian hormones. It is also believed that a like process takes place in the aging male: the adrenal cortex secretes a hormone akin to the male sex hormone. If these theories are correct, it would mean that there may be increased activity of the adrenals during the later years.

What are some of the symptoms that might develop in aging people whose adrenal glands are beginning to function inadequately?

In the female, flushes, inability to properly contract and relax the blood vessels, and a state of general lassitude and weakness may appear. In the male, there may be fatigue, loss of muscle tone, and, occasionally, loss of calcium in the bones. In both sexes, inadequate adrenal-cortex function may lead to faulty mineral metabolism and arthritis.

What condition may result from overactivity of the adrenal cortex?

Cushing's disease may occur. However, this condition is much more common in younger persons. When it is encountered, it presents the following signs and symptoms:

1. A distribution of excess fat in the upper part of the torso, in the neck and shoulders, giving the patient a "buffalo-like" appearance.
2. A moon-shaped face.
3. Pearl-colored streaks in the skin of the abdomen and thighs.
4. In the female, male characteristics may develop.
5. Elevated blood pressure.
6. Elevated blood sugar.

Is there any satisfactory treatment for Cushing's disease?
Yes. X-ray treatment of the pituitary gland in the base of the brain or surgical removal of portions of the adrenal glands will often arrest this condition.

Is failure of adrenal function very common in people past sixty?
Not among healthy individuals. When people in this age group begin to lose weight, tire easily, and complain of loss of appetite and extreme weakness, failure of the adrenal cortex should be suspected.

Is there any satisfactory treatment for underactivity of the adrenal glands?
Yes, but it is important first to determine which hormones are lacking. When this has been determined, the specific hormone—or its controlling hormone manufactured by the pituitary gland—is administered.

What is Addison's disease?
It is a disease in which the adrenal cortex is unable to produce sufficient hormones. As a result, the patient loses his appetite, becomes extremely weak, has exceedingly low blood pressure, and becomes bedridden. Since the widespread use of cortisone, many sufferers from Addison's disease have been maintained in a state of fairly good health for indefinite periods of time.

Do tumors of the adrenal medulla ever occur?
Yes, but rarely. A characteristic tumor, known as "pheochromocytoma," sometimes occurs. This tumor will cause marked elevation in blood pressure, palpitation of the heart, overactive metabolism, diabetes, and mental changes characterized by marked anxiety.

Can pheochromocytomas be treated successfully?
Yes, by surgical removal of the diseased adrenal gland.

Is it safe for older people to medicate themselves with steroids such as cortisone or ACTH when their adrenal glands malfunction?
Absolutely not! These are potent, dangerous drugs, which should be taken only when prescribed by a physician who is fully familiar with both their primary and side effects.

Does cancer ever involve the adrenal glands?
A primary cancer of the adrenals is rare, but not infrequently, a cancer elsewhere in the body will spread to the adrenal glands. When this happens, adrenal function becomes impaired.

How is a primary cancer of an adrenal gland treated?

By surgical removal of the gland.

Are the adrenal glands ever removed in order to slow down the spread of a cancer?

Yes. It has been demonstrated within recent years that in some patients the removal of the adrenal glands will slow down the growth and spread of cancer. Cancers of the breast are particularly influenced by adrenal-gland removal (adrenalectomy). There are now many cases on record in which cancer growth and spread have been arrested for periods of several months to several years following complete removal of both adrenal glands.

If the adrenal glands have been removed, how is life maintained?

By giving cortisone to replace that ordinarily produced by the adrenals. Also, great care is taken to regulate the amount of salt and potassium included in the diet. These substances must be measured precisely throughout the rest of the patient's life so that their metabolism can be maintained within nearly normal limits.

Can special precautions be taken during youth or the middle years so that adrenal-gland function will be maintained in later life?

To a certain extent, yes. More and more investigators feel that excessive strain throughout the middle years will eventually take its toll upon adrenal function. The adrenals are the organs that respond to stress, anxiety, and strain. The draining effect on these glands throughout a long stressful life may lead to premature loss of their ability to secrete the necessary amounts of vital hormones. Therefore, young people should make every attempt to avoid unnecessary stress and should seek a way of life that will minimize anxiety and strain.

ALCOHOL AND ALCOHOLISM

See CIRRHOSIS OF THE LIVER; CORONARY-ARTERY DISEASE; DEGENERATIVE CHANGES OF AGING; DRIVING; GOUT; HEART; HEPATITIS; LONGEVITY.

Do people tend to become more sensitive to the effects of alcohol as they get older?

Yes. With age, the senses of equilibrium, vision, and hearing become less acute and are more easily disturbed. Also, older people are more likely to become confused if they drink too much alcohol.

Are there wide variations in individual sensitivity to alcohol?

Yes. Some people can drink a great quantity of alcohol with little change in their alertness or mental and physical responses. Others are so sensitive that one drink will either exhilarate them inordinately or depress them markedly.

Do people who have taken a moderate amount of alcohol all their lives tend to increase their intake gradually as they advance in years?

Yes, and it would be well if they were aware of this tendency. Addiction to alcohol can be gradual and insidious.

Do people who have done only social drinking in their younger days ever become alcoholics in their sixties?

Yes. In certain older people, the body loses some of its ability to handle alcohol, and addiction results. Furthermore, as emotional problems increase alcohol is used more and more frequently as an escape from reality.

Is there a tendency for people who have been taking one or two drinks before lunch or dinner throughout their adult lives to become addicted as they grow older?

No. If a person limits his drinking to one or two drinks, he will not become an alcoholic. However, people sometimes step up their drinking from one or two drinks before dinner to two or three drinks, then three or four drinks, and so on. Such a practice *can* lead to addiction.

Is alcoholism a disease affecting only some people, or can anyone become addicted?

Although most doctors now believe that alcoholism is related to neurotic personality, it is dangerous to conclude that so-called normal people are immune to addiction. Certain physiological aspects of alcoholism have led several investigators to feel that *all people* are susceptible if they drink enough over a long enough period of time.

What constitutes excessive drinking?

This is almost impossible to answer, but one can safely state that people past sixty should limit drinking to three (one and one-half ounce) drinks of whiskey, or two glasses of wine, or three glasses of beer during any 24-hour period.

Do the various types of alcoholic beverages have different effects on different people?

Yes, but regardless of the type (beer, wine, whiskey, etc.),

ultimate body reactions to alcohol are the same if an excessive
amount is used.

**Do the various alcoholic beverages have different effects if
taken in different dilutions or if taken with meals?**

Yes. A diluted alcoholic beverage is better for older people.
A glass of light wine or beer is much better than a jigger or
two of hard whiskey. In addition, it is wise to eat when one
drinks.

**If a healthy individual has been in the habit of drinking
throughout his adult life, can he continue to do so after
he reaches sixty years of age?**

Yes, provided he has no medical condition that would be
harmed by drinking alcohol. There is no more reason to
prohibit the moderate use of alcohol than there is to ban the
eating of sensible quantities of candy or cake.

**What are the effects of alcoholic beverages on those who
show mental changes due to aging?**

People who show any signs of senility should avoid drinking
any alcoholic beverage, as it may accentuate their mental confusion and the normal weakening of the senses.

**Should people who have ulcers be permitted to drink
alcohol?**

No. Alcohol will cause the stomach to secrete more acid,
which will irritate the ulcer. Hemorrhage or other complications may result.

**Can the drinking of large quantities of alcohol bring on an
inflammation of the lining of a normal stomach?**

Yes. Gastritis (inflammation of the stomach) sometimes results from the drinking of large quantities of alcohol. If
nausea, the vomiting of blood, or marked indigestion follows
the ingestion of alcohol, it is wise not to drink again.

**Can excessive drinking over a long period of time lead to
cirrhosis of the liver?**

Most medical investigators agree that there is a definite
connection between prolonged excessive intake of alcohol
and the development of cirrhosis of the liver. Therefore,
someone who has a known liver disorder, or who at one time
in his life had jaundice or hepatitis, should limit the amount
of alcohol he drinks. (*See* CIRRHOSIS OF THE LIVER.)

How does alcohol cause cirrhosis of the liver in later years?

It is thought that in certain people who drink to excess the
chronic use of alcohol ultimately produces chemical changes
within the lining of the stomach and the intestinal tract.

Such changes may result in the failure of the lining membranes to absorb vital foods and chemicals that the liver needs for its continued normal function. If the liver is so deprived over a period of years, it may undergo cirrhotic changes.

Does the drinking of large quantities of alcohol ever bring on pancreatitis (inflammation of the pancreas)?

Yes. It is thought that bouts of alcoholism, particularly in obese older men, may bring on this serious and dangerous disease. (*See* PANCREAS.)

Should those suffering from gallstones or gallbladder disease avoid alcoholic beverages?

Yes, since alcohol may bring on an attack of gallstone colic or may induce an acute inflammation of the gallbladder.

Does the drinking of alcohol ever bring on an acute attack of gout?

Definitely, yes. People who have gout or a tendency toward gout should give up drinking all alcoholic beverages.

What is the effect of alcohol on those who have arthritis?

Among medical people opinion is divided. If the arthritis is unrelated to gout, in all probability the drinking of a moderate amount of alcohol is harmless. But, as stated above, alcohol is definitely bad for those who have gouty arthritis.

Will drinking large quantities of alcohol ever lead to vitamin deficiencies or nutritional disturbances?

Yes. If people drink excessively in their later years they tend to eat less, and they often fail to vary their diets sufficiently. This practice may lead to malnutrition and vitamin deficiency.

Will the drinking of moderate amounts of alcohol over a period of years lead to the development of kidney disease?

No medical proof has been found that it will if the kidneys have been healthy throughout life.

Should people with known kidney disease avoid the continued use of alcoholic beverages?

Yes, since further damage may result.

Does alcohol, taken in moderate quantities over a period of years, lead to the premature development of hardening of the arteries?

There is no evidence that moderate drinking of alcohol has any bad effect on the arteries.

Can the diabetic who is past sixty drink alcoholic beverages?

Since diabetes is a disease in which diet control is most important, it is necessary to take into account the fact that the average alcoholic drink contains approximately one hundred calories. Therefore, people who have diabetes must include their alcohol calories when making up their diets. People with diabetes should not drink excessive quantities of alcohol, as it may upset their sugar metabolism inordinately.

Is alcohol beneficial for those with poor circulation?

Alcohol can cause some dilatation of the blood vessels and is therefore beneficial, but it is by no means the best medication for this purpose. It is best prescribed in combination with other drugs for the improvement of circulation, and it must be emphasized again that excessive amounts of alcohol are deleterious to those with poor circulation or hardening of the arteries.

What effect does alcohol have on those with high blood pressure?

Most medical men think that alcohol in moderation may actually be beneficial to persons suffering from high blood pressure, as it promotes dilatation of the blood vessels. However, an excessive amount of alcohol will have just the opposite effect.

Is alcohol valuable as a medication for older people who suffer from poor appetite?

Yes, unless the lack of appetite is caused by disease within one of the major organs, for example, the stomach, gallbladder, liver, or kidney.

What effect has a moderate amount of alcohol on the sexual capability of a person past sixty?

One or two drinks may result in beneficial relaxation. However, there is a very thin line of demarcation between moderate drinking and excessive drinking. It is well to remember that excessive drinking will decrease one's ability to function sexually.

Is alcohol useful as medication to induce sleep?

Yes. In certain cases a drink before bedtime will relax a person sufficiently to encourage normal sleep. Older people should be cautioned that more than one drink, or an alcoholic drink in combination with a narcotic or a sedative, can be dangerous, as it may produce a comalike state.

Should alcoholic beverages be taken on a continuing basis to relieve chronic pain?

This is a risky practice, as it may lead to the development of alcoholism. However, if it is used strictly as prescribed by a physician, alcohol can be helpful in relieving certain types of chronic pain—as in some forms of arthritis, for example.

Is alcohol beneficial as a medication for older people who are subject to attacks of angina pectoris (pain in the heart region)?

Yes. A large number of medical practitioners feel that a drink or two before meals may tend to decrease the number of attacks of angina pectoris and may lead to some dilatation of the coronary artery. Here again, the practice should not be encouraged unless a physician prescribes the dosage.

Can people who have recently recovered from coronary thrombosis take alcohol?

Yes, but only on a doctor's prescription and in accordance with his prescribed amounts.

What is the best way to avoid becoming an alcoholic in one's later years?

1. Do not increase the daily intake during the middle years of life.
2. Do not substitute drinking for a well-balanced diet.
3. The family physician or a psychiatrist should be consulted as soon as the tendency to drink too much is noted.

Is there any effective medication to relieve one's desire for alcohol?

No. Since the habit of drinking is largely psychological, this desire cannot be removed solely by the use of medications.

Can Alcoholics Anonymous help alcoholics who are past sixty?

Yes. This is a fine organization and may be particularly good for older alcoholics to join, as it will afford them the companionship they often need so desperately.

ALLERGY

See ASTHMA; DRUGS AND MEDICINES; SKIN.

Do allergies tend to subside as people advance in years?
Some allergies, such as hay fever, do have a tendency to become less intense during the later decades of life. Other allergies, such as skin sensitivity and sensitivity to food and

drugs, are seen more often among older people. It is not at all uncommon for patients who have taken an antibiotic, such as penicillin, for many years to become sensitive to it as time goes on; nor is it uncommon for people to develop sensitivity to certain drugs they had tolerated well throughout their younger years. The skin of people past sixty becomes particularly sensitive, and great care must be exercised in the use of ointments, lotions, soaps, and perfumes. Substances that have been well tolerated in the middle years will sometimes produce marked allergic skin reactions in later life.

There is also increased sensitivity to heat and cold among many people past sixty. Allergic reactions may develop, even though they had not existed earlier.

Do allergies often appear for the first time in people in their sixties, seventies, or eighties?

Such allergies as hay fever or food allergies do not. Other allergies—skin or drug sensitivities, for example—often do begin during the later years of life.

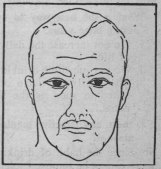

Hives (urticaria) of upper lip

Should people over sixty continue to take hay-fever injections?

If the hay fever has not been severe during the middle years, people in the sixty-or-over age group may experiment by omitting the injections for a season, in order to note whether the hay fever has subsided or disappeared. However, this experiment should be made only on the advice of one's allergist.

Are drug allergies very common in people past sixty?

Yes, particularly in people who had received large doses of such drugs in their earlier years. In other words, a person may develop sensitivity to a medication he had previously tolerated.

Are people past sixty particularly allergic to penicillin?

Yes. Great caution is necessary in the use of penicillin, whether it is applied locally or given by injection. People should tell their doctors if they have ever had a reaction to this drug.

Do people past sixty ever develop asthma for the first time?

Yes, but it is usually a type of asthma different from that seen in childhood or early youth. The asthma of the later years is often associated with bacterial infection in the bronchial tubes or lungs. The asthma seen in childhood or early adulthood is usually due to sensitivity to some allergen (an irritant, such as pollen, dust, or mold) in the environment, rather than to a bacterial invasion.

Do older people tend to become allergic to physical irritants?

Yes, particularly to a good deal of exposure to the sun, to exceedingly hot temperatures, or to extreme cold.

Do food allergies tend to disappear as one grows older?

Some food allergies may subside; others may persist.

Is the female genital area more likely to develop allergic skin reactions in women past menopause?

Yes.

What are the effects of the antihistamine drugs on people past sixty?

These drugs cause a reaction similar to that produced in younger people, as far as allergy is concerned. However, the sedative effect of large doses of this group of drugs and the drowsiness they produce are much more marked in older people.

Are older people more sensitive to antihistamine drugs that are used externally to relieve itching?

Yes. Strangely, older people are often allergic to medications that are commonly used today to relieve allergies. Substances or ointments that contain anesthetic agents or antibiotics should be used sparingly.

How effective are the cortisone drugs in the treatment of allergic conditions among older people?

Although some of these steroids (cortisonelike substances) may be helpful, there are definite limitations to their usefulness for older people. It should be emphasized that these drugs never really *cure* an allergic condition, even though relief from symptoms may result. (An older person who is taking a cortisone drug must be under the constant surveillance of his physician.)

Is there any way to find out whether or not one is allergic to a certain ointment before he uses it?

Yes. A patch test can be made. This will involve putting a very small amount of the ointment on the skin, covering it with adhesive tape, and allowing it to remain undisturbed for forty-eight hours. If the area becomes irritated, burns, or becomes red, an allergy exists and the medication should not be used. (This test is most applicable to those who are known to have allergic tendencies.)

Do older people ever develop reactions to sedatives, the newer tranquilizing drugs, or sleeping tablets such as the barbiturates?

Yes. Allergic reactions are frequent.

Are the eustachian tubes, which connect the throat to the inner ear, ever blocked because of allergic reactions?

Yes. They are often blocked by a swelling of their mucous membranes. This can cause temporary deafness, which is relieved by eliminating the allergen or by prescribing an antihistamine drug.

Are sinus conditions among older people often allergic in origin?

Not often. Sinus conditions resulting from allergic reactions are most often seen among younger people.

Are injections to desensitize one to an allergen as effective in older people as they are in younger people?

No. Allergy in people past sixty is best treated by relieving the symptoms or by removing the person from the source of the irritating factor (allergen).

What general rules for avoiding allergic reactions should be followed by allergic people past sixty?

1. Avoid the eating of all foods that are known to have caused allergic reactions earlier in life.
2. Discontinue any drug or medicine that causes an upset stomach, skin rash, or irritation of the eyes.
3. Do not apply any ointment or liniment to the skin without first consulting a physician. However, if a local application seems to produce greater irritation, discontinue it immediately.
4. Avoid extreme changes in temperature and overexposure to the sun.
5. A persistent cough should be treated by a physician to prevent the development of asthmatic bronchitis.
6. Garments that produce an itch or rash should not be worn.
7. If antihistamine drugs are being taken to combat an allergy, special care must be exercised when crossing streets or driving an automobile. These drugs have a greater tendency to cause drowsiness among older people.

8. One should be cautious about contacts with new substances, such as plants, flowers, clothing materials, ointments, lotions, perfumes, or soaps.

AMPUTATION

See ARTERIOSCLEROSIS; BONES AND JOINTS; CIRCULATION; CLAUDICATION; DIABETES MELLITUS; FEET; REHABILITATION AND PHYSICAL THERAPY.

Does progressive loss of circulation in the legs during the later years endanger the life of the limb?

Yes, but healthy people in their seventies or eighties rarely suffer loss of circulation to such a degree that amputation becomes necessary. However, if diabetes has been present for many years, and if there is marked arteriosclerosis of the arteries in the legs, gangrene may develop. In that case, amputation may be necessary.

Who are most susceptible to gangrene in the legs and feet?

1. Those who have had poorly regulated diabetes for many years.
2. Those with marked hardening of the arteries in the thighs and legs.
3. Those who fail to observe strict hygiene in caring for their feet, thereby permitting infections of the toes and soles of the feet.

Is it possible for people with diabetes to live into their sixties and seventies without developing extensive hardening of the arteries?

Yes. The great majority of those with well-treated, controlled diabetes can avoid the development of premature arteriosclerosis. (Before the use of insulin it was not uncommon for diabetics to develop severe arteriosclerosis in their thirties and forties.)

What tests can be performed to determine the adequacy or inadequacy of circulation in the legs and feet?

1. Noting the color of the legs—unusually pale, red, or blue, or some other deviation from the normal skin color usually denotes trouble.
2. Noting the temperature of the legs and feet. Doctors use very accurate instruments for recording exact skin temperatures.

3. Noting the presence or absence of pulses in the groin, behind the knees, and in the feet.
4. Performing oscillometric readings, which record the extent of the pulsations of the major arteries in the thighs and legs.
5. Taking X rays, which will show the extent of hardening of the arteries in the thighs and legs, and also by injecting various substances into the abdominal aorta that will light up and make visible the arteries in the lower extremities.

How does the physician decide when it is necessary to amputate?

Amputation is recommended only when an infection cannot be controlled, when the life of the patient is endangered by the infection, or when there is insufficient blood supply to nourish the limb.

At what level are amputations of the leg usually performed?

The level at which there is the best possible chance of obtaining good healing of the amputation stump. In many older people with advanced arteriosclerosis or gangrene of the leg, the safest and best site for amputation is *above* the knee.

Why is it often better to amputate the leg above the knee, even though the infection may be limited to the foot or lower leg?

Even though the infection and impairment of circulation may appear to be limited to the foot and lower leg, in most instances they also involve the midleg and upper leg. Therefore, to ensure adequate healing of the amputation stump, above-the-knee amputation is often carried out. Also, an artificial limb fitted to an above-the-knee stump is usually much easier for the patient to manage than one fitted below the knee. Preservation of the knee joint does *not* aid an older person in the use of an artificial limb.

Is amputation of a limb a dangerous operative procedure?

Not if the general health of the patient is satisfactory. Real danger exists when too much time is spent attempting to save a doomed limb. It is much wiser to save the life of the patient by amputating at a time when he can safely undergo surgery.

What steps should be taken by those with arteriosclerosis to avoid infection and gangrene?

1. Scrupulous attention must be paid to cleanliness of the feet. They should be washed daily with a mild soap and water, and dried thoroughly.

2. Toenails should not be cut too short, especially in the corners.
3. Calluses and warts should be cared for by an orthopedist or licensed podiatrist.
4. Well-made, well-fitted shoes should be worn at all times.
5. Walking about barefoot should be avoided because of the danger of splinters and infection.
6. Feet must be kept warm in cold weather.
7. Feet should never be permitted to remain wet or damp for any length of time.
8. A doctor should be consulted immediately if pain, redness, swelling, or other signs of possible infection or impairment of circulation develop.

Can older people learn to walk again after a limb has been amputated?

Yes, in the majority of instances. Rehabilitation experts usually see the patient soon after surgery, and they begin immediately to prepare him for the eventual fitting of an artificial limb.

Rehabilitation techniques have advanced so remarkably in recent years that many people who would formerly have been unable to walk can now be taught to get excellent use out of artificial limbs. It has been discovered that the emotional attitude of older patients is just as important as their physical condition in determining their ability to recover from an amputation and to resume an active life. (*See* REHABILITATION AND PHYSICAL THERAPY.)

ANATOMICAL CHANGES IN ORGANS

See ARTERIOSCLEROSIS; DEGENERATIVE CHANGES OF AGING; FUNCTIONAL CHANGES WITH AGING; LONGEVITY; PREMATURE AGING.

What is meant by "anatomical changes in organs"?

Changes in structure, that is, in the stuff of which the organ is made. For example, the muscle tissue of an organ may deteriorate and be replaced by fibrous tissue as a person ages.

Do anatomical changes in organs always lead to dangerous loss of function in those organs?

No. Fortunately, most organs have sufficient tissue to function even when there has been extensive deterioration. For example, the liver can function satisfactorily when more than half of its normal tissue has been replaced by fibrous tissue.

Do all organs undergo anatomical changes with aging?

Yes. The cells and tissues that make up all organs do deteriorate to some degree.

What are some of the characteristic anatomical changes in the brain during the aging process?

The convolutions of the brain flatten out and the actual quantity of brain substance is decreased. Brain cells may wither and be replaced by fibrous tissue. Brain cells require an extraordinary amount of oxygen and other nutriments for normal function, and if these are cut off or diminished for even a few minutes, cell degeneration may take place. Those anatomical changes that develop over the course of years usually are secondary to hardening of the arteries that supply the brain.

What symptoms may indicate that the brain has been affected by the aging process?

See MENTAL CHANGES.

What are some of the common anatomical changes in the eyes as a result of the aging process?

1. Formation of opacities (cataracts) within the lens of the eye.
2. The development of arcus senilis. (See ARCUS SENILIS AND ARCUS SENILIS LENTIS.)
3. Degeneration of fibers within the optic nerves.
4. Hardening of the arteries of the retina.
5. A shortening of the depth of the eyeball, with possible development of farsightedness.

See EYES for more complete discussion.

What anatomical changes take place most frequently in the ears?

1. A condition known as otosclerosis, which is associated with loss of hearing.
2. Degeneration of fibers within the auditory nerve, which controls hearing.
3. Loss of the elastic fibers that keep open the eustachian tubes, which extend from the throat to the inner ear.

See HEARING AND DEAFNESS for further discussion.

Does the sense of smell tend to diminish and show evidence of aging?

Yes. Some degeneration of the olfactory nerves in the nose is rather common among people in their later years. Also, the mucous membrane lining the nose may become thinned out, and the nerve endings that receive stimuli may lose some of their power to perceive odors.

Does the sense of taste tend to diminish as one grows older?
Yes. As with smell, the power of the taste buds in the tongue to perceive and interpret stimuli decreases. Also, the sense of taste is influenced by the sense of smell, so that taste perception declines with a weakened sense of smell.

What are the characteristic anatomical changes in arteries?
The passageway through arteries becomes narrowed because of thickening of the arterial wall. As the lining membrane thickens it loses its smooth surface. Fibrous tissue replaces the elastic tissue within the wall of the artery, and a deposit of calcium forms. It is this deposit of calcium that gives the vessels the rigidity and hardness that characterize arteriosclerosis.
See ARTERIOSCLEROSIS.

Do veins show the same changes as arteries in aging people?
No. Aging of the veins is often associated with thinning of their walls and malfunction of their valves. Varicosities may result from stagnation of the blood.
See VEINS AND VARICOSE VEINS.

What are some of the anatomical changes that take place in the aging heart?
Heart-muscle tissue is replaced by fibrous connective tissue, which lacks the capacity to expand and contract. When such replacements are extensive, the heart loses much of its ability to function normally. The arteries supplying the heart-muscle wall (the coronary arteries) tend to narrow and harden.
See HEART.

Do the heart valves often undergo anatomical changes as one advances in age?
Yes. The tissue of the valves between the various chambers of the heart also tends to become replaced by fibrous tissue. This results in reduced efficiency in the pumping action of the heart and may lead to heart failure.

What anatomical changes take place within the aging lungs?
1. In some areas, the delicate air cells break down and fuse with other air cells, forming large air sacs. These larger sacs do not absorb sufficient quantities of oxygen from the inhaled air.
2. In a lung showing signs of aging, areas normally containing functioning air cells are replaced by fibrous scar

tissue. This decreases the space from which the lungs can absorb oxygen and expel their waste products, carbon dioxide and water (in the form of vapor).

If the two processes involve the lungs to any great extent, the patient, when exerting himself, will become short of breath.

What evidence of aging is seen in the liver?

The liver can remain an effectively functioning organ throughout one's entire life, even when it is involved in advanced anatomical changes. However, cirrhosis may occur when large portions are replaced by fibrous tissue. It is estimated that normal liver function can be maintained with less than half of the original liver substance present, provided there is no obstruction to the outflow of bile.

See LIVER.

What are some of the anatomical changes in the pancreas during the aging process?

The pancreas is a structure with two major functions:

1. The production of insulin, which is necessary in sugar metabolism.
2. The secretion of enzymes essential to normal digestion in the intestinal tract.

If there is hardening of the arteries that supply blood to the pancreas, there may be deterioration of the cells (called islets of Langerhans) that manufacture insulin, with resultant diabetes. Deterioration of the part of the pancreas that secretes digestive juices will lead to indigestion, weakness, loss of weight, and other symptoms of poor nutrition.

See PANCREAS.

What are characteristic changes in the gastrointestinal tract as one gets older?

The gastrointestinal tract in a healthy individual can function satisfactorily throughout life. Of course, the stomach may secrete less gastric juice and hydrochloric acid, and the intestines may lose some of their absorptive power, but this does not interfere greatly in the life of the normal aging person. He usually compensates for these changes by eating less and chewing his food more thoroughly.

The large bowel often loses a great deal of its muscle tone as one ages and, as a consequence, the intestinal contents are evacuated at a much slower pace. This is the reason for the great incidence of constipation in older people. Also, weakening of the musculature in the bowel wall may lead to the formation of diverticula, little blisters or outpouchings. These may become inflamed and, in rare instances, may rupture.

Another result of aging is the progressive decrease in muscle strength and tone of the anal sphincter (the ringlike muscle that closes the anus).

What are some of the anatomical changes that take place in the kidneys as one ages?

Degenerative change in the kidneys is one of the greatest factors in shortening the life-span. Hardening of the renal arteries, which supply the kidneys, leads to the destruction of kidney cells and decrease in kidney function. Fortunately, kidney function can be maintained when only a small percentage of the tissue is healthy. However, when damage is too extensive, uremia results.
See KIDNEYS.

What are the characteristic anatomical changes that take place in the prostate gland as one ages?

In almost all men this gland tends to enlarge during the sixties, seventies, or eighties. The exact reason for this is not known. Such enlargement of the prostate tends to obstruct the outlet of the urinary bladder.
See PROSTATE GLAND.

What are the usual anatomical changes that occur in the uterus as a result of aging?

The aging uterus shrinks in size and much of its muscle tissue is replaced by fibrous tissue; the lining membrane thins out and becomes nonfunctional. Also, since the ovaries are no longer secreting eggs, the membrane lining the uterus no longer swells each month in preparation for reception of a fertilized egg.
See FEMALE ORGANS.

What anatomical changes take place in the ovaries of aging women?

Eggs no longer mature and hence do not leave the ovaries; the gland structure that produces the sex hormones tends to be replaced by fibrous scar tissue.
See FEMALE ORGANS; OVARIES.

What anatomical changes take place in the vagina and the external female genitals?

There is often considerable loss of the fat beneath the skin in the region of the female genitals in later life and the muscle tone in the region is diminished. Also, the mucous membrane of the vagina flattens out and becomes dry, and much less mucus is secreted.
See FEMALE ORGANS.

What is the anatomical evidence of aging in the male genitals?

There is relatively little replacement of muscle tissue by fibrous tissue in the penis as the male grows older. (Erection is produced by a flow of blood into the organ. This ability may be lost in the later years, but not as a result of anatomical changes.)

The testicles lose their ability to manufacture live sperm and their gland structure may be replaced by fibrous tissue. Normally, the testicles continue to secrete those hormones that are necessary to maintain the male sex characteristics.

What anatomical changes take place within the endocrine glands as one ages?

The so-called endocrine glands (adrenal, thyroid, pituitary, etc.) tend to show some replacement of their former gland structures with fibrous tissue. However, even far into old age, they continue to secrete their hormones and are capable of maintaining normal body metabolism.

It is common medical belief that the process of growing old is due in large measure to the lessening capacity of these vital glands. The adequacy of the blood supply to these structures will determine to a great extent how well they will perform in later life.

See articles about specific glands for further discussion.

What anatomical changes take place within the muscular system of people who are growing old?

The strength of muscles and their ability to contract and expand decrease as one grows older; there may be actual replacement of muscle cells by fibrous tissue. These changes will take place at a much slower pace if one has exercised and used his muscles sensibly throughout life. Muscle size also decreases as one grows older.

The health of the nerves that activate the muscles is an important factor in determining the anatomical changes that may occur within the muscles. In other words, if the nerves associated with the muscles degenerate, the muscles will not function properly.

What are some of the characteristic anatomical changes that may take place in nerves during the later years?

Nerve cells are among the few structures in the body that are not replaced by new cells. They are the same cells from birth to death, and are durable enough to last throughout the entire life-span. Fortunately, the nerves supplying vital organs and structures of the body function satisfactorily throughout life and do not often become seriously diseased. However, aging nerves do undergo replacement by fibrous tissue, but in a healthy older person a sufficient number of nerve fibers within a nerve bundle will survive to maintain satisfactory function.

What are some of the anatomical evidences of aging within the bony skeleton?

Anatomical changes within the bones take place in almost every person as he grows older. The rounded edges near the joints become thickened and sharpened, with little spiny prominences. Another characteristic change is the thinning out of cartilage overlaying the bone. This lessens the efficiency of joint action.

Most bone changes can be discovered by X-ray examination.

Another anatomical evidence of aging within the bone is the narrowing of its marrow. This is of particular importance because both red and white blood cells are manufactured in the bone marrow.

ANEMIA

See BLOOD; HODGKIN'S DISEASE; LEUKEMIA; POLYCYTHEMIA; SURGERY; TESTS.

What is anemia?

Any condition in which there is an insufficient number of circulating red blood cells, or in which the red blood cells are deficient in hemoglobin.

Are there many different types of anemia?

Yes. There are probably thirty to forty different types, each with its own characteristic blood changes. The physician can diagnose the specific type by careful analysis of the blood.

What are the causes of anemia?

There are various causes for the different types of anemia. It may be caused by improper and inadequate diet; by hemorrhage; or as a secondary disease resulting from some other disorder.

Does the treatment of anemia vary with the type?

Yes. For instance, treatment for pernicious anemia includes prescribing large doses of liver, liver extracts, and certain elements of vitamin B to bring about an arrest of the anemic process. Anemia caused by hemorrhage can be corrected by replacement of blood by transfusion. Other anemias, if they are secondary to some other disease, can be corrected by eliminating the primary disorder.

What disorders or conditions may cause secondary anemia among older people?

Kidney disease, heart disease, disturbance of the endocrine glands, metabolic disorders, chronic lung conditions, chronic infections, intestinal-tract disorders, prolonged cancer growth, improper nutrition, arthritis, parasitic infestation, cirrhosis of the liver, obesity, and certain vitamin deficiencies.

Blood diseases such as leukemia, Hodgkin's disease, and lymphosarcoma are also associated with an advanced anemia.

Is anemia more common in the later years of life?

There is no proof that the aging process in itself creates anemia or causes a decrease in the number of red blood cells. The bone marrow, although it may not be as efficient as in youth, is still capable of producing sufficient blood cells and other blood components far into the eighties and nineties if the individual is in good health generally. However, it is true that the illnesses and imbalances of people past sixty are often accompanied by anemia as a secondary condition. In other words, a disorder or disease that might not cause anemia in a young person may cause it in someone in his seventies or eighties. In a study made of several thousand patients over sixty who were admitted to a large general hospital, one out of four was found to be anemic.

What is pernicious anemia?

This is a specific type associated with specific symptoms and characteristic blood findings. It is a serious disease, often affecting people past sixty, in which there is a lack of an antianemic factor produced by the stomach. Such people usually have no hydrochloric acid in their stomach juices.

Before the causes of pernicious anemia were known, most people who had that disease eventually died from it. But it can now be controlled by the daily intake of large quantities of liver and liver extracts. Today, a normal life-span may be achieved despite the presence of pernicious anemia.

Do people with diseases of the kidney, such as nephritis, develop anemia?

Yes, often.

Is it particularly important that people with impaired heart function avoid becoming anemic?

Yes. In order to function properly, the heart requires large quantities of fresh blood carrying an adequate supply of oxygen. In advanced anemic states, insufficient oxygen is carried by the blood to the heart and to the heart muscle.

Do older people ever develop angina pectoris (heart pain) because of anemia?

Yes. Attacks of heart pain in people past sixty are often associated with anemia, and its correction sometimes reduces the number and intensity of these episodes.

Will disease of the bones ever lead to anemia?

Yes. Certain bone conditions among older people, such as osteoporosis, decrease the ability of the bone marrow to manufacture a sufficient quantity of red blood cells.

What is anemia of the brain?

This is a common term used to describe a condition associated with fainting spells, temporary loss of memory, and other mental changes. It is thought to be precipitated by interference with blood supply to the brain.

Actually, the term is no longer used in medical circles because the underlying cause for the symptoms is not true anemia; it is, rather, that the blood vessels supplying the brain have undergone arteriosclerosis and do not permit the passage of sufficient quantities of blood to the brain.

Do older people tend more than younger people to develop anemia secondary to chronic infection?

Yes, because the bone marrow in older people is not as efficient at renewing red blood cells.

What are common symptoms of anemia?

In mild cases, there are frequently no symptoms. However, marked anemia is often associated with the following symptoms:

1. Lack of energy and fatigue.
2. Loss of appetite.
3. Increased susceptibility to changes in temperature.
4. Headache.
5. Muscle weakness.
6. Pallor of the skin and mucous membranes.
7. Increased susceptibility to infections such as boils, abscesses, etc.
8. Increased susceptibility to respiratory infections.
9. Rapid pulse and heart palpitation.
10. Shortness of breath.

Do the symptoms or signs of anemia appear early or late in the course of the condition?

Late. It is very important, therefore, that periodic blood examinations be made in older people.

Can one tell if anemia is present by noting the color of the face and skin?

Not always. Sunburn may hide an anemic state.

How useful are blood transfusions in the treatment of chronic anemia in older people?

Not very useful, since the main value of blood transfusion is the immediate replacement of blood that has been lost suddenly, as, for example, by hemorrhage. The giving of blood to restore red-blood-cell mass is a temporary measure and will not cure anemia. Cure must be brought about by eliminating the underlying cause of the condition, whether it be a disease of the blood-forming organs, tumors, lymph-gland disease, heart condition, liver disorder, or any other ailment.

Do people past sixty ever develop anemia even though they eat a normal diet and take supplementary vitamins and minerals?

Occasionally. If an underlying disease is present, no matter how complete the mineral and vitamin intake in the diet is, anemia may still develop. In such instances, the primary disease must be eliminated before the anemia can be.

Do healthy older people tend to develop anemia when they maintain a well-balanced diet and take supplemental minerals and vitamins?

No. Such people tend to develop anemia no more than younger people.

Is anemia always associated with malnutrition and an underweight condition?

No. Many stout people are anemic because they do not eat a sensible, well-balanced diet containing the appropriate amounts of minerals, vitamins, and other vital nutritive substances.

Can strenuous dieting lead to anemia?

Yes, unless it is very carefully controlled by a physician.

Is anemia always seen in association with cancer and other malignant diseases?

Not in the early stages of these conditions. Many malignancies are accompanied by anemia only in their later stages.

Does anemia ever clear up by itself?

Yes, if the underlying cause is no longer present. For example, if someone is anemic because of a long-standing infection that finally subsides, the anemia will also probably subside. This is not a quick process, however; it may take several weeks or months.

Will extensive exposure to sunshine prevent or cure anemia?

No. The main benefit of sunshine is derived from the absorption of vitamin D. Although vitamin D is an important component of a normal diet, an increased amount will not correct anemia or prevent its onset.

Is it safe for older people to take nationally advertised medications that profess to prevent or cure anemia without first consulting their doctors?

No. Such medication should be prescribed by a physician after a thorough physical examination. Only in this way is it possible for him to uncover the basic cause of the anemic condition.

Is the taking of vitamins over a long period of time sufficient to prevent the onset of anemia in older persons?

No. Even a normal diet with the proper intake of minerals and vitamins cannot prevent anemia if the anemia is due to conditions such as heart disease, kidney disease, diabetes, tuberculosis, cancer, or liver disease.

Will taking liver and iron by mouth or by injection prevent anemia?

Usually, unless there is an underlying disease, as mentioned above.

Is anemia that is caused by iron deficiency any more common in people past sixty than it is in younger people?

No. When it does occur, iron replacement by improved diet and iron preparations are indicated.

What foods are particularly rich in iron?

Egg yolk, green vegetables, liver, red meat, molasses, nuts.

Can all people take iron preparations by mouth?

No. Iron medications sometimes produce intestinal upsets, which necessitates their being given by injection.

Does the taking of iron pills change the color of the stool?

Yes. The stool often turns to green or jet black.

Is it true that older people with anemia tend to recover from infections and other diseases more slowly than those who are not anemic?

Definitely, yes. The presence of anemia may turn an acute condition into a chronic condition.

Do anemic people past sixty require special treatment before undergoing surgery?

Yes. It is essential that they have a sufficient quantity of red blood cells and hemoglobin. To ensure this, repeated blood transfusions are often required prior to surgery. In addition, the chemical makeup of their blood must be close to normal;

especially important is the level of proteins, vitamins B and C, and the amounts of sodium, chloride, potassium, etc.

Do people in their seventies and eighties react as well as younger people to blood transfusions?

Yes.

Does the presence of anemia slow the rate of healing following surgery?

Yes.

How can one tell if he is anemic?

By having a simple blood test made. A drop of blood is taken by pricking a finger and a hemoglobin determination is made.

How often should the blood be checked for anemia?

Once or twice a year or whenever anemia is suspected.

What measures should be taken to avoid the development of anemia?

1. A semiannual physical examination, including a complete blood count, should be made.
2. A well-balanced diet containing adequate amounts of minerals (including iron), vitamins, fresh vegetables, and red meats should be eaten.
3. Strenuous reducing and fad diets should be avoided.
4. Any repeated bleeding, such as that from hemorrhoids or the nasal passages, should be checked and corrected.

Liver-extract pills, iron preparations, vitamins, etc., should not be taken unless prescribed by a physician. By temporarily improving the general sense of well being, they may result in the patient's delaying medical treatment for a serious underlying disease that has caused the anemia.

Can anemia be cured completely in older people?

Yes, if the underlying cause is completely eliminated. In other words, if the anemia is due to diet deficiency and if the diet is then corrected, the anemia will be controlled. But if the anemia is associated with a malignant blood disease (such as leukemia), a permanent cure cannot be effected.

ANESTHESIA

See RESPIRATORY TRACT; SURGERY; TEETH.

Can people past sixty safely undergo surgical anesthesia?

Yes. Anesthesiologists today are well aware of the special problems in operating on older people. If the patient is a good surgical risk, and if the usual techniques of anesthesiology are modified, then anesthesia may be safely administered.

Is there such a thing as being too old to be given an anesthetic?

Not merely because of advanced age. Often, people in their seventies, eighties, or nineties are in remarkably good health and thus can withstand anesthesia without too much risk.

Is it safe to administer local anesthesia to patients past sixty?

Yes, unless there is a sensitivity to the drug used as the local-anesthetic agent, such as novacaine. Older people are no more sensitive to such drugs than younger people.

Is local anesthesia often used for major surgery on people of advanced age?

There are relatively few indications for local anesthesia in major surgery at any age. However, there are certain patients whose general condition will not permit a general anesthesia. For these few, a form of local or regional anesthesia may be indicated. Operations on a strangulated hernia in poor surgical risks in their eighties are occasionally performed with only local anesthesia.

Can intravenous anesthesia, such as Pentothal, be given safely to people in their seventies or eighties?

Yes, as prior to general anesthesia. After the patient has gone to sleep, gas anesthesia is substituted. Intravenous sleep-producing sedatives are most valuable for those who are especially apprehensive about surgery.

Is spinal anesthesia safe for people who are in their later years?

If patients are in good general health, spinal anesthesia is safe at any age. However, if the patient has high blood pressure, hardening of the arteries, or if the operation involves an organ in the upper abdomen (such as the gallbladder or stomach), it is perhaps best to use a general anesthetic.

What gas (inhalation) anesthesia is best to give to people past sixty?

Most older patients can tolerate any of the gases. Special agents are employed only when the patient has an associated condition such as high blood pressure, heart disease, or lung disease. The greatest "all-around" anesthetic is ether.

Can gas anesthesia be given to older people who are known to have bronchitis, emphysema, or some other lung condition?

Yes, but special postoperative precautions are taken to see that accumulating secretions are sucked out of the bronchial tubes at frequent intervals.

Is it safe for older people to receive general anesthesia in a dentist's office?

This is probably not a good idea for anyone, but particularly not for people past sixty. Complications of general anesthesia may arise; if they do, it is much better for the patient to be in a hospital, where all necessary facilities to deal with the problem are available.

Are there any types of anesthesia that should not be given to people past sixty?

No. They can receive any kind of anesthesia if it is given properly and if it is specifically indicated for the particular operation to be performed.

Do complications arising from anesthesia occur more frequently in older people?

Not in those who are in good health and have not yet shown marked signs of aging. However, complications do occur more often in those who have advanced arteriosclerosis, heart damage, chronic lung conditions, or impairment of kidney or liver function.

Should older people take special measures before entering the hospital to ensure smoother anesthesia and milder postanesthetic convalescence?

Definitely, yes.

1. If they are heavy smokers, they should stop smoking several days before surgery. This will cut down on the number of postoperative lung complications.
2. If they are used to drinking large amounts of alcohol, they should decrease the amount before entering the hospital.
3. If they have had a recent cold or other respiratory infection, they should postpone elective surgery.
4. If they have been taking medication to reduce high blood pressure, such medication should be discontinued a few weeks before elective surgery.
5. If they have been taking cortisone, ACTH, or similar drugs prior to surgery, they should inform the anesthetist and surgeon about this.
6. Loose or infected teeth should be removed before entering the hospital for an elective operation.
7. Older people should have plenty of bed rest and nourishing foods for the weeks preceding an elective operation.

What can be done for a very sick older person in order to enable him to receive anesthesia?

1. If the patient is in shock, this condition must be treated by giving blood transfusions, oxygen, and other medications to maintain a satisfactory blood-pressure level.
2. Heart failure or any other form of heart malfunction must be controlled prior to the anesthesia by digitalis or other drugs.
3. If there is marked anemia, blood must be given prior to anesthesia.
4. If the patient is undernourished, he will require minerals, proteins, and vitamins prior to anesthesia. It may be necessary to give these substances intravenously.
5. If the patient is dehydrated or has acidosis, this condition must be corrected by appropriate intravenous injections.

What special measures should be taken to safeguard older people during anesthesia?

1. It is essential that they receive an adequate supply of oxygen. Brain cells are particularly sensitive to deprivation of oxygen. Since older people may have some hardening of the arteries to the brain, which condition reduces the oxygen supply, it is vital that the amount of oxygen be sufficient during anesthesia.
2. People in their later years are particularly sensitive to narcotics, such as morphine, and to sedatives, such as the barbiturates. In medicating older people before anesthesia, it is therefore important that the dosage of these drugs be carefully calculated. As a rule, people past sixty require only about two-thirds of the normal dose of morphine or the barbiturates.
3. Many older people wear dentures; these must be removed before the patient undergoes anesthesia so that they do not become dislodged and block the air passages.
4. Particular care is exercised in choosing the kind of anesthetic agent given to older people. A frank discussion is often held prior to anesthesia to determine the patient's preference and to allay existing fears. In the great majority of instances the anesthetist can vary the method of inducing anesthesia so as to minimize fear.
5. Men past sixty often have enlargement of the prostate gland, which may make urination difficult for the first few days after spinal anesthesia. If the prostatic enlargement is excessive, general rather than spinal anesthesia may be used.
6. Those past sixty have a greater incidence of bronchitis,

emphysema, and other pulmonary conditions that make aeration of the lungs somewhat more difficult. For these people, it is sometimes advisable to choose a local or spinal anesthesia, in order to avoid postoperative lung complications.

7. Since the skin on the face may be thinner and more sensitive, the anesthetist will take special care to protect it during inhalation anesthesia.

8. Teeth in older people are often loose. Therefore, when an airway or other instrument is inserted into the mouth during anesthesia, special precautions are taken not to break or loosen teeth further.

9. The covering membrane of the eyes (the conjunctiva) requires special safeguards when a mask is over the face and when anesthetic gases are being used. Excessive irritation may lead to an ulceration of the lining membrane of the eye (the cornea), which takes a great deal longer to heal in a person past sixty.

What may happen if older people receive insufficient oxygen during anesthesia?

This may cause irreversible damage to brain cells. Of course, it occurs rarely, mainly to those who have advanced arteriosclerosis. Brain damage may be evidenced postoperatively by mental depression, irritability, loss of memory, and other signs of senility.

Does it take older people longer to come out of anesthesia?

Usually, yes. The brain cells take longer to resume normal function in people who show signs of aging.

Do mucous secretions tend to collect in the throat and lungs of older people after anesthesia?

Yes. For this reason, it is essential that they have expert postoperative care. Such care will include the frequent sucking out of mucus from the back of the throat and from the trachea.

In some cases a tracheotomy (making an opening in the trachea) is performed postoperatively in order to assure that the tracheal and bronchial tubes can be thoroughly cleansed of accumulated secretions.

What special precautions should be taken for older people with heart disease who must undergo anesthesia?

A heart specialist or an internist should be in attendance. He will undoubtedly prescribe medications to support the heart before surgery. Cardiac patients, however, should be operated on only if surgery is essential.

Can the heart of an older person withstand extensive and prolonged anesthesia?

Yes, unless there is serious preexisting heart disease. Many people in their seventies and eighties have adequate heart function and will therefore tolerate anesthesia almost as well as those who are many years younger.

Do older people usually have the same fears about receiving anesthesia as younger people?

There are exceptions, but most older people have a more mature attitude about anesthesia and harbor fewer fears than younger people. They tend to be more relaxed and their reflexes are less violent than those of younger patients. All of this is more conducive to a smooth induction of anesthesia. On the other hand, some older people have an extraordinary fear of death and this may be evidenced by a strong resistance to anesthesia. A skilled anesthesiologist can do much to allay such fears if he holds a frank discussion with the patient a day or two prior to surgery.

ANEURYSMS

See APOPLEXY, OR STROKE; ARTERIOSCLEROSIS; BLOOD PRESSURE; HYPERTENSION.

What is an aneurysm?

An aneurysm is a weakness in the wall of an artery, resulting in a bulge in its surface. It can be compared to a blister on an automobile tire. There is also a thinning of the wall, which predisposes to rupture of the artery.

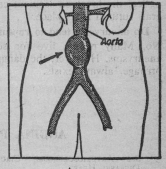

Aneurysm

What causes an aneurysm?

1. The most frequent cause of aneurysm is arteriosclerosis. The normal elastic lining of the arterial wall is replaced by fibrous tissue, which lacks the power of contraction and expansion that normal tissue has. With the continued pressure of the

blood coursing through it, this weakened area in the arterial wall tends to thin out, stretch, and bulge.

2. Decades ago, when many patients with syphilis went for years without treatment, there were many cases of syphilitic aneurysm of large vessels, especially the aorta. Today, syphilis is a rare cause of aneurysm.

3. Aneurysms are occasionally produced by injury to an artery, as from a gunshot or stab wound.

What are common sites for aneurysms?

In the arteries supplying the brain, in the thoracic (chest) and abdominal aorta, or wherever an artery has been injured.

Is there any way to prevent an aneurysm from forming?

Up to the present time, no method has been found for avoiding this phenomenon. When methods of delaying the arteriosclerotic process are discovered, aneurysms will probably be much less common.

What is the treatment for an aneurysm of a major artery?

If a patient has an aneurysm of an artery within the skull and it has been diagnosed prior to rupture, surgery for its correction may be possible. Although considerable brain damage may result from this type of surgery, it must be remembered that a ruptured aneurysm within the skull usually is fatal. If the aneurysm is within the abdominal aorta, the affected segment of the aorta can be removed surgically and a Dacron or Teflon graft can be sutured in its place. Such operations can now be carried out successfully in the great majority of cases. If the aneurysm is in an artery of the arm or leg, the involved segment can be removed and an arterial graft sutured in its place.

Do aneurysms tend to rupture soon after they form?

No. Many people live for several years with unruptured aneurysms. However, the danger of rupture, with fatal hemorrhage, always exists.

ANGINA PECTORIS

See ARTERIOSCLEROSIS; CIRCULATION; CORONARY-ARTERY DISEASE; HEART.

What is angina pectoris?

It is a condition in which there are recurring episodes of severe pain in the chest, usually beneath the breastbone or over the heart region on the left side. The pain often radiates down the left arm and may involve the ring and little fingers. The attacks come on suddenly and last for several minutes.

What causes angina pectoris?

It is thought to be brought on by a spasm of the coronary artery, which supplies blood to the heart muscle. When this important vessel constricts, it delivers an insufficient quantity of blood and oxygen to a segment of heart muscle. As a result, the heart muscle develops a "cramp," which causes pain.

What are some of the major factors underlying a coronary-artery spasm?

1. Arteriosclerosis of the artery. Although the great majority of those suffering from severe angina pectoris do have arteriosclerotic changes within the vessel, many who are afflicted with angina pectoris show almost no arteriosclerosis. A sclerotic artery is more likely to go into spasm than a healthy one.
2. Strenuous physical activity may cause a coronary artery to go into spasm.
3. Emotional upset or severe stress may precipitate a coronary spasm.
4. Strenuous sexual activity may bring on an attack.
5. Walking uphill, especially against the wind or in cold weather, may cause coronary spasm.
6. Eating a very large meal, especially when it is eaten quickly and followed by walking outdoors, may precipitate an attack.
7. Obesity seems to be a factor predisposing to angina pectoris.
8. High blood pressure over a prolonged period of time may cause the coronary artery to spasm.
9. Smoking (especially of cigarettes) may provoke attacks of angina pectoris.
10. There are many other factors that can cause a coronary-artery spasm with the accompanying chest pain.

What is ischemia of the heart muscle?

This term refers to heart muscle that is receiving an insufficient supply of blood.

Does angina pectoris afflict mainly older people?

No. It is not at all uncommon among people in their thirties and forties. However, it is also seen frequently in those who are in their sixties and seventies.

Is the incidence of angina pectoris greater among men than women?

Yes.

When people suffer from this condition, how frequently do attacks come?

There may be one or two attacks a month, or there may be as many as twenty or more attacks each day.

Is angina pectoris frequently a forerunner of coronary thrombosis?

Yes, since most people with angina pectoris have some degenerative changes within the coronary artery.

Is there any satisfactory treatment for the acute chest pain?

Yes. A nitroglycerin tablet dissolved under the tongue will often dilate the coronary artery and relieve the pain within a matter of seconds.

Is it harmful to take nitroglycerin?

No.

Is nitroglycerin habit-forming?

No.

Can one often prevent the onset of an attack of angina pectoris by taking a nitroglycerin tablet before beginning some strenuous activity?

Yes. This is a very good practice to follow.

Are there medications that can be taken daily to prevent an episode of angina pectoris?

Yes. Some long-acting nitrite drugs will, in some cases, maintain the coronary artery in a dilated state and thus reduce the number of attacks of pain.

How can attacks of angina pectoris be avoided?

1. Stay thin, or get thin.
2. Avoid eating large meals.
3. Do not do strenuous physical exercise, especially after eating.
4. Sexual activity should be controlled and moderate.
5. Avoid unnecessary emotional strain.
6. Do not walk rapidly, especially uphill or against a stiff wind.
7. Stop smoking.
8. If anemic, get treatment for the correction of that condition.
9. If blood pressure is very high, get medication to lower it.
10. Take a nitroglycerin tablet *before* doing something that might precipitate an attack.

APOPLEXY, OR STROKE

See ARTERIOSCLEROSIS; BLOOD PRESSURE; BRAIN TUMOR; COMA; CONVULSIONS; EMBOLUS AND EMBOLISM; EPILEPSY; FAINTING; HYPERTENSION; THROMBUS AND THROMBOSIS; VERTIGO AND DIZZINESS.

What are cerebral hemorrhage, cerebral thrombosis, and cerebral embolus?

These terms describe the symptoms resulting from any of the following phenomena:

1. Rupture of a blood vessel, usually of an artery that supplies blood to some portion of the brain (cerebral hemorrhage).
2. A clot, or thrombosis, in a blood vessel—an artery, or vein—within the brain (cerebral thrombosis).
3. A blood clot that has broken away from some distant point, usually the inner lining of the left side of the heart, and has traveled to the brain, where it clogs an artery (cerebral embolus).

Are stroke and apoplexy the same as cerebral hemorrhage, cerebral thrombosis, and cerebral embolus?

Yes. These terms are in general usage and refer to almost all types of blood-vessel accidents within the skull.

Are strokes more likely to affect people past sixty?

Yes. As one might expect, they occur more often in those who have developed hardening of the arteries within the brain and in persons who have developed heart disease.

What is a cerebrovascular accident?

Either a hemorrhage or a clot in a blood vessel within the brain.

What are the symptoms of a cerebral hemorrhage?

If the blood vessel that ruptures is small, only a small area of the brain may be damaged because of the blood-supply deprivation or pressure of the hemorrhage on it. Functions normal to that area of the brain may be impaired. If there has been a sizable hemorrhage, then coma (unconsciousness), loss of speech, and paralysis of one side of the body may ensue. If a major vessel ruptures, then coma, mounting pressure within the skull, and death may occur within a few minutes or hours.

What are common symptoms of cerebral thrombosis?

Coma, loss of speech, partial paralysis, and loss of functions normal to the affected portion of brain often result when a blood clot (thrombosis) involves a vein or artery to the brain.

Degeneration of brain tissue may follow if the blood supply or blood drainage is greatly interfered with. Usually the symptoms are milder and the chances for recovery are greater with a cerebral thrombosis than with a cerebral hemorrhage.

What are common symptoms following cerebral embolism?

They are much the same as those following cerebral thrombosis. Much will depend on the size of the artery that has become clogged by the embolus. As mentioned above, when the heart pumps its blood, a clot is thrown into the circulation and ascends via the blood vessels of the neck into the brain, clogging a vessel within the brain. The symptoms will depend on which particular brain area is deprived of blood by the clot.

Do young people ever have strokes?

Yes, rarely. When they do, the stroke is usually the result of rupture of an aneurysm (*see* ANEURYSMS) in an artery, or is secondary to rheumatic heart disease and the dislodging of clotted blood from the wall of the left atrium of the heart. The clot travels to the brain and causes cerebral embolism.

What are some of the factors that determine whether recovery from a stroke will take place?

First of all, much will depend on the size of the blood vessel involved and how much brain tissue has been damaged. If the coma deepens, if pressure within the skull increases, and if the paralysis extends, the patient will probably not recover. On the other hand, some strokes are so mild that loss of consciousness lasts but a few moments or hours. In such cases the stroke was in all probability caused by the clotting of, or hemorrhage from, a very small blood vessel.

What is hemiplegia?

It is paralysis of one side of the body caused by a rupture or clot of a blood vessel in the *opposite side* of the brain. Thus, if a patient has a stroke on the left side of his brain, his right arm and leg may become paralyzed. This phenomenon is explained by the fact that nerve fibers in the brain cross over to the opposite side before leaving the skull to supply the rest of the body.

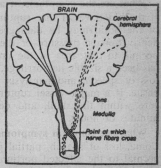

Diagram showing crossing of nerve fibers as they exit from the brain

Do persons ever recover from hemiplegia?

Yes. Recovery often takes place; again, this will depend upon how extensive the brain damage has been.

How long does it usually take to recover from the paralysis of a stroke?

1. If, as occasionally occurs, the paralysis is caused only by spasm of a blood vessel, complete recovery may take place within a few minutes to a few hours.
2. If the paralysis is due merely to the clotting of a small blood vessel, the paralysis may clear up within a few days.
3. If the paralysis is due to hemorrhage within brain substance, or if the thrombosis involves a large vessel, thereby blocking circulation to a large segment of the brain, full recovery will probably never take place. Partial recovery will require several months.

Can rehabilitation aid and speed recovery from a stroke?

Yes. *See* REHABILITATION AND PHYSICAL THERAPY.

How can a physician tell whether or not a patient will survive a stroke?

In all probability, those who survive the first few days will survive. On the other hand, if unconsciousness (coma) continues for more than five or six days, the outlook is poor.

Is the power of speech often lost because of a stroke?

Yes. A common site for cerebral hemorrhage or thrombosis is the area of the brain that controls speech.

Why do some people lose their power of speech following a stroke, whereas others retain it?

In right-handed people, the speech center is located in the *left* side of the brain. If the left side of the brain is affected by a stroke in such people, the likelihood of loss of speech is great. If, however, the right side of the brain is involved, speech will remain unaffected.

The opposite situation obtains for left-handed people.

Can those who have lost their power of speech from a stroke ever regain it?

If the stroke has been mild or moderate, speech may be regained after a period of weeks or months. If damage to the speech area has been great, the power of speech may never be regained, although improved methods of rehabilitation have helped some people to learn to speak again.

Are sight and hearing often lost as a result of cerebral hemorrhage or thrombosis?

No. Fortunately, in the great majority of cases these senses are spared.

Does mental deterioration or insanity usually accompany a stroke?

No. For some interesting, but unexplained, reason, the areas that control one's mental powers are not often affected by cerebral hemorrhage, thrombosis, or embolus. Thus, even though one may have completely lost the power of speech as the result of a stroke, he will usually retain his mental capacities and powers of understanding. Those who attend older people must remember this. Many who cannot speak may be able to write and to make themselves understood by gestures and facial expressions.

Is hemiplegia, paralysis, or stroke ever caused by a thrombosis (clot) in the carotid artery in the neck?

Recent investigations have shown that certain people develop strokes that indicate brain damage as the result of a thrombosis in the carotid artery in the neck, rather than a clot in an artery within the brain itself. In certain cases of this type, where X rays show blockage of the carotid artery, surgery has brought relief. Operations have been performed in which the carotid artery is removed and an arterial graft (usually composed of Dacron or Teflon) has been substituted.

Can most people who suffer strokes be helped by surgery on the carotid artery?

Unfortunately, it is the rare victim of a stroke who can benefit from this type of surgery.

What are the warning symptoms of a stroke?

Frequent severe headaches and dizziness, loss of sense of balance, ringing in the ears, lapses in memory, personality changes, and momentary losses of consciousness should act as warning signals to older people—especially those with exceedingly high blood pressure—that a stroke may be imminent.

What can people past sixty do to lessen their chances of having a stroke?

1. Those who are known to have high blood pressure should visit their doctors regularly—at least every month or two.
2. The onset of any of the symptoms listed above should serve as a warning to cease physical activity and go to bed. If the symptoms persist, the doctor should be summoned, no matter what time of day or night it may be.
3. All possible measures should be taken to avoid emotional strain.

4. Eating, as well as drinking of alcoholic beverages, should be restricted.

APPENDICITIS

See ANESTHESIA; SURGERY.

What is the appendix and where is it located?
It is a wormlike extension of the cecum (the beginning portion of the large intestine), located in the lower right part of the abdomen. It is about the diameter of a lead pencil and measures two to four inches in length.

Does the appendix perform any active intestinal function?
No. It is now thought to be a leftover structure that had specific functions in early man.

Do people past sixty develop inflammation of the appendix?
Yes, but less often than children and young adults do.

Is appendicitis caused by dietary indiscretion?
No.

Are the symptoms and signs of appendicitis different in older people?
In many instances it is much more difficult for the surgeon to make the diagnosis, as the symptoms are less marked. There may be less of a temperature rise, less abdominal pain and tenderness, and less of a rise in the white-blood-cell count, especially in those patients who are in their seventies and eighties.

Is there a greater tendency for an inflamed appendix to rupture or become gangrenous in older people?

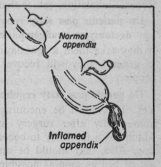

Yes. Arteriosclerosis of the blood vessels supplying the appendix may contribute to a rapid spread of inflammation, with early gangrene.

Can appendicitis be treated safely by antibiotic drugs rather than by surgery among older people?
This is a dangerous proce-

Appendicitis

dure, for if the antibiotics fail to control the infection, peritonitis (inflammation and pus in the abdominal cavity) will result.

Is it just as important to operate on older people who have appendicitis as it is to operate on patients in their middle years?

Yes, and whenever there is doubt as to diagnosis, it is much safer to perform an exploratory operation than to withhold surgery. People in their seventies and eighties are less able to overcome peritonitis, and it is therefore wiser to operate—even if appendicitis is not found—than to take the chance of overlooking an acutely inflamed appendix, which would rupture and cause peritonitis.

Can patients over sixty withstand an appendectomy as well as younger people?

Yes, if their heart, kidneys, and other vital organs are in satisfactory condition. The removal of the appendix is not a dangerous operation. Modern anesthetics and operative techniques have removed most of the hazards of this operation even for elderly patients.

How soon after the diagnosis is made should the operation be performed?

Immediately, or as soon as the patient can be adequately prepared for surgery. Delay carries with it no advantage; it may increase the risk of rupture of the appendix, with resultant peritonitis.

What kind of anesthesia is best for older people who must have an appendectomy?

General inhalation, rather than spinal, anesthesia.

Do patients past sixty recover as quickly from an appendectomy as younger patients?

It may take them a few days longer to get back to normal; in general, they will recover almost as rapidly as younger people.

Do people past sixty require special postoperative care?

Yes. They must be encouraged to resume physical activity immediately after surgery in order to restore circulation, which has a tendency to become sluggish following an operation. Also, they should be made to sit up in bed and to get out of bed as soon as possible after surgery, in order to keep their lungs aerated and to decrease the chances of lung complications.

How long is hospitalization usually necessary following appendectomy?

If the appendix was removed before it ruptured, a hospital stay of approximately 7 to 10 days will suffice. Of course, if the appendix had ruptured, or if peritonitis had set in, several weeks of hospitalization may be required for full recovery.

What special dietary precautions are necessary during recovery from an appendectomy?

One should eat sparingly for two to three weeks after surgery and should avoid fats, greases, spices, and alcohol.

Is there any way for older people to avoid appendicitis?

No.

ARCUS SENILIS AND ARCUS SENILIS LENTIS

See EYES.

What is arcus senilis?

It is a whitish-gray ring that sometimes develops at the margin of the white and colored portions of the eye in people past sixty.

What is the significance of arcus senilis?

It has no clinical significance at all and does not interfere in any way with vision. The ring merely denotes aging.

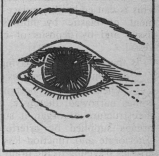

Arcus senilis

What is arcus senilis lentis?

It is an opaque ring occasionally seen in the lens of the eye in older people. It does not interfere with vision and requires no treatment.

Is there any way to prevent the development of arcus senilis or arcus senilis lentis?

No.

ARTERIOSCLEROSIS

See ANEURYSMS; ANGINA PECTORIS; APOPLEXY, OR STROKE; BLOOD PRESSURE; CHOLESTEROL; CIRCULATION; CLAUDICATION; CORONARY-ARTERY DISEASE; DEGENERATIVE CHANGES OF AGING; DIABETES MELLITUS; EMBOLUS AND EMBOLISM; HEART; HYPERTENSION; KIDNEYS; LONGEVITY; MENTAL CHANGES; PARKINSON'S DISEASE; PREMATURE AGING; THROMBUS AND THROMBOSIS.

What is arteriosclerosis, or hardening of the arteries?

The wall of a normal artery is strong, pliable, and elastic. These qualities permit it to expand and contract to accommodate the pulsating stream of blood that passes through it. When it is involved in the arteriosclerotic process, its walls become rigid, pipelike, inelastic, and the passageway is narrowed. This is caused by the replacement of elastic by fibrous tissue and by deposits of calcium within the walls of the vessel.

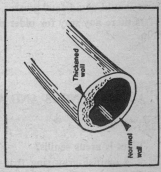

Arteriosclerosis of a blood vessel

Is there truth to the sayings "One is as old as his arteries" or "One is as young as his arteries"?

Yes. When an artery becomes hardened, its passageway becomes narrowed; therefore, it is able to carry less blood to the structure or organ it supplies. For this reason, various organs supplied by arteriosclerotic blood vessels tend to deteriorate and function less effectively. For example, if the arteries traveling to the brain become hardened and narrowed, brain changes will take place and senility will ensue. Similarly, if the coronary artery, which supplies the wall of the heart, becomes hardened and narrowed, heart function will suffer.

Do all people develop extensive hardening of the arteries as they approach the seventies and eighties?

No. Many people show only minor evidence of arteriosclerosis in their sixties—or even in their seventies.

Are all arteries subject to arteriosclerotic changes?

Yes. All arteries are subject to some hardening as time goes on. However, for some unknown reason one set of vessels may demonstrate extensive changes, whereas vessels in other parts of the body will show little or no arteriosclerosis. This phenomenon explains why some elderly people continue to have excellent functioning of one set of organs, such as the heart or kidneys, whereas other organs, such as the brain or liver, may be markedly affected by arteriosclerosis.

Which arteries are particularly susceptible to extensive hardening as one advances in age?

The important vessels such as the aorta and the arteries supplying the brain, heart, liver, kidneys, and the lower limbs.

How does the body react to hardening of its main blood vessels?

There is a slow reactive process, which takes place over a period of time from the middle years onward. When blood flow through the main vessels becomes sluggish, the smaller arteries that make up the so-called collateral circulation tend to take over the function of the main vessels. Thus, someone with marked arteriosclerosis of the major vessels in the legs may continue with adequate circulation because the smaller, collateral, arteries have dilated and can carry a sufficient amount of blood to keep the limb alive.

What is the underlying cause of hardening of the arteries?

If the answer to this question were known, great advances could be made in slowing the onset of aging. We do know that when hardening of an artery takes place, the elastic tissue in the wall of the vessel is replaced by fibrous tissue, and that deposits of a fatlike substance, *cholesterol*, form directly beneath the inner lining of the artery. But we do not know what starts this process; nor have we yet discovered methods to forestall it.

Does everyone develop hardening of the arteries sooner or later?

Yes, if they live long enough. The process goes on in all people, from birth until death—and, to a certain extent, even in the embryo.

However, the arteriosclerotic process does not affect all people in the same way or at the same age; nor does it proceed at an even, measured pace. At certain periods in life the process may be markedly accelerated; at other times the condition may be relatively quiescent.

Does heredity play an important role in the onset of arteriosclerosis?

Yes. Although there are many modifying factors, if one has

a good hereditary background insofar as hardening of the arteries is concerned, then he, too, can anticipate only minor changes. But, if one's parents and grandparents developed arteriosclerosis early in life, the chances are great that the same thing will happen to him.

What causes certain arteries to undergo arteriosclerotic changes while others remain relatively normal?

The answer to this question is not known.

Does kidney disease lead to premature hardening of the arteries?

Indirectly, yes. If there has been serious kidney disease with extensive damage to the organ, blood will have great difficulty passing through it. This will cause a rise in blood-pressure levels and, ultimately, great strain will be placed on the walls of the arteries. If this process continues for many years, arteriosclerotic changes will occur within the walls of those vessels.

Does liver disease lead to premature hardening of the arteries?

Indirectly, yes. The liver is the largest organ in the body and has many functions, including the control of cholesterol metabolism. If this function of the liver is impaired, there will be an increase in cholesterol. Eventually this substance will be deposited in the walls of the blood vessels, and early sclerosis of those vessels will take place.

Does obesity lead to premature hardening of the arteries?

Indirectly, yes. Fat people make inordinate demands upon their heart and blood vessels to pump and carry blood to all the excess fat tissue. Over a period of years, this added burden on the heart and blood vessels will lead to premature arteriosclerosis.

Does diabetes lead to premature hardening of the arteries?

Yes. People who have had diabetes for many years tend to develop premature arteriosclerosis, especially if the diabetes has been neglected and dietary control has been poor.

If diabetes is controlled adequately throughout life, will hardening of the arteries occur?

In all probability it will not. The person whose diabetic condition is well-controlled can anticipate a span of life as long as that of the nondiabetic.

Do certain races tend to develop hardening of the arteries at an earlier age than others?

Although certain peoples do show a greater tendency toward

the development of diseases that are forerunners of arteriosclerosis, for example, diabetes and liver and kidney disease,
hardening of the arteries as a *primary condition* does not
seem to afflict one race more than another. If this were true,
one might expect to find a race of people whose span of life
was greater than others, or a race whose life-span was much
shorter. This is not the case.

**What role do emotional factors play in the onset of harden-
ing of the arteries?**

In all probability, there is a relationship between a life of great
stress and the early development of hardening of the arteries.
For instance, it is more likely that those who live under great
stress will develop high blood pressure and heart disease.
Both of these conditions are forerunners of arteriosclerosis.
There is a current theory that prolonged emotional stress
causes the adrenal glands to secrete an excessive amount of
adrenalin. If this continues for many years, it will ultimately
cause irreversible changes in the heart and blood vessels,
leading to arteriosclerosis.

What effect does gout have on hardening of the arteries?

All disturbances in metabolism, including gout, may lead to
alterations in body chemistry with resultant hardening of the
arteries. It is well known that people with gout are susceptible
to premature arteriosclerosis.

**Does heart disease lead to premature hardening of the
arteries?**

Yes, particularly when the disease forces the heart to work
overtime in order to pump an adequate supply of blood
through the vessels. The converse is also true; that is, hardening of the arteries will cause heart disease.

**What is the effect of hardening of the arteries that supply
the heart?**

1. Angina pectoris may result. (*See* ANGINA PECTORIS.)
2. Coronary insufficiency may result. (*See* CORONARY-AR-
   TERY DISEASE.)
3. Coronary thrombosis (occlusion) may result. (*See*
   CORONARY-ARTERY DISEASE.)

**How can one tell if there is hardening of the arteries that
supply the heart?**

In most instances, this condition will be detected by electrocardiography. But even if the electrocardiogram does not show
it, the physician will be able to make the diagnosis from the
patient's symptoms.

What is the role of strenuous physical exertion in the development of arteriosclerosis?

All other things being equal, it does not appear to play a major role in the onset of hardening of the arteries, provided the individual is in good general health.

Do men tend to develop arteriosclerosis at an earlier age than women?

No. There is no tendency for *healthy* men to develop arteriosclerosis at an earlier age than *healthy* women. However, this statement must be modified by the fact that men are more likely than nonworking women to develop those diseases that lead to early hardening of the arteries. The greater stresses, strains, and physical hazards of the working man predispose him to diseases that lead to hardening of the arteries.

Does hardening of an artery cut down on the amount of blood it supplies to an organ?

Yes. This factor leads to the premature aging of the organ. For example, if a major artery to the brain is markedly sclerotic, that portion of the brain supplied by it will not function properly. If the process involves most of the arteries supplying the brain, senility will result.

Will serious illness in youth or in the middle years cause hardening of the arteries before it normally would have occurred?

Yes. As an example, it is well known that repeated kidney infections in early life may lead to premature arteriosclerosis of the blood vessels of that organ.

Does high blood pressure cause hardening of the arteries?

Actually, the process is just the reverse, in that extensive hardening of the arteries produces elevated blood pressure.

Does arteriosclerosis predispose one to rupture of a blood vessel?

Yes. Loss of elasticity in the artery wall and replacement of normal tissue by fibrous tissue make a blood vessel brittle and more susceptible to rupture.

Can a diagnosis of hardening of the arteries be made from ordinary physical examination?

In many cases this is possible. The physician can feel the sclerotic arteries in the arms, legs, or neck. Furthermore, arteriosclerosis of the blood vessels in the retina of the eye can be seen with an ophthalmoscope.

Will X rays show hardening of the arteries?

Yes, in many areas, such as the arms, legs, and the thoracic and abdominal parts of the aorta. The deposits of calcium in the wall of a sclerotic artery will often show up on X-ray film.

What are symptoms of hardening of the arteries in the brain?

Considerable arteriosclerosis may take place without causing any symptoms. In an advanced stage, there may be dizzy spells, ringing in the ears, headache, episodes of fainting, periods of memory loss, and personality changes. Advanced hardening of the arteries of the brain may ultimately lead to senility. (*See* MENTAL CHANGES.)

If the arteriosclerotic vessel in the brain becomes completely clogged, or if it ruptures, a "stroke" will ensue. (*See* APOPLEXY, OR STROKE.)

What can be done for people who have already developed hardening of the arteries in the brain?

Measures must be taken to ensure that the sclerotic vessels function as effectively as possible. Some of the measures are as follows:

1. The vessels should be kept dilated by giving specific medications that produce this effect.
2. The diet should be low in fats and cholesterol in an attempt to cut down on new deposits of cholesterol in the walls of an already damaged blood vessel.
3. Emotional strain should be avoided as much as possible so that the vessels do not go into spasm. Such spasm may be followed by a thrombosis (clot) in the vessel and further brain damage.
4. In a certain number of cases, it has been found that arteriosclerosis of the carotid artery in the neck is the major factor in insufficient blood supply to the brain. In this type of condition, a graft for replacement of the arteriosclerotic carotid artery may greatly improve the circulation to the brain. At present, the number of patients whose condition lends itself to this type of surgery is limited.

What effect does climate have on hardening of the arteries?

Some medical people feel that extreme cold may lead to earlier arteriosclerosis. However, this theory is not generally accepted. Peoples all over the world, whether they live in the Tropics or in the Arctic, are subject to this disease.

Although climate may not play an important role in bringing on hardening of the arteries, there can be little doubt that a warm (but not hot) climate is best for people who suffer from hardening of the arteries. Warmth stimulates blood vessels to relax and expand; cold predisposes them to constriction and spasm. A relaxed artery, whether involved in arteriosclerosis or not, is able to convey more blood through its passageway.

Should people with advanced hardening of the arteries move to warm climates?

Yes, if they suffer greatly from arteriosclerosis and if they can afford to make such a change.

What effect does strenuous physical exercise have on arteriosclerosis?

If the hardened arteries are called upon to carry more blood than they are able to, they will rebel and go into spasm. Furthermore, the organs and muscles that these arteries supply will receive an inadequate amount of blood and oxygen if the exercise is too strenuous. For this reason, those with marked hardening of the arteries of the legs must limit walking distance and speed. If they fail to do so, severe cramps (intermittent claudication) will occur.

Although strenuous exercise is unwise for those with hardening of the arteries, *moderate* exercise is essential. This will tend to keep the blood vessels open and will increase the blood flow through the narrowed passages. Much more important, however, is the fact that moderate exercise will cause the smaller surrounding arteries (collateral arteries) to dilate and to carry more blood. This collateral circulation allows some people with advanced arteriosclerosis to live healthy, normal lives into their seventies and eighties.

What effect do the endocrine glands, such as the pituitary, the thyroid, and the adrenals, have on the onset of arteriosclerosis?

Some investigators feel that the hormones secreted by these glands play an essential role in the onset of hardening of the arteries. An upset in the chemical balance maintained by these hormones may lead indirectly to premature arteriosclerosis. As mentioned previously, excessive secretion by the adrenal glands may lead to abnormally high blood pressure with eventual damage to blood vessels.

Does eating large amounts of meat lead to premature hardening of the arteries?

No. It is meat *fat* that should be avoided.

Will following a low-cholesterol diet throughout early adult life delay the onset of hardening of the arteries?

It is too early to be able to answer this question positively. Perhaps in twenty or thirty years the answer will become apparent, when people have lived on a low-cholesterol diet for several decades. The best that can be said now is that most physicians recommend such a diet for those who have a tendency toward high blood-cholesterol levels.

How can one tell if he has high blood cholesterol?

By chemical analysis of blood withdrawn from a vein.

What effect does smoking have on the development of hardening of the arteries?

There is no definite proof that smoking causes hardening of the arteries, although it is known that excessive smoking may cause arteries to constrict and go into spasm. The coronary artery, which supplies the heart, and the blood vessels of the legs are particularly sensitive to the constricting effects of nicotine. Over a period of years, smoking may induce earlier changes than would normally have taken place.

What effect does drinking large quantities of alcoholic beverages over a long period of time have on hardening of the arteries?

Excessive drinking of long duration may indirectly stimulate premature hardening of the arteries by upsetting normal metabolism, including cholesterol metabolism. Furthermore, many people who drink excessively may eventually develop fatty degeneration or cirrhosis of the liver. Either of these conditions may predispose one to premature hardening of the arteries.

Does coldness of the hands and feet necessarily mean that one has hardening of the arteries?

No. Such temperature changes may be due to constriction or spasm of completely normal arteries. However, people who do have marked hardening of the arteries also have a tendency toward coldness of hands and feet.

Is there a greater tendency for arteriosclerotic arteries to form clots (thrombi) within them?

Yes. A hardened artery has a narrowed passageway and blood flows through it at a slower rate. These two factors predispose the vessel to formation of blood clots within it.

Why are the arteries and veins more prominent in older people?

As people grow older they tend to lose some of the fat that lies directly beneath the skin. This loss of the fat surrounding the blood vessels makes them more conspicuous. The increased prominence is not essentially due to arteriosclerosis.

If an artery is already involved in arteriosclerotic changes, are there medications that can reverse the process?

No, although some medications can help to keep such an

artery dilated and thus aid the flow of blood through its narrowed passage.

What effect do cortisone and other steroid drugs have in the treatment of hardening of the arteries?

There is no proof that these medications have a beneficial effect, and undesirable side effects may follow their use.

Can anything be done surgically to combat arteriosclerosis?

Yes. Advances in this field have been truly remarkable. In certain cases, circulation can be improved tremendously by one of the following operations:

1. *Endarterectomy.* This is a procedure in which the arteriosclerotic artery is opened and the roughened, sclerotic inner lining is reamed out. This may open up a markedly narrowed artery and permit a new, smooth lining to form. This operation has proved successful in treating certain cases of arteriosclerosis of the abdominal aorta and of the large arteries of the thighs and legs.

2. *Arterial graft.* In this procedure the arteriosclerotic segment of an artery is replaced by a graft made of Dacron, Teflon, or some other plastic substance. There are now thousands of patients who owe many years of their lives to such operations. Arterial grafts are most successful in treatment of the abdominal aorta, major arteries of the legs, and the carotid artery in the neck.

Will the application of heat to a limb in which there are arteriosclerotic arteries be beneficial?

No. As a matter of fact, the application of heat may be harmful. Limbs in which there is decreased blood flow as a result of arteriosclerosis are often less sensitive to the perception of heat and cold and can be burned very easily.

How important is diet in the development of hardening of the arteries?

More and more attention is being given to this predisposing factor. It is thought, by more and more investigators, that a diet high in animal fat will cause high blood-cholesterol levels. There is interesting evidence to support the theory that high blood cholesterol will lead to the deposit of this substance under the lining membrane of the arteries. And, finally, it is thought that cholesterol deposits represent early stages of hardening of the arteries.

What effect does fat intake have on hardening of the arteries?

This is a much discussed question in all medical circles today. Fat, in the form of cholesterol, is presently thought to be one of the most important factors in early hardening of the arteries.

It is thought that if one limits his fat intake (particularly those fats derived from meats, eggs, and dairy products) throughout his earlier years, the cholesterol level will remain low. A low cholesterol level is thought to be the best safeguard against the onset of early arteriosclerosis. Conversely, it is thought that people with a high intake of animal fats will have a high level of cholesterol in their blood and will be more likely to develop premature hardening of the arteries. Much more information on this subject will be necessary before it is generally accepted as fact by the whole medical profession.

Can people live into their eighties and nineties with hardening of the arteries?

Yes. Every adult has some hardening of the arteries. It is the extent of the damage that often determines how long one will live. Furthermore, much will depend upon whether or not vital vessels are extensively involved. For example, if the main arteries to the kidneys are markedly sclerotic, the life-span may be shortened considerably.

What causes arteriosclerotic arteries to form aneurysms or to rupture?

Very few people past sixty have arteries so hardened that they will rupture or form aneurysms (*see* ANEURYSMS). However, when there is marked arteriosclerosis and calcium is deposited in the wall in place of elastic tissue, the blood vessel becomes brittle. Then the blood, which is propelled forcefully by the pumping action of the heart, pounds against a damaged, nonresilient arterial wall and eventually may cause it to give way partially (aneurysm) or to break.

Can one expect that the span of life will be lengthened when better ways are found to delay the onset of hardening of the arteries?

Yes. Although arteriosclerosis and other consequences of aging cannot be eliminated, new ways to slow the changes are being discovered every year.

What can be done to delay the onset of hardening of the arteries?

1. Stay thin.
2. Avoid excessive physical and emotional stress.
3. Have sources of infection treated as soon as they occur. Particularly important are kidney, bladder, and prostate infections and infections involving the nose and throat, the teeth, and the respiratory and intestinal tracts.

4. Avoid excessive alcohol.
5. Avoid excessive smoking of tobacco.
6. Get plenty of rest, recreation, and sleep.
7. Visit a physician for a thorough physical examination once a year, even if you feel perfectly well.
8. Seek medical advice whenever any unusual symptoms appear.

ARTHRITIS AND RHEUMATISM

See ANATOMICAL CHANGES IN ORGANS; BACKACHE; BONES AND JOINTS; CLIMATE; GOUT; PHYSICAL ACTIVITY AND EXERCISE; REHABILITATION AND PHYSICAL THERAPY.

What is arthritis?
Any inflammation or degenerative change within a joint.

What is rheumatism?
This is a vague term used by laymen to describe any of a large number of conditions associated with aches and pains in muscles, tendons, and joints. The term is so nonspecific that it is not used by physicians. (It should not be confused with rheumatic fever, a specific infection involving the entire system.)

Is stiffness in the joints natural as people grow older?
Yes, but this does not necessarily mean that the function of the joint will be so impaired that it will interfere with normal activity.

Regular physical exercise by people past sixty will eliminate much of the stiffness that occurs in their joints. Lessened secretion of the fluid that lubricates the lining of the joint and thinning out of the cartilage that permits friction-free gliding of one bone over another are thought to cause joint stiffness.

Is it natural for people past sixty to develop constant or recurring pains in their joints?
No. Constant or recurring joint pain indicates the need for medical attention. Healthy people in their sixties and seventies should not have severe or repeated joint pain, although fleeting aches and pains do occur occasionally in all people.

Is it true that almost everyone past sixty will show some evidence of degeneration of the tissues of the joints?
Yes. The joint surfaces wear thin as a result of extensive use.

However, it should be emphasized that these changes do not necessarily interfere with joint function.

What are some of the more common types of arthritis?

1. *Rheumatoid arthritis.* Inflammation affecting mainly the middle joints of the fingers and the wrists and knees. It is seen more often in people in their middle years than in those in their later years.

2. *Osteoarthritis.* This is the most common type of arthritis affecting older people. It usually involves the joints nearest the finger tips, the vertebrae of the spine, and such larger joints as the knee, the hip, and the wrist. Osteoarthritis is one of the degenerative changes in the bones and cartilages that take place with aging.

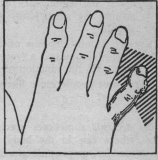

Osteoarthritis, the most common form of arthritis in older people

3. *Gouty arthritis.* This is a form of joint inflammation and inflammation surrounding joints; it is associated with sudden onset of extreme pain. A common site is the big toe, but other joints also may become afflicted. Gout is associated with an upset in uric-acid metabolism and is often seen among older people who eat and drink excessively.

4. *Traumatic arthritis.* This is an inflammation of a joint as a result of injury.

5. *Bacterial arthritis.* This is any infection of a joint caused by bacteria, such as streptococcus, staphylococcus, tuberculosis, or gonococcus.

6. *Metabolic arthritis,* caused by hormonal or chemical imbalance. This type occurs more often among people in their middle years.

7. *Allergic arthritis,* such as that following the injection of vaccines or serums.

What is the incidence of arthritis in people past sixty?

According to reliable statistics, arthritis and allied bone conditions are the most common of all diseases affecting people over sixty.

Is it true that all people past sixty will show some evidence of arthritis?

In a limited sense this is true, inasmuch as X rays of joints will almost invariably show some changes in the bones, even in people who have no joint symptoms whatever. However, this does not mean that active clinical arthritis is present, or that these people will develop pain or limitation of motion in these joints.

What is the significance of the small lumps that appear around the small joints of the hands and feet in older people?

They are usually deposits of calcium or uric acid about the joint. Such lumpiness is a symptom of osteoarthritis. It seldom interferes with the function of the hand or the foot.

Are stout people more likely to develop arthritis than thin people?

Yes.

Is arthritis sometimes precipitated by an infection somewhere else in the body, for example, in the kidneys, bladder, or prostate gland?

Yes. This type of arthritis (usually rheumatoid arthritis) is occasionally encountered in older people, but it seems to be more prevalent in people in their earlier years. When acute inflammation of a joint is accompanied by fever and localized tenderness, an infection elsewhere in the body should be sought.

What is hypertrophic arthritis?

The term hypertrophic refers to the deposits of calcium, urates, or other chemicals that are laid down in certain forms of arthritis occurring in people past sixty. X-ray examination will show these deposits about the involved joints.

Can arthritis be caused by poor diet over the years?

In certain cases, yes. Diets deficient in minerals and vitamins may lead to arthritis.

Is arthritis inherited?

No, but one does tend to inherit his parents' type of metabolism. Thus, if one of the parents had an imbalance in calcium, phosphorus, uric acid, or hormone metabolism, the chance for the offspring to have the same imbalance is great. Of course, the tendency can be modified greatly by the environment and the kind of care he takes of himself.

Can arthritis be caused by overindulgence in alcohol for many years?

It is thought by many medical men that alcohol has some

influence on the incidence of arthritis, but in all probability alcohol alone will not produce arthritis. In combination with other factors, such as chronic mineral and vitamin deficiencies and metabolic imbalance, overindulgence in alcohol may increase the incidence of arthritis.

Is arthritis always accompanied by pain?

No. X rays sometimes show marked evidence of extensive arthritis in people who have no symptoms whatsoever.

What joints are most frequently involved in arthritis?

No joints are exempt from arthritis, although, as mentioned earlier, certain types of arthritis seem to have an affinity for specific joints.

How is the diagnosis of arthritis made?

1. By a history of joint pain and limitation of motion.
2. By careful physical examination.
3. By chemical analysis of the blood.
4. By X-ray examination.

Does arthritis always persist, or does it ever subside spontaneously?

This depends on the type of arthritis. Those cases caused by acute bacterial infection or by injury will subside if properly treated. Some cases of rheumatoid arthritis may be cured, but most people with this disease will continue to have it throughout life. Osteoarthritis, since it is a degenerative process of aging, does not subside; however, its symptoms, for example, pain, will often subside.

Is arthritis always progressive, becoming more severe as the patient gets older?

Not always. Sometimes by discovering and treating the underlying cause of the disease a doctor can arrest arthritis.

Is osteoarthritis painful?

It can be quite painful and is often associated with stiffness in the joints and inability to flex and extend them completely. It is characteristic of this condition that pain and limitation of joint motion are most marked when the arthritic person first gets out of bed. As the joints are used the pain and stiffness tend to subside.

Is rheumatoid arthritis painful?

Yes, in the great majority of cases. It is often associated with swollen, warm, tender joints that cannot be flexed or extended without great pain.

What can be done about stiffness in the joints?

1. Before one gets out of bed in the morning, the joints

should be slowly and easily flexed and extended. After a
few minutes of this exercise, much of the stiffness will
subside.

2. Bedrooms should not be kept too cold at night, since
cold tends to aggravate stiffness of the joints.

3. A hot bath for 20 minutes will help to loosen stiff joints.
Exercises can be conducted while the person is immersed in hot water.

4. Walking is perhaps the best exercise for loosening up
stiff joints in the legs.

5. If one is bedridden or unable to walk, he should be
exercised by his attendant. Even people who must remain in bed can flex and extend their toes, fingers,
wrists, elbows, shoulders, knees, and hips at regular
intervals throughout the day. This is important in order
to prevent further limitation of motion.

**Does arthritis in older people often lead to complete loss
of function of the involved joints?**

In certain types of progressive, advanced osteoarthritis, function may be lost completely. Osteoarthritis in the spinal column
sometimes leads to a fusion of the various vertebrae with loss
of ability to flex or extend the spine. Similarly, advanced
involvement of the fingers, wrists, and other joints, as a result
of rheumatoid arthritis, may result in marked deformity and
loss of use of these structures.

**Do the various spas and resorts, at which special mineral
waters are drunk and baths are taken, help people with
chronic arthritis?**

Many people who take the so-called cures at spas claim to receive great relief from their symptoms. The special baths, hot
packs, and other treatments offered at some of these resorts
tend to make the involved joints less painful. They may
achieve this result by relaxing the muscles and tendons, much
as the Sister Kenny treatment relieved the pain of polio. Also,
the good psychological effects of rest, relaxation, fresh air,
and a healthy diet may have something to do with the
arthritic person's feeling of relief.

Despite the relief of pain and the loosening up of the joints
experienced by the arthritic person after extensive spa treatment, X rays usually show no regression of his arthritis.

**When a person suffers from painful arthritis, should he
treat himself with advertised medications or should he
seek treatment from his physician?**

It is dangerous to medicate oneself for arthritis. Many of the
medications advertised over television and radio can do harm

if taken improperly. At best, self-treatment may waste time that should have been spent following a course of therapy outlined by a physician:

How can one find out if any of the medications advertised on radio and television and in the press are really good for arthritis?

One can conclude that if they are advertised directly to the public, in all likelihood they are not particularly beneficial. Ethical drug companies do not advertise directly to the public.

What are some of the modern methods of treatment for arthritis?

A complete answer to this question would fill several books. Briefly, the following forms of treatment are currently prescribed for arthritis:

1. Measures directed toward the maintenance of general good health. These measures include sufficient rest, the maintenance of a well-balanced diet with adequate intake of vitamins and minerals, and the elimination of infections that might trigger the arthritis.
2. Measures directed toward reducing emotional stress.
3. Local treatment to painful joints: hot packs, whirlpool baths, diathermy, exercises, and other physical therapy.
4. The use of drugs:
   a. The salicylates (aspirin and allied medications) are by far the best group of medicines for the relief of the pain of arthritis. Unfortunately, they rarely cure the disease.
   b. The ACTH and cortisone drugs (the so-called steroids) often cause swelling and pain in an arthritic joint to subside, but they will not, unfortunately, bring about permanent cure. In most cases of arthritis, symptoms return within a few days to a few months after these drugs are discontinued. These drugs should never be taken without the constant supervision of a physician.
   c. Injections of gold salts occasionally are beneficial in the treatment of certain types of rheumatoid arthritis. It is essential that these drugs be administered only by a doctor who specializes in the treatment of arthritis.
   d. Several new drugs, still in the stage of research and trial, are proving beneficial for certain types of arthritis. For their use, one should consult a specialist in arthritis.

**Are rehabilitation techniques helpful to those who are crip-
  pled by chronic arthritis?**

One of the most remarkable developments in medicine in the
past two decades has been the advance made in the field of rehabilitation. With newly devised methods, specialists in this
field are able to teach people who were apparently hopelessly
crippled by arthritis to do most of the things healthy people
can do.

Older people with arthritis should be encouraged to visit a
rehabilitation center or a specialist in physical medicine.
Special training in the use of arthritic limbs may bring about
a great change in the patient's outlook on life and will help
him to live and function more efficiently, despite his condition.

**Does the treatment of arthritis in older people differ greatly
  from that in younger people?**

Yes, to the extent that less strenuous methods are employed in
treating older people. Certain drugs, too, cannot be used as
freely in the treatment of patients past sixty.

**What is the value of physical exercise in the treatment of
  arthritis?**

Physical exercise, as prescribed and administered by specialists
in the field of arthritis, can do much to relieve the pain and
other symptoms of this disease and can increase the range of
motion of an afflicted joint.

**Will the taking of aspirin or one of the other salicylate
  drugs over a long period of time damage the heart or be
  harmful in any other way?**

No. The salicylates do a great deal to relieve pain and spasm
and can be taken for indefinite periods of time. They are
harmful only in the rare instances in which someone is sensitive or allergic to the drugs.

**What can a person do in his middle years to prevent the
  onset of arthritis?**

1. Take regular physical examinations to uncover any
   hidden, chronic infections, such as infected tonsils, infected prostate gland, pelvic infections, infections in the
   urinary tract, infected teeth, and so on.
2. Eat a well-balanced diet, containing adequate minerals
   and vitamins.
3. Avoid excessive use of alcoholic beverages.
4. Avoid physical exertion that places a particular burden
   on one or more joints. (In many occupations, one joint
   or one set of joints carry most of the physical strain.)

5. Take regular physical exercise, such as walking, swimming, or calisthenics.
6. Have a blood chemistry taken once every year to uncover chemical imbalance.
7. If there is joint pain, swelling, or stiffness, consult a physician promptly.

Does arthritis usually shorten the span of life?

Most cases of arthritis do not shorten life. However, if the arthritis is exceptionally crippling, it may cause the patient to become bedridden, and those who are bedridden do have a shortened span of life because of complications that follow.

ARTIFICIAL RESPIRATION

See FAINTING; FIRST AID; GAS AND SMOKE POISONING; INJURIES AND ACCIDENTS.

Under what circumstances should artificial respiration be given?

Whenever breathing has stopped or whenever it is obvious that the patient is having difficulty in breathing. The following is a partial list of such circumstances:

1. Drowning
2. Suffocation
3. Gas poisoning
4. Electric shock
5. When breathing has stopped after a heart attack or stroke
6. Drug poisoning
7. Fainting or convulsions
8. Cold exposure or heat exhaustion

Is artificial respiration ever harmful to people who are having trouble breathing?

Yes, when someone is choking from a foreign body stuck in the throat or trachea (windpipe). In such cases, it is important to dislodge the obstructing object—not to apply artificial respiration. In certain instances, particularly when the mouth-to-mouth method is used, artificial respiration may interfere with the expulsion of the foreign body.

What are the approved methods of administering artificial respiration to older people?

1. The approved Red Cross method, which places the patient flat on his abdomen with the head turned to one

side. The person giving first aid kneels astride the patient and compresses the lower part of the back of his chest rhythmically at the rate of 15 to 20 times per minute.

2. The approved mouth-to-mouth-breathing method:

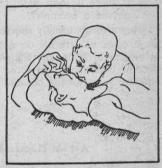

Artificial respiration (mouth-to-mouth breathing)

   a. The patient is stretched out on his back.

   b. Tight clothing about the neck or waist is loosened.

   c. The chin is lifted up and the head tilted back as far as possible so as to straighten out the windpipe and improve the air passage.

   d. The one giving first aid kneels down beside the patient and pinches the nostrils closed with his fingers.

   e. He places his open mouth over the patient's open mouth and blows as hard as he can so as to force air into the patient's lungs.

   f. He withdraws his mouth to permit air to be expelled from the patient's lungs.

   g. The procedure is repeated every 4 to 5 seconds.

   h. When he tires, someone should substitute for him.

   i. If the patient seems to have water or mucus in his throat or chest, tilt him upside down or on his side to permit the fluid to run out from the mouth.

   j. The patient's mouth should be wiped clean of mucus when it collects.

   k. If the person giving first aid is squeamish about mouth-to-mouth contact, he can blow through an open handkerchief. However, this is usually not as effective as direct contact.

How long should artificial respiration be continued?

Until a doctor arrives and ascertains that there is no pulse or heartbeat, even if this means continuing for several hours. As long as there is a heartbeat, there is a chance to save the patient!

Can a disease be caught from the patient by performing mouth-to-mouth breathing?

This is only theoretically possible. If, after the patient has been resuscitated, it is learned that he has a contagious disease, there will be plenty of time for prophylactic treatment.

Do people past sixty respond as well to artificial respiration as younger people?

Usually not, since younger people are better able to withstand oxygen deprivation.

How can one tell if the attempts at artificial respiration are successful?

The patient will at first take an occasional spontaneous breath, and then will resume breathing rhythmically.

Should artificial respiration be stopped as soon as the patient takes his first spontaneous breath?

No. It should be continued until the patient resumes his own regular, deep breathing. This may mean one half to one hour of additional artificial respiration.

What measures should be taken after the victim has resumed spontaneous, rhythmic breathing?

1. He should be covered with coats or blankets and kept warm.
2. He should not be moved for at least half an hour after resuscitation.
3. A doctor should be called.
4. When he regains consciousness, the patient should be encouraged to breathe deeply and to cough up and spit out any accumulated secretions.

Should whiskey or other stimulants be given to people who have just been revived?

No. Wait until expert medical attention can be obtained before giving anything.

ASTHMA

See ALLERGY; BRONCHITIS; CLIMATE; COUGHS; EMPHYSEMA; RESPIRATORY TRACT.

What is asthma?

It is a chronic or subacute condition affecting the bronchial tubes. It may lead to the following:

1. A characteristic type of breathing in which there is no difficulty in inhaling but marked difficulty in expelling air from the lungs.
2. Shortness of breath.
3. Wheezing, with paroxysms of coughing.
4. Difficulty in expelling mucus.
5. Frequent complication by lung infection.

Is asthma in older people usually caused by allergy?

No. Allergic asthma usually affects younger people, although it may persist into the later years. (*See* ALLERGY.)

What is the commonest cause of asthma in older people?

Most often it is secondary to bacterial or viral infection; it may occasionally be due to allergy or such physical factors as the prolonged inhalation of polluted air and fumes.

Is asthma considered to be a form of bronchitis?

Yes. It is associated with swelling, congestion, and inflammation of the lining of the bronchial tubes and production of large amounts of sticky mucus. It is also associated with spasm of the muscles that surround the bronchial tubes, thus making it difficult to expel inhaled air.

Is asthma in older people an acute condition?

No. It is usually a chronic condition lasting a great number of years.

What are the special hazards resulting from asthma in people past sixty?

The difficulty in breathing may be accompanied by inadequate exchange of oxygen and carbon dioxide. This, especially in a person in his seventies or eighties, may lead to serious damage to the heart.

Does an asthmatic attack often cause death among older people?

No. Even though an acute asthmatic attack is a very frightening thing, recovery from the acute episode almost always takes place. Repeated attacks, however, may lead to such serious complications as impairment of lung and heart function.

Should people having an acute asthmatic attack be permitted to sit up in bed or in a chair?

Yes. This position will aid them to breathe. A recumbent (lying down) position is not good for them.

Should older asthmatic patients be permitted to continue to smoke?

Smoking is not good for anyone with a chronic bronchial or

lung condition. On the other hand, if it has been determined that no allergy or sensitivity to tobacco exists, and if the patient is very dependent upon smoking, he may be permitted to do so in moderation.

Should older asthmatic patients give up alcoholic beverages?
An occasional drink will do no harm, but alcohol in large quantities will cause an increase in the secretion of mucus and is therefore harmful!

Do asthmatic attacks tend to come on suddenly and to disappear just as quickly?
Among older people, the sudden acute attack is less common than chronic coughing and wheezing, with difficulty in expelling air and mucus.

Are older people who have asthma more likely to develop complications such as pneumonia or heart failure?
Yes.

Is asthma curable among older people?
It often resists cure and continues as a chronic condition. However, in a great number of instances it can be controlled and its symptoms alleviated.

What is the treatment for asthma and asthmatic bronchitis?
1. If it is suspected that the origin is allergic, the patient should receive treatment from an allergist, who will try to desensitize him against the irritating factors. House dust, animal-fur dust, molds, and pollens provoke asthma; and older people should be tested for sensitivity to these allergens.
2. Antihistamine drugs are often prescribed when it is suspected that the cause is allergic.
3. The acute attack of asthma should be treated immediately by giving antispasmodic drugs, such as epinephrine and ephedrine. These drugs should be kept in the house so that they can be administered by a physician or nurse.
4. Those who are subject to repeated acute attacks should have an oxygen tank available, to be used to relieve oxygen deprivation.
5. Respiratory stimulants, such as Alevaire or other inhalants, should be given for relief of bronchial spasm.
6. Aminophylline is an effective medication for relieving an acute attack and should be kept on hand for injection by a physician or nurse.
7. Inhalation of steam often brings relief and will help the patient to expel mucus.
8. Cortisone and cortisonelike drugs are often helpful for

relieving severe attacks, but these drugs must be used sparingly as a long-term form of treatment.

9. During an acute asthmatic attack, older people are often extremely apprehensive, and must therefore be given a sedative or narcotic.

ATTITUDES TOWARD AGING

See DEATH AND FEAR OF DEATH; FAMILY RELATIONSHIPS; HOBBIES; MENTAL CHANGES; PREMATURE AGING; PSYCHOTHERAPY; RETIREMENT; SOCIAL BEHAVIOR.

What do authorities consider to be a healthy attitude toward growing old?

As they enter their later years people should realize that they face certain limitations of activity and accomplishment that did not exist when they were younger. Mature persons will accept these limitations and devise a mode of life that recognizes them.

No matter how much one might praise the virtues of the sixties, seventies, and eighties, he cannot honestly paint them as being more attractive than youth or the middle years. But, in a very real sense, well-adjusted people over sixty do find new joys and new areas in which to function and serve happily. For example, some of the most rewarding years of life are spent in grandparenthood. Also, many older people discover that some of their most satisfying experiences in life result from the development of hobbies and the adoption of new interests in community activities. If people have the financial means, travel can bring unsurpassed joys to the later decades.

How can a healthy attitude toward growing old be stimulated in people who are approaching their later years?

1. People should be informed that the passage of years does not necessarily mean that their minds and their tissues will lose their ability to function satisfactorily. It is a scientific fact that the minds and bodies of *healthy* people can function normally even into the eighties and nineties.

2. People should be informed that if they maintain good health in their middle years, there is every prospect for their living actively into their eighties and nineties.

3. Aging people should be taught to accept their limitations

and should be encouraged to develop new interests and activities that will conform to their limited capacities. Thus, the man who labored arduously on an assembly line can be taught to work at less strenuous tasks while sitting at a bench. His skilled hands and expert knowledge will still be worthy of utilization.

4. Those who retire should be taught hobbies, many of which can be turned into financially rewarding small businesses.

5. Nothing will make an older person feel young longer than to be placed in a position where he is a useful adviser. Aging people should be encouraged to serve on various union, church, and community committees.

Are depressed states often caused by enforced retirement and the realization that one is aging?

Yes. People often become depressed and inordinately self-concerned when they feel that their usefulness is nearing its end. It is essential, therefore, that members of their family and friends give them tasks and assignments that will make them feel useful and wanted. Retirement should never mean complete inactivity so long as the older person is physically and mentally capable of functioning.

What are some good general rules for children of aging parents to follow?

1. Let them know that they are truly important. Do not let them think that merely because they have stopped earning money their day has passed and their advice and presence are no longer valuable.

2. If aging parents live with their children, the parents should be assigned specific duties to perform.

3. Parents should be dealt with as adults and not talked down to merely because they are old or have retired from active work.

4. Parents' advice should always be sought in areas where they can be helpful—and, perhaps, even when their advice is not so essential. A feeling of participation in the life of the family should be fostered.

5. Older parents should be encouraged to be as physically active as possible. If they are partially incapacitated, those functions that still remain should be utilized.

6. They should be encouraged to make new friends, particularly with older people who are in good health and have happy attitudes.

7. Aging parents should not be forced to live with their children if they prefer to live alone or with other older people.

8. If parents are a financial burden, this fact should be hidden from them as far as possible. Emphasis should be placed on the fact that years ago the reverse situation held.

9. If parents tend to become slovenly or too demanding, they should be told that it is their duty to be a part of family life and that they are not entitled to special privileges merely because they are aging.

10. The advice of physicians who specialize in the care of older people should be sought when necessary. The specialist in geriatrics has much valuable advice to offer those who care for older people.

What are some good general rules for a spouse to follow when his or her mate shows excessive concern over aging?

1. By far the most important thing is for the spouse to let his mate know that he is growing old too. Nothing is more damaging for a wife than the feeling that she is aging while her husband remains young. The converse is equally true!

2. Together, they should develop new interests that will suit their more restricted activities.

3. Mates should realize that they may age at different rates of speed. Thus, one may give up certain physical activities before the other; one may develop changes in appetite before the other; changes in habits may affect one before the other. These differences should be discussed frankly and openly, with full knowledge that the pace of aging is not smooth and even.

4. During their younger years, couples should try to understand that if their interests should diverge because of different rates of aging, they may go in somewhat different directions. This realization will tend to hold them closer together and make each more tolerant of the other.

5. Couples often vary markedly in their sexual desires as they grow older. If they recognize this beforehand, they will tolerate the situation much better.

6. If aging couples tend to lose interest in each other, they should seek professional advice. The objective opinion of a third party, for example, a physician, clergyman, or social worker, may be helpful in directing them toward development of new common interests. (The author knows a husband in his seventies and a wife

in her late sixties who recently discovered that they were immensely interested in sculpture. This new mutual activity, in which the wife became so proficient that she is now a professional sculptress, led to a rejuvenation of their interest in each other. The last few years have proved to be among the happiest of their marriage.)

7. A mate should reassure his or her spouse that the loss in physical attractiveness because of aging has not altered the feeling of love, which still exists.

What are some good rules for a business associate to follow upon discovering that a partner or close associate is showing signs of age that handicap the activities of the business?

1. Do *not* make him feel that he has lost his usefulness to the organization and that he must retire.

2. Discuss, openly and frankly, the future of *all* those in the organization insofar as retirement is concerned.

3. Establish a *mutually* agreeable retirement program.

4. Attempt, by every means possible, to find an area within the business organization where the aging associate can function to better advantage.

5. Whenever possible, enlist the help of members of the aging associate's family in solving difficult business problems.

6. Consult an outside adviser, such as an industrial engineer, efficiency expert, attorney, or even a physician or psychiatrist. Often, the bringing in of an outsider whom both parties respect will avoid unnecessary friction and unhappiness in the business association.

To what agencies should one turn for information concerning part-time jobs for semiretired people, hobbies, volunteer community activities, and other activities that are designed for older citizens?

Church organizations; charitable institutions; sectarian agencies; hospitals; the Community Chest; YMCA; YWCA; YMHA; YWHA; bureaus of social welfare; Veterans Administration; Department of Health, Education and Welfare, in Washington, D.C.; city or county welfare departments; Golden Age clubs and other organizations for elder citizens.

What can be done to help older people who have lost many of their relatives and close friends?

It is interesting and fortunate that as people grow into their seventies and eighties they accept death with much greater equanimity than younger people do. Although this does not alleviate their loneliness, it does make them better able to accept the inevitable. Much can be done to help these people *before* they reach old age. The following is a partial list:

1. They should be encouraged to make new friends.
2. They should be urged to develop hobbies.
3. They should be encouraged to join community and church activities.
4. They should join Golden Age and similar clubs especially organized to interest people who are in their later years.

BACKACHE

See ARTHRITIS AND RHEUMATISM; BONES AND JOINTS; GOUT; MUSCLES; PAGET'S DISEASE; PHYSICAL ACTIVITY AND EXERCISE; REHABILITATION AND PHYSICAL THERAPY; SCIATICA.

What are some of the common causes of backache in older people?

1. Arthritis of the spine and sacroiliac joints.
2. Weakening of the ligaments and muscles that hold the spinal column and sacroiliac joints firmly in place. This leads to instability of the vertebrae.
3. A slipped disk (protrusion of the cartilage lying between the vertebrae).

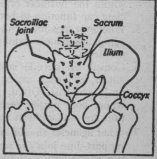

Diagram showing the sacroiliac joint, a very common site of lower-back pain

4. Inflammation of the muscles in the lower back (lumbago).
5. Strain or sprain from lifting heavy objects, a twist or fall, and similar accidents.
6. Improper posture.
7. Osteoporosis (abnormal porousness of the bones) or osteomalacia (softening of the bones with loss of calcium).
8. Sleeping on too soft a mattress.
9. Chronic infections elsewhere in the body.
10. Marked obesity.

Is lower-back pain very common in people past sixty?

Yes, particularly among those who neglect themselves and fail to seek regular medical attention to eliminate ailments and conditions that would cause backache.

Will special physical exercises, whirlpool baths, heat treatments, and massage aid people who suffer from chronic backache?

Yes. Great relief can frequently be obtained from these forms of therapy. The important thing to remember is that the treatments should be prescribed and carried out by specialists. The family physician will usually refer patients with chronic backache to orthopedists or specialists in physical medicine and rehabilitation.

Are corsets and braces helpful in relieving back pain?

Yes. A well-fitted back brace or corset will often give considerable relief. Such appliances should be prescribed by the orthopedist, since there are great variations in types of support and in the benefits derived from them.

Should those suffering from chronic backache sleep on a hard mattress?

Yes, by all means.

Are there specific medicines that can bring about a cure of backache?

No, but many drugs will relieve the symptoms of an acute attack and may relieve much of the severe pain.

Should those with chronic backache take cortisone or similar medications?

Although these medications may alleviate symptoms, they do not produce a cure. Moreover, if these drugs are taken over a long period of time unfavorable side effects are all too frequent. Certainly, cortisone and similar substances should *never* be taken unless they have been prescribed by a doctor.

What can older people do to avoid backache?

1. They should avoid lifting heavy objects, especially from a bending position.
2. They should wear sensible shoes so as to avoid twists or falls.
3. They should have infections such as sinusitis, tonsillitis, kidney or bladder infections, and prostate infections treated promptly.
4. They should not become overweight.
5. Women should wear good corsets.
6. Men who regularly do heavy manual labor should wear back supports or braces.
7. They should sleep on a firm mattress.

BED CARE

See BED-WETTING; BOWEL FUNCTION; HOME-CARE PROGRAMS; HYGIENE; NURSING CARE; NURSING HOMES.

What are some of the items essential to care of a bed-confined older patient?

1. A bedside commode (toilet) to enable the bedridden person to evacuate his bowels without walking to the bathroom. It can be bought or rented from a surgical supply store.
2. A bedpan.
3. A glass urinal (for men).
4. A backrest to enable the patient to sit up in bed. This can be bought or rented from a surgical supply store.

Aluminum and canvas backrest

5. A bedtray for meals.
6. A portable reading lamp that the patient can control.

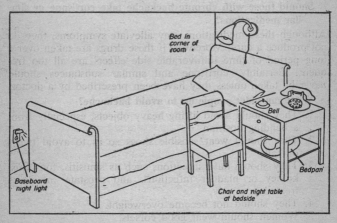

Bedroom specially designed to protect older people

94

7. A simple bell to enable the patient to ring for assistance.
8. A waste basket at the bedside.
9. A night table next to the bed, so that the patient can fill the drawers with things he may want during the day or night.
10. A hand mirror; this often stimulates the patient to take more interest in himself and his surroundings.
11. A box of facial tissues.
12. A telephone within easy reach. It should have a cut-off button so that it will not ring during rest periods.
13. Hand towel and washcloth.
14. "Wash and dry" tissues.

What is the desirable room temperature for older people who are confined to their bedrooms?

Approximately 70° F.

If people are confined to bed and are feeble or ill, should windows be kept closed?

No. Some mechanism for circulation of fresh air should be established. There are methods of getting fresh air into a room without creating direct drafts, which are undesirable.

What can be done to prevent a bedroom from becoming too dry?

Mechanical humidifiers can be purchased if it is known that a patient will be confined for a long time. Also, most radiators have trays or troughs that should be kept filled with water at all times.

Should every effort be made to get older people out of bed, even when they are chronically ill or invalided?

Yes. It is not good for older people to remain in bed any more than is absolutely necessary. Physical inactivity is bad for circulation and may lead to the formation of blood clots within the veins. This can seriously complicate an otherwise mild illness. Moreover, when older people are out of bed, they breathe more deeply and take more oxygen into their lungs. Lying quietly in bed in one position is conducive to the development of pneumonia.

What can be done to prevent skin irritation and chafing?

1. The bedridden patient should be sponged daily with warm water and a mild soap. Sponging with rubbing alcohol after the body has been washed is also beneficial.

2. Care should be taken to dry the body thoroughly after bathing, particularly in the folds and crevices of the skin.

3. The patient should not be covered with blankets so heavy as to make him perspire a great deal. This will result in skin irritation.

4. Body creases should be powdered to prevent moisture from collecting.

5. Position in bed should be changed frequently to prevent excessive pressure on any part of the body.

6. It is important that bed linens be washed only in mild soaps or detergents. Strong soaps may lead to skin rashes and chafing.

7. If ordinary linens cause skin irritation, it may become necessary to purchase other types of bed coverings.

8. Chafing and irritation of elbows and knees can often be prevented by bandaging them or by covering them with satin or silk fabric.

What are bedsores and on what parts of the body do they occur most often?

Bedsores are ulcerations of the skin found at the point of greatest contact between the body and the bed. The most common site is the lower back, where the sacral bones bear the weight of the bedridden patient. A bedridden patient who lies on his side most of the time frequently develops bedsores over the hipbone.

Are bedsores a serious complication in a chronically ill patient?

Yes. They may take months to heal or they may never heal spontaneously. They usually become infected and often require prolonged surgical treatment.

How can bedsores be prevented?

1. The patient's position in bed must be changed frequently to avoid too much pressure on one spot for too long.

2. If it is absolutely essential that the patient lie on his back, a rubber ring should be placed under his buttocks to prevent direct contact between the sacral bones and the mattress.

3. Keeping the patient clean, as described above, is essential for the prevention of bedsores.

4. Since bedsores occur most frequently on people who are undernourished, every effort should be made to prevent this condition. Adequate intake of minerals, vitamins, and proteins is essential.

5. If redness begins to appear in any localized area, the doctor's attention should be called to it immediately. He will then prescribe methods to relieve pressure between the body and the mattress.

6. Antiseptic and antibiotic powders and ointments will not prevent bedsores from forming. Once they have formed, these medications help very little in clearing them up.

On what sites, other than the hip, lower back, and buttocks may bedsores develop?

Any part of the body that remains in constant contact with the bed and bears the weight of the body. Other common sites are the heels and, occasionally, the back of the head.

What are some special measures for people who wet or soil themselves while in bed?

1. Just as a child is taught to inform a parent when he needs to go to the bathroom, so older bedridden people must be instructed firmly and repeatedly to call their attendant when they wish to urinate or evacuate their bowels. If the patient and attendant develop a good system much soiling and wetting can be prevented.

2. Older people should be instructed to use the bedside bell to summon the attendant *before* the need becomes urgent.

3. For male patients, a bedside urinal should always be within easy reach.

4. Some companies manufacture diapers for older people. Diapers should be worn by those who cannot be taught to hold back.

5. Fluids should be withheld for three or four hours before bedtime if there is a tendency for the patient to wet the bed during sleep.

6. All bedridden patients should be encouraged to void and evacuate their bowels just before retiring at night.

7. A rubber sheet should always be placed on top of the mattress.

Is it necessary to get bedridden patients out of bed in order to change the bed?

No. There are satisfactory methods of changing bed linens while the patient remains in bed. A visiting nurse can quickly teach an attendant these methods.

What special precautions should be exercised in feeding bedridden patients?

1. Whenever possible, they should sit up to eat or

drink. It is very difficult
for anyone to swallow
while lying down. More-
over, that position may
cause food or fluid to
go down the windpipe
into the lungs.

2. If the patient cannot
   sit up, a hospital bed
   should be rented or
   bought. Such beds can
   be cranked into a sitting
   position.

3. Some bedridden patients
   may regress to childlike
   habits; this tendency

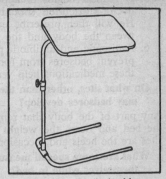

Over-the-side bed table

must be discouraged as much as possible. For example,
it is always best to make a bedridden patient feed and
wash himself if he can.

4. Overfeeding is bad for all people, particularly for those
   who are confined to bed. Food and fluid requirements
   are much less, because of the physical inactivity. Also,
   frequent small feedings are much better than three large
   ones each day.

5. Glass drinking tubes should be used; they make drinking
   much easier and prevent spilling.

6. It is often helpful to the bedridden patient to use un-
   conventional eating utensils. For instance, he may find it
   easier to eat certain foods with a large tablespoon than
   with a "proper" fork.

7. Cutting meat and other foods with a knife and fork may
   be a strenuous effort for some patients, and the very
   thought of having to cut their food may lead to loss of
   appetite. It should be done for them.

**Which is preferable for people who must remain in bed
for long periods of time, a soft or a firm mattress?**

A firm mattress is better for all people. A soft mattress often
causes a person to sink into one position from which movement is difficult. If one lies on a firm surface, he can more
easily change positions.

**Do debilitated older patients ever develop paralysis of an
arm or a leg while in bed?**

Yes. This may occur if they lie on an arm while asleep or
during a lengthy stupor. Also, there is sometimes a tendency
for a foot to drop over the side of the bed; paralysis may
develop if care is not taken to see that the foot is kept at right

angles to the leg and exercised frequently. Bedclothes should not be so snug that they hamper free foot movement.

How often should the position of the patient be changed?
During the waking hours, the position should be changed at least once an hour. It is unusual for older people to sleep straight through a night; they usually awaken every two or three hours. During such periods, their position should be changed.

Is it possible to exercise while in bed?
Yes. It is not only possible but also essential that bedridden people exercise. They must exercise their legs in order to aid circulation. They should also exercise their arms to keep them from getting stiff.

If exercise cannot be performed by the patient himself, the nurse or attendant should exercise his limbs at least once an hour.

What leg exercises will help to keep the muscles and joints limber?
The hip, knee, and ankle joints should be flexed and extended rhythmically, approximately 10 to 12 times each hour. If possible, this should be done by the patient; if the patient is unable to do so, by the attendant.

Should older bedridden people be encouraged to brush their own teeth, wash their own hands and faces, and comb their own hair?
Yes. This is very important from a psychological as well as from a physical point of view. Often, people who have these things done for them begin to think that they are much sicker than they actually are.

How should bedridden men be shaved?
An electric razor should be used. If this is not available and the patient cannot shave himself, the attendant should shave him. There is nothing worse for the morale of a bedridden man than to go unshaven.

What materials are necessary for the bathing of bedridden patients?
1. Washcloths
2. Mild soap
3. An enamel or aluminum basin
4. A rubber sheet to place under the patient so that the bed does not get wet
5. Rubbing alcohol
6. Large bath towels

What is the best bed position for people with heart disease?

People with heart disease are much more comfortable in a sitting or half-sitting position. It is sometimes better for them to sit with their feet hanging down. If they find this to be true, they may sometimes want to sleep in a chair.

How should pillows be placed in order to make bed patients more comfortable?

Most older people like two or three pillows under their head, neck, and shoulders. A pillow in the small of the back is sometimes comforting. In order to prevent sliding down in the bed, a large pillow may be placed under the thighs and knees. A pillow should also be placed at sites where the patient's weight bears down, for example, under the buttocks or beneath the heels.

In what position can bed patients void most easily?

Most older people void readily when they sit up. It is occasionally necessary for a male patient to stand up to void.

What should be done to aid bedridden patients to evacuate their bowels?

A bedside commode should be obtained. This is much better than a bedpan and can be used in a great majority of cases. Laxatives and lubricants should be given only when prescribed by the attending physician.

Are electric pads and hot-water bottles advisable for older bedridden patients?

No. These may cause serious burns. If a patient is cold, more blankets should be used or the room temperature should be raised. Very little relief from pain or from cold comes from using an electric pad or a hot-water bottle. On the other hand, an electric blanket is safe and if one can afford to buy it, one should be used.

Should bedridden people be encouraged to watch television?

Yes, but it should be remembered that if the television set is always in the same place, it will tend to keep the bedridden patient from changing his position frequently. Therefore, a portable television is advisable. A television set the bedridden patient is able to control will also lead to his staying in one position for long periods of time. It is therefore not always advisable to use the newer remote-control appliances.

BED-WETTING

See BED CARE; HYGIENE; NURSING CARE.

Is there a tendency for normal, healthy people past sixty to wet their beds during sleep?

No. Of course, if a woman has a large cystocele (*see* CYSTO-CELE AND RECTOCELE), or if she has loss of sphincteric control, she may wet her bed during the night when she sneezes or coughs. However, this condition is not confined to those who are over sixty.

The desire to void will awaken most older people unless they have been given a narcotic or sedative before retiring.

If there is a tendency toward bed-wetting, what can be done about it?

1. The last act before retiring should be to empty the bladder.
2. If a narcotic or sedative has been given, the patient should be awakened at a specific hour and taken to the bathroom or given a urinal to use.
3. An alarm clock may be set to go off four or five hours after the patient has retired.
4. Fluid intake should be stopped 3 to 4 hours before the patient goes to sleep.
5. Antispasmodic drugs, such as banthine or belladonna, are occasionally prescribed to cut down bladder irritability.
6. Measures should be taken to make it easier for older people to get out of bed and to reach the bathroom. These will include:

   a. a night light, so that the older person will not have to grope in the dark to find the way to the bathroom.

   b. a bedside commode or urinal, if the bathroom is far from the bed.

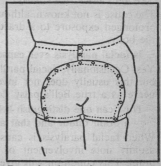

7. There are now companies that manufacture diapers for older people. These diapers should be worn by people who habitually wet the bed.

Pants for those who cannot control urination or defecation

8. A rubber sheet should be placed on top of the mattress.

BELL'S PALSY

See NERVES.

What is Bell's palsy?

It is a condition in which there is paralysis of the facial nerve (the seventh cranial nerve) supplying the muscles of the face.

What are the symptoms and signs of Bell's palsy?

Bell's palsy

1. An abrupt onset, within 24 hours, of facial paralysis on one side of the face.

2. The corner of the mouth droops.

3. Saliva may flow uncontrollably from the paralyzed corner of the mouth.

4. There is inability to use the muscles on the paralyzed side of the face.

5. There is inability to close the eyelid completely on the affected side of the face.

Is Bell's palsy a common condition among people past sixty?

It is much more common among middle-aged adults, but it does occur in older people, too.

What causes Bell's palsy?

The cause is not known, although some scientists attribute it to prolonged exposure to a draft or to an infection elsewhere in the body.

Is facial paralysis ever caused by a tumor within the brain?

Yes. Occasionally, facial paralysis is caused by a brain tumor, but this usually does not involve all of the branches of the nerve as a true Bell's palsy does.

How can one distinguish between facial paralysis caused by a brain tumor and that associated with Bell's palsy?

When facial paralysis is caused by a brain tumor, one will usually note involvement of other nerves arising from the brain. This condition will give additional symptoms, not seen in a typical Bell's palsy.

How long does Bell's palsy last?

A mild case may last only ten days to three weeks, but the

great majority of patients remain paralyzed for six to nine weeks.

Do most patients recover from the facial paralysis?

Yes. Unfortunately, in the majority of cases, some slight residual paralysis remains. In a very small number of cases, recovery from the facial paralysis never takes place.

What is the treatment for Bell's palsy?

Although there are many forms of treatment, in all probability no method substantially alters the course of the disease. In most cases recovery takes place slowly no matter what form of treatment is employed.

Forms of treatment include electrical stimulation to the facial nerve, vitamin B injections, the taking of various cortisonelike medications, and the giving of antibiotics.

Is it necessary to be particularly careful to protect the eye when one has Bell's palsy?

Yes. Sensitivity of the conjunctival membrane of the eye is lost during Bell's palsy and the eyelid cannot be closed completely. Dust and dirt may get into the eye without the patient's knowing it. This may lead to an ulceration of the cornea with permanent damage to vision. To avoid this, an eye patch is often worn. Also, great care should be taken to wash out the eye periodically.

Is there any way to prevent Bell's palsy?

No. Unfortunately, so little is known about the cause of this disease, and its onset is so abrupt, that nothing can be done to prevent it.

BLEPHARITIS

See CONJUNCTIVITIS; ECTROPION AND ENTROPION; EYES; TRICHIASIS.

What is blepharitis?

It is an inflammation of the margins of the eyelids.

Does blepharitis occur very often in people over sixty?

Yes.

What may cause blepharitis?

1. Degeneration or clogging of the tiny glands in the margins of the eyelids.
2. Infection of the glands in the margins of the eyelids.

3. Overexposure to sunlight or wind.
4. Dust or dirt, which clogs the pores of the glands in the eyelids.
5. Allergy to eye shadow, mascara, or other cosmetics.

Is blepharitis an acute or chronic condition?

Some older people have the chronic form of the condition, which may last for years. Others have an acute inflammation, which will subside within a few days.

What is the treatment of blepharitis?

This will depend upon its origin. If it is infectious in origin, antibiotic or other medicated ointments will clear up most cases. Withdrawal of the irritating agent will clear up most cases of allergic blepharitis.

It is important that older people with chronic blepharitis seek care from an eye specialist. Infection of the eyelids may cause them to turn inward (entropion) with the result that the eyelashes will scratch the surface of the eyeball. Also, blepharitis is often accompanied by marked itching, so that the patient may scratch and thereby injure the surface of the eyeball.

BLINDNESS

See CATARACTS; EYES; GLAUCOMA; OPTIC-NERVE ATROPHY; ORGANIZATIONS AND AGENCIES; RETINAL DETACHMENT; RETINAL THROMBOSIS.

What is the incidence of blindness in the United States?

It is estimated that there are between 350,000 and 400,000 blind people in this country.

Is blindness increasing?

It is thought to be *decreasing* insofar as newborn and young children are concerned. However, since an ever-growing number of citizens are living into their seventies and eighties, the total number of the blind has actually increased.

Is blindness among older people increasing?

No. Earlier and better methods of treatment of those conditions that predispose one to blindness have reduced the *relative frequency* among people over sixty.

What are some of the more frequent causes of blindness in people past sixty?

1. Cataract formation (*see* CATARACTS).
2. Glaucoma (*see* GLAUCOMA).

3. Detachment of the retina (*see* RETINAL DETACHMENT).
4. Arteriosclerosis of the blood vessels supplying the eye, occasionally with clot formation in the retinal artery (*see* RETINAL THROMBOSIS).
5. Diseases of the cornea (the thin membrane covering the pupil).
6. Degeneration of the optic nerve of the eye (*see* OPTIC-NERVE ATROPHY).
7. Advanced, severe diabetes.
8. Brain tumor, especially in the region of the pituitary gland.

Is blindness inevitable as a result of aging?

No. The eye is so adaptable that its capacity to function well past the century mark has been postulated. It is estimated that over 85 percent of those in their seventies and eighties are able to function satisfactorily with the vision they possess.

Is there a natural reduction in eye function in older people?

Yes. Visual acuity is reduced, power to accommodate (adjust the eyes to varying conditions of light and dark) becomes weaker, color perception is lessened, and the general efficiency of vision is considerably reduced as one ages.

Can reading in poor light over many years cause blindness?

No, but it can strain the muscles of the eye and may lead to decreased acuteness of vision.

Can overexposure to very bright light over a period of years cause blindness?

No, but it may seriously damage some of the cells in the retina, thereby reducing vision.

Can chronic high blood pressure cause blindness?

It may indirectly cause blindness. Markedly high blood pressure eventually leads to hardening of the arteries, and hardening of the arteries may produce loss of vision.

How can blindness be prevented?

By seeking early treatment for those conditions that predispose one to blindness:

1. Surgical removal of cataracts at the appropriate time.
2. Medical treatment of glaucoma during the years when the disease is in its early stages. Surgical treatment for glaucoma, when it becomes necessary, will prevent blindness in the great majority of cases.
3. Early, expert care of detached retina, with faithful follow-up care for possible recurrences.
4. Regular visits to the doctor throughout the middle years may greatly benefit the patient with elevated blood pres-

sure (hypertension). If this condition can be improved
or remedied, blindness in the later years may be prevented by delaying the onset of extensive arteriosclerosis.

5. Any ulceration or inflammation of the cornea or the
conjunctiva (the membrane lining the eyelid) should be
treated as soon as it appears. This, in most instances, will
prevent loss of vision owing to scarring of the cornea.

6. Atrophy (degeneration) of the optic nerve is often
caused by the toxic effects of prolonged, severe infection
or by the taking of toxic drugs. If infections are treated
promptly and effectively, such damage to the optic nerve
may be avoided. Also, it is important that people abstain
from medications or drugs that may have harmful effects if taken without a doctor's advice. Particularly
dangerous are drugs containing such heavy metals as
arsenic and lead. Wood alcohol can cause blindness by
damaging the optic nerve.

7. Untreated, severe diabetes over a period of years may
lead to blindness. It is therefore important that this
disease be kept under constant control through diet and
medication.

Is surgery effective in curing blindness?

In some instances, yes. Blindness caused by cataract, glaucoma, detachment of the retina, and injury to the cornea can
frequently be overcome by surgery. However, blindness resulting from arteriosclerosis, diabetes, high blood pressure, or
optic-nerve degeneration cannot be helped by surgery.

**Can older blind people be taught to take care of themselves
—to walk about, cross streets, read Braille, etc?**

Yes. Although they may take a little longer than younger
blind people to learn to help themselves, older people can
adapt to this handicap. There are many wonderful agencies
and organizations that will help them to live with this affliction
(*see* ORGANIZATIONS AND AGENCIES).

BLOOD

See ANEMIA; BLOOD PRESSURE; FIRST AID; INJURIES AND
ACCIDENTS; POLYCYTHEMIA; SHOCK; SURGERY; TESTS.

Where is blood formed?

During the life of the embryo, blood is formed in the spleen, in other glands similar in structure to the spleen, and in the marrow of the long bones. After birth, blood is formed almost entirely in the bone marrow.

What are the normal blood-count findings?

Red blood cells	4,200,000 to 5,500,000 per cu. mm. of blood
White blood cells	5,000 to 8,000 per cu. mm. of blood
Hemoglobin	85–100% (12.8 to 15 gm.)
Coagulation time	4 to 6 minutes
Bleeding time	1 to 2 minutes
Prothrombin time	14 to 16 seconds

White blood cell differential count

Polymorphonuclear leukocytes	68-70%
Segmented leukocytes	58-66%
Stab cells	3-15%
Myelocytes	0
Small lymphocytes	20-22%
Large lymphocytes	3- 6%
Eosinophils	1- 2%
Basophils	0.5-1%

What are the normal blood-chemistry findings?

Urea nitrogen	12.0 to 15 mg. per 100 cc.
Glucose (sugar)	80 to 120 mg. per 100 cc.
Uric acid	2 to 4.5 mg. per 100 cc.
Nonprotein nitrogen	25 to 45 mg. per 100 cc.
Creatinine	1 to 2.5 mg. per 100 cc.
Cholesterol	130 to 240 mg. per 100 cc.
Calcium	9 to 11 mg. per 100 cc.
Sodium	137 to 143 milli-equivalents per liter
Chlorides	585 to 620 mg. per 100 cc.
Potassium	4 to 5 milli-equivalents per liter
Phosphorus	3 to 4.5 mg. per 100 cc.
Bilirubin	0.1 to 0.25 mg. per 100 cc.
Phosphatase	1.5 to 4 units per 100 cc.
Icterus index	4 to 6 units
Total protein	6.5 to 8.2 gm. per 100 cc.
Serum albumin	1.5 to 2.5 gm. per 100 cc.
Globulin	2.5 to 3.0 gm. per 100 cc.
Carbon dioxide combining power	55-75 volumes percent
Fibrinogen	0.2 to 0.6 gm. per 100 cc.

What is the average life of a red blood cell?

Approximately 30 to 60 days. They may live slightly longer in young people. In healthy people, there is constant replenishment of blood cells by the bone marrow.

Does the bone marrow lose some of its blood-forming ability as one ages?

Yes. As in all structures, signs of age also occur in the bone marrow. As a consequence, some people in their late seventies, eighties, and nineties may become anemic because the bone marrow is incapable of producing sufficient new blood.

Do chronic diseases, toxic medications, or poisons ever interfere with the ability of the marrow to produce blood cells?

Yes.

How can one tell if he has anything wrong with his blood?

People past sixty should have a complete blood examination every year. This is a simple procedure involving a pinprick of the finger. Such an examination will reveal most blood disorders.

Does bleeding from the gums, nose and throat, or other orifices, such as the vagina or rectum, indicate that there is something wrong with the blood?

Yes. People who bleed spontaneously from several different sites usually have something wrong with their blood. The condition should be investigated without delay.

What is the incidence of anemia and other blood disorders in people past sixty?

About one out of every four people over sixty has some abnormal condition of the blood. Usually it is anemia (*see* ANEMIA).

Do older people who are in good health show blood abnormalities?

No. The majority of older people can live well into their eighties without developing any blood abnormality.

Do healthy older people have blood counts different from younger people's?

No. The blood count remains the same throughout life if good health is maintained.

Is there a tendency for the volume of blood that circulates throughout the body to decrease as people age?

Not in healthy people. However, as people age they often become thin and cut down on their fluid intake. This may lower blood volume somewhat, but not to a great extent.

Does the chemical composition of the blood change as people age?

If they remain in good health, the chemical composition of the blood tends to remain about the same.

How can one tell if blood is deficient in iron?

By testing for the quantity of hemoglobin. This is a very simple test and can be carried out within a few minutes.

Should healthy people past sixty take iron or other tonics to build up their blood?

See ANEMIA.

Do people past sixty show a greater tendency to bleed when they are operated on, lacerated, or cut?

Not if they are in good general health. It is only when they have advanced arteriosclerosis, or are debilitated, or suffer from a deficiency disease that they may have a greater tendency to bleed. Thus, when an older person bleeds from a stomach or duodenal ulcer, he will usually hemorrhage severely. This is because he has lost a certain amount of elastic tissue within the wall of the bleeding vessel, which makes it difficult for the vessel to contract and stop bleeding.

Will physical exercise improve faulty blood circulation in older people?

Yes, to a certain extent. But if there is marked hardening of the arteries, no amount of exercise is going to help circulation. Healthy people in their sixties, seventies, and eighties should be encouraged to carry out regular physical exercise to aid circulation (*see* PHYSICAL ACTIVITY AND EXERCISE).

Are blood vessels more fragile in older people?

Yes, if they have developed advanced arteriosclerosis. (*See also* ARTERIOSCLEROSIS.)

Is low blood pressure an indication that something is wrong with the composition of the blood.

Not usually. People with low blood pressure usually have normal composition of the blood. On the other hand, they may lack a sufficient quantity of blood. (*See also* BLOOD PRESSURE.)

Will high blood pressure cause changes in the composition of the blood?

Not usually, unless there is associated kidney, liver, or heart disease.

Will kidney disease show up when blood is examined under a microscope?

No. The best way to diagnose kidney disease is by *chemical* examination of the blood. (*See also* KIDNEYS.)

Can diabetes be diagnosed by chemical examination of the blood?

Yes, in almost all cases. (*See also* DIABETES.)

Will liver disorders show up on chemical examination of the blood?

Yes, in almost all instances. In addition to blood tests, there are also several urine and stool tests that will uncover liver disorder.

Is the ability of red blood cells to carry oxygen diminished in healthy older people?

No.

Is it especially important for older people to maintain a high oxygen content of their blood?

Yes. If the oxygen content of the circulating blood is high, it will make up for slowed circulation, a frequent sequel to hardening of the arteries. Moreover, as tissues age it is essential that they receive an adequate oxygen supply at all times. Brain cells, particularly, require large quantities of oxygen or they will deteriorate.

Will taking vitamins regularly improve the blood?

It will improve the blood if there is a vitamin deficiency. However, if the vitamin intake in the diet is entirely adequate, taking more will have little or no effect.

Is there a tendency for older people to be more susceptible to blood infections?

Most healthy people in their sixties and seventies have normal resistance to blood infections. However, if they are debilitated or chronically ill, their infection-fighting mechanism is less effective and they become much more susceptible to bacterial infections of the blood (septicemia).

Do cold hands and feet always indicate that one has poor circulation?

Not necessarily. Examination of the pulse is a much more valuable index to adequacy of circulation.

If people are known to have impairment of circulation, skin temperatures have great significance, particularly when the temperature of a healthy area is compared to that of an area involved in circulatory disease. Cold feet and the absence of a pulse are very important indications of impairment of circulation.

Do people past sixty have a greater tendency to form blood clots?

Yes. *See* EMBOLUS AND EMBOLISM; THROMBUS AND THROMBOSIS.

Is it common for older people to develop black-and-blue spots on their body?

Since blood vessels of older people tend to be more fragile, this does occur more frequently.

What are some of the diseases of the blood found in older people?

1. Pernicious anemia (*see* ANEMIA).
2. Polycythemia (*see* POLYCYTHEMIA).
3. Secondary anemia (*see* ANEMIA).
4. Leukemia (*see* LEUKEMIA).

BLOOD PRESSURE

See ANEMIA; ARTERIOSCLEROSIS; CIRCULATION; CONVULSIONS; FAINTING; HEADACHE; HEART; HYPERTENSION; PHYSICAL ACTIVITY AND EXERCISE; VERTIGO AND DIZZINESS.

What is meant by the term blood pressure?

Blood pressure is the result of the force with which the heart pumps the blood through the arteries of the body. It is measured by placing a compression cuff around the upper arm, shutting off the circulation by inflating the cuff, and noting the point at which the pulse returns to the arm below the cuff.

Blood pressure is recorded with two figures: the top one is known as *systolic pressure,* the lower one as *diastolic pressure.*

What is normal blood pressure?

Systolic: 120–140 mm. of mercury.
Diastolic: 80–90 mm. of mercury.

What is meant by systolic and diastolic pressures?

Systolic blood pressure is that which is measured when the heart muscle is contracting. Diastolic blood pressure is that which is measured when the heart muscle relaxes.

Does blood pressure tend to rise as one grows older?

Yes. There is a gradual increase in blood pressure with age, from childhood through to the sixties, seventies, and eighties.

What is normal blood pressure for people past sixty?

Roughly speaking, it should be at the upper limits of that normal for younger people, that is, 140 systolic and 90 diastolic. (This would be read as "140 over 90.")

It used to be said that normal systolic blood pressure was 100 plus the age. Thus, a sixty-year-old should have a systolic pressure of 160; a seventy-year-old should have a systolic pressure of 170; an eighty-year-old, 180, etc. This method of calculation is no longer in use.

How often should older people have their blood pressure taken?

Unless there is known elevation of blood pressure, it need be taken only during the regular semiannual physical examination.

Do geography and climate have an effect upon blood pressure?

Blood-pressure levels tend to be higher in those who live in high altitudes, especially at 5,000 or more feet above sea level.

Blood-pressure levels tend to be lower in people who live in warm or semitropical climates. It must also be stated that there are, nevertheless, many people who live in warm and semitropical climates who suffer from high blood pressure secondary to heart or kidney disease. In other words, climate is not a vital factor in blood pressure.

Does high blood cholesterol lead to high blood pressure?

Not directly, but if a high blood-cholesterol level really does lead to arteriosclerosis (as many doctors now believe), then indirectly it may lead to elevated blood pressure.

Should people in their sixties, seventies, or eighties always receive medications to lower high blood pressure?

No. This is often not good treatment, as it may lessen the amount of blood that is pumped to various vital organs. It must not be forgotten that elevated blood pressure often represents a compensatory effort of the heart to pump adequate quantities of oxygen and nutriments through narrowed, sclerotic arteries.

Does chronic high blood pressure in older people tend to correct itself spontaneously?

Not usually. However, if it is secondary to a kidney infection or some similar condition, it may subside when the infection is controlled.

Can older people with high blood pressure safely undergo surgery?

Modern surgeons and anesthesiologists have learned how to safeguard older patients, even when they have very high blood pressure. It is important that the blood-pressure level not be dropped too precipitously before surgery.

Doctors often tell patients with high blood pressure to discontinue certain medications a week or two before undergoing surgery.

What is the significance of normal or low blood pressure in people past sixty?

It usually indicates that they have relatively little hardening of the arteries.

Does low blood pressure ever produce symptoms?

Symptoms are seldom produced by low blood pressure, unless the person with low blood pressure is suffering from a debilitating condition such as tuberculosis, mental depression, adrenal-gland exhaustion, or widespread cancer.

Does low blood pressure tend to correct itself spontaneously?

As stated above, low blood pressure is usually not an abnormal condition. However, when it is secondary to a disease, it will clear up when the primary condition is brought under control. Thus, when recovery from a mental depression takes place, normal blood-pressure level will return.

What is the significance of a sudden, severe drop in blood pressure?

When it occurs in an older person, it may indicate inadequacy of blood supply to the brain; it may accompany coronary thrombosis; it is often associated with surgical shock.

Is it safe to operate on older people who have low blood pressure?

Markedly low blood pressure may indicate that the patient is anemic or that he has some debilitating disease. If anemia is the cause of low blood pressure, blood transfusions should be given preoperatively.

Can older people with low blood pressure engage in physical exercise?

Yes, if they are in good health otherwise.

Are there satisfactory medications to elevate low blood pressure?

Yes, but most older people do not need them, since low blood pressure rarely produces symptoms.

BONES AND JOINTS

See AMPUTATION; ARTHRITIS AND RHEUMATISM; BACKACHE; BURSITIS; FRACTURES; GOUT; MUSCLES; PAGET'S DISEASE; PARATHYROID GLANDS; PHYSICAL ACTIVITY AND EXERCISE; REHABILITATION AND PHYSICAL THERAPY.

Do the bones tend to become brittle as people age?

Yes, owing to the fact that there is loss of calcium in the bones of people in the late seventies and eighties.

What type of doctor should one consult for aches and pains in the bones and joints?

It is always a good practice to consult the family physician first. If he determines that the bone and joint symptoms are caused by an upset in general health, he will either treat the patient himself or refer him to an internist or rheumatologist. Such conditions as rheumatoid arthritis, osteoarthritis, and gout fall into this category. On the other hand, if he believes the condition requires surgery, he will refer the patient to an orthopedist. Fractures, bone tumors, slipped disks, and sprains fall into this category.

Should an older person whose sense of balance has diminished use a cane?

Certainly. It is regrettable that the cane has gone out of style, for it affords great extra support to older people. The use of a cane should be encouraged.

Is it important that people past sixty take special care of their feet?

Yes. There is a natural decrease in stability and balance in older people. It is, therefore, essential that they not impair these senses further by permitting calluses to develop. It is also important that well-fitting, sensible shoes be worn.

Do people in their seventies and eighties suffer fractured bones more often than younger people?

Yes, because they sustain more falls and accidents and because loss of calcium makes their bones more fragile.

What special precautions should older persons take in order to avoid fractures?

See INJURIES AND ACCIDENTS.

What is meant by pathological fracture?

This is a fracture in a diseased segment of a bone, for example, a bone that contains a cyst or a cancer.

Are bone infections, such as osteomyelitis, commonly seen among older people?

No. Bacterial infections of the bone are much more frequently seen in younger people.

What is osteomalacia?

Osteomalacia is a bone disease thought to be brought on by vitamin D and hormone deficiencies. The affected bones become softer and more susceptible to fracture. Older patients with this condition may experience severe aches and pains in their bones and joints. Unless the vitamin and hormonal deficiencies are rectified, the patient becomes extremely debilitated and often develops severe complications in other vital organs of the body.

What is osteoporosis and what causes it?

It is produced by the slowing down of normal bone-cell replacement by the aging body. It is also thought to be linked to hormone deficiencies that accompany the aging process. Osteoporosis is a bone disease seen very often in people in their seventies and eighties. It is characterized by decalcification, increased porosity, and weakening of the bony structure to such an extent that fractures often take place. When it affects the spine, it may cause great pain.

What hormone affects calcium in the body?

Normal function of the parathyroid glands is essential for normal calcium metabolism. Insufficient or excess secretion of the hormone of these glands (parathormone) will lead to such bone diseases as osteomalacia, osteoporosis, and cystic disease of the bone.

What treatment will benefit older people afflicted with osteomalacia or osteoporosis?

If the parathyroid glands are secreting insufficient amounts of their hormone, this substance should be given. If intake of calcium or vitamin D is inadequate, they must be given. It should be stated, however, that complete cure is not easy if the general health of the patient is poor.

Is it true that people in their sixties, seventies, and eighties are shorter than they were in their middle years?

Yes. People do lose height during the later years. This is due to a decrease in the amount of cartilage between the vertebrae in the spinal column. As the cartilage thins out the vertebrae come closer together, which causes the individual to become shorter.

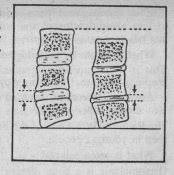

Narrowing of spaces between vertebrae, seen often in older people

Other important factors in the loss of height are (1) tendency to assume poor posture and to stoop; (2) the development of curvature of the spine.

What measures can older people take to avoid becoming round-shouldered and to avoid curvature of the spine?

Little can be done, since these conditions usually result from arthritis of the spine. However, people in their middle years should take every measure to delay the onset of arthritis. (*See* ARTHRITIS.)

Can braces or special physical exercises help older people who have curvature of the spine?

Unfortunately, by the time curvature of the spine has taken place physical aids, such as braces and corsets, can do very little to remedy the situation. There are, however, specialists in physical medicine who may be able, to a limited extent, to rehabilitate people with this condition.

BONE TUMORS

Are bone tumors very common in people past sixty?

No. It is a condition found primarily in children, adolescents, and young adults.

What is one of the most frequently encountered bone tumors in people past sixty years of age?

Multiple myeloma (Kahler's disease). It affects all the bones, especially the marrow of the bones. Although it is a disease that may last several years, eventually most people succumb to it. Recently, some of the anticancer chemicals have been helpful in slowing down the progress of this disease.

Is primary cancer of the bone very common in people past sixty?

No. This disease is rare in older people.

Does cancer tend to spread from other organs to the bones?

Yes. One of the most common places for cancer to spread is to bone. Since cancer of such organs as the stomach, breast, prostate gland, uterus, and lungs is seen more frequently in people past sixty, it is only natural that incidence of bone cancer in older people should also be high.

What is metastatic bone cancer?

It is a cancer that has spread from some other organ to the bones.

Can metastatic bone cancer be treated successfully?

Very few cases can be cured. It should not be forgotten, however, that cancer has a tendency to grow very slowly in older people. Often, cancer that has spread from some other organ can be arrested by administering certain ovarian or testicular hormones, by treatment with anticancer chemicals, or by giving X-ray or cobalt treatments.

BOWEL FUNCTION

See BED CARE; CONSTIPATION; DIARRHEA; INTESTINES; LAXATIVES; RECTUM AND ANUS.

Should people past sixty undergo a rectal examination every year?

Yes, because tumors of the rectum and lower bowel occur frequently during the later years, and they can often be discovered in the early stage if examination is made regularly. Often, tumors can be spotted before they have become malignant.

Is it natural for the bowels to function sluggishly as one gets older?

There are many people whose bowels will function normally throughout their lives, but a sizable number of people will develop constipation as they age.

Is it necessary for older people to have a daily bowel evacuation?

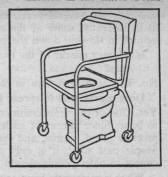

A chair commode for bedside use

No. This is a common misconception. Many healthy people in their sixties, seventies, and eighties regularly evacuate their bowels every two or three days. It should be mentioned, however, that people who do not have bowel movement every two or three days may develop an impaction (hardening of the stool within the rectum). This can be an extremely painful condition to relieve.

Should a sigmoidoscopic examination be part of a routine rectal examination?

Yes. In this procedure a hollow metal instrument is inserted for a distance of ten or more inches into the rectal canal, thus enabling the surgeon to note the presence or absence of a tumor or other abnormal condition. This test is especially important for someone who has been bleeding from the rectum.

What is the significance of a change in the appearance of the stool?

One of the first signs that something is wrong in the large bowel is a change in the character of the stool. An older person who notices that his stool has become stringy, has changed in consistency, or contains blood should consult his physician so that a rectal examination can be made.

What is the significance of an abrupt change in bowel habits, such as the onset of constipation or diarrhea in one who has always had normal movements?

If the change continues for several weeks, it may indicate the presence of a tumor in the bowel. In any event, such a change should be the basis for a thorough rectal and bowel investigation.

How does a physician determine whether or not there is a tumor in the bowel?

1. By examination with a finger, the doctor can tell whether or not there is a tumor in the last 4 or 5 inches of the rectum.
2. By using a sigmoidoscope, a physician will be able to tell whether or not there is a tumor within the last 10 or 12 inches of the bowel.

3. A barium enema X ray will reveal the presence of a tumor anywhere in the large bowel. This examination is carried out by injecting barium (an opaque substance) into the rectum and then taking an X ray.

Are psychological factors important in determining efficiency of bowel function?

Yes. For some reason, older people tend to pay considerable attention to the functioning of their bowels. If they are emotionally disturbed about an upset in bowel function, their concern seems to aggravate the malfunction. Doctors usually relieve this apprehension by informing their patients that it is not absolutely essential to have a daily bowel movement.

What are good rules for older people to follow in order to assure regular elimination?

1. Form regular habits. People should sit on the toilet at the same hour each day, preferably immediately after breakfast.
2. They should be instructed not to strain. If the bowels do not move readily, one should abandon the effort.
3. It is essential that older people drink at least eight to ten glasses of liquid daily. This may prevent the stool from becoming too solid. (An exception to this rule exists for those people who must limit fluid intake because of a heart condition.)
4. If one tends to be constipated, he should take a lubricant such as mineral oil each day. (Mineral oil is not absorbed from the intestinal tract, nor is it habit-forming. Furthermore, for those who eat a full, normal diet, mineral oil will in no way interfere with the absorption of vitamins.)
5. If mineral oil does not aid evacuation, a laxative should be prescribed by the family physician.
6. If neither lubricants nor laxatives result in normal bowel function, a small enema may be taken if it is prescribed by the physician. Perhaps the best enema is a quart of warm tap water. No more than a glass or two may be required to start an evacuation. It is not usually necessary to add soap, salt, bicarbonate of soda, or other substances to the water.
7. Suppositories are sometimes employed to stimulate bowel evacuation (*only on advice of a physician*).

What is the significance of inability to pass gas through the rectum?

This condition is often associated with bowel obstruction. It demands immediate investigation.

What is the significance of blood in the stool?

Blood in the stool is an indication that something is wrong in the lower intestinal tract. This condition should be reported to the doctor.

What are some of the causes of blood in the stool?

1. By far the most common cause of blood in the stool is hemorrhoids (piles).
2. Constipation, with excessive strain, can cause a crack in the lining membrane of the anus. This will result in blood in the stool.
3. A fissure or fistula will cause blood in the stool. (*See* RECTUM AND ANUS.)
4. Colitis or dysentery (inflammation or infection of the lower intestinal tract) will cause blood in the stool.
5. A nonmalignant (benign) polyp of the rectum or bowel will produce blood in the stool.
6. A malignant tumor of the bowel usually causes blood to appear in the stool.
7. Inflammation of a diverticulum (an outpouching of the bowel wall) in the large intestine sometimes causes blood in the stool. (*See* DIVERTICULOSIS AND DIVERTICULITIS.)

What causes undigested food to appear in the stool?

This is often a sign that the pancreas and small intestines are not functioning properly. If this occurs frequently, it should be investigated. However, it should be mentioned that bolting food or improper chewing habits may cause some substances (kernels of corn, for example) to pass through the intestinal tract undigested.

What is the significance of mucus in the stool?

Some forms of colitis are associated with the discharge of mucus in the stool. If no blood accompanies the mucus, there is no reason to become too concerned.

BRAIN TUMOR

See APOPLEXY, OR STROKE; BLINDNESS; CANCER AND OTHER MALIGNANT GROWTHS; COMA; CONVULSIONS; EPILEPSY; HEADACHE; MENTAL CHANGES; PITUITARY GLAND.

Are brain tumors common in people past sixty?

They do occur, but their incidence is greater among younger people.

What are some of the signs and symptoms of a brain tumor?

1. Headache, usually severe and progressive.
2. Disturbance in sight, with double vision and limitation of the field of vision.
3. Weakness, numbness, or paralysis in one or more limbs.
4. Convulsions involving the whole body or a convulsion involving jerky, involuntary spasms of an arm or leg.
5. Coma (loss of consciousness with inability to be aroused).
6. Personality changes in someone who has had no apparent emotional crisis.
7. Episodes of spontaneous, forceful vomiting without nausea.
8. The smelling of strange odors that do not actually exist.

Is it difficult to diagnose the presence of a brain tumor?

Not usually. Neurologists and brain surgeons have many excellent techniques for making a precise diagnosis of the location and size of a brain tumor. Various X rays, employing the injection of dyes into the blood vessels to the brain or the injection of air into the spinal canal, will demonstrate accurately the presence and location of most brain tumors. The electroencephalogram (a test in which the brain waves are recorded) is also helpful in localizing the tumor site.

Can people with a brain tumor be helped by surgery?

Yes. Modern surgery on the brain is relatively safe, with good promise of operative recovery. Well over 90 percent of persons undergoing brain surgery will recover from the immediate effects of the operation.

Do brain tumors in older people tend to be of a type that can benefit from surgery?

Yes. Many of the brain tumors found in people in their sixties and seventies are more amenable to surgical treatment than those found in younger patients.

What types of brain tumors are most susceptible to cure?

1. Tumors of the coverings of the brain (called *meningiomas*). Fortunately, meningiomas constitute about 20 percent of all brain tumors.
2. Tumors of the pituitary gland in the base of the brain. These growths constitute about 10 percent of all tumors within the skull.

How are brain tumors approached surgically?

After the head is shaved, an incision is made beneath the hairline and a bone flap is cut. The surgeon severs the membranes covering the brain (the dura, arachnoid, and pia), exposing the brain itself. After he removes the tumor, he replaces the bone flap and stitches the tissues covering the skull. When the hair grows back, almost no scar is visible.

Can brain tumors be helped by X ray, radioactive cobalt, or treatment with other radioactive substances?

Yes. In certain cases, for example, some pituitary tumors, X-ray or cobalt treatments can bring about a cure. In the majority of cases, however, these measures merely delay the progress of a malignant brain tumor.

Does mental deterioration usually follow an operation on a brain tumor?

Usually not. Although there may be partial paralysis as a result of removal of the tumor-bearing portion of the brain, mental faculties are often not impaired. Peculiarly, relatively few brain tumors are located in those sections of the brain that control thinking and emotions.

BREATS

BREASTS

See CANCER AND OTHER MALIGNANT GROWTHS; ENDOCRINE GLANDS AND HORMONES; FEMALE ORGANS; PLASTIC SURGERY; SEX HORMONES.

When do a woman's breasts start to show signs of aging?

At about the time of menopause (change of life). The changes consist mainly of loss of the breast gland tissue and its replacement by fibrous tissue. Since the ovaries are no longer actively secreting hormones, breast tissue undergoes a certain amount of atrophy (degeneration). There is also a loss in fat tissue of the breast.

Do the contour and appearance of the breasts in women past menopause change?

Yes. Breasts tend to become flatter and to sag. This is caused by degeneration of gland and fat tissue and their replacement by fibrous tissue. In addition, the ligaments that hold up the breasts on the chest wall become lax.

Is there any way to prevent breasts from sagging and becoming flabby as one grows older?

To a limited extent. If a woman takes the following measures during her twenties and thirties, her breasts will have a better chance of retaining a more youthful appearance.

1. Avoid getting too stout. An overweight condition will cause the skin of the breasts to stretch. When weight is lost the skin becomes streaked and has less elasticity.
2. Avoid undernourishment. This will cause the fat tissue to disappear and will weaken the tissues that hold the breasts in their proper position.
3. Special care of the breasts should be taken during pregnancy and during the nursing period. The obstetrician's instructions should be followed carefully. The contour of the breasts is often unnecessarily altered by failure to take proper care of them at this time.
4. A well-fitted, uplift brassiere should always be worn.

Creams, hormone ointments, and other such preparations are of doubtful value. Certainly, hormone ointments should be used only on a doctor's prescription. Breast pumps and the so-called exercisers are valueless.

Can plastic surgery on the breasts be successfully performed on women past sixty?

Yes. With the longer life-span and the increased desire of older women to retain their youthful appearance, plastic surgery on the breasts is being performed increasingly. Although vanity usually stimulates a woman's decision to undergo this operation, there are frequently medical advantages. Older women with heavy pendulous breasts receive great relief through plastic surgery.

How often should women past sixty have their breasts examined?

Twice each year. If this practice is adhered to, tumors can be discovered during the early stage. (Four out of five cancers of the breast can be cured if discovered before they have spread to surrounding lymph glands.)

Should older women depend on self-examination of the breasts?

No! This is very unwise if it is substituted for examination by a physician.

What is the significance of a lump in the breast of a woman who has passed the menopause?

Unfortunately, the majority of lumps that develop in the breasts of women past menopause are malignant. However, there are benign tumors, such as fatty tumors and areas of fat necrosis (degeneration), which develop after menopause. In addition, older women who lose a great deal of weight may discover in the breast a deep lump that has gone unnoticed for many years. Such lumps are almost always benign.

What is the significance of a discharge of blood or another substance from the nipple in a woman past sixty?

This usually indicates that there is a tumor within the ducts of the breast. In many such cases, the lump cannot be felt. Secretion from the nipple occasionally takes place when a patient has been having intensive hormone treatment. This is, however, uncommon.

What causes painful breasts in women past sixty?

They occur in women who are markedly obese and whose breasts are pendulous. They also occur in older women who are receiving large doses of female sex hormones. Another cause is an inflammation within the breast (mastitis), occasionally appearing as a complication of a virus infection that has traveled throughout the body. Finally, pain in the breasts may sometimes be brought on by improperly fitting brassieres.

Is cancer of the breast usually associated with pain?

No. Most malignant breast tumors are painless.

What is the significance of a chronic ulcer or sore on the nipple?

This often indicates the presence of a malignant tumor in the breast. The appearance of such an ulcer should stimulate a woman to seek medical advice promptly.

Can a blow or injury to the breast cause cancer to develop?

No. Many women relate the onset of a breast tumor to a blow or injury they received. The explanation is as follows: A woman is unaware that she has a lump until she receives a blow on the breast. The pain occasioned by the blow causes her to examine the breast and to discover a lump that has been there for some time.

Is acute inflammation of the breast common in women past sixty?

No. It is rare.

Are malignant diseases of the breast more common in women past sixty than they are in younger women?

No. Statistics show that cancer of the breast occurs more often in women between the ages of forty-five and sixty than in those over sixty. However, there is too great an incidence of this disease in women of all ages.

Is cancer of the breast in older women curable?

Yes. As a matter of fact, malignant tumors tend to grow

more slowly in older women, thus giving them a better chance for cure than many younger women. Of course, they must seek medical care early in the course of the disease. (*See* CANCER AND OTHER MALIGNANT GROWTHS.)

Is it safe for women past sixty to undergo extensive surgery for the removal of a breast cancer?

Yes. Even the most radical breast-removal operation can be tolerated by older women, provided they are in a satisfactory state of general health. Only when someone is debilitated or has severe heart, liver, or kidney disease will less extensive surgery be proposed.

What is the significance of enlargement of the breasts in older women who are receiving hormone therapy?

Large doses of female hormone may cause a senile breast to become active again. The glands will respond to the influence of the hormone and the breasts will increase in size. When the hormones are discontinued, the breasts return to their quiescent state.

Can older women tolerate X-ray or cobalt treatments for breast cancer?

Yes.

THE MALE BREAST

Does the male breast ever become enlarged in men past sixty?

Yes. For some reason, the gland tissue in the male breast (which is essentially the same tissue as in the female) often enlarges and may become tender to the touch. This condition is known as adenomatous disease of the breast, or gynecomastia.

What can be done about enlargement of the breasts in stout men?

Obviously, the best advice for them is to lose weight. However, despite weight loss, some men do have large, pendulous breasts, which causes them considerable embarrassment. They can undergo surgery for the removal of excess breast tissue if they so desire.

Is diffuse enlargement of one or both male breasts usually a sign of malignancy?

No. Male breast cancer, a rare disease, is usually characterized by an irregular, firm lump in one segment of the breast beneath the nipple.

Is enlargement of the male breast in older men usually associated with loss in virility?

No. Enlargement of the male breast is no indication whatever of degree of virility.

What is the treatment for adenomatous disease of the male breast?

Because it is not always possible by external examination to distinguish between this benign condition and a malignant growth, surgery is often recommended. This may consist of removal of the nipple and underlying breast tissue in order to obtain sufficient material for microscopic analysis.

What is the significance of an isolated lump in the male breast?

It may be caused by an inflammation, or it may be caused by a tumor. Whatever the cause, surgery should always be performed so that the tissue can be subjected to microscopic examination.

Are operations on the male breast dangerous?

Even radical surgery for cancer can be tolerated if the patient is in satisfactory health.

Does the nipple always have to be removed when the underlying breast tissue is excised?

No. If the operation is for adenomatous disease and not for cancer, the nipple can often be left in place.

How common is cancer of the male breast?

It is not at all as common as the incidence of this disease in females. When it does occur, it often affects men who are in their sixties and seventies.

What is the treatment for cancer of the male breast?

It differs very little from the surgery for cancer of the female breast. The entire breast, underlying muscles of the chest wall, and lymph glands in the armpit are removed.

BRONCHIECTASIS

See ASTHMA; BRONCHITIS; COUGHS; EMPHYSEMA; INFLUENZA AND GRIPPE; PNEUMONIA; RESPIRATORY TRACT.

What is bronchiectasis?

It is a chronic disease in which the smaller bronchial tubes are widened, either in small localized areas or throughout the lungs. Usually, infection and pus formation are associated with these changes.

Does bronchiectasis affect older people very often?

Yes. There is a congenital form of the disease. However, the acquired type is much more common in older people.

What are some of the symptoms and complications of bronchiectasis?

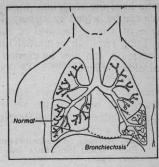

Bronchiectasis showing dilated air spaces

1. Chronic cough.
2. Expectoration of large quantities of infected sputum.
3. Attacks of asthma.
4. The development of pneumonia or a lung abscess.

How does the physician diagnose bronchiectasis?

It is usually necessary to perform a bronchoscopic examination (the insertion of a hollow, lighted metal tube into the bronchial tubes). An opaque dye is then injected and an X ray is taken. The smaller bronchial tubes are outlined on the X-ray picture, thus permitting an accurate diagnosis to be made.

Is bronchiectasis more serious for older people?

Yes, because it can lead to lung infections and to impaired respiratory function. Ultimately, the heart will suffer.

What is the treatment for bronchiectasis?

1. Making sure that there is adequate drainage of the mucus secreted by the bronchial tubes. To accomplish this, cough mixtures are given to make the secretions easier to cough up.
2. If infection is superimposed on bronchiectasis, antibiotics should be given to prevent complications such as pneumonia or lung abscess.
3. The general health of the patient should be maintained at a high level to prevent development of complications. Nourishing diet and adequate mineral and vitamin intake are essential.
4. If there is difficulty in breathing, oxygen should be administered. Also, various drugs are helpful in aiding respiration and in drying up excess secretions.

Is surgery for bronchiectasis helpful in people past sixty?

Although it is more frequently indicated for younger people

who have the congenital form of the disease, some older people can be helped by surgery. If the condition is limited to one lobe of a lung, removal of the lobe will bring about a cure.

Lung removal, or partial lung removal, although a serious operation, can now be carried out safely in the vast majority of older patients.

BRONCHITIS

See ASTHMA; BRONCHIECTASIS; COMMON COLD; COUGHS; EMPHYSEMA; INFLUENZA AND GRIPPE; PNEUMONIA; RESPIRATORY TRACT.

What is bronchitis?

It is an inflammation of the bronchial tubes. It may be an acute infection or it may exist in a chronic form.

What is acute bronchitis?

It is a severe infection caused by a virus or bacteria. Onset is rather abrupt, with the development of fever and a cough and the expectoration of infected sputum.

What is the usual course of acute bronchitis among older people?

Acute bronchitis, which is less common in older people than the chronic form, usually lasts about a week before it subsides.

What is the treatment for acute bronchitis?

1. Bed rest, usually in a semisitting position, to make breathing easier.
2. Large amounts of fluid (water, fruit juice, tea, carbonated drinks, etc.).
3. Cough mixtures to aid the patient to bring up sputum. These medications are best prescribed by the family doctor rather than bought over the drugstore counter.
4. Room air should be kept moist and warm. Cold, dry air will often bring on spasms of coughing.
5. If there is fever and if it is feared that complications such as pneumonia might set in, antibiotics should be prescribed. Also, drugs such as aspirin will often relieve discomfort and lower the temperature.

Do people usually recover from acute bronchitis?

Yes.

Do older people often develop chronic bronchitis?

Yes. It is one of the most common afflictions of people past sixty. Chronic bronchitis has its origin in earlier life. It is usually secondary to repeated respiratory infections, heavy smoking, or breathing pollens, dust, and chemicals for long periods.

Miners and people who work in plants where the air is polluted or who live in congested city areas are more likely to develop chronic bronchitis.

What are the signs and symptoms of chronic bronchitis?

The outstanding symptoms are coughing and the expectoration of infected mucus. Other symptoms may include shortness of breath, coughing up blood, wheezing on respiration, and a progressive enlargement of the chest cage. (*See* EMPHYSEMA.)

What is the treatment of chronic bronchitis?

This will depend largely on the origin of the disease. Every attempt should be made to eliminate the factors that have brought on the condition or are associated with it. For example, people with chronic bronchitis should stop smoking. They should wear masks and other protective equipment if they work in plants where the air is polluted by chemicals, dust, or smoke. If protection is impossible, they should give up this kind of work. If an allergy is responsible for the bronchitis, an attempt should be made to eliminate the irritating allergens. If people with bronchitis live in areas where air pollution is great, they should make every attempt to move. Older people with chronic bronchitis should take every precaution to avoid acute infections.

When acute bronchitis is superimposed on the chronic form of the disease, the acute symptoms should receive the same treatment as that outlined above for acute bronchitis.

Does chronic bronchitis ever develop from acute bronchitis?

Yes. The usual sequence of events is that repeated attacks of acute bronchitis will cause the condition to become chronic. People in their middle years who are subject to attacks of acute bronchitis can prevent the development of chronic bronchitis by eliminating the causes of their acute attacks.

BURNS AND FROSTBITE

See CLIMATE; CLOTHING; FIRST AID; INJURIES AND ACCIDENTS; SMOKING; TRAVEL.

Are older people more likely than younger people to get burned?

Yes, because many older people are slower in reacting to situations in which there is danger of burns. Kitchen accidents, burns from cigarettes, electrical burns, etc., may result because of a slowing down of protective mechanisms. In addition, decreased sensitivity of nerve endings in older people—in the finger tips, for example—may result in failure of the individual to be warned that he is being burned.

Are burns more serious to older people?

Yes, because the older the patient the more likely it is that the burn will produce shock, an upset chemical balance, or an overwhelming infection.

What first aid should be given for burns?

1. If a burn is superficial (first degree) it can be self-treated, unless it involves a large area of body surface. The burned areas should be placed under running, cold, tap water for 5 to 10 minutes. This will relieve pain and will separate clothing that may have become stuck to the burned areas. If dirt is in the wound, it should be removed by gentle wiping with cotton and soapsuds. Plain Vaseline ointment and a sterile gauze dressing should then be applied.

2. If the burn has caused marked blistering or seems to have penetrated deeper than the superficial skin layers (second-degree burn), it should be seen as soon as possible by a doctor. Immediate first-aid measures will include the following:

   a. Holding under cold running tap water for 5 to 10 minutes.

   b. Washing gently with mild soap and water.

   c. Covering with a sterile dressing. (Ointments or butter should *not* be applied.)

   d. Seeing that the patient drinks large quantities of water.

   e. Giving pain-relieving medications, such as aspirin or codeine.

If the burn has gone through the skin into the deeper layers of tissue, a sterile dressing or, if this is not available, a clean handkerchief should be placed over the wound and the patient transported immediately to a doctor's office or a hospital. If the patient shows signs of shock, with rapid pulse, shallow breathing, and cold perspiration, he should be covered with warm blankets, placed on a stretcher, and taken to the emergency room of a hospital. No ointments should be applied to the burned areas. (*See* SHOCK.)

Should the blisters that form in second-degree burn be opened?

Not by the patient, for infection may follow. If eventually the blisters must be opened, this should be done by a doctor.

When should ointments be applied to burns?

Only when the burn is superficial. Whenever the burn is deep or extensive, it is best not to apply an ointment.

Do chemical burns require special treatment?

Yes. Since membranes such as the mucous membrane of the eye, the nose, and the mouth are more sensitive in older people, it is particularly important that first aid be given quickly when this type of burn exists. Such treatment consists of flushing the area thoroughly (for 5 or 10 minutes) with a steady flow of cold water. This will dilute the chemical and eliminate any that has not become fixed in the tissues.

Are people past sixty more likely than younger ones to develop frostbite?

Yes. The circulation to the fingers, toes, the tip of the nose, and the ears is diminished somewhat in older people. For this reason, these areas are especially susceptible to frostbite.

What is the major complication of frostbite?

If it is severe and lasts for several hours, the frostbitten tissue may become gangrenous. Consequent loss of fingers or toes is not unusual in older people.

What is the first-aid treatment for frostbite?

1. The person with frostbite should be warmed gradually, not placed immediately in a hot room.
2. If pain is severe, codeine or aspirin should be given.
3. Warm liquids and hot foods should be given.
4. All wet or frozen clothing should be removed, and the patient should be wrapped in warm blankets.
5. The frostbitten areas should be permitted to warm spontaneously in a room heated to about 72° F.
6. A sterile dressing should be placed over the frostbitten areas, but no antiseptics should be applied.
7. As soon as circulation returns, the part should be gently exercised.

Should frostbitten areas be massaged in order to restore circulation?

No! This can do much harm and no good.

Is it good practice to rub snow into a frostbitten area?

No!

Can one tell immediately whether or not permanent damage has been done by frostbite?

No. Gangrene may set in several days after the exposure. Conversely, tissue that looks as if it might become gangrenous may recover after a few days.

BURSITIS

See ARTHRITIS AND RHEUMATISM; BONES AND JOINTS; MUSCLES; PHYSICAL ACTIVITY AND EXERCISE; REHABILITATION AND PHYSICAL THERAPY; X RAY.

What is bursitis?

It is an inflammation of a bursa. A bursa is a pad of fat lying beneath muscles and tendons in the vicinity of joints. Its function is to promote smooth, gliding movements of the muscles and tendons as they expand or contract over the rough edges of underlying bones or joints.

Where is bursitis most likely to occur?

In the shoulder, elbow, hip, and knee regions.

Do people past sixty often develop bursitis?

Yes.

What are the signs and symptoms of bursitis?

Pain and extreme tenderness about the involved bursa and inability to move the joint without excruciating pain. The symptoms are, for some reason, much worse at night.

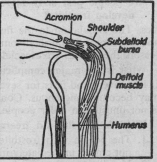

Subdeltoid bursitis, one of the most prevalent types

X rays will often reveal a calcium deposit in the inflamed bursa.

What brings on bursitis?

The most common cause is injury from a twist, a fall, or a strain in the region of the joint. Also, infections elsewhere in the body (teeth and sinus, for example) are thought to trigger this painful condition.

What are the types of bursitis?

1. *Acute bursitis.* This comes on within a few hours or a day or two, and is associated with severe pain and tenderness.
2. *Chronic bursitis.* This may represent the remnants of an acute bursitis that has not completely subsided, or it may be an independent condition not preceded by an acute condition. In the chronic form of this condition there is a nagging, aching pain in the region of the bursa, with

stiffening of the underlying joint. Frequently, chronic bursitis, if untreated, may lead to permanent limitation of motion of the involved joint.

What is the treatment for bursitis?

There are several methods of treatment, depending on whether the bursitis is acute or chronic and on the severity of the condition.

1. The best treatment for the severe case is to inject the inflamed bursa with a mixture of procaine (novocaine) and a cortisonelike medication. The bursa is washed out with this solution and any liquid calcium is removed through the needle. Often, a dramatic cure will take place within a day or two. If initial treatment does not relieve the condition, it should be repeated every third or fourth day.

2. Chronic cases are also treated by the injection method, but it may take several weeks to months to obtain relief. The stiffness about the involved joint is often due to muscle spasm, which will be relieved by the injections.

3. X-ray treatments have helped many cases of bursitis, but it is perhaps best to reserve this form of treatment for cases that fail to respond to injections.

4. In stubborn cases, it is occasionally necessary to operate and remove the diseased bursa. This is not a serious operation, even for those who are in their later years.

Does bursitis ever recur?

Yes, if there is another injury to the bursal region.

CANCER AND OTHER MALIGNANT GROWTHS

See BRAIN TUMOR; BREASTS; INTESTINES; KIDNEYS; LEUKEMIA; LEUKOPLAKIA; LUNG TUMORS; MOLES AND MELANOMAS; MOUTH, LIPS, AND TONGUE; ORGANIZATIONS AND AGENCIES; POLYPS OF THE LARGE BOWEL; PROSTATE GLAND; RECTUM AND ANUS; STOMACH AND DUODENUM; THYROID GLAND; URINARY BLADDER AND URETHRA.

What is cancer?

It is a disorderly growth of tissue cells. If the process continues unchecked, the normal structure and function of an organ will be destroyed. Cancer cells may be compared to weeds in a well-kept garden. If the weeds are not eradicated, eventually the entire garden will die.

Is the incidence of cancer greater in older age groups?

Yes. Although cancer is encountered in all age groups, there *is* increased incidence among people over sixty.

What is the incidence in the United States of the various types of cancer, and what are the chances for cure?

The following statistics have recently been published by the American Cancer Society:

INCIDENCE OF CANCER EACH YEAR IN THE UNITED STATES*

		Number of Cases	Cured	Potential Cures**
Skin	Males	41,000	90%	92%
	Females	25,000	95%	96%
		66,000		
Breast		63,000	58%	82%
Lungs	Males	38,000	4%	13%
	Females	5,700	9%	31%
		43,700		
Mouth, Pharynx, and Larynx		18,500	36%	45%
Stomach	Males	16,000	12%	37%
	Females	10,000	11%	36%
		26,000		
Colon and Rectum	Males	35,000	37%	65%
	Females	35,000	42%	71%
		70,000		
Kidney and Bladder	Males	17,000	25%	33%
	Females	8,500	23%	32%
		25,500		

*Courtesy of the American Cancer Society, 1961.

**A "potential cure" is one that could be obtained if the patient received treatment during the very early stages of the disease.

		Number of Cases	Cured	Potential Cures
Prostate		31,000	38%	52%
Uterus	Cervix of Uterus	29,000	61%	79%
	Body of Uterus	11,000	75%	87%
		40,000		

TOTAL CANCERS EACH YEAR..........................383,700

Is it true that the number of people with cancer is greater today than it was years ago?

Yes. This can be explained partially by the fact that more people today are living into their seventies and eighties. Since there are more cancers in this age group, the incidence of cancer for the total population is increasing. Despite this consideration, statistics do show an actual increase in *all* age groups. Moreover, better diagnostic methods have uncovered cancers that, years ago, would have gone undiagnosed.

Is cancer in older people always a progressive disease?

No. In a small number of instances, the cancer grows so slowly that it almost appears to be stationary. The patient lives out his normal life-span, succumbing to some totally unrelated condition. Although this occasionally occurs, no one should omit active treatment; for the great majority of malignant growths, unfortunately, do end fatally if they are untreated.

Do most tumors tend to grow more rapidly and to spread more quickly in younger people?

Yes.

Are cancer-detection examinations advisable for people past sixty?

Yes, but a *cancer*-detection examination is no substitute for a thorough, complete examination, which seeks out all abnormalities. It should be remembered that there are many serious conditions other than cancer that require attention.

Are there any disadvantages in a cancer-detection examination?

Not in the examination itself, but in the reaction of some

people who, on learning that they are free of cancer, proceed to neglect themselves thereafter. At some later time, if they do develop symptoms of cancer, they recall only the clean bill of health they once received and, instead of seeking immediate advice, do not visit their doctors until it is too late.

Should women past the menopause have vaginal smears taken yearly?

Yes. Since cancer of the uterus is curable in the great majority of cases, and since examination of a vaginal smear will almost always uncover the condition even in its early stages, all women should have it done once a year.

What are some of the early warning symptoms of cancer?

SKIN

1. Change in color, repeated bleeding, or growth of a mole or wart.
2. Any skin sore that fails to heal after 3 to 4 weeks, especially if it is on the nose, face, or an area that is exposed to repeated irritation.

BREAST

1. Any change in the size of the breast.
2. Bloody, yellow, or green discharge from the nipple.
3. Any lump in the breast, usually painless.
4. Any dimpling or change in the texture of the skin of the breast.
5. Any persistent irritation, scaling, or ulcer of the nipple.

LUNGS

1. Pain in the chest.
2. Chronic cough.
3. Spitting up of blood, or hemorrhage.
4. Unexplained weight loss.
5. Unexplained pallor or anemia.

MOUTH, PHARYNX, AND LARYNX

1. Hoarseness that last more than 3 weeks.
2. Ulcerations, sores, whitish plaques, lumps—anywhere on the lips, tongue, cheeks, throat, etc.—that fail to disappear within 2 to 3 weeks.
3. Repeated bleeding from the tongue, cheeks, or throat.

STOMACH

1. Loss of appetite for more than 2 weeks.
2. Indigestion, especially after eating, if it persists for more than 2 to 3 weeks.
3. Bloody or "coffee-ground" vomit.
4. Tar-black stool from someone *not* taking iron-containing pills.
5. Weight loss, weakness, and lethargy (often late symptoms).

COLON AND RECTUM

1. Change in ordinary bowel habits.
2. Change in appearance, size, and consistency of stool.
3. Bleeding on moving bowels.
4. Dark red blood in stools; tarry stools.
5. Increasing difficulty in moving bowels.
6. Distention of abdomen.
7. Abdominal cramps, often colicky.
8. Episodes of vomiting, sometimes of fecal material.
9. Unexplained anemia.

KIDNEY, BLADDER, OR PROSTATE GLAND

1. Blood in the urine.
2. Burning on urination.
3. Increased frequency of urination.
4. Inability to urinate.

UTERUS AND CERVIX

1. Vaginal bleeding in women past the menopause.
2. Unusual vaginal bleeding, especially when the menstruation period is not expected.
3. Unusual vaginal discharge.
4. Vaginal bleeding after intercourse.
5. In younger women, excessive bleeding during menstruation.

Does smoking play a role in the development of cancer?

Two or three types of cancer have been attributed to smoking. For many years, the medical profession has indicted pipe smoking as a strong contributory factor in the development of lip and tongue cancer. Within recent years, most physicians agree that there is a very close relationship between heavy cigarette smoking over a period of years and the development of lung cancer.

Are lip and tongue cancer caused by smoking now as much as they used to be?

No. Modern pipes filter out much of the hot smoke and tar, which are thought to be the cancer-stimulating factors.

Should those who have been smoking for thirty or forty years stop smoking in order to avoid the possible development of lung cancer?

Unfortunately, if they have been smoking for that long, most of the damage has already been done. Therefore, if people in their later years want to continue to smoke, perhaps it would be unwise to force them to stop. On the other hand, young cigarette smokers would be wise to study the statistics just given and then come to their own decision.

Is weight loss an early symptom of cancer?

No. Weight loss is a rather late symptom in most cases of cancer

What precautions can people take in their middle years to diminish their chances of getting cancer in the later years?

1. Stay thin or get thin! It has been demonstrated statistically that there are more cases of cancer in fat people than in thin ones.
2. Stop smoking!
3. Have all benign (noncancerous) growths removed. Tumors of the skin, breasts, mouth, throat, intestinal tract, rectum, thyroid, urinary tract, or genital organs can, if neglected, undergo changes to cancer. Their removal when the patient is still in the middle years is usually a simple, safe operation.
4. Have a thorough, complete physical examination performed at least once a year.
5. Report bleeding or discharge from any orifice as soon as it is noted.
6. Avoid handling irritating substances without adequate protection. Certain petroleum and tar products and radioactive chemicals have been shown definitely to induce cancer if they are in day-to-day contact with the skin over a period of years. If one's occupation requires that he handle such substances, he should take every possible precaution.

Do older people respond as well as those in their middle years to cancer surgery?

Although younger patients do have more stamina and ability to withstand extensive surgery, modern technical and physio-

chemical advances place even the oldest cancer patients in
a highly favorable position to recover from surgery. Medical
and surgical specialists have learned a great deal about how to
support the aging heart, liver, kidney, and other vital organs
so that they can survive radical cancer surgery.

**Should people past sixty be given forms of cancer treat-
ment different from those given to younger and stronger
people?**

As a general rule, cancer patients of all age groups should
be given the advantage of the latest and most radical forms
of treatment, including extensive surgery. Earlier in this book
it was stated that the span of anyone's life cannot be predicted
with accuracy. Therefore, there is no justification for withholding any type of treatment in the expectation that "the
patient doesn't have many years left anyway." An individual
in his early seventies may have a potential life-span of eighty-
five to ninety years; his cancer should therefore be treated as
if, on removal of the growth, he will live the full time allotted
to him.

**Are the chances for cure of a cancer improved because of
the slower growth and spread of tumors in people past
sixty?**

Paradoxically, in many instances, the outlook is better in older
patients because of this peculiarity of cancer behavior.

**Are X-ray treatments, cobalt treatments, and treatments
with other radioactive substances beneficial and safe for
cancer patients of advanced age?**

Yes. They are just as effective for older people, although they
may sometimes cause a somewhat more severe reaction.

**Are chemical agents effective in treating older people with
cancer (chemotherapy)?**

To a certain extent, yes. Some of these drugs can slow the
growth and spread of certain types of cancer. Fortunately,
newer and more effective chemicals are being developed with
each succeeding year.

**Can one look forward to a cure for cancer at some time
in the near future?**

Cancer is *not one disease;* it is perhaps fifty or more—some
having entirely different characteristics and life cycles from
others. It is therefore highly improbable that one cure will be
found for all forms of this disease. Despite this fact, new
methods of treatment are curing a greater and greater percentage of cases each year. And as one can see from the preceding

statistical table, improved methods of treatment can now bring about cure in more than 90 percent of certain types of skin cancer, 75 percent of certain types of cancer of the female organs, and in 58 percent of breast cancers!

CATARACTS

See BLINDNESS; DEGENERATIVE CHANGES OF AGING; EYES.

What is a cataract?

It is an opacity (loss of transparency) of the lens, which condition interferes with normal passage of light rays to the retina.

Do all people past sixty lose this transparent quality of the lens?

Although there is a tendency for the lens to become somewhat less transparent with age, only a small percentage of people develop true cataracts, which interfere with vision.

How common are cataracts?

It is estimated that 5 percent of all people eventually develop cataracts.

What causes cataracts to form in some older people and not in others?

The cause is not yet fully understood, but the following are thought to be important in producing this condition:

1. Heredity seems to play an important role.
2. Long-standing diabetes predisposes one to cataracts.
3. An upset in calcium metabolism, which is rather common in older people.
4. Arteriosclerotic changes in the blood vessels of the head, eyes, etc.
5. Neglected glaucoma.
6. Direct injury to or infection of the eyeball, especially the anterior portion of the globe.
7. The taking of certain toxic drugs over a long period of time.

If a diabetic individual develops a cataract, will control of the diabetes influence its progress?

In a few cases, early treatment of the diabetes may arrest the growth of the cataract before it interferes with vision.

Do people always develop cataracts in both eyes simultaneously?

No. Cataracts sometimes develop only in one eye. More often, this condition involves both eyes, although many years may separate cataract formation in one eye from the onset of that condition in the second eye.

What percentage of people who have a cataract in one eye will eventually develop a cataract in the other eye?

Approximately 90 percent.

Can anything be done to prevent cataract formation?

Yes. Conditions that predispose one to the formation of cataracts should be treated early and vigorously. A diabetic patient, for example, should be treated promptly and continuously throughout the earlier years. On the other hand, even if no predisposing condition is present, healthy people may develop cataracts if they have an inherited tendency to do so.

Is there any satisfactory medical treatment for cataracts?

No. When cataracts are ripe they must be removed surgically.

What is the meaning of the statement that cataracts must be "ripe" to be removed?

Certain cataracts are so young in their development that their removal is not indicated. In other instances, removal is not as easy in the early stages

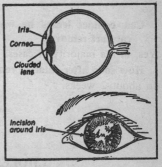

Diagrams showing cataract and location of incision for removing a cataract

of cataract development. The eye surgeon will make the decision as to the proper time for removal.

How long does it take for an immature cataract to become ripe?

Usually a year or two, but some may never mature.

How effective is surgery in the treatment of cataracts?

Surgery is very effective in the treatment of cataract and the operation is a safe, simple one to perform. In a great majority of cases, vision will be restored following cataract removal, although the wearing of powerful eyeglasses will be required.

If someone has cataracts in both eyes, will the surgeon recommend removal of both cataracts?

Yes, but in many instances they are not removed during the same operation.

What is the usual interval of time between removal of cataracts?

Usually 4 to 6 months.

What is the main indication that surgery on a cataract is needed?

Interference with vision.

What, exactly, is done during a cataract operation?

Under local anesthesia, a small incision is made at the junction of the white and colored portions of the eye. The lens is grasped with a special forceps and is removed. The incision is then sutured.

Is there a visible scar after cataract removal?

No.

Can contact lenses be worn instead of eyeglasses after cataract removal?

Yes, in the majority of cases.

How soon after cataract removal will vision be restored?

In about 2 weeks.

CHOLESTEROL

See ANATOMICAL CHANGES IN ORGANS; ARTERIOSCLEROSIS; BLOOD PRESSURE; CORONARY-ARTERY DISEASE; DIET; GALL-BLADDER AND BILE DUCTS; HEART; TESTS.

What is cholesterol and where it is found?

It is an important constituent of all animal fats and oils; it is found in such body substances as blood, bile, liver, kidneys, and adrenal glands. Cholesterol is a major component of gallstones and arteriosclerotic plaques in arteries.

Do people normally have cholesterol in their bloodstream and tissues?

Yes.

What is the normal amount of cholesterol that should be found in the blood?

150-250 mg. per 100 cc. of blood.

How is cholesterol associated with the aging process?

A large number of medical investigators now feel that an increase in blood cholesterol during the younger and middle years will lead to premature hardening of the arteries.

Is there a tendency for blood-cholesterol levels to rise as people get older?

Yes, unless the intake of animal fats and other foods containing large quantities of cholesterol is greatly curtailed.

Do cholesterol deposits tend to form in the coronary arteries and the valves of the heart as one advances in age?

Yes.

Do high blood-cholesterol levels over a long period of time increase the chances of a person's having a coronary thrombosis?

Yes, but it must be remembered that many other important factors can alter this tendency.

With advancing age, is there a tendency for cholesterol metabolism to become unbalanced?

Yes. As a result, cholesterol may be deposited in the walls of arteries. Once it is deposited in the wall of a blood vessel, it causes narrowing of the passageway and diminished blood flow.

Should people limit the amount of cholesterol in their diet?

From present-day investigations it can be inferred that it is a good practice for all people, regardless of age, to limit the amount of *animal fats* and dairy products they eat.

What foods contain the greatest amounts of cholesterol?

Egg yolk, butter, and animal fats. *Animal fat* means any fat derived from animal matter rather than from vegetable matter.

What is meant by saturated fats?

Saturated fats (animal fats) are those that have a high cholesterol content.

What is meant by unsaturated fats?

These are the fats that contain low amounts of cholesterol; they are vegetable fats, such as corn oil.

What specific foods contain large quantities of cholesterol?

Fatty meats, such as bacon, corned beef, and ham.
Sweet or sour cream, butter, cheese.

Fish processed in oils and fish oils.
Egg yolks.
Lard, suet.
Ice cream, whipped cream.
Pastry, pies.
Candy made with butter, cream, chocolate, or cocoa.
Whole milk.
Meat gravy, cream sauce.

What foods are low in amount of cholesterol?

Breads made without eggs, butter, or milk.
Cereals.
Soups without milk or meat stock (vegetable soups, for example).
Lean beef, ham, lamb, veal.
Chicken without skin.
Fish not processed in oil.
Egg white.
Cottage cheese, farmer's cheese, pot cheese.
All vegetables, provided they are cooked without fats and served without cream sauces.
Vegetable oils.
Fruits.
Gelatins.
Ices prepared without cream.
Jellies and jams.
Sugar.
Hard candies.
Buttermilk (there is no butter in buttermilk).
Skim milk.
Coffee.
Tea.
Carbonated beverages.

Will a low-cholesterol diet, followed over many years, delay the onset of arteriosclerosis?

Since so many factors are involved in the onset of arteriosclerosis, it cannot be stated with certainty that a low-cholesterol diet will delay the process. However, it can be conjectured that high-cholesterol intake predisposes one to development of arteriosclerosis.

Does lowering of cholesterol intake always lead to a lower blood-cholesterol level?

No. In certain people the blood-cholesterol level remains high, even though the cholesterol intake is low.

Do high cholesterol levels tend to run in families?

Yes, there seems to be a familial tendency to high blood cholesterol. People from such families may retain high blood-cholesterol levels even when they have a low cholesterol intake.

In certain cases, will the lowering of cholesterol intake improve heart symptoms such as angina pectoris?

Insofar as it may delay further arteriosclerotic deposits, lowered cholesterol intake may help to relieve symptoms. However, diet alone usually does not relieve heart symptoms.

What types of people are most likely to have high blood-cholesterol levels?

Those who have diabetes and those who are markedly over-weight.

What can people do to prevent the onset of arteriosclerosis resulting from high blood-cholesterol levels?

They must begin early in life to eat low-fat diets and to remain thin. Only when people abstain from eating animal fats for a period of twenty or more years will they maintain a significantly low cholesterol level.

Do diets high in cholesterol tend to lead to the development of gallbladder disease?

Yes. One of the main constituents of gallstones is cholesterol.

Are yellowish spots about the eyelids evidence of a high blood-cholesterol level?

Although these deposits do have a chemical composition somewhat similar to that of cholesterol, they are not necessarily an indication that a high blood-cholesterol level is present. They do indicate, however, that a blood-cholesterol determination should be made.

Do high blood-cholesterol levels tend to lead to high blood pressure?

One of the greatest causes of high blood pressure is hardening of the arteries; since high blood-cholesterol levels over a period of years predispose one to hardening of the arteries, it follows that a high level of blood cholesterol is associated with high blood pressure in many instances. However, the relationship is not that simple. Many people with high blood-cholesterol levels do *not* have high blood pressure and many with high blood pressure have a normal blood-cholesterol level.

Will a low-cholesterol diet help an older person who already has marked arteriosclerosis?

Once the blood vessels have undergone marked arteriosclerosis very little will be gained through diet. Nevertheless, people with arteriosclerosis should maintain a low cholesterol diet so that they do not make matters worse. It must be emphasized that people past sixty who are overweight should lose weight, and that one of the best ways to lose weight is to adhere to a low-fat diet.

Do certain diseases predispose one to the development of high blood-cholesterol levels?

Yes. Certain kidney conditions, such as nephrosis, and thyroid conditions associated with underactivity of the gland are frequently associated with high blood-cholesterol levels.

Are there effective means of lowering blood cholesterol through medication or hormone treatment?

Yes, but the effect lasts only as long as the treatment is continued. Moreover, occasionally there are undesirable side effects from these methods of treatment.

What medications or hormones will lower the cholesterol level?

1. *Nicotinic acid,* a vitamin, will often bring down a high cholesterol level, but it often leads to increased stomach acidity and is therefore not to be given to those with an ulcer or a tendency to ulcers.

2. *Methionine, choline,* and similar chemicals are sometimes effective, but they frequently cause bad reactions when taken for long periods of time.

3. *Heparin* lowers blood cholesterol, but it must be used only under strict medical supervision. It delays blood clotting and may lead to hemorrhage, especially in older people.

4. *Estrogen,* the female sex hormone, will lower blood cholesterol when given in large doses. However, when administered to men for prolonged periods, it may lead to enlargement of the breasts and loss of potency. When women past menopause take estrogen steadily in large doses, it may cause them to bleed vaginally or may activate a dormant tumor in the female organs.

5. *Thyroxine* hormone can lower blood cholesterol, but when administered in large doses for several weeks or months, it may accelerate body metabolism too greatly. This is particularly undesirable in older people who suffer from angina pectoris or other heart conditions.

CIRCULATION (BLOOD FLOW)

See AMPUTATION; ANGINA PECTORIS; ARTERIOSCLEROSIS; BLOOD PRESSURE; CIRRHOSIS OF THE LIVER; CLIMATE; CORONARY-ARTERY DISEASE; EMBOLUS AND EMBOLISM; HEART; HYPERTENSION; SHOCK; THROMBUS AND THROMBOSIS; VEINS AND VARICOSE VEINS.

Is there a tendency for circulation to slow down as one advances in age?

Healthy older people will continue to maintain normal or near-normal circulation. However, since there may be a decrease in the extent of physical energy expended, the body will demand less of a blood flow. Under such circumstances, circulation may slow down.

If there is advanced arteriosclerosis—and this condition does occur in many people in their later decades—then blood flow will be curtailed by the narrowed arteries.

How can a physician tell if circulation is adequate?

There are several tests that demonstrate quite accurately the adequacy of circulation. The simplest, of course, is to feel the pulses in the wrist or feet. If these are adequate, the chances are that blood flow throughout the body is adequate. More precise tests for the degree of adequacy are:

1. *Oscillometric* readings. The oscillometer is an instrument that measures very accurately the amount of blood flow through the thigh and leg.
2. An *arteriogram* is a procedure in which an opaque dye is injected into an artery and an X ray is taken showing the passage of the dye through the vessels. An arteriogram will often demonstrate whether a particular artery is blocked or whether it is the site of an aneurysm (*see* ANEURYSMS).
3. Circulation tests are performed by injecting substances into a vein in the arm and noting the length of time it takes the injected substance to course throughout the body.
4. The adequacy of circulation through the coronary artery of the heart can be gauged to a certain extent by taking an electrocardiogram.

Is there a tendency for the volume of blood that circulates throughout the body to decrease as people age?

The blood volume tends to remain the same in normal people. It must be remembered, however, that as people age their

147

weight and their fluid intake tend to decrease; this may lower blood volume somewhat, but not significantly.

Can diminished blood flow to the brain cause fainting spells or convulsion?

Yes. This phenomenon is seen quite often among older people who have hardening of the arteries to the brain, especially the carotid artery in the neck.

What can be done to improve poor circulation?

1. A general physical examination should be performed with special emphasis on discovering a hidden, chronic infection. Such an infection may impair circulation.
2. It is important that people with impaired circulation eat a good diet, with ample vitamins and essential minerals.
3. If anemia is present, appropriate medications to correct it should be prescribed (*see* ANEMIA).
4. People with impaired circulation should not wear constricting garters around their legs, as this practice may further decrease blood flow.
5. Medications may be prescribed to dilate the blood vessels or to prevent the arterial spasm seen so frequently among older people with hardening of the arteries.
6. If circulation to the lower limbs is impaired, an operation to cut the nerves that initiate arterial spasm can be performed. This operation, known as lumbar sympathectomy, may improve circulation in those in whom spasm is a major factor in impaired circulation.
7. If the main arteries to the lower extremities are clotted, an arterial graft is sometimes inserted to replace the diseased blood vessel. This operation is applicable mainly to those whose main arteries to the lower extremities are so arteriosclerotic that very little blood can pass through them.

What is meant by collateral circulation, or collateral blood flow?

Some older people may have to depend heavily upon their collateral circulation. As discussed elsewhere (*see* ARTERIO-SCLEROSIS), there is a tendency for large arteries to harden in the later years of life. This condition cuts down greatly the amount of blood that flows through them. If circulation of blood to any organ is greatly impaired, interference with normal function of that organ is inevitable. In the legs, gangrene may result. Nature, however, combats the closing down of the major arteries by causing alternate channels to develop through which the blood may flow. These smaller, alternate channels become dilated and carry much more blood than they did when the person was young. This flow of blood through the smaller, formerly little-used arteries, is called *collateral circulation*. Often, an entire extremity will come to depend for its survival upon the adequacy of collateral circulation.

What can be done to improve collateral circulation?

Little can be done to improve collateral circulation, but much can be done to preserve remaining circulation. For example, it is essential that the individual avoid infection and take particular care of his general health. Some doctors feel that physical exercise, such as walking or doing calesthenics, will improve collateral circulation.

Is smoking bad for circulation?

Yes, if the patient is in his sixties or seventies and has arteriosclerosis. Nicotine causes arterial spasm.

CIRRHOSIS OF THE LIVER

See ALCOHOL AND ALCOHOLISM; ESOPHAGUS; GALLBLADDER AND BILE DUCTS; HEPATITIS; JAUNDICE; LIVER; VEINS AND VARICOSE VEINS; VITAMINS.

What is cirrhosis of the liver?

It is a condition in which there is destruction of liver tissue and replacement by fibrous tissue. This process may eventually obstruct the flow of blood through the portal vein into the liver and may also obstruct the exit of bile from the liver. Such obstruction may result in jaundice and may cause fluid to accumulate in the abdominal cavity. The obstruction of free blood flow through a cirrhotic liver usually leads to the formation of large varicose veins in the esophagus. Often, these swollen, enlarged veins will rupture, leading to a serious or fatal hemorrhage.

What causes cirrhosis?

Any condition that seriously affects the liver may eventually lead to cirrhosis. Among these are:

1. Hepatitis, whether caused by virus or bacteria, especially if full recovery does not take place or if the patient fails to observe special precautions for several months afterward.

2. Liver damage as a result of taking drugs or poisons.
3. Alcohol.
4. Marked obesity, with fatty liver.
5. Chronic severe infection of the gallbladder and bile ducts.
6. Chronic obstruction of the flow of bile from the liver.
7. Other generalized infections and chronic conditions.

Does drinking excessive quantities of alcoholic beverages for many years lead to cirrhosis of the liver?

It is thought that excessive alcohol plays an important role in the development of cirrhosis, although it is acknowledged that alcohol is not the sole factor. In most cases chronic alcoholism is accompanied by chronic dietary insufficiency, and the combination of the two factors is probably responsible for the onset of cirrhosis. It is also thought that for those without a predisposition to cirrhosis, alcohol alone will not initiate the process.

Is cirrhosis of the liver more common in people past sixty?

No. It is a disease usually having its onset in the forties or fifties.

How can the diagnosis of cirrhosis of the liver be made?

1. By noting enlargement of the liver.
2. By noting an upset in liver function, which can be detected by a blood analysis.
3. By noting an accumulation of fluid within the abdominal cavity (ascites).
4. In advanced cases, by the presence of nausea, vomiting, weakness, weight loss, loss of appetite, and listlessness.
5. In later stages, by hemorrhage of blood from the mouth, owing to ruptured varicose veins in the esophagus. Special X-ray examination will usually demonstrate the presence of these varicose veins.

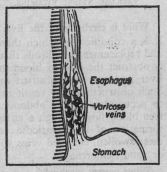

Esophageal varicose veins

6. In certain cases, jaundice is present. This is due to obstruction of the bile ducts.

What is the treatment of cirrhosis of the liver?

1. If there are toxic influences on the liver, such as might

arise from a severe systemic infection or from harmful drugs or medications, these should be eliminated.

2. A diet rich in vitamins, proteins, and carbohydrates, but low in fat should be taken.
3. Anemia must be overcome by giving appropriate medication.
4. In recent years, some cases of cirrhosis of the liver have been successfully treated by surgery to relieve the obstruction of blood flow through the portal vein. In one operation, the large portal vein, which brings blood from the intestinal tract to the liver, is connected to the vena cava. This will cause blood from the intestines, which would ordinarily flow *through* the liver, to *bypass* the liver and go directly into general circulation. Such an operation relieves a great part of the load on the liver and allows it to handle more adequately the amount of blood that will reach it through its artery. Although this operation does not actually cure cirrhosis, it allows the patient to live much longer and removes most of the hazard of a fatal hemorrhage from ruptured varicose veins in the esophagus.

What can be done to prevent cirrhosis and maintain normal liver function?

1. Avoid excessive drinking of alcoholic beverages or taking drugs that may cause liver damage.
2. Stay thin so as to avoid excess fatty deposits in the liver.
3. If the gallbladder is infected, it may have to be removed.
4. Maintain an adequate diet containing ample quantities of protein, sugar, vitamins, and minerals.
5. If hepatitis (jaundice caused by infection) is present, the patient should have it treated thoroughly and should remain inactive for a period of several weeks to several months. It has been shown that failure to recover fully from an attack of hepatitis may eventually result in the development of cirrhosis several years later. It is particularly important that those who have recently had hepatitis should refrain from excessive drinking and should avoid taking potentially dangerous drugs.

Does cirrhosis of the liver always end fatally?

No. Many older people have a mild form of cirrhosis that never really interferes with normal living. In such cases, liver destruction is mild, and true obstruction to blood and bile flow never really takes place.

CLAUDICATION

See ARTERIOSCLEROSIS; CIRCULATION; CLIMATE; DIABETES MELLITUS; FEET; MUSCLES; PHYSICAL ACTIVITY AND EXERCISE; SMOKING.

What is claudication or intermittent claudication?

These terms refer to the symptoms often occurring in people who have marked hardening of the arteries in the legs. When people so afflicted attempt to take a walk (even for a few short blocks), their narrowed arteries fail to deliver sufficient blood and oxygen to the muscles of their legs. Such oxygen shortage will cause a severe cramp. The pain is usually so intense that walking must be halted for several minutes until the muscles once again receive a sufficient supply of oxygen.

How can the diagnosis of claudication be made?

1. The symptom of pain in the legs as a result of walking or exercising is characteristic of this condition.
2. Loss of pulsation of arteries in the ankles or feet often is present in people who have claudication.
3. X rays of the arteries of the legs will often reveal arteriosclerosis in people who have claudication.

Is claudication more common in men than in women?

Yes.

Does claudication ever occur among younger people?

Yes. Although it is seen most often in the later years, younger people with sclerotic arteries or vessels that tend to go into spasm can have this disease. Diabetics and heavy smokers tend to develop claudication.

Is claudication caused solely by hardening of the arteries?

No. A combination of hardening of the arteries plus spasm of the arteries produces claudication. The symptoms are thought to result from spasm of the narrowed arteries precipitated by walking or exercise.

What is the medical treatment for claudication?

1. Since tobacco tends to cause spasm of arteries, it should be discontinued.
2. People with known arteriosclerosis of the arteries in the legs should walk slowly and halt at the first signs of pain. They can resume walking after the pain has subsided completely.

3. Antispasmodic medications are often helpful in combating the tendency of arteriosclerotic arteries to go into spasm.
4. Moderate amounts of alcohol, as prescribed by a physician, should be given daily in order to promote dilatation of the arteries.
5. Whirlpool baths may be given to stimulate the circulation and to aid in the dilatation of arteriosclerotic arteries.
6. Baking-lamp treatments and other forms of heat are of limited value, but they may help to lessen arterial spasm.
7. People with claudication should avoid extreme cold because it induces arterial spasm. When out in the cold, they should wear long underwear and heavy wool stockings.

What surgical treatment may benefit older people with claudication due to hardening of the arteries in the legs?

1. A *lumbar sympathectomy* may be performed to overcome the tendency of the arteriosclerotic arteries to go into spasm. This is a rather simple operation in which the sympathetic nerves are severed in an area just behind the abdomen alongside the vertebral column. Cutting these nerves destroys the ability of the arteries to contract or become spastic. In this way, some relief from claudication may be obtained.
2. If the main artery in the thigh or leg is so completely involved in arteriosclerosis that it carries little or no blood, then an arterial graft connecting the functioning artery in the lower abdomen with the functioning artery in the lower leg is inserted. In many instances, this operation has restored circulation to an otherwise doomed limb.

Can anything be done in the middle years to prevent the onset of claudication in later life?

1. If one has a high blood-cholesterol level (and, therefore, a possible tendency toward the development of arteriosclerosis), he should go on a low-fat diet.
2. If smoking tends to cause spasm of the arteries, it should be discontinued.
3. Sensible exercise and regular long walks during the younger years will tend to maintain good circulation in the legs and will help toward the development of good collateral circulation (*see* ARTERIOSCLEROSIS).

CLIMATE

See BURNS AND FROSTBITE; HOTELS, APARTMENTS, AND COM-MUNITIES FOR THE AGING; LONGEVITY; RETIREMENT; TRAVEL.

Does climate affect the rate at which aging proceeds?

This is a very difficult question to answer. Statistics do not seem to support the contention that climate has a significant effect on the process of aging. It is true that people who live in extreme climates have a greater struggle for survival. This struggle is often associated with increased incidence of disease, poorer nutrition, and greater damage to the vital organs. Thus, premature hardening of the arteries and other degenerative changes may ensue rather early in such climates.

What climates are conducive to longer life?

The temperate climates. However, many other factors play more important roles and the role of climate cannot be called decisive.

Is it better for people who show premature signs of aging to live in a warm climate?

Yes, provided the warmer area has sanitation and all the other modern improvements of civilization.

Why is a warmer climate beneficial to older people?

In a warm climate, narrowing and hardening blood vessels will dilate more readily. Moreover, older people are particularly subject to respiratory infections, and the major respiratory diseases (pneumonia, bronchitis, sinus infections, and so on) are less prevalent in warmer climates.

Is extreme heat detrimental and even dangerous to people in their seventies and eighties?

Yes. Extreme heat often results in marked dehydration, with loss of valuable body fluids and minerals. Older people cannot readily tolerate upsets in their fluid and mineral balance.

Should people in their seventies and eighties be especially protected against extreme cold?

By all means, yes. Since there is a narrowing of their blood vessels, especially those in the extremities, it is essential that older people be kept out of extreme cold. Cold will cause these narrowed blood vessels to contract more and thus further diminish the amount of blood that can pass through them. Also, the coronary artery in older people is often somewhat narrowed, and extreme cold may cause this vital blood vessel to go into spasm.

Will living in a wet, damp climate affect older people adversely?

Wet, damp climates are often associated with a high incidence of upper respiratory infections. Since older people are less able to handle upper respiratory infections, wet, damp climates should be avoided if possible.

Is a semitropical climate beneficial to older people who have high blood pressure?

People who live in semitropical climates tend to perspire greatly and to lose large quantities of body fluids. This will reduce blood volume to a certain extent and may therefore help those with high blood pressure. However, it is by no means a decisive factor in the care of people with hypertension.

What is the effect of climate on older people with arthritis?

Arthritics are definitely benefited by warm or semitropical climates.

Are warm climates better for older people who have advanced hardening of the arteries?

Yes, for the same reason that they are better for those who have high blood pressure.

Is it safe for people in their seventies and eighties to change conditions abruptly by taking long plane trips?

Flying from a very warm climate to a frigid one should be avoided whenever possible. When they must make such an abrupt switch, older people should take special precautions on arrival in the cold climate. They should be particularly careful to avoid people who have respiratory infections.

Are older people ever affected by a sudden change from a cold to a warm climate?

Yes. They may develop a condition known as "tropical fatigue," which is characterized by lassitude and shortness of breath and which lasts a few days. Whether this is an actual physiological phenomenon or a psychological one is hard to say.

Is it true that people who have had arthritis or rheumatic conditions for many years can often foretell when damp or rainy weather is on the way?

Although there is no scientific basis for this, it does seem to be true.

Do people who live at very high altitudes tend to age prematurely?

No. Although there are changes that take place in the circulation of people who live at very high altitudes, the body makes the necessary adjustments.

Should people in their seventies and eighties avoid living at the seashore?

No. There are usually no detrimental effects unless the climate happens to be exceptionally damp. If it is, the incidence of infections of the sinuses, nose, throat, bronchial tubes, and lungs may be greater.

Should older people avoid overexposure to the sun?

Yes. Sunstroke and heat exhaustion are more common among older people, particularly those in their seventies or eighties.

Should older people avoid walking in high winds or severe cold?

Yes. Walking under such conditions places an extra load upon the heart and may precipitate a spasm of the coronary artery.

What room temperatures are best for older people?

Room temperature should be about 70° F. If the person is undressed, temperature should be maintained at about 80° F. People in their late seventies or eighties tend to become uncomfortable when room temperature falls below 62° F.

CLOTHING

See SOCIAL BEHAVIOR; TRAVEL.

Do manner of dress and attention to neatness often change in people who approach the later years?

Most active, healthy people past sixty will continue to dress in much the same way as they have throughout their adult lives. For this group, clothing presents no problem. There is, however, a significant group of people who tend to lose interest in their clothing and in their appearance as they get older. They may cause concern and embarrassment to their families.

What special advice should be given to older people concerning clothes and dressing habits?

1. Healthy older people should take special care to dress in

an up-to-date fashion. Nothing shows advancing age quite so much as old-fashioned clothing. Special attention must be given to a tendency among some older persons to become sloppy and uninterested in their wearing apparel.

2. As people get on in years, they tend to feel changes in climate more acutely. They need, therefore, to dress very warmly in cold weather and to dress lightly in warm weather. It is the responsibility of those who care for older people to see that their clothes are changed when the seasons change.

3. People in their seventies and eighties sometimes have less secure footing. It is important, therefore, that particular attention be paid to well-fitting shoes that provide good support, although special orthopedic shoes are often unnecessary. Women, as a general rule, should avoid spike heels. This does not mean that they should purchase ugly, old-fashioned shoes.

4. It is important for those who care for older people to see that their clothing is not stained. Moreover, it is often important to urge older men to have their suits pressed at frequent intervals.

5. People who attend older people should see that their undergarments, socks, and handkerchiefs are changed daily.

6. Older men and women should be discouraged from wearing garters that encircle the thigh or leg. Garters often interfere with circulation.

7. Clothing accessories add much to one's appearance. Older women should be encouraged to wear cheerful costume jewelry and men should wear happy, colorful ties and cuff links.

8. Bright, new clothes usually have a favorable effect upon older people, even if they are in their eighties or nineties.

Should the family or the attendant buy the clothing for older people?

Whenever possible, the older person should be encouraged to shop for himself rather than to have someone else make the purchases.

Are elastic or elastic-nylon stockings often recommended for older people?

Yes. There is a natural tendency for the veins of older people to function less efficiently and for blood to stagnate in the legs. For this reason, even if there are no marked varicose veins, many older people will derive benefit from wearing elastic stockings. This practice will lead to better return blood flow from the veins in the legs and may benefit heart function considerably.

Should older people wear hats when out in the sun?

Yes, since they are particularly susceptible to sunstroke and heat exhaustion.

Should older women wear brassieres?

If they have pendulous breasts, they should certainly wear a well-fitted brassiere. There is no greater concession to old age than for a woman to allow her figure to appear slovenly.

Should older women wear corsets?

Yes, if they are obese and wish to wear something that will improve their appearance. Also, a good corset will give support to the spinal column.

COMA

See ALCOHOL AND ALCOHOLISM; APOPLEXY, OR STROKE; BRAIN TUMOR; CONVULSIONS; DIABETES MELLITUS; EMBOLUS AND EMBOLISM; EPILEPSY; FAINTING.

What is coma?

A state of unconsciousness from which a patient cannot be aroused.

What are some of the more commonly encountered causes of coma among older people?

1. A stroke. (*See* APOPLEXY, OR STROKE.)
2. Uremia, with failure of kidney function.
3. Severe diabetes that has gone untreated.
4. Brain tumor.
5. Brain infection or inflammation of its coverings—encephalitis or meningitis.
6. A fall or a blow upon the head causing concussion or skull fracture.
7. Extensive liver damage with cholemic poisoning.
8. Overdose of a sedative, narcotic, or hypnotic drug.
9. Alcoholism.
10. Gas poisoning, as from inhaling carbon monoxide.

How can one discover whether an older person is merely in deep sleep, has fainted, or is in an actual state of coma?

Firm, steady pressure with the thumb just under the eyebrow will cause a person who has fainted or is sleeping to grimace or show some other signs of consciousness. Similar pressure over the bone just behind and below the ear will also cause a reaction if the patient is not in coma.

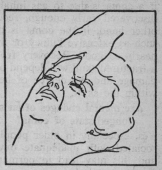

Application of pressure over eye to determine if patient can be aroused or is unconscious

If the patient *is* in coma, such maneuvers will not arouse him.

What first-aid measures should be carried out for someone who is found unconscious and cannot be aroused?

1. Collars, belts, and other tight clothing should be loosened. If breathing seems labored or shallow, the chin should be lifted up so that the neck is extended.

2. Artificial respiration should be started if breathing has stopped or is obviously inadequate. Bluish lips and skin will indicate the need for artificial respiration (*see* ARTIFICIAL RESPIRATION).

3. If there is choking or vomiting, the neck should be extended and the head turned to one side. Mucus should be wiped out of the mouth.

4. If the patient is found in a sitting position, he should be placed in a lying-down, face-up position, and a pillow should be placed under the shoulders.

5. No attempt should be made to revive the patient by slapping, pouring cold water on him, or attempting to force whiskey or other liquids into his mouth.

6. A doctor should be summoned. If a doctor is unavailable, the patient should be transported by ambulance to the nearest hospital.

Can people who have been in a coma for several days recover?

Yes, but the longer one is in a coma the less his chances are for recovery. Much will depend on the underlying cause of the coma. If the coma is due to diabetes and the diabetes is brought under control, recovery is the general rule. Similarly, if a coma is due to gas inhalation and the patient has been discovered early enough, recovery may take place. On the other hand, if the coma is due to an irreversible situation such as extensive kidney or liver damage, the outlook is not nearly so good. Recovery from brain injury associated with a fractured skull will depend on the extensiveness of the brain damage and the degree of hemorrhage that has taken place within the skull.

Are mental changes often seen after recovery from a prolonged state of coma?

Yes, especially in older people. Prolonged coma is often associated with inadequate oxygen supply to the brain cells and this may lead to permanent brain damage with consequent mental changes.

COMMON COLD

See ASTHMA; BRONCHITIS; CONTAGION AND CONTAGIOUS DISEASES; COUGHS; INFLUENZA AND GRIPPE; PNEUMONIA; RESPIRATORY TRACT.

Do people develop an immunity to the common cold and to other respiratory infections, such as sinus infections, as they grow older?

It is thought that some immunity may be developed, inasmuch as the common cold and sinus infections are more prevalent in younger people. But one should not count too much on this increased immunity, since it is not of great significance.

Does air conditioning predispose older people to the development of colds?

It is not the air conditioning itself that may cause people to catch cold, but rather the associated abrupt change in temperature and humidity. If older people remain in an air-conditioned environment and do not go in and out of it, they will have no increased tendency to catch cold.

Should special precautions be taken to protect older people from the common cold and other upper respiratory infections?

Yes. Contagion from other people is just as likely to take place in people past sixty, and isolation should therefore be strictly enforced. It is particularly important to prevent such contagion, since the common cold and respiratory infections tend to be more severe and are accompanied by greater incidence of complications in those who are in their later years.

What measures should older people take to avoid the common cold?

1. They should stay away from people who have acute respiratory infections. (Older people are susceptible to respiratory contagion.)
2. They should avoid exposure to wet, damp climates.
3. If exposed to wetness and dampness, they should dry themselves thoroughly and stay in a warm, dry room.
4. They should avoid exposure to cold drafts.
5. Fatigue and overexertion should be avoided. For some reason, people who are overtired and get insufficient rest are more susceptible to colds.
6. Although the reasons have not been scientifically established, supplemental vitamins may give added protection.
7. Influenza vaccine should be given to older people in the fall of each year. The value of this vaccine against the common cold has not been proved, but it does afford added protection against the development of complications.

Does it usually take longer for an older person to recover from an ordinary cold?

Yes, just as it takes longer for him to recover from any infection. This is especially true of people in their late seventies and eighties. Healthy people in their sixties and early seventies usually have the same reaction to colds as people in their middle years.

What complications may develop if a cold is neglected?

1. Bronchitis.
2. Bronchial pneumonia.
3. Lobar pneumonia.
4. Viral pneumonia.
5. Impairment of heart function.

What special treatment should be given people in their late seventies or eighties when they have a common cold?

1. They should be seen by a doctor and should not treat themselves.
2. They should go to bed.
3. They should remain in bed so long as they have a temperature and for approximately 48 hours thereafter.
4. They should rest in bed in a semisitting position, rather than lying flat.

5. Oxygen should be supplied if they are short of breath or show evidence of heart-function impairment.
6. Although the antibiotic drugs will not specifically affect the cold, an antibiotic may be prescribed by the doctor in order to protect the patient against the development of complications.
7. Adequate fluids should be taken unless the physician limits the quantity because of a coexisting heart condition. Water, fruit juice, and tea are the best liquids to take.
8. Keep the room at about 70° F. and arrange for good circulation of air. Do not permit a direct draft.
9. Give light foods; avoid heavy meals.
10. Give pain-relieving medications, such as aspirin, if necessary.
11. If there is an accompanying cough, cough mixtures may be given. (Heavy sedation or large doses of codeine, which suppress the cough reflex, should be avoided.)

Should antibiotics be taken by all older people when they have a common cold?

No! Antibiotic drugs should never be given unless specifically ordered by the attending physician.

Should whiskey or other alcoholic beverages be given in the treatment of the common cold?

No. There is a common misconception that alcohol will help a cold. It does not.

Can younger people catch an upper respiratory infection from an older person as readily as the older person can from them?

Yes.

Are there any medications, such as those advertised on radio and television, that can prevent a cold or break it up before it becomes severe?

No. Most of these drugs do have helpful ingredients, but they do not significantly alter the course of the common cold. The antihistamine ingredients in these drugs are thought by some doctors to be helpful, but it is generally recognized that they do not stop a cold from developing and running its usual course.

What is the difference between the common cold and the grippe?

The common cold is a virus infection usually limited to the mucous membranes of the nose and throat. Grippe causes symptoms that are felt throughout the body. Although both of these conditions may be caused by the same virus, the common cold is more limited in nature and does not cause symptoms throughout the body.

Does the common cold often lead to the development of grippe?
Yes. This is especially true when treatment, as outlined above, is neglected.

What is the difference between grippe and influenza?
Ordinarily, grippe is thought to be a milder form of influenza.

Should people in their seventies and eighties take vaccine injections against grippe and influenza?
Yes, although the effectiveness of these vaccines is not always as great as one might wish.

CONJUNCTIVITIS

See ALLERGY; BLEPHARITIS; EYES; TRICHIASIS.

What is conjunctivitis?
It is an inflammation of the mucous membrane lining the eye.

What can cause conjunctivitis?
An infection, injury, or allergy. Infection may be caused by many kinds of bacteria. Injury may be caused by dust, scratching, overexposure to the sun, excessive wind, etc. Allergy may be secondary to direct irritation by pollen, a drug, cosmetic, or other allergen.

Are people past sixty particularly susceptible to conjunctivitis?
Yes. For this reason, they should wear protective eyeglasses to safeguard themselves. This is especially important when they are out in the sun, in high wind, or in an automobile.

Why are older people more susceptible to conjunctivitis?
In some instances, they lose some of the sensitivity of this membrane and are therefore less aware when a foreign particle enters the eye. They may also be less aware of excessive sunlight or the presence of an infection.

How can a diagnosis of conjunctivitis be made?
The eye becomes reddened, tears readily, and itches.

What complication of conjunctivitis is most likely to affect older people?
An ulceration of the cornea (that part of the membrane

covering the colored portion of the eye) may develop. Such ulcerations may take a long time to heal and may leave behind scar tissue, which will interfere with vision.

What is the treatment for conjunctivitis?

This will depend on its origin. It should be stressed that whenever an eye irritation persists for 24 hours, an ophthalmologist should be consulted.

If the conjunctivitis is caused by infection, antibiotic eyedrops or ointments will, in most cases, be prescribed.

If it is caused by burn due to overexposure to the sun, astringent drops and compresses are applied.

If it is due to an allergy, the irritating factor must be removed and an antihistamine medication is given.

Should an ulcer of the cornea develop, antibiotic and cortisonelike medications are often employed.

Regardless of cause, in all cases of conjunctivitis the eyes should be rested, kept clean, and further irritation avoided. Expert medical attention should be sought in all cases occurring in old people.

CONSTIPATION

See BED CARE; BOWEL FUNCTION; DIARRHEA; INTESTINES; LAXATIVES; RECTUM AND ANUS.

Is it natural for the bowels to function less efficiently and for constipation to develop as one advances in age?

Yes, although there are many people whose bowels function normally throughout their lives.

Why does constipation tend to become more common during the later years?

Much of one's ability to evacuate the bowels depends on the muscle tone of the abdominal muscles and the muscles surrounding the rectum and anus. As people enter the seventies and eighties there is a tendency for these muscles to lose tone. Furthermore, older people tend to drink less fluids, and this practice results in harder stools, which are more difficult to expel.

Are psychological factors important in constipation?

Yes. For some reason, many older people seem to be inordinately concerned about their bowel function. When they are disturbed about this matter, their concern often leads to even greater difficulty with evacuation.

Is it necessary for older people to evacuate the bowels every day?

No. This is a common misconception. The important thing is to develop some regular system for bowel evacuation. Many healthy people in their sixties, seventies, and eighties normally evacuate their bowels every other day or every third day. It should be understood, however, that people who go more than two or three days without moving their bowels may develop an impaction. This condition is often painful to correct.

What is meant by an impaction?

It is a collection of a large quantity of hardened stool within the rectum—so large that it cannot be spontaneously evacuated.

What is the treatment of an impaction?

1. A nurse instills several ounces of warm mineral oil into the rectum.

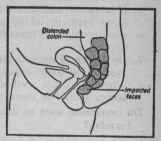

Hard fecal masses, as seen in impaction

2. Lubricants such as mineral oil are given by mouth.
3. If there is no contraindication, laxatives are given.
4. If the bowels do not then move spontaneously, a soap-suds enema is given.
5. If the bowels are not evacuated after the enema, the nurse or physician may have to break up the hard stool in the rectum with the fingers. Occasionally, general anesthesia must be given before such removal of an impaction.

How can an impaction be prevented?

Vigorous treatment of constipation is the best method of prevention.

What are good rules for older people to follow in order to assure regular elimination?

1. Form regular habits. Older people should be instructed to sit on the toilet at the same time each day, preferably directly after breakfast.
2. Older people should be taught not to strain. If the bowels do not move within a 15-minute period, they should abandon the effort rather than remain for long periods on the toilet.

3. It is essential that older people maintain an intake of at least eight to ten glasses of fluid daily. This will prevent the stool from becoming too solid. (There may be exceptions to this rule for those who must limit their fluid intake because of a heart condition.)

4. If one tends to be constipated, he should take some lubricant each day. The best lubricant to take is a tablespoon or two of mineral oil.

5. If a lubricant does not work, there should be no hesitation in taking a laxative. The specific laxative should, however, be prescribed by the family doctor.

6. If lubricants and laxatives do not move the bowels, there is no harm in taking a small enema once or twice a week provided permission is first obtained from the family doctor.

7. On advice of one's doctor, certain suppositories may be used to aid bowel evacuation.

8. When the usual methods are not effective, the family doctor should be consulted.

Do lubricants, such as mineral oil, tend to become habit-forming?

No.

Is it harmful to take lubricants, such as mineral oil?

No. There is an erroneous idea that taking mineral oil will prevent absorption of vitamins from the intestinal tract. If the patient is on a normal diet and has a normal digestive system, this is not true.

Are colonic irrigations helpful in aiding bowel function?

As a one-time procedure, colonic irrigation can be helpful. As a routine procedure, it is definitely not indicated.

Certainly, if colonic irrigations are to be taken regularly, they should be prescribed by the physician.

Is it safe to take bulk-forming medications?

These are sometimes an aid to bowel function, but they should be prescribed only by a doctor. In undernourished older people, bulk-forming substances may interfere with appetite and cause further undernourishment.

Is it safe for older people to take enemas regularly?

Yes, if they are prescribed by a doctor.

If an older person is forced to take enemas on a regular basis, how often should they be given and what do they contain?

Twice a week is usually often enough. Plain tap water, one or two glasses, is perhaps the best enema. Soap sometimes irritates the lining membrane of the rectum, as do other substances.

How should enemas be given?

The patient should sit on the toilet; the enema bag should be located no more than two feet above the level of the rectum. (It is not a good practice to place the bag higher, as this will cause the fluid to rush into the intestinal tract too forcefully.) Older patients may prefer to take an enema while lying down in bed or in the bathtub. If this is done, the fluid should be allowed to flow in gently, with the bag no more than two feet above the level of the body. Someone should be in attendance to help the patient from the bed or bathtub to the toilet.

Does regular physical exercise aid normal bowel evacuation?

Yes. For people in their seventies and eighties, regular walking is by far the best exercise.

Is it safe to use suppositories regularly in order to aid bowel evacuation?

Most suppositories contain glycerin and this tends to be irritating to the lining of the rectum if used regularly. For this reason, suppositories should be used only on the advice of a physician.

Should an older person consult a doctor if he has never been constipated but becomes so abruptly?

Yes. The abrupt onset of constipation may be caused by an obstruction in the bowel.

What is the significance of inability to pass gas from the rectum?

This is frequently associated with bowel obstruction and should be investigated immediately by the family doctor.

Should older people who are constipated and have abdominal pain take laxatives or enemas?

No! Whenever abdominal pain accompanies constipation, the family doctor should be called. It is extremely dangerous to take a laxative when there is abdominal pain.

Is it safe for older people to take laxatives?

Yes, but these should be prescribed by the family doctor. Certain laxatives can produce an irritation of the lining of the intestinal tract and these should be used sparingly. It should be emphasized that laxatives are best avoided whenever it is possible to regulate the bowels by other means, and also when there is abdominal pain.

Do people tend to become accustomed to laxatives so that they lose their effectiveness?

Yes. It is often necessary to switch from one laxative to another in order to obtain the desired effects.

What can be done by older people to prevent the onset of constipation?

1. Eat a hearty breakfast, preferably at the same hour each morning.
2. Develop regular habits, as indicated above.
3. Eat plenty of fresh fruits, vegetables, and roughage, such as bran products.
4. If coffee is permitted by the doctor, this will often stimulate bowel evacuation.
5. An adequate intake of fluids (8 to 10 glasses daily) is essential.
6. Use lubricants when prescribed by the physician.
7. If hemorrhoids exist, they should be treated by a surgeon.

What foods tend to be constipating?

Those that leave behind very little roughage, such as meats, starches, and sweets.

What can one do to encourage regular bowel function in older people?

Healthy older people in their sixties and seventies rarely need any training in this regard. However, those who are well into their seventies and eighties, or are invalids who require nursing care, must be retrained to move their bowels in much the same way as infants are trained.

A nurse attending an older, ill patient usually develops her own system for encouraging bowel function, much as a baby's nurse does. It is important not to overemphasize the need for daily bowel evacuation, and no threats should be posed for failure to accomplish it!

Do certain medications tend to cause constipation?

Yes, many medications will cause the bowels to act sluggishly. The more important of these are codeine and the morphine-derivative drugs. In certain people, iron medications (which are often given for anemia) tend to be constipating.

Do such foods as prunes, apricots, and bran aid bowel evacuation?

Yes. However, their effect varies markedly from one individual to another.

CONTAGION AND CONTAGIOUS DISEASES

See COMMON COLD; INFECTIONS; INFLUENZA AND GRIPPE; PNEUMONIA; RESPIRATORY TRACT; TUBERCULOSIS.

Are the contagious diseases of childhood a hazard to people past sixty?

No. Only in rare instances do older people develop mumps, whooping cough, chickenpox, measles, or other diseases of childhood. If people are susceptible to these diseases, they usually develop them long before they reach sixty.

Are people past sixty as susceptible as younger people to other contagious diseases such as pneumonia, common cold, and influenza?

Unfortunately, people do not develop true immunity to these conditions. As a matter of fact, with age there is increased susceptibility to pneumonia and other respiratory infections.

What are older people's chances of developing one of the following contagious diseases?

Disease	Rare	Infrequent	Same as Others	More Frequent
Chickenpox	*			
Diphtheria	*			
Dysentery			*	
Gonorrhea		*		
Hepatitis			*	
Infectious mononucleosis	*			
Measles	*			
Meningitis	*			
Mumps	*			
Pneumonia				*
Poliomyelitis	*			
Scarlet fever	*			
Smallpox	*			
Tuberculosis		*		
Typhoid fever		*		
Whooping cough	*			

Should people past sixty be vaccinated against the various contagious diseases?

With very few exceptions, vaccination is unnecessary. However, if there is an epidemic (of smallpox, for example), older people should also be vaccinated.

Is it advisable to give older people gamma globulin to avoid developing contagious diseases to which they have been exposed?

No.

Should people over sixty be vaccinated against polio?

Most investigators think this is unnecessary.

Should people past sixty be immunized to or vaccinated against yellow fever, cholera, plague, typhus fever, typhoid fever, and smallpox before traveling to countries where such diseases might be prevalent?

Yes. Older people have no special immunity to these particular diseases, with the possible exception of smallpox.

Are cold vaccines and influenza vaccines effective when given to older people?

They are just as effective for them as for younger people. None of these vaccines has proved to be as effective as the medical profession would wish them to be. However, during an epidemic of influenza, older people should definitely be given influenza vaccine.

Should people past sixty take the same precautions in guarding against contagious diseases as younger people do?

Very definitely, yes. Although they themselves may not develop the contagious disease, they may act as carriers and transmit it to others.

When an older person does develop a contagious disease is it treated in a manner different from treatment of the same disease in younger people?

The possibilities of complications from the ordinary contagious diseases are much greater in older people. This is because their organs may be less able to resist the infection. It is therefore essential to treat these diseases more vigorously and to keep the patient in bed longer. It is well known that even a common cold can become a serious illness to a debilitated person in his eighties or nineties.

CONVULSIONS

See APOPLEXY, OR STROKE; BRAIN TUMOR; COMA; EPILEPSY; FAINTING; NERVES.

What are some of the more common causes of convulsions?

1. An overdose of insulin in a diabetic. The convulsion

in these cases is called "insulin shock" and can be overcome by giving the patient sugar.

2. Rupture of a blood vessel in the brain or clotting (thrombosis) in a blood vessel in the brain. Such convulsions occasionally accompany apoplexy, or stroke.

3. A brain tumor.

4. Heart disease associated with inadequate oxygen supply (hypoxia) to the brain.

5. Hemorrhage beneath the covering of the brain (subdural hematoma) as the result of an injury.

6. Fractured skull.

7. Advanced uremia, with failure of kidney function.

8. Various poisons.

9. Epilepsy.

Can a doctor usually isolate the particular cause of a convulsion?

Yes, but diagnosis may require a thorough investigation involving many specific tests.

Do convulsions tend to recur?

When they are caused by an underlying organic disease that has not been treated and controlled, they tend to recur.

Do convulsions tend to leave permanent defects, or does the patient return to a normal state after the convulsion has ended?

If the convulsion was caused by hemorrhage or thrombosis of a blood vessel in the brain, there may be permanent disability. On the other hand, if the convulsion is due to epilepsy, overdose of insulin, or inhalation of carbon monoxide, there will usually be no permanent aftereffects. It is the doctor's task to establish the exact cause of the convulsion and to see if it can be eliminated.

What first-aid should be given to an older person who is having a convulsive seizure?

1. A spoon, stick of wood, or rolled handkerchief should be placed between the teeth to prevent the patient from biting his tongue. (Be careful, for a convulsing patient may involuntarily bite.)

2. The patient should be placed on his back with a pillow under the shoulders and the chin held up.

3. Tight collars, belts, and other clothing should be loosened to aid breathing.

4. If breathing is inadequate, artificial respiration should be started (*see* ARTIFICIAL RESPIRATION).

5. The patient's clothing should be searched. If he is an epileptic or has recurring convulsive seizures from another cause, he will probably have a card somewhere on him that gives full first-aid instructions in the event of an attack.

CORONARY-ARTERY DISEASE

See ANGINA PECTORIS; ARTERIOSCLEROSIS; CHOLESTEROL; CIRCULATION; HEART; SMOKING; THROMBUS AND THROMBOSIS.

CORONARY INSUFFICIENCY

What is coronary insufficiency?

Failure of the coronary artery to carry a sufficient amount of blood to the active heart muscle. Coronary insufficiency is almost always brought on by arteriosclerosis of the coronary artery plus spasm of the vessel.

Is coronary insufficiency encountered very often among people past sixty?

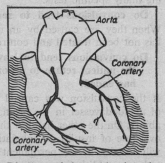

Diagram of heart showing the two main coronary arteries

Yes. Since this condition reflects hardening of the coronary artery, one would expect it to be prevalent in those who are getting into their later years.

Will coronary insufficiency result in attacks of angina pectoris?

Yes, in the great majority of instances (*see* ANGINA PECTORIS).

What is the treatment for coronary insufficiency?

More or less the same as that for angina pectoris.

What is the relationship between cholesterol and the development of angina pectoris and coronary insufficiency?

The exact role of cholesterol has not as yet been fully determined. It is thought, however, that a high blood-cholesterol level over a period of years may lead to the premature development of arteriosclerosis of the coronary artery.

Will adherence to a low-cholesterol diet during young adulthood and the middle years delay the development of hardening of the coronary arteries?

Medical teaching within the past few years advises young and middle-aged people to eat low-cholesterol diets. Whether or not this advice will lower the incidence of coronary disease remains to be seen. Certainly, it can be stated that there are no known harmful effects from following a diet low in cholesterol.

CORONARY THROMBOSIS

What is coronary thrombosis?

A blood clot has formed in the passageway of the coronary artery of the heart. This obstruction will prevent the artery from supplying a certain segment of the heart-muscle wall with adequate amounts of oxygen and nourishment.

Is coronary occlusion the same as coronary thrombosis?

Yes.

Is coronary thrombosis very common in people past sixty?

It is one of the most common causes of death in the later years.

Are men and women equally affected by coronary thrombosis?

No. In the younger age groups, coronary thrombosis is three times as common in men. In people past sixty years of age, this disease is almost as common in women.

What types of older people are susceptible to coronary thrombosis?

1. Those with marked arteriosclerosis.
2. Those with chronically elevated blood pressure.
3. Diabetic patients.
4. Fat people.
5. People who have had high blood-cholesterol levels for many years.
6. People who live unordered lives and who subject themselves to excessive physical and emotional stress.

What are the symptoms and signs of coronary thrombosis?

1. Severe pain located beneath the breastbone. It may last for several hours or may be so severe that it is not relieved even by an injection of morphine.

2. Spread of pain to the left-shoulder region and down the left arm.
3. Ashen-gray skin, with cold sweat.
4. A rapid, small, thready pulse.
5. A sense of apprehension and fear.
6. Rapid, shallow breathing.
7. Mild fever developing a day or two after the attack of pain.
8. On the electrocardiogram will be shown characteristic changes developing on the second or third day after the attack of pain.
9. Characteristic changes in the blood chemistry with elevation of some of the enzymes, such as transaminase.
10. A soreness with residual pain beneath the breastbone lasting for several days after the initial attack.
11. In severe cases, heart irregularity and signs of heart failure.

How often is the initial attack of coronary thrombosis fatal?

It is estimated that four out of five people survive the initial attack of coronary thrombosis and recover from it.

Are older people as able to survive coronary thrombosis as younger people?

Yes. Paradoxically, many of those past sixty are better able to withstand coronary thrombosis. This is because through the years they have developed circulation through smaller, collateral, arteries. Thus, although the main coronary artery is clotted, the heart muscle is less deprived of blood and oxygen.

What is meant by the development of collateral circulation?

The heart muscle has a network of blood vessels traveling to it. When the main coronary artery becomes arteriosclerotic or has a clot in it, the blood will reach the heart muscle by traveling through the smaller arteries, which become dilated in order to carry more blood. This dilatation of the smaller arteries and the resulting increased capacity to carry blood constitute collateral circulation. It is, in a sense, a compensatory system.

Is it common for people to have a second coronary thrombosis?

This does occur, but not in all cases.

What is the treatment of coronary thrombosis?

1. Bed rest and withdrawal of all possible sources of irritation or excitement.

2. Medication is given to relieve the pain.
3. Sedatives are given to relieve the fear and apprehension that usually accompany a coronary attack.
4. The patient is placed in a semisitting position to make breathing and heart action easier.
5. Oxygen is given to make breathing easier and to spare the heart muscle too much activity.
6. Anticoagulant medications are given to keep the blood in a fluid state and to decrease its tendency to clot. (Such medications as heparin or dicoumarol are given for this purpose.)
7. Salt intake is restricted so as to avoid extra fluid accumulation.
8. Diuretic medications to increase excretion of excess fluids are given.
9. If heart action falters, digitalis is given.
10. A light diet containing adequate protein, sugars, minerals, and vitamins is given. If the patient is overweight, caloric intake is restricted.

What is the long-term treatment of coronary thrombosis?

The patient is kept at rest for a period of two to four weeks, depending on the severity of the attack. From time to time, he is permitted to dangle his feet at the side of the bed, and after a few days he may be permitted to take a few steps about the room. If he is overweight, caloric intake is strictly limited and salt restrictions are continued. Anticoagulant medications are continued for months to years after recovery from coronary thrombosis in an attempt to avoid another episode.

Is heart surgery ever advocated for people who have had a coronary thrombosis?

Yes, but people past sixty years of age are not as good candidates for it as younger people.

What surgery is occasionally recommended for people who have a coronary thrombosis?

An operation known as *poudrage* is performed. This means that talcum powder is introduced into the pericardial sac, which surrounds the heart. The talc causes an irritation in the pericardial sac with subsequent formation of new small blood vessels that will supply the heart wall. This procedure has limited application but has helped many people, particularly those who continue to have severe heart pain after recovery from coronary thrombosis.

Can one ever resume usual activities after recovery from coronary thrombosis?

Usually. Recent study has shown that physical exercise, when performed in moderation, is often beneficial after recovery from coronary thrombosis. Exercise stimulates the circulation and allows the heart to function more normally than if the patient were to be kept physically inactive after it is no longer necessary.

If an older person has recovered from coronary thrombosis, will he be able to return to sexual activity?

Yes, in moderation.

How can one tell if a complete recovery has been made from coronary thrombosis?

After a person has recovered from an acute attack, he should have periodic examinations, including electrocardiograms. The electrocardiographic tracings will show the course of recovery.

How long does it usually take an older person to recover fully from an attack of coronary thrombosis?

Approximately 4 to 6 months.

How can a damaged heart muscle repair itself?

The part of the heart-muscle wall that has been destroyed by the thrombosis is replaced by fibrous scar tissue. Usually the scar tissue does not interfere with return to normal heart function.

What is the relationship between cholesterol and the development of coronary thrombosis?

The exact role of cholesterol has not yet been fully determined. It is thought, however, that a high blood-cholesterol level over a period of years will lead to the development of premature arteriosclerosis of the coronary artery. Since arteriosclerosis is a forerunner of thrombosis, a definite relationship may exist.

Can people over sixty do anything to prevent coronary thrombosis?

Yes, although most of the factors that predispose one to develop this condition are fixed and cannot be remedied. Nevertheless, people can control obesity; if they have diabetes they can regulate it; they can take medication to lower their blood pressure; and they can reorder their lives so as to minimize physical and emotional stress.

COUGHS

See ALLERGY; ASTHMA; BRONCHIECTASIS; BRONCHITIS; COMMON COLD; CONTAGION AND CONTAGIOUS DISEASES; EMPHYSEMA; INFLUENZA AND GRIPPE; PNEUMONIA; RESPIRATORY TRACT; TUBERCULOSIS.

Do older people have a greater tendency than younger ones to develop coughs?

Yes. As people advance in age some of the elastic tissue in the lungs is replaced by fibrous tissue. As a consequence, mucous secretions tend to collect in the base of the lungs and vigorous coughing may be necessary to expel them. Moreover, a condition known as emphysema often develops: the air spaces become dilated and lose their ability to expel secretions. This, too, will result in increased coughing.

What are some of the common causes of coughing?

1. Irritation of the back of the throat.
2. Irritation or inflammation in the larynx or in the trachea (windpipe).
3. Inflammation in the bronchial tubes or in a lung.
4. Irritating gases, smog, tobacco and other kinds of smoke, etc.
5. Exposure to extremely cold air.

Does persistent coughing ever have a serious effect on the health of an elderly person?

Yes. Violent, persistent coughing may result in the expenditure of a great deal of physical energy. Such coughing may weaken an older person who is already ill with a respiratory or other type of infection.

Is coughing ever helpful?

Yes, when it is accompanied by the bringing up of secretions that have accumulated in the bronchial tubes or lungs. As a matter of fact, physicians encourage people who have bronchitis or pneumonia to cough moderately if it results in bringing up accumulated secretions.

What is the significance of blood in the sputum?

1. It may be caused merely by a severe coughing spasm and may not indicate the presence of serious disease.
2. It may be caused by an infection in the nose, sinuses, or throat.
3. It may be found in cases of bronchitis or pneumonia.
4. It can occur in patients with lung abscess.

5. It may indicate tuberculosis.
6. It is seen in cases of lung tumor.

Should older people be X-rayed if they cough up blood?

Yes, by all means. Actually, it is a good practice for all people past sixty to have a chest X ray taken every year, whether or not they cough blood. In this way tuberculosis, lung tumors, and other serious conditions may be spotted *before* other symptoms develop.

What is the significance of foul-smelling sputum?

It may indicate the presence of a lung abscess. Chest X rays should be taken in all such cases.

How soon after the onset of a cough should medical attention be sought?

Any cough that persists for several days should be a signal for medical consultation.

What procedures are carried out if a cough persists and chest X rays are negative?

The nose, throat, sinuses, larynx, trachea, and bronchial tubes are investigated. Examination with a bronchoscope also may be made.

What is a bronchoscope?

It is a long, hollow, tubular, metal instrument with a light at its end. A bronchoscope is inserted through the mouth into the trachea and down toward the bronchial tubes.

What is the value of a bronchoscopic examination?

It may demonstrate the presence of a tumor in the trachea or in one of the bronchial tubes. It may also make visible a foreign body that has been swallowed or show the origin of pus from a lung abscess.

Is smoking harmful to those who have a chronic cough?

Yes, definitely. It is difficult to cure many infections of the respiratory tract if one continues smoking.

Is there such a thing as "smoker's cough"?

Yes. Many older people will develop a chronic cough as a result of smoke irritation.

If one has a cough that originates from an infection in the respiratory tract, what measures can be taken to relieve it?

1. The air of the room in which the patient lives or works should be kept warm and moist.
2. Steam inhalations from a croup kettle or electric inhalator should be taken. Tincture of benzoin may be added to the inhalant.

3. Medications to aid in bringing up sputum may be prescribed.
4. Medications may be given to dry up excessive secretions.
5. When coughing causes sleeplessness, sedatives are prescribed.
6. If the cause of the cough is an infection that will respond to antibiotics, then these medications should be prescribed by the physician.

Are mustard plasters and other counterirritants helpful in relieving a cough?

They may have some beneficial psychological effect, but they are of little value otherwise.

In what position should older people who suffer from coughing spells rest in bed?

The semisitting position. This position will make it easier for them to bring up secretions that have collected in the bronchial tubes or lungs.

Do warm poultices, hot-water bags, or electric pads aid in bringing up sputum?

No. These are of little or no value.

Is it advisable for an older person to medicate himself with cough medicines?

This is not a good practice. There are so many serious causes for chronic cough that it is far better to seek a physician's advice. In hiding the cough, one may be unwittingly hiding a serious underlying condition.

Will the inhalation of oxygen and carbon dioxide help persons with chronic cough?

When people are older and seriously ill, breathing a mixture of 95 percent oxygen and 5 percent carbon dioxide will often greatly help to relieve a cough. Of course, it must be prescribed by the attending physician.

Does coughing spread disease?

Yes, definitely. Whenever one coughs, a spray of droplets travels a distance of 8 to 10 feet. If a person has a contagious disease, such as tuberculosis, pneumonia, or influenza, he can spread it to those around him if he fails to cover his mouth when he coughs.

Can excessive coughing damage the heart?

If the coughing is severe, continuous, and characterized by strong spasms, it can strain a heart that is already weakened by old age or disease. In the average healthy patient past sixty, permanent bad effects rarely result from coughing.

CYSTITIS AND INTERSTITIAL CYSTITIS

See CYSTOCELE AND RECTOCELE; GONORRHEA; KIDNEYS; PROSTATE GLAND; URINARY BLADDER AND URETHRA.

CYSTITIS

What is cystitis?

It is an inflammation of the wall of the urinary bladder. Cystitis may arise from infected urine, which drains down from the kidneys, or it may result from an infection that ascends through the urethra from the outside.

Does cystitis often occur in older people?

Yes, since urinary infections are very common in those in the older age groups. The incidence in men is even greater, as a result of the obstruction of the bladder outlet that accompanies an enlarged prostate gland. In women, a cystocele (*see* CYSTOCELE AND RECTOCELE) or stricture of the outlet of the bladder often causes urine to become stagnant and infected, which ultimately produces an inflammation of the bladder wall.

Does urine become more easily infected in older people?

Yes, because older people tend to develop an obstruction to the bladder outlet and this prevents complete emptying. Stagnant urine often becomes infected.

What types of germs may cause cystitis?

The same ones that occur in infections elsewhere in the body, such as the streptococcus, the colon bacillus, the bacillus Proteus, the staphylococcus.

What are the symptoms and signs of acute cystitis?

1. Frequent urination, with a sense of urgency.
2. Pain and burning on urination, felt at the outlet of the urethra and sometimes in the region of the bladder in the lower abdomen.
3. Rise in temperature, occasionally with chills.
4. Cloudy urine, which, on examination, shows pus and, in some cases, blood cells.
5. After voiding, the feeling that the bladder has not been fully emptied.

Are bladder infections contagious?

No, except in the rare instances when the infection has been caused by gonorrhea or tuberculosis.

What is the treatment of acute cystitis?

1. Taking large quantities of fluids, mainly water.

2. Bed rest.
3. A bland diet, with no highly seasoned foods or alcohol.
4. Sedatives to relieve pain, spasm, and a sense of urgency to void.
5. Taking antibiotic drugs, sulfa drugs, or urinary antiseptics *after* it has been determined to which specific medication the infecting organism is sensitive. To discover this, the physician may recommend that a urine culture be made in order to identify the bacteria. When they have been identified, the bacteria are then checked for sensitivity to various antibiotics.

What is the best way to avoid a serious bladder infection?

1. A physician should be consulted as soon as any symptoms appear. Increased frequency of urination is usually one of the earliest signs of bladder trouble.
2. Such conditions as cystocele in a woman or enlargement of the prostate in a man should be corrected.

What is chronic cystitis and does it occur often in older people?

Chronic cystitis is similar to acute cystitis, except that it lasts for several weeks to months. It represents an uncured case of acute cystitis. Many of those who suffer from chronic cystitis have associated disease in other parts of the urinary tract, for example, the kidney, the ureter, the urethra, the prostate gland.

What associated conditions can cause acute or chronic cystitis?

1. Obstruction to the outlet of the bladder.
2. A stone in the kidney or in the ureter.
3. A tumor in the kidney or ureter.
4. A stone in the bladder.
5. A tumor in the bladder.

Is cystitis curable when it occurs in older people?

Yes, but it often entails eradicating an associated condition as well as local treatment of the bladder. Thus, a woman may have to be operated on for a coexisting cystocele or a man may have to have his prostate gland removed before the cystitis is completely cured.

INTERSTITIAL CYSTITIS

What is interstitial cystitis?

It is a chronic inflammation and thickening of the wall of the bladder, usually without an associated infection of the urine. It is seen most commonly in older women; it is rare in men.

What causes interstitial cystitis?

The cause is unknown.

What are the symptoms and signs of interstitial cystitis?

1. The thickening of the bladder wall is associated with a loss in its ability to expand greatly. Thus, the capacity of the bladder to hold large amounts of urine is markedly reduced. Frequency of urination results.
2. There may be frequent episodes of bladder spasm with the sensation that one must void immediately. At voiding, only a few drops of urine are passed.
3. As elastic tissue is lost in the bladder wall, areas of ulceration and thinning of the musculature may take place. The ulceration further increases bladder irritability and inability to hold urine.

How does the urologist make a diagnosis of interstitial cystitis?

The most characteristic findings are increased frequency of voiding, both by day and by night, with pain above the pubic bone in the lower abdomen. When the urine is examined, it is usually found to be free of pus and infection.

The diagnosis can be made certain by cystoscopic examination of the interior of the bladder; the wall lining has a characteristic appearance.

What is the treatment for interstitial cystitis?

Unfortunately, this condition is very difficult to cure and usually persists for a number of years. Irrigations of the bladder with various medications are of some benefit. Antispasmodic drugs are also helpful in relieving symptoms. Cauterization of the ulcerations of the bladder wall through a cystoscope may bring about some healing.

CYSTOCELE AND RECTOCELE

See CYSTITIS AND INTERSTITIAL CYSTITIS; FEMALE ORGANS; URINARY BLADDER AND URETHRA.

What is a cystocele?

It is a protrusion of the urinary bladder down into the vagina. The condition is produced by a relaxation, weakening, or degeneration of the ligaments that normally hold the bladder in its proper position.

Is cystocele ever caused by a tear resulting from childbirth?

Yes, but that condition is not very common today because of improved obstetrical methods. Cystocele is more likely due to weakening of the ligaments resulting from multiple childbirth. However, many women who have never borne children develop cystocele in their later years.

How common is cystocele in older women?

It is one of the most frequently encountered gynecological conditions in older women.

What are the usual symptoms of cystocele?

1. A small cystocele may produce no symptoms.
2. Protrusion of the bladder into the vaginal canal and an uncomfortable feeling.
3. Frequency of urination.
4. Losing urine when coughing, sneezing, or laughing.
5. The sensation after voiding that the bladder is not completely emptied.
6. Symptoms of cystitis brought on by an infection of the urine (*see* CYSTITIS).

How is the diagnosis of cystocele made?

By a simple pelvic examination.

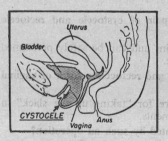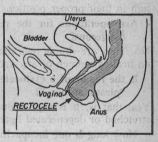

Diagrams showing cystocele and rectocele

What is a rectocele?

It is a protrusion of the rectum into the vaginal canal.

How common is rectocele?

It is one of the most common gynecological conditions found in women past sixty.

What causes a rectocele to develop?

Laxity, stretching, or degeneration of the ligaments that normally hold the rectum in place.

Is rectocele ever caused by a tear resulting from childbirth?

Yes, but modern obstetrical methods now prevent this from taking place. Most cases now encountered are among older women and are unrelated to childbearing.

What are the symptoms of rectocele?

1. A bulge from the rectal area into the vagina, with accompanying discomfort.
2. Increasing constipation, with a feeling that the stool is just at the exit but cannot be expelled because of lack of muscle power.

Are cystocele and rectocele usually seen together?

Yes. Since these conditions have a similar origin, one usually finds both of them present.

Are cystocele and rectocele often associated with prolapse of the uterus (fallen womb)?

Yes.

What is the treatment for cystocele and rectocele?

Mild cases may be controlled by the use of a pessary, an appliance inserted into the vagina to maintain normal position of the bladder and uterus. More advanced cases are treated surgically.

Surgery consists of repairing and shortening the ligaments and surrounding fibrous tissues that hold the bladder and rectum in their proper positions.

Are operations for the repair of cystocele and rectocele dangerous?

No. They are simple operations and can be safely performed on healthy women of any age.

Is the repair of a cystocele and rectocele a form of vaginal "plastic surgery"?

Yes; that is, it is a procedure for "taking up the slack" in stretched or degenerated ligaments.

How long is one incapacitated by such an operation?

Today, with modern surgical methods and techniques, patients usually get out of bed the day after surgery and leave the hospital within 5 to 10 days.

Is it possible for an older woman to have marital relations following surgical repair of a cystocele or rectocele?

Yes.

If cystocele, rectocele, and prolapse of the uterus are present at the same time, will all three conditions be repaired during one operation?

Yes.

Can anything be done to prevent the development of cystocele, rectocele, or prolapse of the uterus?

No, but if they are present during the younger years, it is a good idea to have them repaired at that time.

To avoid surgery, can a pessary be worn instead?

Most cases of advanced cystocele, rectocele, or prolapse of the uterus cannot be held in place satisfactorily by the use of a pessary. (It is somewhat similar to a man's wearing a truss to hold in a hernia, in that it may work for a short time, but not indefinitely.)

If a pessary does satisfactorily retain a cystocele, rectocele, or prolapse, it must be removed, cleansed, and reinserted at regular intervals. This must be done by the gynecologist. Failure to do so may lead to infection, ulceration, or even tumor formation in the vagina. In some instances, pessaries have been known to grow into the vaginal tissues, requiring surgery to remove them.

DEATH AND FEAR OF DEATH

See ATTITUDES TOWARD AGING; LONGEVITY; MENTAL CHANGES; SLEEP AND REST; SOCIAL BEHAVIOR; WIDOWHOOD.

Do most people have an increasing fear of death as they enter their later decades of life?

Although some people do, the majority do not. Most people are so constituted that they develop a more mature attitude and accept the idea of death as they come closer to it.

What kind of individual usually demonstrates excessive fear of death?

The poorly adjusted, neurotic person. If someone has faced the vicissitudes of living in a mature manner during his middle years, he will in all probability demonstrate the same maturity later.

What advice will help the elderly person who does dwell inordinately on the subject of death?

1. He should be encouraged to be active and should not be permitted to remain free of responsibilities.
2. His interests and thinking should be directed toward others, with emphasis on service to those who may need his help and advice. In other words, the aging individual must be aware that he is still useful!
3. He should be induced to keep up on current events and

should be encouraged to look ahead, rather than back. When he dwells too much on the past, it will accentuate fear of death.

4. He should be helped to make new friends, particularly among those who have a happier outlook. He may then identify with these people.

Should people be told when death is imminent?

Most people who are nearing the end of life know it without being told. More and more, today, the accepted philosophy is to tell people when they are approaching the end. This is important; it helps them to meet death with equanimity and gives them an opportunity to take care of important matters. It is perhaps best not to force those who have been unstable and emotionally unable to handle crises during their younger days to face the inevitability of death.

Does loneliness contribute to an increased fear of death?

Yes. This is another reason why older people should be helped to keep in contact with friends and encouraged to make new friends and develop new interests.

Are there medications or drugs that can calm those who dwell inordinately on death?

The tranquilizers have been used for this purpose, but they are of questionable value. Most of these people are experiencing emotional upsets that require psychiatric advice.

Should older people who are aware of impending death be permitted to discuss their problems with family and friends?

Very definitely, yes. It is common knowledge that older people often wish to talk about death only to find that their family and friends refuse.

Does sleeping alone increase fear of death?

This is very often the case. In such instances, older people should have a nurse or attendant sleep in the same room with them. If this is not feasible, they should sleep with their bedroom door open so that they have some means of communication with others in the household.

Is sleeplessness (insomnia) ever an indication of an exaggerated fear of death?

Yes.

What can be done to combat sleeplessness that appears to arise from fear of dying?

Perhaps the best treatment is a frank and open discussion. This talk can be held with members of the family or the family physician. The air is often cleared to the extent that fears are reduced greatly. Of course, there are also many sleep-producing medications that can be prescribed.

Do social contacts with other older people tend to allay fear of death?

Yes. Older people often discuss the subject among themselves and so reduce some of their anxiety.

What steps should be taken when a member of the family dies?

1. The family physician should be notified so that a death certificate can be made out.
2. If the deceased has not been under the care of a private physician within the last few days, weeks, or months before death, it is necessary to notify the police. They will send an investigator, who, after satisfying himself that death resulted from natural causes, will authorize the filing of a death certificate.
3. An undertaker should be notified. He will arrange for the processing of the death certificate and will remove the body of the deceased to his establishment. (This cannot be done until the death certificate is signed and accepted by the local health and police authorities.)
4. The undertaker should be told the type of funeral service desired, the type of burial, and the cemetery to which the body of the deceased will go. Finances should be thoroughly discussed prior to the funeral.
5. A member of the family should be assigned to notify other relatives and friends of the deceased.
6. Someone should be assigned to notify the obituary department of the local newspaper so that an announcement can be placed.
7. The attorney for the deceased should be notified.
8. Clubs and organizations to which the deceased belonged should be notified.
9. Close business associates of the deceased should be notified.
10. The insurance policies that the deceased possessed should be checked. Such policies should be located and the insurance companies notified.
11. About 8 to 12 photostatic copies of the death certificate should be obtained through the undertaker.
12. Acknowledgment cards for expressions of sympathy may be purchased from the funeral director.
13. The will should be located so that it may be read at some later date.

14. Arrangements should be made for settling the outstanding debts of the deceased.

**What precautions should be observed by a family that has
lost one of its members?**

1. They should remember that there are many different
prices of caskets, funeral services, etc. There should be
no hesitation in asking for a less costly funeral if funds
are limited.

2. It is not necessary to buy a burial plot at the time of
burial. Too often, they are sold at a higher price because
the family is unaware that arrangements can be made
at a later date.

3. It is wise to turn over all financial matters of the deceased to an attorney. All too often, false claims are
made by so-called creditors against the estate of the
deceased.

DEGENERATIVE CHANGES OF AGING

See ANATOMICAL CHANGES IN ORGANS; ARTERIOSCLEROSIS;
FUNCTIONAL CHANGES WITH AGING; LONGEVITY; MENTAL
CHANGES; PREMATURE AGING.

What are degenerative changes?

The basic structures of the body, the cells and tissues that
make up the organs, undergo deterioration. For example, a
degenerative change in the wall of an artery is the replacement of its elastic tissue by fibrous tissue. Such a change prevents the artery from contracting and expanding as it should,
which leads ultimately to the narrowing and hardening of the
blood vessel. Another example is nephrosclerosis, or degeneration of the kidney. In nephrosclerosis, the glomeruli, which
filter out waste materials from the bloodstream, undergo degeneration, and are replaced by fibrous tissue. If this process
involves many glomeruli, kidney function will be markedly
impaired.

**Do all cells and consequently all organs undergo some de-
generative changes as one ages?**

Yes.

**What is considered to be the underlying cause of the de-
generative changes that take place in the various organs?**

The exact mechanism behind this degeneration is not known.
We do know that certain organs may show almost no changes

until late in life, whereas other organs may undergo complete degeneration. For example, the intestinal tract in a ninety-year-old person may function quite efficiently, with the stomach and intestines continuing to secrete their juices and digest food normally; that same person may suffer complete loss of sight, loss of hearing, and marked degeneration of brain cells. Once the cause for the degenerative process is discovered, ways will be found to lengthen the life-span.

Is it true that "aging" begins before birth?

Yes. For example, during certain stages of the human embryo's development, it has fishlike gills. These gills degenerate completely by the time the child is born, and only fibrous tissue remains in their place. This process is degenerative. Similarly, the blood vessels in the umbilical cord (which attaches the embryo to its mother) undergo degenerative changes during the latter part of embryonic life.

Is it true that certain organs might be able to live for 150 or 200 years?

Yes. Post-mortem examinations of people who have lived for more than a hundred years often show structures that have undergone only minor changes. Also, almost all of us have known people whose minds were alert and young in their nineties or whose vision was nearly perfect throughout a long life.

What brings on the premature degenerative changes seen in certain organs?

See PREMATURE AGING.

Is there such a thing as a normal rate of degeneration?

Not really. The rate varies from organ to organ within the same person and from person to person. However, the average life-span today is about seventy years. A century from now the present limit may be extended to ninety years by slowing down the degenerative process.

What are some of the factors thought to play a major role in determining the rate of degenerative changes?

1. Heredity.
2. The mode of living.
3. Injuries that various organs have sustained.
4. Infections and diseases that have affected the various organs.
5. Chemical and hormonal changes.
6. Psychological factors.

Will leading a physically inactive life tend to retard the degenerative changes of aging?

This is a very difficult question to answer. A certain amount of physical activity is required to maintain bodily health, but overexertion may be especially harmful to older people.

Is there a tendency for certain organs to show signs of degeneration at specific ages?

Yes. For instance, the uterus and ovaries show degenerative changes at the menopause (anywhere from forty-five to fifty-five years of age). The thymus gland, in the chest or at the base of the neck, degenerates normally in early adult life.

Why is it that certain body tissues can regenerate, whereas others are incapable of regeneration?

This is a biological fact that is not fully understood. It is known that muscle and nerve cells, once destroyed, will not regenerate. The cells of the skin will regenerate after being repeatedly destroyed.

Can the lining of the intestinal tract regenerate after it has once been destroyed (by an ulcer, for example)?

Yes.

Do older people usually show degenerative changes in the cells of the lining of the intestinal tract?

In the healthy individual, degeneration of the lining of the intestinal tract is not great, and those cells can digest and absorb food normally throughout that person's life. It should be stated, however, that the capacity of the stomach and the intestines to absorb large quantities of food is decreased as people enter their later decades.

Do the stomach and small intestines tend to secrete less digestive juice as one ages?

Yes, but most people can still function satisfactorily.

Does the heart undergo degenerative changes?

Yes. The heart is a muscular organ that contracts and relaxes continuously. It is no small wonder, then, that this muscle will eventually show replacement of its muscle fibers by fibrous tissue.

Is there any way to protect the heart muscle so that it will not undergo premature degenerative changes?

Yes. One should avoid those things that make excessive work for the heart. In brief:

1. Stay thin. Since the heart muscle has to pump blood to every single cell in the body, the more cells it has to serve, the harder work it has to do.
2. Avoid excessive smoking or drinking.
3. Avoid excess physical strain.
4. Treat all infections as soon as they appear. Toxins from

bacterial infection affect the heart adversely. For instance, rheumatic fever may cause severe heart damage.

5. Avoid repeated emotional stress. This may cause spasm of the coronary arteries with a consequent decrease of oxygen and nutriments going to supply the heart muscle.

Is it true that samples of heart muscle have been kept alive in test tubes for many years, and that these samples show very little evidence of degeneration?

Yes. It must be remembered, though, that these experiments do not parallel what goes on in the human body. However, the experiments do show that when heart muscle is not subjected to undue tension and physical strain, or is not influenced by infections or toxins, it can live for many extra years.

Is there any way to slow down the degenerative processes that take place in the blood vessels?

Arteriosclerosis is thought to be associated with deposits of cholesterol in the wall or lining of the blood vessels. It is therefore suggested that an individual keep his blood-cholesterol level as low as possible. (*See also* ARTERIOSCLEROSIS.)

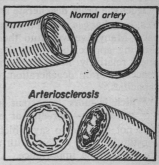

Typical degenerative changes seen in arteries of aged people

Do the lungs undergo degenerative changes as people get older?

Yes. The elastic tissue is replaced by fibrous tissue, and the walls of the air cells break down. Both processes lessen the capacity of the lungs to extract oxygen from the air.

Can anything be done to slow down the degenerative processes that take place in the lungs?

Yes. Some recommendations are:

1. Rooms should be well ventilated so that fresh air can replace old, stale air.
2. Inhalation of dust, chemicals, and fumes should be avoided whenever possible.
3. Smoking should be stopped.
4. Any respiratory infections should be treated as soon as they appear, in order to prevent a chronic condition from developing.

Do the endocrine glands secrete less hormones and degenerate as one ages?

Yes. Many scientists feel that the degenerative process has its origin in changes that take place in these glands. The pituitary gland, the adrenal glands, the thyroid gland, the ovaries, and the testicles all show degenerative changes in the later years, and the age at which those changes occur probably influences the onset of the entire aging process.

Do the kidneys undergo degenerative changes as one advances in age?

Yes. This is very important, since the maintenance of kidney function is essential to life. Arteriosclerosis of the arteries supplying the kidneys is common in older people.

Does the brain degenerate as one ages?

Yes, but changes within the brain usually take place at a slow pace. Many live well into their eighties and nineties without showing appreciable brain degeneration. Peculiarly, there is often relatively little correlation between the physical evidences of brain degeneration and the maintenance of mental capacities.

Which is more important in determining the rate of degeneration—heredity or environment?

It is not possible to say which is more important. Both the constitution one is born with and the kind of life one leads are of extreme importance.

Does overwork accelerate degenerative changes?

Yes. Excesses of any kind, when continued for many years, will accelerate degenerative changes. However, in a person trained and adjusted to hard physical labor, in all probability it will not cause degenerative changes to speed up.

Do overeating and obesity lead to earlier degenerative changes?

Yes.

What effect does physical inactivity have on degenerative changes?

It is now thought that physical inactivity is almost as bad as physical overactivity. Moderation in all things seems to be the best approach toward slowing degenerative changes.

Is it true that most forms of animal life have a rather fixed life-span and that little can be done to alter it?

This is essentially true, but few humans live out their full life-span. It is the aim of the medical profession to get more people to live out their entire natural life. This "entire natural life" may approach one hundred years if we can control all of those factors that shorten life.

Are there ways to discover early signs of degenerative changes in a healthy person?

Yes. For instance, an electrocardiogram may demonstrate early evidences of heart-muscle changes even though the patient feels perfectly well. X rays of the intestinal tract may uncover degenerative changes in someone who is free of gastrointestinal difficulties. Blood-chemistry analyses may give evidence of degenerative changes in the liver and kidneys long before the patient shows outward signs of impairment of function.

Is it possible that degenerative processes may be caused by a virus that has not yet been discovered?

This possibility is highly unlikely, and research tends not to support such a theory.

Is there a progressive decrease in the body's ability to replace old cells by new ones?

Yes, but this may not influence general health materially, since the *need* for cell replacement decreases with age.

Is there a decrease in the ability of the skeleton to replace worn-out bone cells as one ages?

Yes. This leads to increased brittleness and possibility of fracture.

Is there a decrease in the ability of the bone marrow to manufacture blood cells and to replace worn-out elements as one ages?

Yes. This is responsible for the high incidence of blood disease and anemia among older people.

Is there any way to stop the degenerative changes that take place in the ovaries?

No. Taking female sex hormones will not delay such changes appreciably. This form of treatment merely replaces temporarily the hormones secreted by the ovaries. As soon as the hormone treatment is stopped, the menopause will begin and the natural degenerative changes will soon follow.

Is there any way to stop the degenerative processes in the testicles?

Taking male sex hormones does not delay appreciably the degenerative changes that normally take place here. When hormone therapy is discontinued, the degenerative processes continue.

Will taking pituitary, thyroid, pancreatic, or adrenal extracts stop the degenerative changes that may take place in these glandular structures?

No. But, as stated above, hormones may substitute for the normal activity of these glands. As soon as the hormone treatment is discontinued, the degenerative processes will proceed.

DERMATITIS

See ALLERGY; HERPES ZOSTER; LEUKOPLAKIA; SKIN; SYPHILIS; VEINS AND VARICOSE VEINS.

Is there an increase in the incidence of dermatitis as one gets older?

Yes, because the skin tends to be more sensitive as one advances in age. Also, there is less resistance to irritations and infections.

What are some of the more common types of dermatitis in people past sixty?

1. Contact dermatitis, resulting from contact between the skin and an irritating agent. Some of the agents that may cause this kind of dermatitis are:
   a. Cosmetics.
   b. Soaps or detergents.
   c. Flowers and plants.
   d. Clothing fabrics, such as wool, cotton, nylon and plastics.
   e. Medications and lotions.
2. Allergic (atopic) dermatitis, from an allergen in foods to which one is sensitive.
3. Dermatitis from drugs or medications taken (dermatitis medicamentosa).
4. Dermatitis secondary to an upset emotional state (neurodermatitis).

What are some of the signs and symptoms of dermatitis?

1. A rash, either localized or spread over the entire body. A favorite site for a rash is the folds of the skin, where perspiration is greatest.
2. Itching, usually worse at night or when the skin is damp from sweat.
3. Discharge or oozing from the irritated skin areas.

4. Flaking of the skin.
5. Loss of superficial skin cells, with rawness.
6. Loss of sleep, loss of appetite, and irritability when the condition persists for any length of time.

Are there many different types of dermatitis?

Yes. There are dozens of various kinds of skin inflammations, each precipitated by a different causative agent. The skin specialist will concentrate on determining whether the dermatitis is of local origin, such as contact with an irritant, or is due to a general upset or disease.

Will the cause of the dermatitis dictate the type of treatment required?

Yes. Dermatitis of systemic origin must be treated generally, whereas that brought on by local irritants can often be cured by local treatment.

What is the treatment of dermatitis?

It varies tremendously according to the specific type. Lotions, baths, ointments, dusting powders, specific medications by mouth or injection may all play a part in the treatment of these conditions. It must be remembered that most cases of dermatitis, of whatever origin, have a tendency to persist for weeks or months.

Is it safe for older people to take cortisone or cortisonelike medications for long periods of time in an attempt to cure a chronic dermatitis?

There are many dangerous side effects from these drugs, and anyone taking them must be under the constant surveillance of a dermatologist.

Can chronic dermatitis be cured?

Most cases can be, although a cure may require several weeks or even months.

DIABETES MELLITUS

See CIRCULATION; CLAUDICATION; COMA; DIET; FEET; INFECTIONS; PANCREAS; TESTS; VITAMINS.

What causes diabetes?

It is thought to be caused by an upset in carbohydrate metabolism owing to lack of insulin production by the insulin-producing cells of the pancreas (islets of Langerhans).

How prevalent is diabetes?

It is thought that almost 1 percent of the population has diabetes.

Is there a tendency for people past sixty to develop diabetes?

Yes. The disease develops characteristically in the middle and later years of life, especially from sixty-five to seventy-five.

Is diabetes that begins in later life usually milder than a case beginning in childhood or young adulthood?

Yes. Many of the symptoms seen in younger people, such as inordinate thirst, extreme hunger, frequency of urination, etc., are often absent. Moreover, diabetes seen in the later years is more readily kept under control.

What are the usual symptoms of diabetes in older people?

Many people develop diabetes in their later years without knowing it. If symptoms do occur, they take the form of itching skin, excessive thirst, increased appetite and desire for sweets, excessive urination, loss of weight, and anemia.

What are the complications of diabetes in older people?

Approximately one-half of those over sixty who have diabetes will show evidence of heart disease and arteriosclerosis, especially of the blood vessels in the legs. One-half will have high blood pressure. One out of four will develop some degree of impairment of eyesight due to inflammation of the retina. Kidney disease, secondary to arteriosclerosis of the smaller arteries in the kidney, is also a common complication of diabetes.

How can one tell if he has diabetes?

By examination of the urine. If sugar is found in the urine, a blood-sugar analysis should be made. A blood sugar in excess of 120 mg. per 100 cc. of blood usually indicates the presence of diabetes. If there is still doubt, a glucose-tolerance test is made.

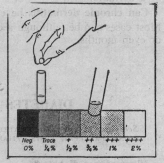

Self-testing for sugar by dropping specially prepared pill into test tube containing small quantity of urine

Does sugar in the urine always indicate the presence of diabetes?

In most cases, it does. However, in certain instances a test for sugar will be positive even though the person is not diabetic. This is particularly true for those persons who take salicylate drugs for arthritis or chloral hydrate for sedation. Taking these medicines in large quantities will cause a positive reaction the same as when there is sugar in the urine.

It is therefore essential to test for the amount of sugar in the blood whenever a urine test is positive.

Do people with diabetes have a tendency to develop more hardening of the arteries than nondiabetics?

Yes, but this tendency can be lessened by continuous control of the diabetes.

What complications of hardening of the arteries are sometimes seen in severe diabetes?

1. Angina pectoris and coronary thrombosis.
2. High blood pressure (hypertension).
3. Impaired vision.
4. Impaired kidney function and, possibly, uremia.
5. Cerebral hemorrhage (stroke).
6. Claudication, with walking accompanied by severe pain in the legs.
7. Gangrene of a limb owing to clotting in arteriosclerotic arteries in the legs.

What advice should be given to diabetics about special care of their feet?

1. Feet must be kept meticulously clean by washing daily with warm water and a bland soap.
2. Socks should be changed daily.
3. The feet, especially between the toes, should be dried thoroughly after washing.
4. Toenails should be cut straight across, leaving an ample amount of nail at the corners, where infections are most likely to take place.
5. If there is an infection, prompt medical treatment is indicated.
6. Calluses and corns should be treated by a podiatrist.
7. Care should be taken to avoid injuries, since feet with impaired circulation heal very slowly.
8. Well-fitting shoes are essential to avoid blisters and pinching.

Is diabetes in people in their seventies and eighties associated with gangrene of the leg, and does it ever require amputation?

Yes. Actually, it is not the diabetes alone that causes this sequence of events. It is diabetes plus arteriosclerosis. Many older people with diabetes do develop this type of infection and do eventually have to have a limb amputated.

Are elderly diabetics especially susceptible to neuritis and other diseases of the nerves?

Yes. Neuritis, as evidenced by tingling, numbness, burning, and shooting pains in the arms and legs, especially at night, is very common in diabetics. These symptoms increase during cold weather.

What can be done about the neuritis associated with diabetes?

Treatment does not always bring relief from symptoms. Large doses of vitamins, particularly vitamin B_{12}, and careful regulation of the diabetes are perhaps the best approach.

Does diabetes that has existed for many years often clear up as one grows older?

No. It might become milder as one ages, but it seldom disappears by itself.

What diet should older diabetics follow?

The precise diet should be prescribed by the physician. It should be emphasized that the diabetic patient requires a well-rounded diet, containing measured amounts of protein, carbohydrates, fats, and vitamins. The exact amount of each dietary constituent will be determined by the physician after frequent examinations of the patient, especially of his blood and urine. From time to time, the quantities of each constituent are varied.

Should a diabetic make regular visits to his physician?

Yes, by all means. Only in this way will the doctor be able to follow the course of the diabetes and treat it as required.

Does diabetes tend to run in families?

Yes, predisposition to diabetes is thought to be inherited.

How often should the diabetic examine his urine?

Daily. He should take the first specimen in the morning, *before* breakfast.

Are there satisfactory ways for the older diabetic to examine his own urine?

Yes. Simplified methods (such as the Clinitest) make it easy even for those in their seventies or eighties to test their own urine.

Must the older diabetic patient always maintain a sugar-free urine?

No. Consultation with one's physician about this is important.

As a general rule, it can be stated that there is no danger in the average diabetic's having a small amount of sugar in the urine, provided there is no accompanying acidosis.

What is acetone?

Acetone is a chemical found in the urine of persons whose diabetes is not properly controlled. It is a sign of acidosis.

What is acidosis, or ketosis?

This is a condition that results when diabetes is not properly controlled. Certain chemical products of metabolism known as ketone bodies are present in the blood in excessive quantities, causing the blood to become too acid. Severe acidosis (ketosis), unless corrected, may lead to diabetic coma.

Is diabetic coma encountered frequently in patients over sixty?

It is seldom seen unless the diabetes has gone untreated.

What is glycosuria?

The presence of sugar in the urine. Normally, the urine contains no sugar.

What is hyperglycemia?

An excessive amount of sugar in the blood.

What is hypoglycemia?

Less than a normal amount of sugar in the blood, a condition encountered when an overdose of insulin has been taken.

Do all diabetics have to take insulin?

No. Dietary control is often sufficient, especially for the older patient with mild diabetes. But only a doctor should decide this.

Can patients over sixty take the newer antidiabetic medications, which are administered by mouth?

Yes, the "oral hypoglycemic" drugs are effective in a large percentage of cases.

Are the oral antidiabetic drugs just as effective for older patients as for the younger diabetics?

Yes. As a matter of fact, they may be even more effective.

Can most older diabetics learn to give themselves insulin injections?

Yes. However, when there is impairment of eyesight or some accompanying physical handicap, it may be necessary for a nurse, attendant, or some member of the family to prepare the insulin dose for them. If such older diabetics live alone, the insulin dosage for several days should be prepared in advance (by buying several syringes and needles and filling them with the proper amount of insulin) and stored in a refrigerator.

Modern methods of taking insulin often make it possible to limit injections to one a day.

By and large, is it a wise policy for the older diabetic to use as little insulin as possible?

Yes, but only on advice of the physician. It is no longer thought essential that the dia-

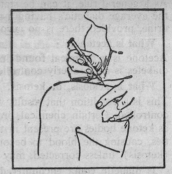

Self-administration of insulin into thigh

betic's urine be completely free of sugar at all times, nor that he always maintain a normal blood-sugar level. Excessive doses of insulin may do more harm than allowing a diabetic to have a little sugar in the urine.

What harm can an overdose of insulin do?

It will cause hypoglycemia (too little sugar in the blood). Hypoglycemia will deprive such organs as the heart and brain of sugar, which they must have for normal functioning. Also, hypoglycemia may set off spasm of the coronary arteries.

What is insulin shock?

This is a reaction to an overdose of insulin.

Is insulin shock very common in older diabetics?

No, because someone who has been taking insulin for a long time knows what to do when he feels symptoms of shock approaching.

How does the diabetic know that insulin shock is approaching?

He gets a jittery feeling, sees spots before his eyes, has tingling in and tremor of his hands, and feels tight in the throat and abdomen. Diabetics know these warning signs and will immediately take sugar, candy, orange juice, etc., to prevent the shock.

What happens if the overdose of insulin is untreated?

A full-blown episode of insulin shock may follow, which includes loss of consciousness and convulsions.

Do older people usually recover spontaneously from insulin shock?

Yes. Unless a very large overdose has been taken, the patient will recover within a few minutes to a few hours.

Is insulin shock to be avoided by older diabetics particularly?

Yes, because it may cause permanent brain damage or coronary thrombosis.

What treatment should be given when a patient is discovered unconscious from insulin shock?

An intravenous injection of glucose (sugar) should be given. This will usually remedy the shock within a few minutes to an hour.

How is it determined when to give a patient medication for his diabetes?

The patient's blood is examined on several occasions for the quantity of sugar present; a blood test known as the "glucose-tolerance" test is performed; and the urine is tested frequently for sugar and acetone. After evaluating all of these findings, the doctor may prescribe a trial diet without insulin or antidiabetic drugs. If the trial diet does not regulate the diabetes, then either insulin or oral antidiabetic drugs are given.

Is there a tendency for the older diabetic to develop vitamin deficiency?

Yes. For this reason, supplemental vitamins are often prescribed.

Is anemia seen often in older diabetic patients?

Yes, if the diabetes is not well controlled. Even in cases in which it is well regulated, there is a tendency for diabetics to become anemic.

What effect does obesity have on diabetes?

Obesity aggravates diabetes and makes it more difficult to regulate.

Does diabetes always affect eyesight in older people?

No. Although hardening of the arteries and inflammation of the retina are seen in a certain number of cases, the majority of well-controlled diabetics do not suffer from marked impairment of vision.

Is the incidence of cataracts greater in diabetics?

Yes, but mainly in those who have a severe form of the disease or who have not had it well regulated throughout life.

What is the effect of diabetes on the incidence of infections?

Diabetics appear to be more susceptible than nondiabetics to the development of infections. It is therefore essential that they protect themselves insofar as possible against infection at all times.

Does the diabetic have greater difficulty overcoming infections once they have developed?

Yes.

What special precautions should be taken when the diabetic patient develops an infection?

1. Medical advice should be sought immediately, even for a simple boil or abscess.
2. The patient should be instructed never to squeeze, open, or try to treat an infection himself.
3. Large doses of antibiotics should be prescribed.

Does diabetes that has been present for many years make the patient more susceptible to the development of coronary thrombosis?

Yes, since the diabetic has more of a tendency to develop arteriosclerosis. However, it should be emphasized that with good management, the diabetic can lessen this tendency considerably.

Does the diabetic have a greater tendency to develop gallbladder disease?

Yes.

What effect does emotional stress have on the diabetic?

Excessive emotional stress will tend to aggravate the existing diabetes, or it may possibly activate a case of latent diabetes.

Can diabetics who are past sixty safely undergo surgery?

Yes. With modern techniques and added knowledge of how to control diabetes, there is very little extra hazard. The predilection to infection can be overcome by giving antibiotic drugs, and blood sugar can be regulated by administration of insulin.

Can a well-controlled diabetic look forward to living as long as the nondiabetic?

It is estimated today that a well-controlled diabetic has almost the same life-span as that of the nondiabetic. This may be due to the fact that the diabetic seeks medical advice much more often than the average nondiabetic. Therefore, coexisting diseases are discovered in their earlier stages, when they can be more readily corrected.

Should the well-controlled diabetic be told to live a normal life and to engage in all of his usual physical activities?

Yes. If a diabetic is well controlled, he should not treat himself as an invalid.

What are the main aims of treatment in the older diabetic?

1. To see that he maintains a normal nutritive diet.
2. To maintain a normal intake of vitamins and minerals.
3. If he is underweight, attempts should be made to bring him up to normal.
4. If he is overweight, he should reduce.
5. If there is anemia, medications to remedy the anemia should be taken.
6. To maintain a blood-sugar level below 180 mg. per 100 cc. (normal blood-sugar levels are 80 to 120 mg.).
7. To use the oral antidiabetic drugs if these will suffice to maintain a satisfactory blood-sugar level.
8. To prescribe insulin if it is necessary to control the blood-sugar level.
9. To keep the urine free of acetone so as to prevent acidosis.
10. Perhaps most important is to take all possible measures to avoid the complications of diabetes.

DIAGNOSIS OF DISEASE

See TESTS; TREATMENT; X RAY.

Is it more difficult to diagnose disease in older people?

No. The physician uses the same diagnostic methods.

Is it important for a physician treating an older person to have a thorough familial history of disease?

Yes. Certain diseases have a tendency to run in families, and this information may help to establish a diagnosis in a difficult case.

Is there a tendency for some older people to be excessively modest and to resist physical examination?

Yes. Extreme modesty, a remnant of older notions of decorum, is evident in many people in their seventies and eighties. The physician should overcome this shyness before examining the patient.

Does the physician usually proceed at the same rate in making diagnostic tests on elderly patients as on younger people?

No. It is wiser to give an older patient more rest between tests. X rays, examinations of various body cavities, the taking of blood, and other tests are more wearing on the older patient.

Are many diagnostic tests designed particularly for older patients?

No. By and large, the same diagnostic methods are used for all adults.

Is there a tendency for older patients to conceal their symptoms?

Unfortunately, yes. Many people in their seventies and eighties erroneously decide that a particular illness will be their last illness, that nothing much can be done to help them. This thought motivates them to conceal symptoms and to avoid medical care. Doctors are aware of this tendency and will therefore question older patients more carefully than they would younger ones.

Do older patients often exaggerate their symptoms?

This tendency does exist in some older people, especially in those who crave attention. Also, there is an increasing fear of the seriousness of disease as one gets older, and this may lead to exaggeration of symptoms.

Is it important for the physician to have a thorough history of the past illnesses of an elderly patient?

Yes, because the diagnosis of an obscure present condition may depend on uncovering the history of a condition that existed forty or fifty years before. Older people's memory for childhood diseases or diseases that occurred in their youth is often faulty. When such a history is unreliable, the children or other relatives of the patient should be questioned.

Do symptoms and signs of disease differ greatly when they are present in patients of advanced age?

No. Pain, tenderness, burning, nausea, numbness, etc., in people of all ages, are interpreted in much the same way.

Should vaginal and rectal examinations be done routinely on older people?

Yes. In older people, the genital tract in females and the rectum in both sexes are likely sites of malignant disease.

Should a chest X ray be included in a routine physical examination of an older person?

Yes, because pulmonary conditions, such as tuberculosis, bronchitis, emphysema, bronchiectasis, and lung cancer, do occur in the older age groups.

Is it harmful to take a large number of X rays of people past sixty?

No. Actually, it is much safer for them than for younger people since they need not fear overexposure or sterilization.

Should an electrocardiogram be taken routinely on older people?

Yes. A thorough physical examination should include an electrocardiogram.

Should a urine examination, blood count, and blood-chemistry analysis be done as part of a thorough physical examination?

Yes. These tests will reveal the state of health of the kidneys, liver, pancreas, and other organs and will show the presence of anemia, diabetes, and other conditions.

Should cancer-detection tests be made on people past sixty?

A thorough physical examination will include a search for evidences of cancer. To undergo a cancer-detection test without an accompanying thorough physical examination is not a wise procedure. Information about the presence or absence of cancer does not include information about other serious disorders that may be present.

Are special tests necessary to determine whether or not elderly patients are satisfactory surgical risks?

Yes. For example, it is especially important to learn about cardiac and respiratory reserve and the state of liver and kidney function.

Why is it so important to learn about the state of the patient's blood chemistry before he undergoes surgery?

Today, operative techniques are so well developed that the average person, no matter what his age, can withstand actual surgery. Postoperative mortalities in older people are not necessarily due to a failure of the operative technique, but rather to a failure of function in organs such as the adrenal glands, the liver, or the kidneys. Extensive surgery can greatly affect the function of these organs, and it is therefore important to make sure, through chemical analysis of the blood, that they are in good working order *before* surgery is undertaken.

DIARRHEA

See BED CARE; BOWEL FUNCTION; CONSTIPATION; INTESTINES; LAXATIVES; RECTUM AND ANUS.

What are the most common causes of diarrhea in older people?

1. Colitis or dysentery (inflammation of the mucous membrane lining the large intestine).
2. An allergy, or sensitivity, to certain foods.
3. Taking drugs that irritate the lower intestinal tract.
4. Taking strong laxatives.
5. Emotional upsets of an acute nature.

What dietary rules should be followed by those who have episodes of frequent diarrhea?

1. Avoid excessive use of spices and highly seasoned foods.
2. Do not drink alcoholic beverages.
3. Eat fresh fruits and fresh vegetables sparingly, and only after the skins have been removed; avoid other kinds of roughage, such as bran.
4. Avoid fatty, fried foods.
5. Have the attending physician check the medications that are being taken to make sure that they are not causing bowel irritability.
6. Make a daily list of the foods that are being eaten. It may be that there is a sensitivity to one specific food. It should be removed from the diet.

What medications tend to cause diarrhea?

1. Medications containing iron or such other metals as mercury and arsenic.
2. Some of the mycin group of antibiotic drugs.
3. Laxatives, of course.
4. Overdoses of almost any medication.

What is the treatment of diarrhea?

1. If it is due to colitis, an intensive investigation must be made to discover the cause. Colitis may be of bacterial origin; it may be secondary to upset in metabolism; it may be of emotional origin. Many cases are extremely resistant to cure.
2. If it is secondary to a parasite or a specific germ, it can be cured in most instances by giving the drug that will kill the specific invading organism.
3. Diarrhea secondary to food sensitivity can be controlled by eliminating the particular food from the diet. An allergist is often needed to discover the irritating food.

4. Diarrhea caused by drug sensitivity will usually subside spontaneously soon after the medication is stopped.
5. Diarrhea of emotional origin may require psychotherapy by a trained psychiatrist.

Are all physicians equipped to treat chronic diarrhea?

No. It is wisest to refer an older patient who has been suffering for several weeks with diarrhea to a specialist in diarrheal diseases. He will know many things about such conditions that the family doctor will not know.

What medications will help to stop the ordinary acute type of diarrhea?

1. Paregoric or other opium derivative drugs. (These medications should be taken only on a doctor's prescription.)
2. Kaopectate or other chalky, inert medications.
3. Antibiotic drugs to combat specific intestinal infections. (These drugs should be taken only on a doctor's prescription, as some of them may aggravate rather than stop the diarrhea.)
4. Specific medications such as Entero-Vioform and Carbarsone, to rid the intestinal tract of parasites. (These drugs tend to be toxic and should be taken only on a doctor's advice.)
5. Antispasmodic and sedative drugs. These are especially helpful in cases in which the diarrhea is of emotional origin.

DIET

See ANEMIA; CHOLESTEROL; DIABETES MELLITUS; GASTRITIS; HEPATITIS; JAUNDICE; LIVER; STOMACH AND DUODENUM; TEETH; ULCERS OF STOMACH AND DUODENUM; VITAMINS; WEIGHT.

What dietary advice should be given to people past sixty?

In general, healthy older people require no advice different from that given younger people. However, certain dietary rules should receive more emphasis as people grow older. Some of these are:

1. Stay thin or get thin.
2. If there is doubt about whether or not the diet contains sufficient vitamins, multiple-vitamin capsules should be taken daily.

3. If there is a tendency toward anemia, medications containing iron and other substances to elevate the hemoglobin content of the blood should be taken.
4. Large meals should be avoided. It is much better to eat smaller quantities more frequently.
5. Rich, greasy, and highly seasoned foods should be omitted from the diet.
6. Few sweets and fats (whether animal or vegetable) should be eaten.
7. Drinking of alcoholic beverages should be moderate.
8. Heavy meals are to be avoided especially before retiring.
9. Raw fruits and raw vegetables should be peeled and washed thoroughly before eating.
10. Healthy older people should maintain a fluid intake of six to eight glasses of liquid daily.
11. Excessive salt should be avoided, unless the weather is very humid and hot.

Is there a difference between older and younger people in the amount of food absorbed from their intestinal tracts?

No. The aging process seldom interferes with the absorption of the necessary quantities of food from a normal intestinal tract.

Is it necessary for all people over sixty to limit their salt intake?

Not if they are in good health and show no evidence of high blood pressure, heart disease, or other conditions that would be adversely affected by salt. On the other hand, it is necessary to take extra salt if the climate is hot and humid and perspiration has been profuse.

Are there fewer calorie requirements as one advances in age?

Usually. Older people are less active physically and therefore require fewer calories.

Do most people have smaller appetites as they get older?

Yes. With the decrease in caloric need, there is a decrease in desire for food.

Should older people take medicines to curb excessive appetite?

See DRUGS AND MEDICINES.

Are "crash" reducing diets dangerous for older people?

Yes, they can be. Sudden changes in caloric intake are not tolerated too well by people in their seventies and eighties. When people go on starvation diets, they deprive their systems of needed carbohydrates, which are needed to nourish the heart muscle, brain cells, and other vital organs. The organs of younger people can endure this deprivation, whereas great harm may come to older people who attempt it.

Is it true that as one advances in age certain foods that have never caused upset may become poorly tolerated?

Yes. Young people are much better able to tolerate rich, fatty, fried, and highly seasoned foods.

Is the stomach less able to handle large meals as one ages?

Yes. Overdistention of the stomach causes much greater discomfort as one gets older and may, in some people, precipitate angina pectoris (heart pain).

What foods are most difficult for older people to digest?

1. Fried foods.
2. Foods containing large quantities of fat.
3. Gravies and heavy sauces.
4. Foods containing large quantities of carbohydrates.
5. Highly seasoned food.
6. Some raw fruits and some raw vegetables.

Can permanent harm result from eating highly seasoned and spiced foods?

No, except that it can produce an acute stomach or intestinal upset.

Will eating foods rich in fatty substances tend to elevate the blood cholesterol?

Yes, in some people. (*See also* CHOLESTEROL.)

Should people in their later years cut down on those foods containing large quantities of cholesterol?

Yes. Although the relationship has not been proved conclusively, there is a great deal of evidence to indicate that a high cholesterol intake leads to a high blood-cholesterol level. The latter may be conducive to earlier and more extensive arteriosclerotic changes.

What foods are particularly rich in cholesterol?

All foods with a high fat content; e.g., meat, fish, fowl, game, butter, cream, cheese, and egg yolks.

Will eating foods low in cholesterol tend to decrease the arteriosclerosis present in elderly people?

In all probability, this will *not* help very much because the hardening of the arteries has already taken place. The time to start a low-cholesterol diet is in youth and the early middle years.

Are animal and vegetable fats equally responsible for elevating the cholesterol level?

No. The vegetable fats, such as those found in corn oil, do not cause elevation of the blood-cholesterol level.

Are the chances of getting coronary thrombosis increased by eating diets rich in cholesterol throughout one's younger years?

Cholesterol is thought to be a factor in this disease, but there is no conclusive proof.

Will the eating of large quantities of fat cause disturbance in gallbladder function?

If there is existing disease in the gallbladder or bile system, fatty foods may precipitate an acute attack. It has not been proved that gallbladder disease can be caused merely by ingesting large quantities of fatty or fried foods.

Can healthy people past sixty continue to drink alcoholic beverages?

See ALCOHOL AND ALCOHOLISM.

Can people past sixty drink carbonated beverages?

Yes, if there are no harmful results.

What is the best time of day for people in their seventies or eighties to eat their main meal?

Midday.

Is it essential that three meals be eaten each day?

No. Many older people do much better with two meals a day with smaller feedings in between. A good breakfast should be eaten, as this will aid bowel evacuation. Also, it will supply sufficient calories for the most active hours of the day.

Is it good practice for older people to eat just before going to bed at night?

No.

Are stimulants, such as coffee and tea, safe to take?

Yes, in moderation. As we know, when coffee is taken during the evening it may interfere with sleep. There are, in addition, certain medical conditions that make the use of coffee and tea inadvisable. Large quantities of either tea or coffee can be injurious because of the high caffeine content.

Should specific times be set aside for meals each day?

Yes. Older people respond best to regular habits and routines.

Is it important for older people to be particular about chewing their food thoroughly?

Yes, because digestive processes may be somewhat slower, and well-chewed food aids digestion.

What foods tend to be constipating?

Those foods that contain little roughage or residue, such as carbohydrates and starches.

What types of foods aid bowel evacuation?

Foods containing large amounts of roughage, such as fresh fruits and vegetables, bran products, and cereals.

Do healthy people in their seventies and eighties continue to secrete sufficient saliva and gastric and intestinal juices?

Yes, although the quantities of these food-digesting secretions may be somewhat diminished.

What happens if there is an insufficient secretion of saliva?

When food has to be swallowed in too dry a state, there may be difficulty in swallowing, with possible choking and regurgitation.

What takes place if an excess of saliva is secreted?

This is a most uncomfortable abnormality affecting some older people. It necessitates constant swallowing in order to prevent drooling from the sides of the mouth and often is associated with nausea.

Can medications be given to control excessive secretion of saliva?

Yes. Medications in the belladonna group will tend to decrease the amount of secretion. However, such medications should be given only by a doctor, since there may be bad side effects from this group of drugs.

Do the stomachs of some older people tend to secrete too little gastric juice (stomach juice) and too little acid?

Yes, particularly in people in their seventies or eighties. This is one reason for advising older people to eat less at one time.

Do older people show a tendency to gag, choke, and have difficulty in swallowing their food?

Yes. For this reason, older people should be advised to avoid large bites and to chew thoroughly before attempting to swallow. They should also be cautioned not to talk while chewing.

Is there a tendency for older people to regurgitate food that they have already swallowed?

Occasionally. Spasm of the lower end of the food pipe (a condition called achalasia) is responsible for this symptom.

Does a defect in the swallowing mechanism itself ever develop with advanced age?

Occasionally, particularly in those who are in their late seventies or eighties. It must be remembered that the swallowing mechanism is a complicated one demanding great timing and muscle control. The ability to retain this coordination is decreased with age.

Is it a good practice for older people to count their daily caloric intake?

This is usually not necessary unless there is obesity or under-nourishment. Healthy people do a great deal of unnecessary calorie counting. By the time most people reach their sixties, they know how much to eat without having to calculate the number of calories in their food. However, if the individual is an invalid or is markedly debilitated, a physician should pre-scribe a diet, including an adequate number of calories. And, of course, if the person is diabetic, calorie counting may be necessary.

Should diets be changed according to the season of the year?

Yes, but this usually happens naturally, because of the avail-ability of different foods. It is a good idea, though, to eat lightly in hot weather and to eat more nourishing foods dur-ing colder weather.

What are some of the more easily digested foods?

1. Well-cooked foods.
2. Foods that do not demand a great deal of chewing.
3. Boiled or baked foods.
4. Foods that are low in fat content.

Should people past sixty who are in good health take vitamins?

See VITAMINS.

Is vitamin D deficiency sometimes associated with osteo-malacia?

Yes. This is one important reason why elderly people should have an adequate intake of vitamin D.
(*See also* BONES AND JOINTS.)

Should minerals be added to the diet of people past sixty?

Not if they are in good health and eat a well-rounded diet. If, on the other hand, they are debilitated or anemic, minerals should be added. Many of the vitamin capsules on the market also contain the essential minerals, such as iron, magnesium, calcium, and phosphorus.

What can be done to stimulate the appetite of an under-nourished older person?

1. His favorite foods should be included in the diet fre-quently.

2. It should be ascertained how the patient likes his food prepared, and every effort should be made to conform to this desire.

3. A pleasant atmosphere should be created at mealtime:
   a. The dining area should be clean and quiet, and the table should be set prettily—if possible, with flowers.
   b. Soft, pleasant music often encourages appetite.
   c. The patient should be exposed to the aroma of good smelling foods while they are being cooked.
   d If possible, the foods should be seen while they are being prepared.
   e. Appetite can sometimes be stimulated by looking at pictures of exciting and interesting foods in magazines.

4. Small amounts of alcohol or appetite-stimulating medications can be given a half hour or so before mealtime.

Are psychological factors important in stimulating the appetite?

Yes, they are of the utmost importance. Many elderly, debilitated people act just like children. They must, therefore, be excited, stimulated, and persuaded to eat, even when it means playing games with them, as one might with a small child. Attempts to force food usually are met by rebellion.

What is the significance of sudden loss of appetite if it persists?

It may or may not indicate the presence of disease, but it is important enough to warrant an X-ray investigation of the intestinal tract.

Is repeated indigestion an indication that a physician's advice should be sought?

Yes. Unfortunately, some of the most serious gastrointestinal diseases cause no symptoms until they are in their late stages. For example, cancer of the stomach may be present for several months without causing any indigestion whatever. It is therefore important that indigestion be investigated when it recurs often. However, one should not conclude that he has a serious disease merely because he has repeated indigestion. It may be completely functional and may disappear as soon as dietary habits are better regulated.

Is it harmful for people to drink large quantities of water or other fluids while eating?

No. For generations people have thought that it is unwise to drink fluids while eating. This is not true. On the contrary, digestion is aided by liquid intake.

Is it harmful for people to combine certain foods in one meal, such as frankfurters and ice cream, seafood and alcohol, etc.?

This is a superstition of the past. Although for various reasons people do not usually combine certain foods, there are no medical grounds for such prohibitions. It is *not* true that certain foods, when eaten together, will combine to form a poison.

Is it essential that older, undernourished people have their teeth and dentures checked carefully?

Yes. One of the most frequent causes for poor appetite is difficulty in chewing.

Is adequate calcium in the diet important for older people?

Yes, it is very important. Osteomalacia and osteoporosis are among the most common conditions found in people in their later decades. These are disorders in which there is a calcium deficiency in and a weakened condition of the bones. Although taking large quantities of calcium in the diet will not necessarily cure these conditions, it is nevertheless essential that the intake of that mineral be adequate.

Are foods rich in phosphorus important for people in their later years?

Yes, for the same reason given in the answer above. However, most diets contain a sufficient quantity of this mineral.

Should older people with high blood pressure avoid eating red meat?

No. It was formerly thought that red meat was conducive to the development of high blood pressure and also that it would cause kidney damage. We now know that this is false.

How can one make sure that the diet contains a sufficient amount of protein?

Older people should eat at least one liberal portion of meat daily. (*See* the diet lists below for diets rich in protein.)

Is it safe for older people to fast during their religious holidays and throughout religious periods?

Yes, if they are in good health otherwise. People in their late seventies or eighties who are debilitated or who are chronically ill had best forgo fast periods. (Most religions make allowances for those who are ill.)

1. NORMAL DIET FOR PEOPLE OVER 60

(A total of approximately eight glasses of liquids should be consumed during each twenty-four hours.)

Breakfast	Lunch	Dinner
1 piece of any fruit, or several prunes or figs, or fruit juice.	1 meat or egg sandwich, or any meat, fish, vegetable or fruit salad, or 1 portion of meat.	1 portion of meat, fowl or fish.
½ cup of any cereal with sugar and milk, or 2 eggs, any style.	1 or 2 vegetables.	1 or 2 vegetables. Green salad.
1 slice of bread or toast with ½ pat of butter.	1 slice of bread.	1 or 2 slices of bread.
Tea, coffee or milk (sugar and milk may be taken with tea or coffee).	1 piece of fruit or canned fruit, stewed fruit, etc.	Dessert: Fruit, cake, pie, ice cream, etc.
	1 glass of milk, tea, or coffee.	Tea, coffee or milk.

2. ELIMINATION DIET (for allergic persons)*

Foods	Include	Avoid
Breads	Quick bread, yeast bread, crackers—if made without eggs.	Bread or rolls containing eggs or nuts.
Cereals	All, except ———→	Chocolate-flavored cereals.
Soups	All	None
Meat, fish, eggs or cheese	Any meat or fowl except fresh pork. Cottage cheese.	Fresh pork, fish, seafood, eggs, all cheeses except cottage cheese.
Vegetables	All, except ———→	Corn, tomatoes.
Potato or substitute	Potato, hominy, rice, macaroni.	Noodles containing eggs.
Fats	Butter, cream, French dressing without pepper, lard, margarine, oil.	Salad dressings containing eggs or pepper.
Fruits	All fruits, except ———→	Fresh strawberries, raspberries, huckleberries, blackberries, melon.
Desserts	Cakes, cookies, gelatin, puddings, ice cream—if prepared without eggs, chocolate, cocoa or nuts.	Baked custard, desserts containing eggs, chocolate, cocoa or nuts.
Sweets	Candy, jelly, sugar, honey, syrup.	Chocolate, nuts, candy containing eggs.
Beverages	Carbonated beverages, decaffeinated coffee, milk.	Cocoa, chocolate, coffee, tea.

*Courtesy of *The New Illustrated Medical Encyclopedia for Home Use*, Abradale Press, N.Y.

3. GOUT DIET*
(Low Purine)

Foods	Include	Avoid
Breads	All	None
Cereals	All	None
Soups	Milk soups made with vegetables.	Bouillon, broth, consommé.
Meat, fish, eggs or cheese	Fish, fowl, shellfish, meats (except those listed), eggs, cheese.	Kidney, liver, meat extracts, sweetbreads, roe, sardines, anchovies, gravy, broth, bouillon.
Potato or substitute	White potato, sweet potato, hominy, macaroni, rice.	Fried potato, potato chips.
Fats	Butter	None
Vegetables	All (except those listed)	Asparagus, beans, lentils, mushrooms, peas, spinach.
Desserts	Simple cakes, cookies, custard, gelatin, pudding, etc.	Mince pie.
Sweets	All	None
Beverages	Carbonated beverages, coffee, milk, tea.	None
Miscellaneous	Spices, cream sauces, nuts, salt, condiments.	Alcohol, gravy, yeast.

4. HIGH CALORIC
DIET FOR UNDERWEIGHT OR UNDERNOURISHED PEOPLE

Breakfast	Lunch	Dinner
Fruit juice with sugar or grapefruit with sugar.	1 (or 2) meat or egg sandwich, or 1 large portion of meat or fowl.	1 plate of cream soup.
1 cup of cereal with cream and sugar.	2 vegetables with butter.	1 large portion of meat, fish or fowl.
2 scrambled or fried eggs.	1 potato, or portion of spaghetti or noodles.	1 potato, or portion of spaghetti or noodles.
2-3 slices of bread or toast with butter and jam.	2-3 slices of bread and butter.	2 vegetables with butter.
		2-3 slices of bread and butter.

*Courtesy of *The New Illustrated Medical Encyclopedia for Home Use*, Abradale Press, N.Y.

4. HIGH CALORIC
DIET FOR UNDERWEIGHT OR UNDERNOURISHED PEOPLE
(Concluded)

Breakfast	Lunch	Dinner
Tea or coffee with cream and sugar.	Dessert: Fruit, cake, pie, ice cream, etc. Milk with cream.	Green salad with Russian or Roquefort dressing. Dessert: Same as for lunch.
	Midday Snack Malted milk, ice cream soda, eggnog, with cake or crackers.	**Bedtime Snack** Sandwich or delicatessen and milk, tea or coffee with cream and sugar.

5. LIQUID DIET

Broths, strained cream soups.
Tomato juice, carrot juice, fruit juice.
Raw eggs in beverages.
Custards, gelatins, junket, sherbet, ice cream.
Water, tea, milk, milk drinks, coffee, carbonated beverages.

6. LOW CALORIC
DIET FOR OVERWEIGHT PEOPLE

Breakfast	Lunch	Dinner
Orange juice or ½ grapefruit (no sugar)	Vegetable, meat, fish or fruit salad with juice of lemon and/or vinegar, or 1 portion of lean meat.	1 portion of boiled or broiled lean meat, fish or fowl.
1 boiled egg		2 vegetables such as: spinach, lettuce, tomato, celery, cucumber, cabbage, onion, peppers, asparagus, string beans, etc.
1 slice of toast	Dessert: 1 portion of fresh fruit or low-sugar canned fruit.	
1 cup of tea or coffee with saccharin and milk.	Tea, coffee, with saccharin and skimmed milk.	Dessert: Jello, fresh or stewed fruit. Tea, coffee or skimmed milk.

Avoid
Bread, rolls, crackers, butter, cream, cheese, beans, potato, noodles, spaghetti, cereals, sugar, nuts, cake, pie, pastry, ice cream, candy, gravies, sauces, fried foods, meat fats, etc.

7. LOW CARBOHYDRATE (SUGAR) DIET

Breakfast	Lunch	Dinner
1 portion of fruit, canned or stewed without sugar.	Meat, fish, seafood, vegetable or fresh fruit salad.	Clear soup.
2 soft or hard boiled eggs.	2 salt crackers.	1 portion of any meat, fish, seafood or fowl.
1 slice of bread or toast.	Gelatin sweetened with saccharin.	Any 2 of the following vegetables: asparagus, string beans, water cress, celery, cucumber, cabbage, tomato, lettuce, eggplant, beets, carrot, endive.
Coffee or tea with saccharin, or milk.	Tea, milk or coffee.	Unsweetened canned fruit, or fresh fruit or gelatin.
		Tea, milk or coffee with saccharin.

Avoid

More than 1 slice of bread, potato, noodles, spaghetti, macaroni, lima beans, baked beans, corn, rice, gravies, sugar, cake, pie, pastry, ice cream, carbonated beverages, sweetened canned fruits, nuts, cream sauces, beer.

8. LOW FAT, LOW CHOLESTEROL, HIGH PROTEIN DIET*

Foods	Include	Avoid
Meat and other protein foods	Lean meats (trim off fat): veal, beef, ham, chicken, turkey, lamb. Non-oily fish: haddock, cod, halibut, fresh water fish, flounder, blue fish, bass. White of egg only.	Fried meats, fat meats, fresh pork, egg yolk, fish canned in oil, mackerel, herring, salmon, shad, brains, tuna, liver,† sweetbreads,† shellfish,† bacon,† kidney.†
Fats	Margarine, corn oil, peanut oil, vegetable shortening used sparingly.	Butter, lard, suet and other animal fats.

*Courtesy of U.S. Vitamin and Pharmaceutical Corp.

†Note: The following foods are of high nutritive value, but are omitted from the diet because of their moderate cholesterol content. Any one (but not more than one) of these foods may be eaten once a day in amount not to exceed that suggested:

Liver — 3 ounces   Lobster — 3 ounces
Kidney — 3 ounces   Canadian bacon — 3 ounces
Sweetbreads — 3 ounces   Peanut butter — 1 tablespoon
          Whole milk — 1 glass (6 oz.)

8. LOW FAT, LOW CHOLESTEROL, HIGH PROTEIN DIET*
(Concluded)

Foods	Include	Avoid
Cereals	Any cereals (preferably whole grain), bread, wheat cakes made without eggs, macaroni, spaghetti, noodles made without eggs.	Noodles made with eggs, breads and hot breads made with eggs.
Dairy products	Skim milk, buttermilk, cheese made from skim milk (dry cottage cheese).	Whole milk, cream, most cheeses, ice cream.
Fruits	Any fruit or juice.	Avocado.
Vegetables	Potatoes, baked without butter, or mashed with water or skim milk, any vegetable prepared without oil or fat.	None.
Desserts and sweets	Gelatin desserts, ices and sherbets, tapioca and rice puddings made with fruit and juices. Plain cookies, angel food and other cakes made without egg yolks and butter. Jams, jellies, honey, candy made without butter or cream.	Rich desserts made with fat, cream, egg yolks. Rich candy made with butter. Ice cream, pastry, chocolate.
Beverages	Tea, coffee, cereal drinks, buttermilk, skim milk, soft drinks.	Whole milk, alcohol.
Soups, etc.	Clear broth, vegetable soup made without whole milk or fat.	Cream soups, gravies, cream sauce.
Miscellaneous	Salt, spices, vinegar, popcorn without butter, relishes, pickles, catsup, low fat yeast extracts	Olives, mayonnaise, oily dressing, fried foods, potato chips, brewer's yeast.

9. LOW ROUGHAGE, LOW RESIDUE DIET*

Foods	Include	Avoid
Breads	White, enriched or fine rye bread, crackers, toast.	Whole wheat, graham, dark rye bread.
Cereals	Refined cereals, corn, rice, wheat, dry cereals prepared from cooked oatmeal.	Whole grain cereals.
Soups	Bouillon, broth.	Cream soups, vegetable soup.

*Courtesy of *The New Illustrated Medical Encyclopedia for Home Use*, Abradale Press, N.Y.

9. LOW ROUGHAGE, LOW RESIDUE DIET* (Concluded)

Foods	Include	Avoid
Meat, fish, eggs or cheese	Bacon, tender meat, fish, fowl, canned fish, eggs, cheese.	Tough meat.
Vegetables	None.	All.
Potato or substitute	Potato, macaroni, noodles, refined rice.	Hominy, unrefined rice.
Fats	Butter, cream, margarine.	None.
Fruits	None.	All.
Desserts	Plain cakes, cookies, custard, gelatin, ice cream, pie, pudding, all without fruits or nuts.	Desserts containing fruits or nuts.
Sweets	Hard candy, jelly, syrup, honey.	Candy containing fruits, jams or nuts.
Miscellaneous	Cream sauce, gravy, peanut butter, vinegar.	Nuts, olives, pickles, popcorn, relish.

10. LOW SALT (Low Sodium) DIET*

Foods	Include	Avoid
Meat and meat substitutes	Lamb, beef, pork, veal, rabbit, liver, chicken, turkey, duck, goose, fresh cod, halibut, fresh salmon, fresh water fish, one egg daily.	Salted, canned, smoked meats, frankfurters, bacon, ham, sausage, liverwurst and other spiced meats, brain, kidney, tongue, salt or canned fish, haddock, shellfish (oysters, clams, lobster, shrimp), salt pork.
Vegetables	Fresh, frozen or specially canned without salt: asparagus, string beans, broccoli, Brussels sprouts, cabbage, cauliflower, corn, cucumber, eggplant, endive, lettuce, mushrooms, okra, onions, parsnips, peas, peppers, potato, rutabaga, soy beans, squash, sweet potato, tomato, lima beans.	All canned vegetables and relishes, beets, beet greens, chard, kale, celery, spinach, sauerkraut, rhubarb, potato chips, pickles.
Fruits	Any raw, cooked, canned fruit or juice, apricots, avocado, banana, blackberries, blueberries, cranberries, dates, grapes, grapefruit, lemons, oranges, peaches, pears, pineapple, plums, raspberries, strawberries . . . and other fresh and frozen fruits.	Dried fruits containing benzoate of soda, raisins, prunes.

*Courtesy of U.S. Vitamin and Pharmaceutical Corp.

10. LOW SALT (Low Sodium) DIET* (Concluded)

Foods	Include	Avoid
Cereals and bread	Salt-free cereal: barley, farina, oatmeal, pettijohn's, ralston, rice, wheatena, puffed wheat or rice, shredded wheat, macaroni, spaghetti, noodles, yeast bread prepared without salt.	Most commercially prepared cereals, bread, crackers, pretzels, hot bread, etc., made with salt, baking powder or soda.
Desserts	Ice cream or puddings made with milk allowance, unsalted fruit pies, gelatin desserts, custards.	Those prepared with salt, baking powder or soda, or egg white.
Soups	Unsalted soups and broths, cream soups out of milk allowance	Canned soups, and those made with bouillon cubes.
Dairy products	Whole milk—1 pt. per day (dialyzed milk may be used more freely, if available), unsalted cottage cheese—1 oz. per day, unsalted butter, homemade ice cream, cream—⅓ cup per day.	All hard cheeses, all salted cheeses, salt butter, oleomargarine, buttermilk, commercial ice cream.
Beverages	Coffee, tea, cocoa, wine, fruit juices; beer and soft drinks—8 oz. per day.	
Fats	Lard, oil, vegetable fat.	Salted shortening, bacon fat, salad dressing.
Seasonings, condiments	Pepper, garlic, paprika, vinegar, herbs, dry mustard, onion, vanilla, lemon, cinnamon.	Catsup, chili sauce, prepared horse radish, pickles, relishes, steak sauce, salad dressings.
Miscellaneous	Sugar, syrup, candy, jam or jelly made without benzoate of soda, unsalted nuts, popcorn.	Olives, salted nuts and peanut butter.

11. DIET FOR PEOPLE WITH ULCER OF STOMACH OR DUODENUM

Foods Permitted

Soups	White toast, crackers, rolls.
Meats, fish, eggs or cheese	Farina, cream of wheat, rice.
	Cream soups, such as asparagus, tomato, beets, pea.
Vegetables	Scraped beef, minced white meat of chicken, lamb chops, broiled liver, sweetbreads, fresh fish, salmon, eggs, cottage or cream cheese.
Potato, etc.	Cooked beets, asparagus, carrots, peas, beets, squash, string beans.
Butter	Baked or mashed potato, corn purée, lima bean purée, macaroni, noodles, rice.
Breads	
Cereals	Butter, margarine, cream.

11. DIET FOR PEOPLE WITH ULCER
OF STOMACH OR DUODENUM (Concluded)

Foods Permitted

Fruits	Avocado, banana, canned or stewed apples, apricots, cherries, peaches, pears. Dilute orange juice, prune juice, prune whip.
Desserts	Sponge cake, crackers, cookies, custard, jello, rice or bread pudding, ice cream, sherbet.
Sweets	Jellies, plain candies, sugar, honey.
Beverages	*Milk,* milk drinks, tea, decaffeinated coffee.

GENERAL INSTRUCTIONS

1. Eat, or drink milk every 2 to 3 hours.
2. Drink milk and eat lightly before retiring at night and if you wake up during the night.
3. Eat slowly and chew food thoroughly.
4. Adhere strictly to diet and *AVOID* the following: SMOKING; ALCOHOL; COFFEE; and mustard, chili sauce, horse radish, other spices and condiments. Also avoid gravies, hot sauces, nuts, pickles, etc.

DIVERTICULOSIS AND DIVERTICULITIS

See BOWEL FUNCTION; DIET; INTESTINES.

What is a diverticulum of the large intestine?

It is a protrusion of a small portion of the mucous membrane that lines the large bowel through the muscle wall of the bowel. The outpouching, or protrusion, gives the appearance of a pea or grape. Diverticula are analogous to blisters on an automobile tire.

What is diverticulosis?

It is a condition in which there are many diverticula protruding from the wall of the large bowel.

What causes diverticula to form in older people?

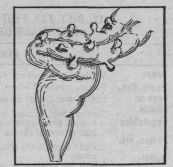

Diverticulosis of large bowel

They are thought to be caused by a progressive weakness in the musculature of the bowel, aggravated by chronic constipation.

How frequent is diverticulosis in people in their later years?

It is estimated that approximately 10 percent of all people in their late sixties or seventies will develop some diverticula of the large intestine.

Does diverticulosis always produce symptoms?

No. The great majority of people with diverticulosis have no symptoms and the diagnosis is made incidentally during the course of a routine X-ray examination of the lower intestinal tract.

What is diverticulitis?

It is an inflammation of a diverticulum.

What causes a diverticulum to become inflamed?

Usually, inflammation is caused by the accumulation of hard stool in the diverticulum.

Is diverticulitis very common in older people?

It is estimated that approximately one in ten of those who have diverticulosis will at some time or other develop diverticulitis.

What are the symptoms of diverticulitis?

Since the left portion of the colon is most frequently involved, there is usually pain in the lower left part of the abdomen. When pressure is applied to this area, there is pain and spasm of the abdominal muscles. The patient may also have temperature, constipation, nausea, and vomiting. In some cases, there is bleeding from the rectum. Occasionally, an inflamed diverticulum will rupture, causing peritonitis or the formation of an abcess within the abdominal cavity.

Do most cases of diverticulitis subside spontaneously or do they require surgery?

Most cases subside with medical treatment over a period of a week or two.

What medical advice should be followed by those who have diverticulosis?

1. They should make every attempt to have regular bowel movements. Lubricants or laxatives should be taken when necessary.
2. Food containing large amounts of roughage, highly seasoned foods, and large quantities of alcoholic beverages should be avoided.
3. If abdominal pain develops, the doctor should be consulted.

Do people with diverticulosis ever hemorrhage from a diverticulum?

Yes, once in a while. This is not a common occurrence, however.

How can one distinguish between diverticulitis and a tumor of the large bowel?

A barium enema X ray will make the distinction in the great majority of cases. Also, some tumors of the area can be seen directly through a sigmoidoscope.

What is the treatment for diverticulitis?

If a diverticulum is mildly inflamed, or if several of them are mildly inflamed, the patient is taken off food by mouth and is fed intravenously. Antibiotics are given to control the infection. As the inflammation subsides, usually after hospitalization, the patient recovers spontaneously. If, on the other hand, an abcess has formed, or if the inflammation does not subside, surgery becomes necessary.

What surgery is recommended for diverticulitis that does not respond to medical treatment?

1. If the patient is in satisfactory general health, the inflamed segment of bowel is removed and the bowel's continuity is reestablished.
2. If peritonitis has resulted from the diverticulitis, it is necessary to drain the abdominal cavity and to perform a temporary colostomy (opening of the bowel onto the abdominal wall) rather than to attempt removal of the bowel segment in the presence of severe infection.
3. When a drainage procedure and colostomy have been performed, it is necessary to wait several weeks for the peritonitis to subside. Then the patient is brought back to the hospital for removal of the diseased segment of bowel.
4. Several weeks after the second operation, the patient is again operated on to close the colostomy, thus reestablishing the normal continuity of the bowel.

Is recovery usual after surgery for diverticulitis?

Yes. In a great majority of cases, the patient makes complete recovery from this type of surgery, although three major operations over a period of several weeks or months may be required.

DRIVING

See ALCOHOL AND ALCOHOLISM; EYES; HEARING AND DEAFNESS; TRAVEL.

Should people past sixty be allowed to drive?

Yes, if they are in possession of all their faculties. Most older people can drive efficiently until far into their seventies and eighties. Statistical reports from the American Safety Council show that healthy people in their sixties and seventies are actually safer drivers than young men in their twenties. This is probably due to the fact that those in their later years have learned the wisdom of driving at safe speeds and know that alcohol and driving do not mix.

Should people past sixty take special care while driving?

Yes, because there may be some diminution in reaction time and in muscular coordination. However, this is more than compensated for by the added wisdom and safety habits people develop as they get along in years.

What special precautions should older people take when driving an automobile?

1. If there is impaired eyesight, glasses should always be worn.
2. If there is impairment in hearing, hearing aids should be used.
3. It is best not to drive when there is heavy rain or snow. Older people should pull over to the side of the road until the rain stops. If a snowstorm looks as if it will continue for a long time, the car should be put in the nearest garage.
4. Cars should not be driven in a thick fog.
5. A window of the car should always be kept open at least an inch or two, to ensure adequate air circulation.
6. The radio should not be played loudly in a heavily traveled area, as it may interfere with hearing a car horn or the sound of an approaching car.
7. Whenever the driver is sleepy, he should pull off to the side of the road and go to sleep. A rest of a half hour will often restore him to a fully wakened state.
8. On a superhighway all drivers tend to become hypnotized by the monotony of the road. A rest should therefore be taken at least once an hour.
9. Older people should be particularly careful to see that their cars are in good shape. The driver's slowed reac-

225

tion time may result in greater demands being made upon brakes, accelerator, and steering mechanism.

Is the car-accident rate greater among people past sixty?

No. It is smaller.

Should older people restrict the rate of speed at which they drive?

Yes. Safe driving involves not going beyond the posted speed limits. In most instances, older people can drive safely at those speeds, although perhaps it would be best if they held to a 50-mile-an-hour limit on the superhighways.

Can an older person who drives too slowly become a menace to himself and others?

Yes. Overcautious drivers may cause accidents by forcing those behind them to take undue risks. Excessive slowness in driving is almost as dangerous as excessive speed.

At what times during the day is it advisable for older people not to drive?

1. When the sun is setting and the driver is traveling toward it.
2. At night, if there is heavy traffic on the roads. Many older people do not adjust well to the glare of oncoming headlights.

DRUGS AND MEDICINES

See ANESTHESIA; FIRST AID; PAIN; SMOKING; SURGERY; TESTS; TREATMENT; VITAMINS.

Is it permissible for people past sixty to take drugs and medicines that have not been prescribed by a doctor?

Whenever possible, this practice should be avoided. The source of information as to the value of drugs should be one's own physician—not the radio, television, newspapers, or neighbors. This is particularly important for people who are entering a period of their lives in which serious illness is prevalent.

Are patented drugs obtainable without prescription, and are they safe to take?

Some are obtainable over the drugstore counter; others are not. Many drugs that are sold without a doctor's prescription can be harmful when taken for the wrong condition. Moreover, some people may be sensitive to a seemingly harmless medication. The best policy is to ask the family doctor to do the prescribing.

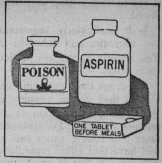

Labeling of medicines in large letters so that they can be read even by people with impaired vision

Should older people exercise particular care insofar as sensitivity to drugs is concerned?

Yes. Older people tend to develop sensitivity to drugs toward which they were not sensitive in earlier years. Also, the liver, kidneys, and other organs of older people are particularly sensitive to the toxic effects of certain drugs.

What are some of the evidences of drug toxicity that should warn a patient to stop taking it?

1. Nausea and vomiting.
2. Wheezing or shortness of breath.
3. Inflammation of the eyelids and reddening of the whites of the eyes.
4. Itching skin or hives.
5. A skin rash.
6. Blood in the urine.
7. An agitated or upset emotional state.
8. Diarrhea.

Should older people contact their physician immediately on noticing any of these toxic reactions?

Yes. It is dangerous to continue taking a drug to which one is sensitive.

Is it possible for people to be just as sensitive to an ointment as to a drug taken internally?

Yes. There are just as many sensitivity reactions to ointments.

Is the skin of older people usually more sensitive than that of younger people?

Yes.

Are the doses of medications given to people past sixty usually the same as those for younger adults?

If the person is healthy, the dosage varies very little. However, if the patient is thin and debilitated, the dose should be reduced.

Is it particularly important to give smaller amounts of narcotics and sedatives to older, debilitated people?

Yes. Elderly people are particularly sensitive to the effects of these drugs.

Do drugs have the same chemical effect on older patients as they do on younger patients?

Yes. The specific action of a drug on the organs or tissues remains the same. For instance, if a drug helps to bring down fever and relieve aches and pains (aspirin, for example), it will have that effect regardless of the person's age. The only difference is that in small, thin, or ill older people, the drug may have a more powerful effect.

Do people past sixty react to antibiotic drugs in ways they formerly did not?

No, except that if they received treatment repeatedly with these medications earlier in their lives, they may have developed a sensitivity to them.

What unfavorable reactions in older people may follow the prolonged use of antibiotics?

1. Signs of sensitivity, as mentioned above, may develop. These include nausea, vomiting, skin rashes, and inflammation of the eyes.
2. Some antibiotics may cause diarrhea that will take several weeks to subside.
3. If the antibiotic kills off too many of the bacteria that are normally present in the intestinal tract, a growth of fungi may develop that will be very difficult to control.
4. The prolonged taking of antibiotics by mouth may allow the staphylococcus, which is not sensitive to some antibiotics, to outgrow all other organisms. This can result in a dangerous form of colitis (staphylococcal enterocolitis).
5. Certain antibiotics must be used with care, as they may adversely affect the nerves controlling the sense of balance. Permanent damage to equilibrium from the prolonged use of these drugs has been noted in some cases.

Can people past sixty safely take medications to curb appetite?

Yes, but only under the supervision of a doctor. The ingredients in some of these preparations can be injurious to older people. Such medications often contain ingredients that will harm those with hardening of the arteries, elevated blood pressure, or heart disease. Other diet-curbing medications contain bulk-forming substances that may interfere with the normal passage of food through the intestinal canal.

Should older people take heart medications or stimulants without medical supervision?

No. An overdose of most of the medications that aid the heart, such as the digitalis group of drugs, can cause severe damage.

Can medications to relieve angina pectoris (pain in the heart region) be taken without a doctor's supervision?

No. The most widely used medications for this purpose are nitroglycerin (small tablets allowed to dissolve beneath the tongue), amyl nitrite (which comes in a small glass ampule that is broken and the vapor inhaled through the nose), and longer-acting nitrite tablets, which are taken regularly every few hours to stave off an attack.

After the doctor has instructed the patient in the use of these medications, he is permitted to medicate himself.

Are medications for the heart, such as digitalis, nitroglycerin, and amyl nitrite, habit-forming?

No.

Do people past sixty tend to react in the same ways as younger people to pain-relieving medications?

These drugs have essentially the same effect on older people as they do on younger ones. It may be necessary, however, to vary the amount of the drug, depending on the severity of the symptoms and the person's reaction to those symptoms.

Are pain-relieving drugs, such as aspirin, safe for older people to take on their own?

Yes, unless they are allergic or sensitive to such drugs.

Do pain-relieving drugs, such as aspirin, have a bad effect on the heart?

No. This is an erroneous idea.

How do older people react to an overdose of narcotics?

1. Blood pressure usually drops markedly.
2. Heart beat and pulse slow to 40 to 50 beats per minute.
3. Breathing becomes very slow, 6 to 10 respirations per minute.

Although these symptoms are not alarming in a younger person, they may produce severe damage in an elderly person. Slowed heart rate may result in impaired circulation; lowered blood pressure may induce clotting in narrowed blood vessels; slowed respirations may lead to inadequate aeration of the base of the lungs, with resultant pneumonia. Finally, permanent damage to the brain may result because of oxygen deprivation.

Is the danger of addiction to drugs greater in older patients?

Yes. Older patients are past the stage in life when they must prove to themselves their ability to withstand suffering. They may, as a result, rely more on pain-relieving and sleep-producing drugs and become addicted to them. The attending physician must balance this greater tendency toward addiction with his knowledge of the patient and his disease. If the patient is in his eighties and is suffering severely from an incurable condition, it is perhaps better to give than to withhold narcotics, even if the price is addiction. On the other hand, if the patient is a healthy, robust sixty- or seventy-year-old, the doctor will be more careful about prescribing potentially habit-forming drugs.

Can a patient become addicted after three, four, or five injections of a narcotic?

No! Narcotics, such as morphine, must be given every few hours for a period of several weeks before true addiction takes place.

Is it wise to use narcotics to produce sleep?

No. The narcotics (morphine, codeine, dilaudid, and demerol, for example) should not be used regularly to produce sleep. Sedatives such as the barbiturates and some of the newer sleep-producing medications are much better to use than narcotics.

What are some general rules to follow in the use of sleeping pills by elderly patients?

1. They should not be withheld from someone who has demonstrated, over a period of weeks or months, that he is unable to get a good night's rest without them.
2. The smallest dose that will produce sleep should be used.
3. The sedative should be given approximately an hour before the patient goes to sleep, so that there will be time for it to act.
4. Excitement should be avoided before bedtime; a sleeping pill will work much better when one is calm.
5. Every few nights the sleeping pill should be withheld to see if the patient can fall asleep without it.
6. If the patient notes that the pill is losing its effectiveness, the family physician should be contacted so that he may prescribe something else.
7. If the pill produces such deep sleep that the patient

does not awaken in the morning, or if he feels groggy on awakening, a less powerful medication should be prescribed.

8. The patient should be instructed not to use two pills merely because one fails to work. Even though one pill may fail to work, two pills might amount to a harmful overdose.

ECTROPION AND ENTROPION

See BLEPHARITIS; CONJUNCTIVITIS; EYES; TRICHIASIS.

What is ectropion?

It is a condition in which the lower eyelids tend to drop away from the eyeball. As a result, tears, which normally bathe the surface of the eyeball, run out onto the cheek. People with ectropion look as if they are always crying.

Ectropion is harmful because it leads to insufficient lubrication of the eyeball; when dust particles enter the eye, they are not washed away by the tears. Conjunctivitis or ulcerations of the cornea may ultimately result.

Is ectropion common in older people?

Yes, it affects them much more often than young people.

What is the treatment of ectropion?

A simple operation, performed under local anesthesia, in which a portion of the inside of the eyelid is removed so as to cause the lid to turn inward.

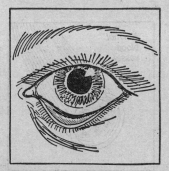

Ectropion

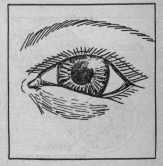

Entropion

What is entropion?

Entropion is a condition in which the margins of the eyelids, more commonly the lower, tend to turn in toward the eyeball. This may be serious, as it results in the continuous scratching of the surface of the eyeball by turned-in eyelashes.

Is entropion very common in older people?

Yes. It affects them more often than young people.

What is the treatment of entropion?

It is corrected by an operation, performed under local anesthesia, in which a portion of the inside of the eyelid is cut away in such a manner as to cause the lid to bend outward. The procedure is successful in almost all cases.

In addition to surgery, the eyelashes are plucked to make sure that they do not rub against the eyeball.

EMBOLUS AND EMBOLISM

See APOPLEXY, OR STROKE; CIRCULATION; HEART; THROMBUS AND THROMBOSIS; VEINS AND VARICOSE VEINS.

What is an embolus?

An embolus is a piece of clotted blood that has become detached from the lining of the heart or a vein or artery. The embolus travels through the bloodstream and lodges in some other part of the body, where it obstructs the normal blood flow.

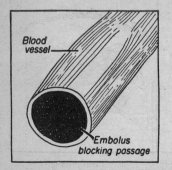
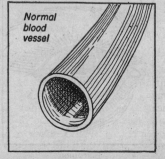

Embolism

What is an embolism?

It is a condition caused by obstruction of the blood flow by an embolus.

What are the symptoms of embolism?

1. If a major vessel is blocked, sudden death (within seconds) may result. This occurs most often in pulmonary embolism.

2. If death does not follow the blockage of a major vessel, shock may ensue. The patient will become cold, clammy, and perspire freely; heart action will weaken; pulse will become rapid; and blood pressure will go down.

3. If the embolus has lodged in the brain, a stroke will result. (*See* APOPLEXY, OR STROKE.)

4. If the embolus has lodged in the lungs, the result will be shock, severe chest pain, difficulty in breathing, and spitting of blood.

5. If the embolus lodges in the aorta at the site where that vessel divides to send arteries to each leg, then pain, coldness, and loss of pulsations will be noted in both legs. This type of embolus is often associated with shock.

6. If the embolus lodges in an artery in the thigh or leg, that limb will become cold and blue and will lose its pulsations.

Do older people display a greater tendency to develop embolism than younger people?

Yes, because impaired heart function, seen so often in older people, permits blood clots to form in the chambers of the heart. Also, blood circulation in the veins in the legs and pelvis tends to become sluggish, thus permitting blood to clot in the veins. When either of these conditions prevails, the chances are great that a piece of this clotted blood will break away and travel to some distant part of the body.

In what sites are emboli most likely to originate, and where are they most likely to lodge?

Many originate from the left atrium (auricle) or from the valves of the left side of the heart as a secondary condition to impaired heart function or rheumatic heart disease. When emboli from this site break away, they may lodge in the arteries of the legs or in a

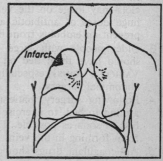

Area of lung blocked by embolus, resulting in an infarct, an area of dead or dying tissue

vessel in the brain. Gangrene of one or both legs or a stroke may be a consequence. If the embolus should go to a kidney or some other organ, the function of that organ will be seriously impaired.

If the embolus originates from a vein in the leg or pelvis (as sometimes occurs as a postoperative complication), it usually travels to the lungs and causes a pulmonary embolism.

Can surgery help when an embolus has lodged in one of the main arteries in the thigh or leg?

Immediate surgery is necessary to save the limb. An operation is performed in which the obstructed artery is opened and the embolus is removed (embolectomy). If this procedure is carried out within a few hours after the embolization has taken place, circulation may be restored and the life of the limb preserved.

Can surgery help when an embolus has traveled to the brain?

It is often difficult to locate the exact site at which the embolus has lodged when it affects one of the small arteries in the brain. For this reason, it is seldom feasible to operate for the removal of an embolus to the brain.

Can surgery help when a pulmonary (lung) embolus has occurred?

Usually not, although there are a few cases on record in which immediate surgery has saved the patient's life.

Are there methods of preventing an embolism?

Yes.

1. Medications to improve heart regularity and function will decrease the chances of blood clots forming in it.

2. In cases of rheumatic heart disease where infected blood clots may lodge on the valves (subacute endocarditis), huge doses of antibiotic and anticoagulant drugs may prevent an embolus from breaking away.

3. Older people with large varicose veins in their legs should have them tied off or stripped (*see* VEINS AND VARICOSE VEINS), especially if they are to undergo future abdominal surgery.

4. Following surgery, patients should be made to move around in bed, to exercise their legs, and to get out of bed as soon as possible. This will help to prevent clots from forming in the veins of the legs and pelvis.

5. Anticoagulant drugs should be given those who appear to be in danger of getting blood clots. Such medications

keep the blood more fluid, thus reducing the possibility of clot formation. This type of treatment is frequently carried out both before and after surgery.

6. If embolism has already occurred, treatment with anticoagulant drugs may prevent the extension of the clot and may help to preserve fluidity of blood that is on the point of clotting. (Anticoagulant therapy must be carried out only under the constant supervision of a specialist, as severe hemorrhage may result unless the treatment is carefully regulated.)

What are some of the anticoagulant drugs, and how do they work in cases of embolism?

The two main drugs are heparin and dicoumarol. They work by prolonging the clotting time of the blood, thus reducing its tendency to clot.

Does spontaneous recovery ever take place after a patient has sustained a pulmonary embolus, cerebral embolus, or embolus to a major artery at other sites?

Yes. However, unless the underlying cause of the embolus is eliminated, the chances of recurrent, eventually fatal, emboli are great.

EMPHYSEMA

See BRONCHITIS; RESPIRATORY TRACT.

What is emphysema?

It is a lung condition affecting a great number of older people. Emphysema results from the loss of elastic tissue in the lung and resultant overstretching of the tissues. This process eventually leads to a decrease in the aerating surface of the lungs. People with emphysema have limitation of chest expansion and, sooner or later, develop shortness of breath and a barrel-chested appearance.

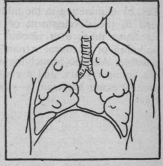

Overdistention of lung, as seen in emphysema

Who is most likely to develop emphysema?

People with chronic lung infections, such as bronchitis, or those who have had asthma for many years.

Why is emphysema so often seen in older people?

Actually, emphysema is part of the aging process in the lungs.

Does emphysema always produce symptoms?

No. A certain amount of emphysema is present in almost all people who are in their seventies or eighties, and in most instances there are no symptoms. However, when this condition is associated with chronic bronchitis or with a dilatation and rupture of a large number of air cells, symptoms will be manifested.

What are the symptoms of chronic emphysema?

1. Shortness of breath and a consequent desire to sleep in a semisitting position.
2. Difficulty in expelling air from the lungs.
3. Coughing, with the expectoration of large amounts of mucous secretions.
4. Bluish discoloration of the fingertips and the lips, owing to inadequate amounts of oxygen in the circulating blood.
5. An increase in susceptibility to respiratory infections.
6. Frequent asthmatic attacks.
7. In very severe cases, heart failure.

What is the treatment of emphysema?

The main treatment is directed toward keeping the patient free from respiratory infections. Even a minor respiratory infection in one who has emphysema may progress to a serious lung complication.

Is there any way to prevent the onset of emphysema?

Yes, by eliminating in the middle years those things that may lead to the development of chronic bronchitis or asthma. Excessive tobacco or alcohol and excessive exposure to air pollution or chemical irritants should be avoided whenever possible. Allergic bronchitis should be treated vigorously in the younger years, and every precaution should be taken to control acute bacterial or viral infections of the respiratory tract.

ENDOCRINE GLANDS AND HORMONES

See ADRENAL GLANDS; DIABETES MELLITUS; LONGEVITY; OVARIES; PANCREAS; PARATHYROID GLANDS; PITUITARY GLAND; SEX HORMONES; THYROID GLAND.

What are the important endocrine glands?
1. The pituitary gland, in the base of the brain.
2. The thyroid gland, in the neck.
3. The pancreas, in the abdomen.
4. The adrenal glands, above the kidneys.
5. The ovaries.
6. The testicles.

Do gland secretions decrease in amount with aging?
Yes. Gland tissues show the same effects of aging as other structures do. The secreting portion of the gland is replaced by fibrous tissue. Fortunately, sufficient secreting substance remains active to maintain normal body functions. In addition, the lowered metabolism of advanced age makes fewer demands on the glands.

Does decreased glandular secretion play an important role in the aging process?
It is not possible to state categorically that this is true, but there is a very definite interrelationship between gland activity and aging. Whether aging causes decreased gland activity or vice versa has not yet been decided.

Do all endocrine glands produce hormones?
Yes. All endocrine glands produce hormones, which are secreted into the bloodstream. A hormone is a chemical substance having a specific effect on other structures located in other parts of the body. For example, the pancreas manufactures insulin and secretes it into the bloodstream, where it acts to convert circulating sugar into energy. Similarly, the thyroid gland manufactures the hormone thyroxine, which it secretes into the bloodstream for the regulation of metabolism.

Which glands do not produce hormones?
The lymph glands are believed not to produce hormones; nor do such glands as the spleen and thymus.

What are the major body hormones and what are their main functions?
1. The anterior and posterior pituitary hormones, which regulate growth and control such other glands as the thyroid, adrenals, ovaries, and testicles.

237

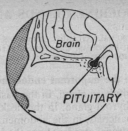

PITUITARY

Brain

PARATHYROIDS

THYROID

IMPORTANT
ENDOCRINE GLANDS

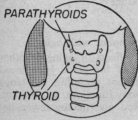

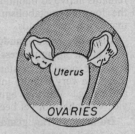

Uterus

OVARIES

ADRENAL

Kidney

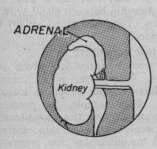

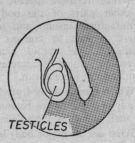

TESTICLES

Important endocrine glands

2. The thyroid hormone, which regulates metabolism.
3. The parathyroid hormone, which controls calcium metabolism.
4. Insulin, which is manufactured by the pancreatic cells, controls sugar metabolism.
5. The adrenal hormones, which control blood pressure, fluid balance, salt and mineral metabolism, and other functions. Cortisone is manufactured by the cortex of the adrenals; adrenalin, in the interior of the gland.
6. The female sex hormones, which are manufactured by the ovaries, control menstruation, development of secondary sex characteristics, pregnancy, and other female functions.
7. The male sex hormones, which are manufactured and secreted by the testicles, control development of male secondary sex characteristics, the production of sperm, and other male functions.
8. In addition to these hormones, there are others, which are secreted by the liver, stomach, and other organs. Each has a specific chemical action that influences the function of some other part of the body.

Do continued health and vigor into the sixties and seventies indicate that the glands are continuing to secrete normal amounts of hormone?

People who stay young longer probably continue to manufacture unusually large amounts of hormones.

Is it possible to delay the onset of aging by giving hormones during the middle years?

No!

Will the taking of female sex hormones delay the onset of menopause (change of life)?

It may extend the menstrual cycle some time, and it may delay signs of aging in the breasts, but these reactions are temporary. On the other hand, there may be harmful consequences from taking female sex hormones for years in order to delay the natural processes of aging.

Will the taking of male sex hormones delay the onset of aging?

No. However, in certain cases where impotence is caused by a decrease in the amount of male sex hormones being secreted, the condition may be remedied by the taking of the synthetic hormone. (It should be mentioned that there may be harmful consequences from taking male hormones for long periods of time.)

Can "youthfulness" be preserved by taking a combination of hormones?

No. Innumerable experiments have been carried out by investigators throughout the world to discover some method of rejuvenation. They have all failed!

Should older people take hormones without a doctor's permission?

No.

What is replacement therapy?

Giving a hormone to replace a natural hormone that is not being produced in normal amount. For example, if an older person has inadequate thyroid secretion, giving the thyroid substance will make up for the deficiency.

What are the dangers of taking hormones for a long time?

1. It is thought, although not definitely proved, that large doses of female sex hormones may stimulate a dormant tumor in the breast or ovary to become active and grow.

2. It is thought, although not definitely proved, that large doses of male sex hormones may stimulate a dormant tumor in the prostate gland to become active and to grow.

3. It is well known that occasionally the taking of large doses of hormone for long periods may have the effect opposite of that desired. Instead of stimulating the gland to function more normally, synthetic hormones may cause it to undergo degeneration. For example, large doses of thyroid hormone in a healthy individual in the sixties or seventies may cause the thyroid gland to secrete less of its own hormone than it otherwise would. Even after the synthetic hormone is discontinued, the gland may not regain its ability to manufacture its own hormone.

Will giving large doses of hormones cause cancer?

No, but as mentioned above, there is the distinct possibility that large doses of male or femae sex hormones may activate a dormant tumor.

Can transplanting of glands bring about rejuvenation?

No. Many attempts have been made to rejuvenate people through surgery. For example, glands from animals or from younger humans have been transplanted to the bodies of aging persons. To date, these attempts have not been successful.

There are cosmetic operations that can restore some of the youthful *appearance*—operations to eliminate wrinkles, plastic operations on the breasts, etc.—but these are not truly rejuvenation procedures.

Do hormones influence the time at which hardening of the arteries begins?

This question will require much more investigation before it can be answered with any degree of certainty. It is known that there is a correlation between the secretion of the female sex hormone (estrogen) and the deposit of cholesterol in the walls of arteries. It may be, although it has not yet been proved, that the continued secretion of female sex hormones in some way protects the blood vessels from developing arteriosclerosis. Some support is lent to this theory by the statistical fact that women tend to develop arteriosclerosis at a later age than men.

Can giving female sex hormones or any other hormone prevent or delay the onset of arteriosclerosis?

No. Someday, however, science may discover some hormone or chemical that can do this all-important job.

EPILEPSY

See APOPLEXY, OR STROKE; COMA; CONVULSIONS; DRIVING; FIRST AID; NERVES.

Is epilepsy common in those over sixty?

No, but if they have had epilepsy during most of their lives, they will in all probability continue to have it in old age. A very small number of people develop this condition for the first time during later life.

Are convulsive seizures or other symptoms of epilepsy different in older people?

The symptoms of epilepsy are pretty much the same for all. However, convulsive seizures may be brought on by factors other than epilepsy. Spasm of arteriosclerotic blood vessels within the brain, overdose of insulin, tumor of the insulin-producing cells of the pancreas, brain tumors, and other factors may be the underlying cause of convulsions. These must be ruled out before a diagnosis of epilepsy is made.

What are the symptoms of epilepsy?

There are two main forms of epilepsy: that associated with convulsive seizures—*grand mal;* and that associated with slight momentary lapses in consciousness without convulsion—*petit mal.*

The symptoms of grand mal are:
1. Loss of consciousness.

2. Shaking convulsions, involving the arms and legs particularly.
3. Frothing at the mouth and muscle spasms, which may cause the epileptic to bite his tongue.
4. Involuntary passing of urine or feces.
5. Mental confusion for several minutes after emerging from an episode.

How long does the average convulsion last?

Only a few minutes. If the convulsions continue for more than an hour, they are, in all probability, due to something other than epilepsy.

What is the treatment of epilepsy?

People who have epileptic seizures should take sedatives regularly. The older the patient, the smaller the dose of sedative that has to be given to keep him free of convulsions.

What special precautions should the older epileptic take?

1. He should limit fluid intake to four glasses of liquid daily.
2. He should never skip his medication.
3. He should avoid emotional and physical stress.
4. He should not drink alcoholic beverages.
5. He should give up driving.

ESOPHAGUS

See HERNIA; STOMACH AND DUODENUM.

Does spasm of the lower end of the esophagus (food pipe) ever prevent swallowed food from entering the stomach?

Yes. When the spasm is brief, it is called *cardiospasm;* when the spasm is prolonged or constant, it is called *achalasia.*

Does cardiospasm occur in older people?

Yes. It is usually brought on by stress, nervousness, or an inflammation of the lower end of the esophagus.

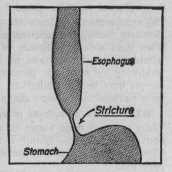

Achalasia

Does achalasia often develop in older people?

No. It almost always begins during young adulthood, but it may persist beyond sixty.

What course does achalasia usually follow?

Achalasia is a chronic condition associated with a more or less constant obstruction to the free passage of food into the stomach. It is thought to be caused by failure of development of those nerves in the lower end of the esophagus that cause the muscles to relax. When the obstruction persists over a period of years, it leads to a marked dilatation of the esophagus above the obstruction. It also results in the regurgitation of food that fails to pass through into the stomach.

What are the symptoms of spasm of the lower part of the esophagus?

1. Distress and pain beneath the breastbone (lower end of the sternum).
2. Regurgitation of swallowed foods.
3. Loss in weight, owing to inadequate quantities of food entering the stomach.
4. A characteristic appearance of the esophagus, with narrowing of the lower end and dilatation of the upper portion. This condition may be diagnosed by having the patient swallow barium and then taking X rays of the esophagus.

What is the treatment of cardiospasm?

This condition, since it is transient, can usually be relieved by giving medications to allay the underlying stress and nervousness that have caused it. In addition, there are several effective antispasmodic drugs that will relax the esophageal muscles and allow food to pass on into the stomach.

What is the treatment of achalasia?

Since most cases of achalasia are chronic and exist for a period of years, it will usually require surgical correction. An incision is made in the chest cavity; the outer muscular coats of the esophagus are cut, thereby allowing it to dilate and permit the free passage of food. Most operations of this type are highly successful, and although they are major operations, they do not endanger life.

Are tumor growths common in the esophagus?

Approximately 1 percent of all cancer is cancer of the esophagus.

Does cancer of the esophagus affect people over sixty?

Yes. It is most frequently encountered in this age group.

What are the symptoms of a tumor in the esophagus?

1. Difficulty in swallowing.
2. Regurgitation of undigested food.
3. Loss in weight, owing to undernourishment.

How does a doctor diagnose a tumor in the esophagus?

If the patient has the symptoms listed above, the doctor will
have him X-rayed. Barium X ray will reveal the presence of a
tumor.

What is the treatment of cancer of the esophagus?

Surgical removal of the tumor-bearing portion of the esophagus. The portion above the tumor is then sutured (stitched)
to a loop of bowel, which is brought up from the abdomen
and is used as a substitute food pipe.

**Is operation for removal of part of the esophagus very
serious?**

Yes. It is one of the most formidable kinds of surgery. However, cancer of the esophagus is one of the most lethal of all
diseases, and surgery offers the main hope of cure.

Is X-ray treatment ever helpful in cancer of the esophagus?

Yes. It may delay the cancer's growth and spread for several
months—occasionally, for years.

What is a hiatus hernia?

It is an opening (rupture) in the diaphragm alongside the
lower end of the esophagus as it passes from the chest to the
abdominal cavity. Through such an opening, a portion of the
stomach may protrude into the chest cavity.

Do older people often develop hiatus hernia?

Yes, it is extremely common in those past seventy. However,
it causes symptoms only in a small number of cases.

What symptoms can hiatus hernia cause?

1. Pain beneath the lower end of the breastbone.
2. Difficulty in swallowing.
3. Bleeding from the lower end of the esophagus or
   stomach.

**Is surgery indicated for older people who have hiatus
hernia?**

Only if there is hemorrhage from the esophagus, if nutrition
is interfered with by obstruction to passage of food, if the
pain is unbearable, or if a portion of the stomach becomes
caught in a hernia sac.

**Can most older people get along without surgery for hiatus
hernia?**

Yes.

Do varicose veins ever occur in the esophagus?

They occur in older people who have obstruction to blood flow through the liver, as in cirrhosis. (*See* CIRRHOSIS OF THE LIVER; VEINS AND VARICOSE VEINS.)

Are varicosities of the veins in the esophagus serious?

Yes. They can rupture and may cause a fatal hemorrhage.

What is the treatment of varicose veins in the esophagus?

The underlying cirrhosis of the liver must be treated. In special cases, treatment will involve a *portocaval shunt*. In this major operation the portal vein leading to the liver is stitched to the vena cava. Much of the blood can then bypass the obstructed liver, and the circulatory load on the esophageal veins will be lessened.

EYES

See ARCUS SENILIS AND ARCUS SENILIS LENTIS; BLEPHARITIS; BLINDNESS; CATARACTS; CONJUNCTIVITIS; ECTROPION AND ENTROPION; GLAUCOMA; OPTIC-NERVE ATROPHY; PTERYGIUM; PTOSIS OF THE EYELID; RETINAL DETACHMENT; RETINAL THROMBOSIS; TRICHIASIS; XANTHELASMA.

Does vision usually become poorer as people age?

Yes, although many people retain near-normal vision well into their seventies and eighties.

Will extensive use of the eyes throughout the middle years lead to poorer vision later in life?

No. The belief that the eyes can be hurt by extensive use is false. Of course, they definitely can be damaged by use under improper lighting conditions, or by neglect in getting corrective eyeglasses. In other words, eyes that are properly cared for will not be harmed by use.

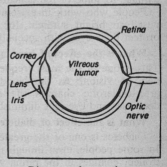

Diagram of normal eye

It should be remembered that the eyes are rested each night during sleep. Under normal conditions, this rest is sufficient to restore them for the tasks of the next day.

How is it that some people who have always worn glasses no longer need them in the later years?

These people have been only moderately nearsighted. In nearsighted people the eyeball is longer, more egg-shaped than normal. As they grow older their eyeballs tend to become rounder and less ovoid. A time may therefore be reached when the nearsightedness will disappear, and glasses are no longer required.

Is there a tendency for the eyes to change color as one reaches the later years of life?

Yes. The pigment in the iris of the eye does tend to fade as one enters the later years. Thus, someone with very dark brown eyes may find that they have turned a few shades lighter. Similarly, those with steel blue eyes may discover that the hue fades somewhat. Also, there may be a loss of pigment just around the outside edge of the colored portion of the eye. (*See* ARCUS SENILIS AND ARCUS SENILIS LENTIS.)

Can reading in poor light for many years cause permanent damage to the eyes?

Yes. Eye-muscle strain and loss of acuteness of vision can occur as a result of abusing the eyes throughout the early and middle years.

Can overexposure to very bright light or to sunlight do permanent damage to the eyes?

Yes. The retina, the important light-receiving portion of the eye, is very sensitive to excessive light. Overexposure to light is particularly dangerous, since it may cause permanent damage to some of the delicate cells in the retina.

People who work in extremely bright light or who are exposed to bright sunlight for long periods of time should protect their eyes with specially designed glasses or shields.

What is the effect of hardening of the arteries on eyesight?

This is one of the most frequent causes of decrease in acuteness of vision. As the blood vessels in the eyes undergo arteriosclerotic changes the efficiency of the retinal cells decreases and eyesight diminishes.

What is the effect of diabetes on eyesight?

Diabetes is one of the greatest causes of decrease in vision. In some people, even though the diabetes has been well controlled, changes in the retina will take place.

Does chronic high blood pressure (hypertension) affect the eyesight?

Yes, because high blood pressure that has been present for

many years is almost always associated with hardening of the arteries in the eyes.

Can eyestrain cause headaches?

Yes. It is a very common cause of headaches.

Do older people find it more difficult to adjust their eyes when going from light to darkness, or from near to far vision?

Healthy older people have very little limitation of this eye function (called *accommodation*). Nevertheless, muscle reactions, including those of the eye muscles, are slower in people who are in their seventies and eighties. Because of the slowed reactions, older people should take their time in judging distances, and they should be particularly careful when going from a light to a dark place, and vice versa.

Is there a tendency for the eye lens to become less translucent with age?

Yes. (*See* CATARACTS.)

Should people over sixty take special precautions against dust particles?

Yes. This is very important because a foreign body in the eye of an older person is more likely to cause an ulceration of the cornea, the thin membrane covering the pupil and colored portion of the eye. Moreover, an ulceration of the cornea may not heal as quickly in an older person.

It is wise for older people to wear goggles or some other type of protective eyeglasses while outside on a windy day or when riding in an automobile with the windows open.

Is there a tendency for older people to develop conjunctivitis?

Yes. (*See* CONJUNCTIVITIS.)

What special eye hygiene should older people practice?

1. The ophthalmologist should be visited twice a year, even if there are no eye symptoms. In this way, conditions such as cataracts, glaucoma, and retinal detachment may be diagnosed and treated in their early stages.
2. Eyes should be washed out morning and evening. An eyecup can be used for this purpose.
3. The eyewash should be prescribed by an eye specialist.
4. Any foreign particle that gets into the eye should be removed promptly. No one should permit such a particle to remain in the eye overnight, even if he must get the doctor out of bed to remove it.
5. Any signs of eye inflammation, crusts on the eyelids,

excessive tearing, or other unusual condition should be treated promptly.

6. Dark glasses should be worn in bright sunlight.
7. Good over-the-shoulder light should be used when reading, sewing, or working.

Is there a tendency for older people's eyes to tear?

Yes, because the lower eyelid tends to adhere less snugly to the eyeball, thus permitting some of the tears to run out onto the cheeks. In some people, the duct that drains the tears away from the eye may be blocked. This condition allows tears to collect within the eye and to spill over.

What can be done for those whose eyes tear excessively?

People with this condition should see an eye specialist. It may be necessary for him to probe and open the nasolacrimal duct, which leads from the eye to the back of the nose.

Will the wearing of properly prescribed eyeglasses tend to preserve vision?

Unfortunately, the wearing of eyeglasses cannot stop degenerative processes in the eye. However, it will help to preserve vision by counteracting chronic eyestrain.

Will the wearing of properly prescribed sunglasses tend to preserve vision?

Since excessive light can do marked damage to the retina, wearing good sunglasses can be helpful.

Is the wearing of sunglasses ever harmful?

Yes. Older people should *not* wear sunglasses indoors or in dim light. In these situations, sunglasses will obscure vision.

Is a visit to an optometrist a satisfactory substitute for going to an eye specialist (ophthalmologist)?

No. Although optometrists perform a useful and necessary function in filling prescriptions and fitting eyeglasses, they are not trained to diagnose and treat diseases of the eyes.

What is the significance of "seeing double"?

This may be secondary to a serious condition, either in the eyes or in the brain. A doctor should be consulted.

What is the significance of spots before the eyes?

Although "spots before the eyes" are often not significant, the condition sometimes indicates disease. If it is a recurring phenomenon, a physician should be consulted.

Will older people hurt their eyes permanently by looking at television for long periods of time?

No. However, it should not be forgotten that riveting the

eyes on any bright object for a long time is not a good thing and may cause temporary eyestrain.

What special steps can people take to preserve their vision?

1. They should seek medical treatment promptly for any minor condition, such as an inflammation of the eyelids, turning in or out of the eyelids, inflammation of the conjunctiva (membrane covering the eyeball).
2. They should protect their eyes against direct exposure to excessively bright light.
3. They should not expose themselves without protection to strong winds, dust, chemical vapors, or other potential eye irritants.
4. They should avoid working or reading in poor light.
5. They should check their general health regularly and have conditions such as diabetes, gout, arthritis, and high blood pressure cared for on a continuing basis.

Are eye operations safe for people in their seventies and eighties?

Yes. No matter how old the patient is, he can usually withstand eye surgery. In most cases, only a local anesthetic is given.

It must be emphasized, however, that the chances of obtaining good results from eye surgery will depend in large measure on the state of general health. Many a brilliant surgical performance has been to no avail because the patient was in poor general health.

TUMORS IN THE EYE

Are tumors in the eye very common in older people?

No. They are rare.

What are some of the symptoms of an eye tumor?

1. Blurred vision in one eye.
2. Lightning flashes shooting across the field of vision of one eye.
3. Patchy loss of vision, possibly shifting in position, in one eye.
4. Blindness developing in an eye that previously had good vision.

How can a diagnosis of an eye tumor be made?

The ophthalmologist will look into the interior of the eye with various instruments and will be able to make his diagnosis by the characteristic appearance of these tumors. The diagnosis is not difficult to make.

Where are most eye tumors in older people located?

Behind the retina in the back of the eyeball. As the tumor grows, it usually causes the retina to become detached.

Are most eye tumors in older people malignant?

Yes.

Are most of these malignant tumors curable?

Yes, provided they are discovered at an early stage.

What is the treatment of a malignant eye tumor?

Removal of the entire eyeball and the contents of the orbit.

FAINTING (SYNCOPE)

See ANEMIA; APOPLEXY, OR STROKE; ARTIFICIAL RESPIRATION; BLOOD PRESSURE; CIRCULATION; CONVULSIONS; NERVES; VERTIGO AND DIZZINESS.

What is fainting?

It is loss of consciousness, lasting for a few minutes, precipitated by inadequate blood and oxygen supply to the brain cells.

Is fainting very common among older people?

Yes. Inadequate heart function and spasm of arteriosclerotic arteries that go to the brain predispose older people to fainting spells.

What are some of the factors that tend to cause fainting spells?

1. A sudden drop in blood pressure, as when an older person who has been lying down stands up abruptly.
2. Sudden changes in heart rhythm, as seen in conditions such as *tachycardia* (extremely rapid heart beat) and *heart block* (extremely slow heart beat).
3. Marked arteriosclerosis, with the involved arteries tending to go into periods of spasm.
4. Inadequate respiration, with low intake of oxygen and the accumulation of carbon dioxide in the body.
5. Fasting, with resultant weakness and low blood-sugar level.
6. An overdose of insulin, which occasionally happens to diabetic patients.
7. Prolonged standing, as in a crowded bus or train.
8. Marked fatigue.

9. Extreme pain.
10. Severe emotional upset.
11. Severe states of anemia.
12. Very high blood pressure.
13. Markedly dehydrated states, as in heat stroke or heat exhaustion.
14. Severe infections accompanied by high temperature.

Is it more serious when older people faint?

Yes, because they are more likely to hurt themselves when they fall. Younger people have quicker reflexes and can protect themselves better when they get a warning that they may be going to faint. Also, the brain cells in older people are less able to withstand even a momentary deprivation of oxygen.

How can one distinguish between a simple fainting spell and a more serious condition, such as a stroke or coma?

1. In a fainting spell unconsciousness lasts only a few minutes; unconsciousness may last for several hours or days after a stroke or during a coma.
2. In a faint the skin becomes white or greenish gray; this may not happen in a stroke or coma.
3. In a faint the pulse becomes rapid and weak and may even disappear for a moment or two; during a stroke or coma the pulse beat may be slow, strong, and pounding.

What should be done for someone who has fainted?

1. The patient should be stretched out flat, with the head lower than the rest of the body. However, if he is a cardiac, his head and shoulders should be elevated, rather than flat, since this position permits easier breathing.
2. All tight clothing—girdle, collar, tie, brassiere, belt, etc.—should be loosened in order to aid deep breathing.
3. Windows should be opened so that there is plenty of fresh air.
4. Place an ear against the left part of the chest to make sure that the heart is beating.
5. If the heart beat has stopped, closed-chest cardiac massage should be carried out (*see* FIRST AID).
6. If breathing has stopped, artificial respiration should be started. (*See* ARTIFICIAL RESPIRATION.)
7. Do not move the patient until he has fully recovered; he should be mentally oriented, his pulse should be regular and bounding, and his breathing deep and regular.

What measures should be avoided when someone has fainted?

1. Do not throw cold water on his face.
2. Do not slap him to revive him.
3. Do not attempt to get him on his feet or to walk him about.
4. Do not try to pour water or whiskey down his throat while he is unconscious.

Is it advisable to give nourishing fluids, tea, coffee, or an alcoholic beverage after someone has recovered fully from a fainting spell?

Yes, provided the fainting spell was an isolated episode and not a recurring condition. Recurrent fainting spells demand thorough medical investigation.

Should an older person be put to bed after he has recovered from a fainting spell?

Yes, and a physician should be notified.

How long does it take for an older person to recover from a fainting spell?

It may take as long as a half hour. If he is moved too soon, a second period of fainting may take place.

Is fainting more serious when it affects someone in his seventies or eighties?

Yes, since it may indicate the presence of a serious underlying disease or may be a forerunner of a stroke. Also, during the period of unconsciousness there is an inadequate supply of oxygen to the brain and the brain cells of older people may suffer permanent damage.

FAMILY RELATIONSHIPS

See ATTITUDES TOWARD AGING; HOME-CARE PROGRAMS; HOTELS, APARTMENTS, AND COMMUNITIES FOR THE AGING; INSTITUTIONAL CARE; MARRIAGE AFTER SIXTY; NURSING HOMES; RETIREMENT; SOCIAL BEHAVIOR; WIDOWHOOD.

If one member of a couple dies, is it better for the survivor to live alone or to move in with his or her children?

Many older people are still active, both in business and socially, and therefore will prefer to live alone and preserve their independence. It is most often when the surviving member is dependent and unable to care for himself or herself that a real problem arises. If he has a choice, it is usually wiser for the widowed member to live alone! This will remove the need for making new adjustments and giving up established habits of living. If the widowed person desires to live with his or her children, and the children truly want the parent to do so, then the move should be made.

If one member of a couple dies, what is the children's responsibility to the surviving parent if he cannot care for himself?

A family conclave is needed in an instance such as this. All too often the children have grown apart from one another. Therefore, each may have his own idea as to what should be done about the remaining parent. Personal hostilities should be submerged at such a time in order to smooth the path for the surviving parent. In democratic fashion, the decision of the majority of the children should prevail. Many families have great difficulties simply because they have followed the advice of only one child.

When a parent moves in with his children and grand-children, what steps should the family take to preserve his independence?

1. Whenever possible, a room (or rooms) should be set aside to give him the maximum amount of privacy.
2. Whenever possible, a private bathroom should be provided. Older people are very dependent on bathrooms and they use them a good deal.
3. If eating habits differ markedly from those of the family, if possible, arrangements should be made for the older person to eat alone. Many older people will want to fix their own food even though they have moved in with their children. This practice should be permitted.
4. An older person should be encouraged to clean and care for his own room if he is capable of doing so. This not only fosters independence but also lessens the feeling of obligation.
5. Sleeping habits of older parents are usually different from those of their children and it is possible that they will want to retire and rise earlier. Every effort should be made to allow them to follow their usual practice.
6. Children should inform the parent explicitly about the living arrangements *before* he comes to live with them. This is essential to avoid future misunderstanding.
7. Children should continue to lead their own social lives

and it should be made clear to the parent that his presence will not alter their usual pursuits.

8. Children should interfere as little as possible in the life of the older person. His independence should be encouraged and advice, unless it is solicited, should be given sparingly.

How should one handle a dispute between a parent and a son-in-law or daughter-in-law, or between the parent and the grandchildren?

If all attempts to resolve the dispute fail, the son or daughter should side with the spouse—even if not in complete agreement with the spouse's point of view. It is best that the parent be made to understand that this will take place, even *before* a dispute arises.

What are some good rules for older people to follow when they live with their children, and in their contacts with them?

1. If it is obvious that the children genuinely desire their company, then they should not withdraw. Many parents, in an attempt to be obsequious and circumspect, hold themselves much more aloof than their children want them to be.

2. Contrariwise, an older person should not intrude into the social life of his children unless he is asked to participate.

3. Parents who live with their children must refrain from giving unsolicited advice, especially to the grandchildren. Even though the child of the older person might willingly accept such advice, the "child-in-law" may resent it.

4. Parents should do their share of the household chores if they are physically able to do so. They should also contribute financially to the home if they have sufficient means.

5. Parents who live with their children should develop their own social life with people of their own choosing.

6. "Adult children" should be reproached as little as possible for neglect of their parents. Each reproach is usually followed by a longer interval between contacts! It must be remembered that the "adult children" are in the full bloom of their middle years and lead extremely full lives of their own. Their lack of contact does not necessarily indicate lack of love, but perhaps a preoccupation with problems that they must face.

7. Parents should refrain from taking sides when there is a dispute between husband and wife.

8. "Adult children" retain many of their earlier attitudes toward parents, no matter how old they may be. Recognizing this, an aging parent should respond. For example, a wealthy aging parent should offer financial assistance when he knows it is needed. Furthermore, an aging parent should recognize that his children will one day be his heirs and he should, if it is feasible, permit them to enjoy—during his lifetime—the things they will inherit later on.

What steps should be taken when a parent lives with a child and the arrangement is not a happy one?

1. A discussion of existing problems should be held with the parent before difficulties have mounted and attitudes have become fixed.

2. If problems are not readily resolved, and if there are other children, a family conference should be held.

3. If the family fails to come up with an acceptable solution, the family physician, the religious adviser, or a family-counseling agency should be consulted.

4. When harmony within a family unit is threatened, it is up to the parent to make other living arrangements. Nothing is worse for a marital relationship than strife over a mother- or father-in-law. Furthermore, the grandchildren in the home may suffer grave emotional upset from the arguments and conflicts.

Do older people have difficulty in adjusting to new family situations and relationships?

Yes. A characteristic of aging is decrease in ability to adjust to new situations. Older people often forget their own earlier conduct and develop great intolerance toward behavior they once condoned.

Is there a tendency for aging people to become more jealous in their family relationships?

Yes. Although it is difficult to generalize about this, nevertheless it does appear to be true. As people grow older they seem to try harder than ever to hold on to what remains of their family relationships. It should never be forgotten that the answer to jealousy is love.

Should grandparents live with grandchildren if they are invited?

Yes. It is well known that relationships between grandparents and grandchildren are often closer than those between parents and children.

Are there rules for grandparents to follow when they live with grandchildren?

Yes. They must realize that their adult grandchildren are fully capable of leading their own lives and that they are mature, despite their youth. The grandparents must therefore exercise unusual restraint when tempted to give unsolicited advice.

Should a parent who lives with his children permit them to handle his financial affairs?

Usually this is a poor idea, unless the parent is incompetent.

How should one handle the aged parent who can no longer take care of himself?

If he is mentally alert and therefore able to understand his physical problems, a full, frank discussion should be held with him. He should be asked how he wishes his problems solved. Children, no matter how well intentioned, should never make decisions for their parents without first consulting them.

The following questions should be asked of the parent:
1. Do you wish to maintain your own home?
2. Do you wish to move to another home, apartment, hotel, or community?
3. Do you wish to live alone?
4. Is there someone with whom you would particularly wish to live?
5. Can you afford to maintain your own home?
6. Can you afford to hire someone to look after your physical needs at home?
7. Do you wish to go to a nursing home?
8. Do you wish to go to a home for the aged?

Wherever possible, the parent should be allowed to remain in his existing living quarters if they are satisfactory. If new arrangements must be made, a community agency should be consulted. (*See* ORGANIZATIONS AND AGENCIES.)

What agencies should be consulted for advice on dwelling places for older people?

See ORGANIZATIONS AND AGENCIES; INSTITUTIONAL CARE.

Is it wise for older couples who cannot get along with each other to separate, or should they stay together?

All too often, family and friends advise older people to stay together, despite the fact that they make each other miserable and may have within them the possibility of happiness if they separate. Of course, they should do their best to reconcile their differences, but it is poor advice to urge them to remain together merely because they are getting on in years. It should be remembered that the healthy man or woman of sixty can expect to live another fifteen or more years.

FEET

See AMPUTATION; ARTHRITIS AND RHEUMATISM; BACKACHE, BONES AND JOINTS; BURNS AND FROSTBITE; CLAUDICATION; DIABETES MELLITUS; PHYSICAL ACTIVITY AND EXERCISE; SMOKING.

Do older people have increased susceptibility to foot infection?

Yes. Circulation is poorer because of hardening of the arteries in the legs, and foot infection may be a result.

Should people over sixty open a blister, abscess, or other infection in the foot by themselves?

No, they should not even remove a splinter! It is essential that they see a physician in order to prevent spread of infection, which may complicate even the most minor infection.

Is it particularly important for elderly diabetics to take special care of their feet?

Yes, because the average diabetic has more arteriosclerosis and less resistance to infection.

What special care of the feet should older people take?

1. The feet should be kept meticulously clean by daily washing with warm water and a mild soap.

2. After washing, the feet should be dried thoroughly, (particularly between the toes) so that no moisture remains.

3. If there is a tendency to perspire, medicated talcum powder should be used; moist feet are

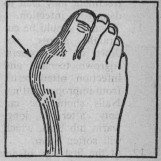

Bunion

more susceptible than dry feet to infection.

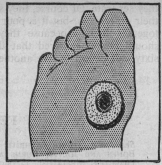

Corn pad for plantar wart

4. Tight garters around the legs or thighs should not be worn. It is harmful to restrict circulation.

5. Older people should avoid standing in one position for long periods of time; for this makes it more difficult for blood in the veins of the legs to return to the heart.

6. Regular daily walks should be taken, unless the doctor has restricted exercise.

7. Avoid walking barefoot. This is the easiest way to pick up a splinter or to get athlete's foot or some other infection.

8. Avoid going out in the rain or snow without rubbers. Damp feet are subject to spasm of arteries that are already arteriosclerotic. This may further impair circulation.

9. Feet should not be permitted to get cold or frozen. Warm stockings, heavy shoes, and overshoes should be worn during the winter months. Frostbite often leads to gangrene.

10. Calluses and corns should be treated by a physician or licensed podiatrist only. Self-treatment may lead to dangerous infection.

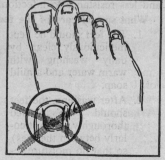

Properly and improperly cut toenails

11. Toenails should be cut straight across, not down in the corners. Ingrown toenails and infection often result from improper cutting. Nails should be cut only after a long, warm tub bath, which will soften them.

12. At the first sign of any discoloration of a toe, a physician should be consulted.

13. Well-fitting shoes should be worn at all times. The feet are so important during the later years that one should spend as much money as necessary for good shoes. Poorly fitting, cheap shoes may cause blisters or pressure points to form, and these may start a gangrenous process.

14. Toes and feet should be rubbed periodically with cocoa butter or lanolin to keep them soft and pliable.

15. If there has been a scratch, cut, or splinter, do *not* use a strong antiseptic such as iodine. This may cause more harm than good by burning the laceration. Cleanse with soap and water; this is a sufficient antiseptic. Then cover the area with a clean bandage.

16. If toes overlap, separate them with a wisp of cotton or lamb's wool.

17. Cotton stockings are better than wool stockings for covering the feet. If it is very cold, wear wool stockings *over* the cotton stockings.

18. Cotton stockings, preferably white, should be boiled every day.

19. If the feet are cold at night, wear socks to bed. Do not use hot-water bottles or heating pads.

What is the significance of swelling of the feet and ankles?

In people over sixty, such swelling may indicate that the heart is not functioning as efficiently as it should. Such a condition is known popularly as "dropsy." The family physician should be consulted in all such cases. However, swelling of the feet does not always denote heart trouble. Constricting garters, excessive heat in tropical climates, varicose veins, sprains, and other conditions may cause the feet or ankles to swell.

What is the significance of a toe or foot that becomes cold and starts to turn blue?

It may mean that an artery has become clogged with a blood clot. It may be a forerunner of gangrene. Immediate medical attention is essential.

What causes the soles of the feet to feel as if they are burning?

Usually it indicates a vitamin deficiency or the onset of a circulatory disturbance.

What is the significance of tingling and numbness in the toes and feet of older people?

This may be a symptom of impaired circulation or it may indicate a vitamin deficiency.

Does the shape of the foot tend to change as one grows older?

Not usually in the sixties. However, those in their seventies or eighties may find that their ligaments become lax and their arches tend to fall. This is another reason why it is so important to buy well-fitting shoes with adequate arch supports.

How can one tell if the circulation of the feet and toes is adequate?

1. There are pulses in the foot just as there are in the wrist. A physician can easily test circulation by noting the presence or absence, and the caliber, of these pulsations. Absent pulses are a sure sign of impaired circulation.

2. Feet with diminished circulation are usually cold. Comparing the temperature of the two feet in a well-heated room will often demonstrate the adequacy or inadequacy of circulation.

3. A physician will have other instruments, such as an oscillometer or a skin-temperature machine, that will accurately gauge the degree of damage to circulation.

4. X rays of the arteries of the legs will also help to show the adequacy or inadequacy of circulation.

Does climate have any effect on the circulation in one's feet?

Yes. People with impaired circulation do not fare nearly as well in cold climates. Warm climates minimize spasm and aid dilatation of blood vessels.

Are foot baths advisable for older people who have painful feet?

Yes, provided there is no impairment of circulation. It can do harm to take hot foot baths when circulation is impaired. Serious burns may result because of decreased sensitivity to the sensation of heat.

Will elevating the feet while in bed improve circulation?

Usually it will aid return of blood through the veins to the heart, but it will not help arterial blood supply to the feet.

Will wrapping feet in warm bandages improve circulation?

In all probability, this does no good. Room temperature with warm socks will do more good.

Are there medications to improve the circulation of the feet?

Yes. Some of these medications will help the arteries to remain dilated.

Are there surgical operations that can improve the circulation to the feet?

Yes. More and more people are being helped by operations to replace arteriosclerotic arteries.

Will the application of hot-water bags and heating pads improve circulation to the feet?

No. Furthermore, they may cause serious burns to feet with diminished sensation.

Should older people wear arch supports for flat feet?

Only if their feet are painful.

What advice should be given to older people about purchasing shoes?

1. Women should avoid high spike-heeled shoes.
2. Women should have leather supporting the sides of the shoes.
3. There should be a rubber pad on the heel.
4. Shoes should not be so pointed that they cramp the toes.
5. Shoes should not rub the heels.
6. Shoes should be well ventilated. Heavy rubber soles may produce excessive perspiration.
7. Slippers should not be worn about the house as a substitute for shoes.

FEMALE ORGANS

See BREASTS; CYSTOCELE AND RECTOCELE; ENDOCRINE GLANDS AND HORMONES; OVARIES; SEX AFTER SIXTY; SEX HORMONES.

What are the normal changes that take place in the female organs after menopause (change of life)?

1. Menstruation stops.
2. The ovaries stop maturing eggs. In other words, ovulation no longer occurs and pregnancy is no longer possible.
3. The uterus decreases in size and its lining membrane thins out.
4. The mucous membrane of the vagina becomes thinner and its cells secrete less mucus. This leads to increased dryness of the vaginal tract.
5. The lips of the external genitals become thinner as they lose some of the fat that lies beneath the skin.

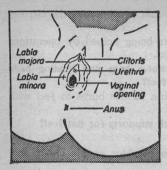

Diagram of normal external female organs

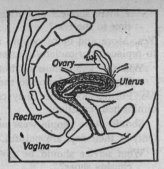

Diagram of normal internal female organs

What is the normal age for the onset of menopause?

This varies considerably from country to country and from
individual to individual. For women living in temperate
climates, the average age for change of life is between forty-
five and fifty-two years. This can vary two or three years in
either direction and still be within normal limits.

**Do women ever continue to menstruate after sixty years of
age?**

No.

**How can a woman know positively that she has passed the
menopause?**

Toward the end of the normal female cycle, menstrual periods
become irregular, either increasing or decreasing in frequency.
When menstruation has stopped completely for a full year,
she can be sure that menopause has taken place.

**Should someone who has not bled vaginally for a full year
seek medical advice if bleeding recurs?**

Definitely, yes.

**What may cause vaginal bleeding in women in their late
fifties or sixties?**

1. An inflammation of the vagina or external genitals.
2. Scratching secondary to itching.
3. A tumor in the cervix.
4. A tumor in the uterus.
5. A malignant tumor in an ovary.

Will taking female sex hormones for several months ever cause vaginal bleeding in a woman past sixty?

Occasionally this will occur. However, it is more common for the bleeding to take place after the hormones have been stopped. This is called "withdrawal bleeding." The bleeding may be due to other conditions, such as a tumor, and not to the sex hormones.

How often should women past sixty undergo a pelvic examination?

A complete pelvic examination is part of the regular yearly medical checkup. However, whenever vaginal bleeding, pain, or discharge appears, a pelvic examination is indicated.

Should a pelvic examination include the taking of a smear?

Yes. The Papanicolaou smear test may reveal the presence of a tumor in the cervix or uterus before any symptoms appear. When this happens, the tumor is in the very earliest stages of its growth and thus can be removed with excellent prospects for complete cure.

Should older women douche?

Yes, if there is discharge or unpleasant odor from the vagina it is good practice for them to douche every second or third day. Douching, if properly done, is not harmful.

Is it natural for older women to have a vaginal discharge?

No. If there is a discharge, a doctor should be consulted.

What may produce vaginal discharge in older women?

1. A fungus infection.
2. A bacterial infection.
3. A vaginal tumor.
4. A prolapse (fallen womb).

What should be used in the ordinary cleansing douche?

Many different ingredients can be used, but a good, safe douche is one or two tablespoonfuls of white vinegar dissolved in one to two quarts of warm tap water.

Do the genitals tend to become dry and itchy in women past sixty?

Yes. This is part of the aging process.

Is it harmful for healthy women over sixty to have sex relations?

No.

What is senile vaginitis?

It is an inflammation of the mucous membrane of the vagina, which is brought on by the changes that accompany the aging process. The cells lining the vagina become thinner, secrete less mucus, and are more likely to become inflamed or infected.

What are the symptoms of senile vaginitis?
1. Itching in the genital region.
2. Discharge, with odor, from the vagina.

Is senile vaginitis common in older women?
Yes, particularly in people in their seventies or eighties.

What is the treatment of vaginal discharge and itching?
It must be determined first that the symptoms are caused only by senile vaginitis. A complete examination, including the Papanicolaou smear test, is performed to rule out the possibility of a tumor in the reproductive tract.

If the vaginitis is due to a fungus infection, antifungal tablets are taken by mouth and local medications are applied. (There are many effective powders, suppositories, and ointments that can control this type of infection.)

If the vaginitis is bacterial in origin, antibiotic medications are often given by mouth and applied locally. Also, medicated douches may be prescribed.

Will taking female sex hormones control senile vaginitis?
Hormones may bring the condition under control for a short period of time, but it will return soon after treatment is stopped. Today, most gynecologists feel that hormone treatment should not continue for more than a few weeks.

Why should an older woman not be given female sex hormones for long periods of time?
Because the hormones might create an artificial situation in which the ovaries would be stimulated to become active again. It is thought, although not proved conclusively, that such ovarian stimulation may contribute to the activation of a dormant tumor. Another reason why prolonged hormone therapy is not generally advocated is that the symptoms of senile vaginitis recur soon after the treatment is discontinued.

Will the giving of cortisone or cortisonelike medications control senile vaginitis?
Yes, for a short time. Again, these medications may have harmful effects if taken too long.

Is itching around the female genital region ever caused by allergic conditions?
Yes. This is a very frequent cause of itching, especially when one is sensitive to nylon, rubber, or other materials. If this is the case, cotton underclothing should be worn.

How common in older women is a bacterial infection in the vaginal tract?

Not very common, even though the membranes are somewhat less resistant to infection as one gets older.

How can one tell if a fungus infection is present?

A smear is made from the vaginal discharge and is placed under a microscope. The fungus can easily be seen by microscopic examination.

How does the physician make a smear to test for cancer?

It is an extremely simple office procedure. The patient is placed in position for pelvic examination; a vaginal speculum is inserted into the vagina; the vaginal wall and cervix are swabbed with a cotton applicator. The cells so obtained are then rubbed onto a glass slide. This procedure produces no pain whatever.

What is then done with the slide?

It is sent to a laboratory, and technicians there will prepare and examine the slide under a microscope.

How can the laboratory tell whether the smear indicates that a cancer is present?

The cancer cells will be seen under the microscope.

Can any laboratory perform these tests?

Yes, but it is much better to send a "Pap" smear to a laboratory that specializes in this type of analysis.

What is leukoplakia of the vulva?

It is a precancerous lesion affecting the skin of the external genitals.

Does leukoplakia always turn into cancer?

No, but it must be watched carefully and biopsies must be made from time to time.

Can measures be taken to prevent leukoplakia from becoming cancerous?

Yes. Surgical removal of the involved areas will control the situation adequately.

Does cancer of the external genitals occur frequently in older women?

It is seen quite often, particularly in women in their seventies or eighties.

How can a woman know if she has cancer of the vagina?

A routine pelvic examination reveals it immediately. Also, the appearance of blood or other discharge, and itching in the area are clues that something is wrong.

Is cancer of the external genitals or vagina curable?

In about 90 percent of cases, if the cancer is detected early enough, it can be cured by surgery. An operation known as *vulvectomy* is performed.

Is the entire vagina removed when a vulvectomy is performed?

Not unless the cancer is very extensive. In most cases only the superficial tissues are removed.

Is it possible for a woman to have sexual intercourse after a vulvectomy has been performed?

Yes, unless the entire vagina has been removed. This operation is done only occasionally for advanced cancer.

PROLAPSE

What is prolapse of the uterus?

Fallen, or dropped, womb.

What is a fallen womb?

It is a condition in which the ligaments and fibrous tissues that hold the uterus in place have become lax and weakened. As a result, the uterus tends to sink down or protrude through the vaginal outlet.

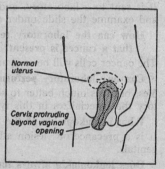

Prolapsed uterus (dropped womb)

How common is prolapsed uterus in women past sixty?

It is a very common condition, although often it causes few symptoms.

How does a woman know if she has a prolapse of the womb?

She will sense that her organs are protruding through the vagina and she will experience a general feeling of discomfort in the area. If it is an advanced case, there may be considerable back pain and difficulty in voiding.

What is the treatment of prolapsed uterus?

1. If it has not reached an advanced state and if the patient is not in her seventies or eighties, medical management should be tried rather than surgery. Treatment

will consist of the insertion of a pessary into the vagina. (A pessary is a ring-shaped plastic substance molded to fit the size of the vagina.) It will help prevent the uterus from descending too far into the vaginal canal.

2. If the uterus protrudes beyond the outlet of the vagina and the symptoms are marked, surgery will become necessary. This usually involves removal of the uterus through an incision into the vagina (vaginal hysterectomy).

How serious is an operation for the repair of a prolapsed uterus?

Today, with greater knowledge of the preoperative preparation of older people for surgery, with improved surgical techniques, and with efficient new safeguards against postoperative complications, operations for prolapse can be performed safely even on those who are in their late seventies or eighties. Of course, the operation is not done on patients who are markedly debilitated or who have serious heart ailments.

Can a woman past sixty have intercourse after surgery for prolapsed uterus?

Yes.

Is it dangerous for older women to wear a pessary?

No.

What precautions should older women take if they wear a pessary?

1. They should make sure that the pessary fits well. There should be no sensation of pressure if it is well fitted. Discomfort when wearing a pessary means that it does not fit properly or has been inserted improperly. A return visit to the gynecologist is indicated in such instances.

2. The pessary should be removed, cleaned, and reinserted every four weeks. This is done to make sure that there is no irritation or inflammation of the vaginal membranes.

3. The patient should take cleansing douches every second or third day, as prescribed by the gynecologist.

4. Any bleeding or discharge from the vagina should be reported to the physician.

What is atrophy of the uterus?

It refers to the shrinking of the muscles that make up the body of the uterus and the thinning out of the membrane that lines the cavity of the uterus. It occurs in all women who have passed the menopause. During pelvic examination, the doctor will note that the uterus is smaller than normal.

Do fibroids of the uterus develop often in women past sixty?
No. It is most unusual for women past sixty to develop new fibroids of the uterus.

If fibroids have been present for many years, what happens to them after sixty?
There is a tendency for them to become smaller, just as there is a tendency for the normal uterine muscle to shrink. However, if they are very large, they will not disappear entirely.

What is the significance of an enlarging uterus in a woman past sixty?
It indicates, in almost all instances, the presence of a malignant tumor.

Will a smear test demonstrate the presence of a malignant tumor in the uterus?
Only in some cases.

Will the material obtained from scraping the lining of the uterus (dilatation and curettage) reveal the presence of a cancer?
Yes, in almost all instances. Wherever there is doubt about the presence of a malignancy, this procedure should be carried out.

Is a smear test effective in detecting the presence of cancer of the cervix?
Yes.

Is a smear test effective in detecting cancer of the ovaries?
Not usually.

What are an older woman's chances for survival after surgery for cancer of the uterus?
Unless the malignancy has already spread beyond the confines of the uterus, approximately 90 percent of all women can be cured of cancer of the uterus.

What are the chances for cure of cancer of the cervix?
The majority of women past sixty can be saved if the cancer is detected in the early stages. As happens all too frequently, by the time it is detected the cancer has already spread to other structures. In such instances, only one out of three can be saved. This is a major reason for all women past menopause to have a pelvic checkup at least once a year.

What changes normally take place in the ovaries of women past menopause?

The ovaries stop maturing eggs. It should be remembered, however, that the ovaries may continue to secrete hormones that help to retain feminine appearance and characteristics.

If older women should lose some of their feminine characteristics and develop a deep speaking voice, should female sex hormones be given?

No. The normal processes of aging should not be disturbed, as there are no adequate methods for reversing that trend. Taking female hormones will not rejuvenate and may, in certain cases, have harmful effects.

What are some of the effects in aging women from taking female sex hormones?

Their breasts may become swollen and painful. They may start to bleed vaginally.

Is it true that taking female sex hormones for long periods of time can actually cause cancer?

This has not been proved. The danger is more that an existing, although dormant, tumor in the female organs will be activated by the stimulating effect of the hormones.

What is the significance of an enlarging ovary in an older woman?

It indicates the presence of a tumor or cyst.

What is done when a tumor in an ovary is discovered in a woman past sixty?

Both ovaries, the fallopian tubes, and the uterus are removed. This operation is not dangerous and will eliminate the possibility of tumor growth in the uninvolved female structures.

Are all ovarian tumors in older women malignant?

No. Some are benign, but all of them are potentially malignant.

What are the warning signs of a tumor in an ovary in older women?

The majority of women may have no symptoms. It is therefore especially important that a pelvic examination be made each year.

Is cancer of the ovary curable?

Yes, if it has not spread to adjacent structures and if the cancer cells have not migrated to the abdominal cavity.

Will radioactive substances, such as radioactive gold and phosphorus, or anticancer chemicals, such as nitrogen mustard, increase the possibility of a cure of cancer of the ovary?

Yes. These substances have been most helpful in certain types of ovarian cancer.

Are there changes in the physical appearance of an older woman after her ovaries have been removed?

None whatever.

FIRST AID

See ARTIFICIAL RESPIRATION; BURNS AND FROSTBITE; CONVULSIONS; EPILEPSY; FAINTING; FRACTURES; GAS AND SMOKE POISONING; INJURIES AND ACCIDENTS; SHOCK.

When should first aid be given?

When a person is suffering from an injury or other condition that demands immediate treatment. It must be clearly understood that first aid is merely a form of emergency treatment until the doctor arrives. If a doctor is not readily available, call the police.

Do first-aid measures for people over sixty differ from those for younger people?

In general, the same principles are followed. It should be understood, however, that the heart and brain of older people are more sensitive to the effects of injury. Therefore, first-aid measures must be carried out more quickly.

Is there a tendency for wounds or lacerations to bleed more profusely in older people?

Yes. Their blood vessels have lost some elasticity and therefore do not contract as readily after they have been severed.

Must special precautions be taken when putting a tourniquet on an older person?

Yes. Their blood vessels are more fragile and can be damaged more easily by a

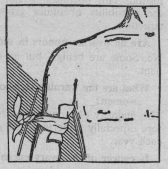

Tourniquet

tight tourniquet. Furthermore, most old people have diminished blood supply in their limbs as a result of hardening of the arteries. They are less able to withstand the temporary shutting off of blood supply that a tourniquet produces. For this reason, tourniquets should be used only when no other method will do and it should be released every few minutes. A tourniquet should be made just tight enough to stop bleeding. This can be judged by slowly loosening it and noting the point at which bleeding barely stops.

What first-aid measures should be taken when someone bleeds or hemorrhages?

1. Have patient lie down flat.
2. Place sterile gauze pad, sanitary napkin, or clean handkerchief directly over the wound.
3. Apply direct, firm pressure (with your fingers or hand) over the wound; continue pressure for 5-15 minutes.
4. If bleeding does not stop with prolonged direct pressure, and the wound is in the arm or leg, apply a tourniquet for 10-15 minutes. Release it to see if bleeding has stopped. If not, reapply tourniquet and transport patient to nearest doctor.
5. Do NOT apply a tourniquet until you have first tried pressure upon arteries supplying the arm and leg. This will often stop the bleeding and make the use of a tourniquet unnecessary. (These pressure points are located on the inner side of the upper arm and just below the groin.)
6. Most bleeding, unless from a major vessel, will stop within a few minutes. Clean wound thoroughly with plain soap and water. If bleeding is too active, apply a tourniquet for 10 minutes in order to thoroughly cleanse the wound.
7. Bandage to stop bleeding should NOT be applied so tightly that it will interfere with circulation. If the patient feels it is too tight, or if the tissue below the bandage turns blue in color, cut the bandage down the middle and apply new bandage material more loosely *over* the original bandage.
8. Take patient to doctor for possible further cleansing and stitching of the wound.
9. Internal bleeding will usually evidence itself by the coughing up or vomiting of blood or "coffee ground" appearing material. Bleeding from the urinary tract will show itself upon passage of bloody urine. Bleeding from

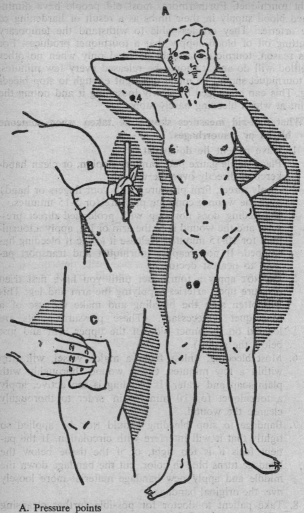

A. Pressure points
   1. To stop bleeding from front of scalp
   2. To stop bleeding from face
   3. To stop jugular-vein bleeding
   4. To stop bleeding from arm and hand
   5. To stop bleeding from thigh and leg
   6. To stop bleeding from leg
B. Tourniquet applied to stop bleeding from arm and hand
C. Diagram showing direct pressure to stop local bleeding

the intestinal tract will show itself by blood in the stool or by passage of black, tarry stools. Have such a patient lie flat and breathe deeply. Transport him as soon as possible to a hospital. Do NOT attempt to give medicines to such patients.

10. Bleeding from areas where tourniquets cannot be applied, such as the neck, should be treated by applying direct finger pressure over the wound. Keep pressure in place until doctor arrives.

Do older people fall more often than young ones?

Yes. It has been estimated that approximately four out of five accidental deaths in the home involve falls by people over sixty-five years of age.

Do older people have a high incidence of hip fractures?

Yes. These are the most vulnerable bones in the body for people in their late seventies and eighties.

What first aid should be given to someone who has suffered a severe fall?

1. No attempt should be made to move the patient until the location of the injury has been determined. As accurately as possible, one should try to determine whether or not a bone is broken. If there is extreme pain, an abnormal contour to the bone, severe tenderness localized to one bony area, and rapid swelling, it is almost certain that there is a fracture. The injured area should be moved as little as possible, since older people tend to go into severe shock if disturbed too much.

2. If an arm or leg has been injured, great care must be taken to straighten it slowly, never forcefully. If it is apparent that there is a fracture, the limb should be splinted to limit motion as much as possible.

3. If the head has been injured, the same first-aid measures should be carried out as for fainting or unconsciousness. (*See* FAINTING; COMA.)

4. If there is injury to the neck, special attention should be paid to the patient's breathing. The chin should be raised from the chest. Artificial respiration should be begun if breathing is difficult. (*See* ARTIFICIAL RESPIRATION.)

5. If the abdomen has been injured, the patient must be given nothing to eat or drink.

6. Most people recover from the ordinary fall within a ten- to fifteen-minute period. If the patient is still unable

to get up and move about after that period of time, it is wise to call the doctor or see that he is taken to a hospital. Transporting an older person after a severe fall requires the use of a stretcher. If none is available, an overcoat, blanket, or sheet can be used. Four people are needed to carry the patient.

What first-aid treatment should be carried out when the heart suddenly stops beating?

Closed-chest cardiac massage should be started at once. The patient should be placed on his back and the first aider kneels and straddles him, with one knee on either side at the level of the patient's abdomen. He then places the flat of his left hand over the patient's breastbone, then takes the palm of his right hand and presses down on his left hand so that the breastbone is depressed about an inch toward the chest cavity. This is done rhythmically, with pressure and release, about sixty to seventy times

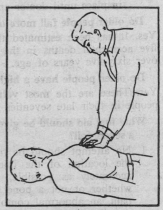

Closed-chest method of cardiac massage applied when heart stops beating

per minute. This procedure should be continued until it is obvious that the patient is reviving. Do not discontinue massage if response is not immediate, for in some cases a heart has resumed beating after 20 to 30 minutes of this type of cardiac massage.

If another person is available, mouth-to-mouth artificial respiration should be given at the same time as the closed-chest cardiac massage.

What first aid should be carried out when a person has a heart attack and the heart continues to beat?

1. The patient should be placed in a semisitting position.
2. Tight clothing should be loosened.
3. If there is difficulty in breathing, artificial respiration should be started.
4. Cardiac patients often know that they are subject to

heart attacks and so they may carry medications with instructions for use. This should be ascertained before starting first-aid measures.

5. The patient should not be moved until instructions to do so have been received from a doctor.

6. Whenever possible, ambulance transportation is best. If it is not available, the patient should be transported in a sitting position. This will make breathing easier. (Four people can easily carry a patient who sits in a chair.)

Can the newer methods of artificial respiration, such as mouth-to-mouth breathing, be used on older people?

Yes.

Are older people more susceptible to heat than younger people?

Yes. Their heat-regulating mechanism does not work as efficiently in the later decades.

What is the first-aid treatment for heat stroke or heat exhaustion?

See Heat Stroke and Heat Exhaustion below.

Should people in their seventies and eighties avoid staying in the sun or in very hot areas because of the danger of heat stroke or heat exhaustion?

Yes. No one in his seventies or eighties should permit himself to be exposed to the sun or hot temperatures for long periods of time.

What are first-aid procedures for specific emergencies?

ANTIDOTES AND EMERGENCY MEASURES FOR POISONING

1. Find the poison container. Most containers of poisonous substances have printed directions pasted on them.

2. If the poisoned person is fully conscious, induce vomiting. This should be done only when the person is not in a stuporous condition and there are no convulsions.

3. When vomiting and retching begin, place the person face down, with head lower than the rest of the body, so that the vomit will not enter the lungs and cause further damage.

4. Save the poison container or some of the vomit for the doctor's inspection. This may help him to decide on the appropriate treatment.

Substances	Procedures*

Acids
  Sulfuric
  Nitric
  Hydrochloric
  Chromic
  Carbolic
	1. Cause vomiting.†
	2. Give milk, raw eggs, jello, gelatin.
	3. Gargle with solution of bicarbonate of soda.

Alcohol	1. Cause vomiting.† 2. Have stomach washed out, preferably at hospital. 3. Keep body warm. 4. Give several cups of black coffee.
Alkalies	1. Give vinegar diluted in water, wine, lemon or apple juice. 2. Cause vomiting.† 3. Have stomach washed out as soon as possible. 4. Give milk.
Arsenic	1. Cause vomiting.† 2. Have stomach washed out at nearest hospital. 3. Give milk.

Barbiturates
  Phenobarbital
  Seconal
  Amytal
  Luminal, etc.
	1. Cause vomiting.†
	2. Have stomach thoroughly washed out as soon as possible.
	3. Apply artificial respiration.‡
	4. Give laxative.
	5. Give strong coffee.

Belladonna (*Atropine*)	1. Cause vomiting.† 2. Give strong coffee. 3. Give charcoal tablets. 4. Sponge body with cold water.
Benzine	1. Cause vomiting.† 2. Have stomach washed out. 3. Give milk.

Botulism
  (*and other*
  food
  poisoning)
	1. Cause vomiting.†
	2. Have stomach washed out as soon as possible.
	3. Give enema with soapsuds and water.
	4. Give large dose of castor oil.
	5. Give charcoal tablets.

Bromides	1. Give strong coffee. 2. Have stomach washed out.
Chloral hydrate	1. Give oxygen. 2. Apply artificial respiration.‡ 3. Give black coffee, strong. 4. Sponge head with cold water.
Cocaine	1. Cause vomiting.† 2. Have stomach washed out. 3. Apply artificial respiration if necessary.‡ 4. Give any available barbiturate, such as phenobarbital, amytal, etc.

*Adapted from "Poisons," a chart compiled by U.S. Vitamin and Pharmaceutical Corp.

†To cause vomiting: 1. Add baking soda or salt to drinking water. 2. Give large quantities of warm water. 3. Put finger in back of throat and tickle.

‡For method, see ARTIFICIAL RESPIRATION.

Substances	Procedures
Copper	1. Cause vomiting.* 2. Have stomach washed out. 3. Give white of egg every 4 hours. 4. Give charcoal tablets. 5. Give milk.
Corrosive sublimate	*See* Mercury poisoning.
Cyanide	1. Cause vomiting.* 2. Have stomach washed out as soon as possible. 3. Apply artificial respiration.† 4. Obtain oxygen from police or fire department as soon as possible. 5. Give strong coffee.
Digitalis	1. Cause vomiting.* 2. Give charcoal tablets. 3. Give small doses of alcoholic beverage. 4. Give tea or coffee. 5. Rest in bed.
Insulin	1. Give sugar or any available candy. 2. Give orange juice, grape juice.
Iodine	1. Cause vomiting.* 2. Have stomach washed out. 3. Give flour or starch in a paste or solution. 4. Give white of raw egg. 5. Give milk. 6. Give bicarbonate of soda solution. 7. Give laxative.
Kerosene	1. Cause vomiting.* 2. Have stomach washed out. 3. Give milk.
Lead	1. Cause vomiting.* 2. Have stomach washed out as soon as possible. 3. Give dose of epsom salts. 4. Give white of raw egg and milk. 5. Give charcoal tablets.
Lysol	1. Cause vomiting.* 2. Give milk. 3. Give raw eggs, Jello, gelatin. 4. Gargle with solution of bicarbonate of soda.
Meat poisoning	1. Cause vomiting.* 2. Have stomach washed out as soon as possible. 3. Give enema with soapsuds and water. 4. Give large dose of castor oil. 5. Give charcoal tablets.

*To cause vomiting: 1. Add baking soda or salt to drinking water. 2. Give large quantities of warm water. 3. Put finger in back of throat and tickle.

Substances	Procedures
Mercury	1. Wash out the mouth with sodium perborate solution or other available mouthwash. 2. Cause vomiting.* 3. Have stomach washed out as soon as possible. 4. Give white of eggs and milk. 5. Give sugar. 6. Give bicarbonate of soda.
Methyl alcohol	*See* Wood alcohol poisoning.
Morphine	1. Cause vomiting.* 2. Have stomach washed out. 3. Give strong tea or coffee. 4. Give charcoal tablets. 5. Apply artificial respiration.†
Mushrooms	1. Cause vomiting.* 2. Have stomach washed out as soon as possible. 3. Give starch or flour paste. 4. Give charcoal tablets. 5. Give strong tea.
Narcotics	1. Apply artificial respiration.† 2. Cause vomiting.* 3. Give strong coffee or tea. 4. Give charcoal tablets.
Nicotine	1. Have stomach washed out. 2. Give any sedative medication available. 3. Give charcoal tablets.
Opium	*See* Morphine poisoning.
Phenol	*See* Acid poisoning.
Phosphorus	1. Cause vomiting.* 2. Have stomach washed out as soon as possible. 3. Give large dose of epsom salts. 4. Give dose of bicarbonate of soda. 5. Do *NOT* give milk or eggs.
Poison ivy or Poison oak	1. Wash thoroughly with soap and water immediately after contact. 2. Wash with rubbing alcohol to relieve itching.
Snake bite	1. Immediate sucking out of wound. 2. Crisscross incision with knife in area of bite. 3. Place tourniquet above the site of the bite. Release every 20 minutes for a few minutes in order to permit some circulation to return. 4. Keep patient as quiet and still as possible.
Strychnine	1. Cause vomiting.* 2. Have stomach washed out as soon as possible. 3. Give any sedative available. 4. Give moderate dose of alcoholic beverage. 5. Apply artificial respiration if breathing is poor.†

*To cause vomiting: 1. Add baking soda or salt to drinking water. 2. Give large quantities of warm water. 3. Put finger in back of throat and tickle.
†For method, *see* ARTIFICIAL RESPIRATION.

Substances	Procedures
Sulfur	1. Apply artificial respiration.†
	2. Give salt water to drink.
Tobacco	*See* Nicotine poisoning.
Wood alcohol	1. Cause vomiting.*
(*methyl alcohol*)	2. Have stomach washed out.
	3. Keep body warm.
	4. Apply artificial respiration if necessary.†
	5. Give strong coffee.
Zinc	1. Cause vomiting.*
	2. Have stomach washed out.
	3. Give white of egg and milk.
	4. Give strong tea.

BITES

Animal or Human Bites

1. Scrub wound thoroughly for 5-10 minutes with soap and plenty of water.
2. Apply a sterile gauze bandage or, if this is not available, use a clean handkerchief.
3. Take patient to a doctor, who may give tetanus antitoxin, tetanus toxoid, or, possibly, antibiotics. If the bite has been caused by a dog, cat, rat, or other animal, your physician may recommend antirabies injections.
4. Do NOT pour strong antiseptics, such as iodine, on a wound caused by a bite.

Insect Bites

1. If a stinger (bee, wasp, etc.) has been left in place, pluck it out. Do so gently, in order to avoid breaking the stinger.
2. If a great deal of swelling is present, this indicates a marked sensitivity to the bite poison. In such cases, place a tourniquet above the bite area so that the poison will be more slowly absorbed.
3. If the bite is caused by an insect that burrows under the skin, such as a chigger, or by one that attaches itself to the skin, such as a tick, wash the area thoroughly with soap and water. A drop or two of turpentine

---

*To cause vomiting: 1. Add baking soda or salt to drinking water. 2. Give large quantities of warm water. 3. Put finger in back of throat and tickle.
†For method, *see* ARTIFICIAL RESPIRATION.

     may dislodge a tick or kill a chigger. Cover with Vaseline so that the insect cannot breathe.

4. Antiallergic (antihistamine) medications may be prescribed by your physician to reduce the swelling and itching.
5. Do NOT scratch a bite area, as that may lead to greater absorption of the poison or to infection.
6. If the bite has been caused by a black widow spider, treat like a snake bite.

Snake Bites

1. Treat all snake bites as if they have been caused by poisonous snakes, unless you are thoroughly familiar with the various types of snakes.
2. A tourniquet should be placed above the site of the bite. Do this immediately.
3. Crossed incisions *through* the skin should be made over the two fang marks. A penknife may be used. Do not wait to sterilize it. The incisions should be ¼ inch long.
4. The bite should be sucked out thoroughly. (No harm can come from swallowing or taking into the mouth the venom of a poisonous snake.)
5. The tourniquet should be loosened every 20 minutes for 2-3 minutes and then reapplied.
6. Suction to the wound should be repeated every 5 minutes for an hour.
7. Have victim lie down and keep quiet, so as to reduce circulation.
8. If ice or running cold water is available, immerse the bitten area so as to reduce circulation.
9. Take victim to nearest hospital so that the appropriate antivenin can be administered.
10. If possible, kill the snake and take it to the hospital so that it can be identified. (A particular antivenin is effective against a specific snake venom only.)

BURNS

1. *First-degree burns* extend only to the top layers of the skin. They can usually be self-treated by applying plain Vaseline or any other mild ointment that soothes the reddened area and prevents the skin from becoming too dry. (Sunburn, without blister formation, is the most common type of first-degree burn.)

2. *Second-degree burns* extend deeper into the skin than first-degree burns but do not involve the very deepest layer, the corium. They can be diagnosed by noting blisters and destruction of the top layers of skin.
   1. Such burned areas should be immediately placed under cold running water for 10-15 minutes and, if dirty, mild (soap) cleansing should be carried out.
   2. A clean, sterile gauze dressing should be applied.
   3. The patient should drink large quantities of fluids.
   4. Blisters should NOT be opened.
   5. The patient should be taken to a physician for further treatment.
3. *Third- and fourth-degree burns* extend to or through all the layers of the skin. First aid should include:
   1. Place area under cold running water.
   2. Gently clean away dirt. If clothes can be removed from the burned area without pulling away tissue, this should be done.
   3. Do NOT put butter or ointments on deep burned areas.
   4. Patients should be given large quantities of fluids.
   5. If patient is in shock, he should be covered with blanket and transported, on a stretcher, to the nearest hospital.
4. *Chemical burns* should be immediately flushed with cold running water to wash away the chemical. Cover the burned area with a sterile dressing. Patient should then be taken to a doctor.
5. *Eye burns* should be flushed with large amounts of water. The eye should then be covered with a sterile dressing and the patient taken to a physician.

CARBON MONOXIDE (GAS) POISONING

Carbon monoxide gas has no odor. It may originate from the exhaust of an automobile or from defective stoves burning wood, coal, or oil.

1. Open all windows and doors to permit fresh air into the area.
2. Start artificial respiration if the patient is not breathing spontaneously or regularly. Continue until a doctor arrives.
3. Encourage deep breathing of fresh air.
4. Keep patient lying down quietly.
5. Keep patient warm.

6. Notify the police or fire department, who will respond with emergency equipment.

CHOKING

1. Encourage coughing.
2. If obstructing object is not expelled, place index finger in mouth and sweep it around back of throat. This may dislodge the foreign body.
3. If the victim turns blue and cannot breathe at all, and if a doctor is not available—*and only when it is obvious that death will ensue*—an emergency tracheotomy may be performed. This is done by stabbing a hole with a knife into the windpipe below the adam's apple. The hole is kept open, so that air can pass in and out of it, by twisting the knife blade.
4. If patient continues to choke but is able to breathe, take him immediately to the nearest doctor or hospital.
5. If the offending object has not been coughed up, take patient to doctor even if the choking has subsided. Some foreign bodies go deep into the bronchial tubes, where they will eventually cause infection.

COLD
(*See below,* Exposure; Frostbite.)

CONVULSIONS

1. Prevent self-injury by protecting the patient, particularly the head.
2. Place patient on the floor or ground and give him plenty of room.
3. Loosen clothing around the neck and lift up the chin so that breathing is unobstructed.
4. If possible, place a folded handkerchief between the teeth to prevent tongue biting. (Keep your own fingers away from patient's teeth to avoid being accidentally bitten.)
5. Do NOT throw cold water on these patients in an attempt to revive them.
6. Do NOT try to restrain their convulsive movements.
7. Most convulsions last only a few minutes. After re-

covery, comfort the patient, keep him quiet, and send for a physician.

8. Do not leave a patient alone after he has emerged from a convulsion, for at least one half hour. (They are often confused and it may take this length of time for them to fully regain their normal mental and physical senses.)

9. Search the patient's clothing for information. Epileptics and diabetics often carry instructions on what should be done for them.

DISLOCATIONS

1. Do NOT try to replace a dislocation yourself.
2. If a doctor is nearby, transport patient with as little movement of the joint as possible.
3. If you are a long distance from a hospital or doctor, bind the dislocated limb with a towel, bandage, etc., so that it does not move.
   a. Gently tie dislocated ankle, knee, or leg to the normal limb on the other side.
   b. Bind the arm, in which there is a dislocation, to the chest and abdomen.
4. If neck dislocation is suspected, firmly pull on head and hold it in a straight position without permitting movement.

DROWNING

1. If patient is breathing, place him on his abdomen with head turned to one side.
2. Do NOT place him over a barrel or attempt to hold him upside down. Water from the lungs will be brought up spontaneously if the patient is breathing.
3. If the patient is not breathing, place flat on his *back*, lift up the chin, and commence artificial respiration.
4. If mouth-to-mouth breathing does not get air into the lungs, it indicates a severe spasm of the larynx. Continued spasm may require an emergency tracheotomy (*see* Choking *above*), *but this should be done by someone other than a doctor only when it is obvious that the patient is not getting air into the lungs and is dying.*
5. Call a doctor or the police or fire department as soon as possible.
6. Continue artificial respiration until a doctor arrives.

ELECTRIC SHOCK

1. Do NOT touch a person who is still in contact with an electric current.
2. Separate electric contact and patient as quickly as possible.
   a. Use a *dry* stick to shove away wire or to move the patient.
   b. Cut off the source of current, such as a live wire, if this is possible, or use an ax with a wooden handle to chop the wire bearing the current.
   c. Do NOT attempt to remove a victim from the electric contact unless your body and hands are dry and you are standing on dry ground or on a dry surface.
3. If victim is not breathing, start mouth-to-mouth artificial respiration. Continue until a doctor arrives.
4. Keep victim warm.
5. Call a doctor or the police or fire department for additional help in resuscitation.
6. Give first aid to any burned area on body. (*See* Burns *above.*)

EXPOSURE TO COLD
(*See also* Frostbite *below.*)

1. Wrap patient in blankets.
2. Place in warm room.
3. Place in tub of warm (not too hot) water.
4. Dry body and place in warm bed.
5. Give warm drinks.
6. Do NOT give alcoholic beverage.
7. If necessary, start mouth-to-mouth artificial respiration.

FAINTING, DIZZINESS, AND VERTIGO

1. Place patient in a lying-down position with face up and head at body level or slightly lower.
2. Elevate legs to slightly above level of rest of body (use pillow, coat, blanket, etc.).
3. Loosen collar or any tight clothing that might interfere with breathing.
4. If breathing is shallow or stops, apply mouth-to-mouth method of artificial respiration.
5. Keep in lying-down position at least 15 minutes after consciousness is regained.
6. Do NOT throw cold water in face.

7. If patient fell during faint, examine head to make sure he did not injure himself.
8. If patient has merely had dizziness or vertigo, do not permit him to arise until the symptoms have completely disappeared.
9. If the fainting, dizziness, or vertigo persists for more than a few minutes, call a physician.

FOREIGN BODIES

Eyes

1. Blink eyelids repeatedly to stimulate flow of tears, which may wash out foreign body.
2. Do NOT rub eye. (This merely makes foreign body embed itself deeper.)
3. Wash out eye by dropping in drops of lukewarm water.
4. Draw down lower lid. If foreign body is embedded in lower lid, take moistened edge of clean handerchief and gently wipe it off.
5. Bend up upper lid. If foreign body is embedded in upper lid, take moistened edge of clean handkerchief and gently wipe it off.
6. If foreign body is embedded in the pupil or in the colored portion of the eye, do NOT try to remove it. See a doctor.
7. If foreign body has been removed, irritation of the eye can be relieved by dropping in a drop or two of mineral oil or castor oil.

Ears

1. No lasting harm can come from a foreign body in the ear. Therefore, do NOT get excited or put a sharp instrument into the ear canal.
2. Have patient lie down and pour in sufficient mineral oil, castor oil, or olive oil to fill the canal. Permit it to stay there a few minutes. This will usually float out or dislodge a foreign body.
3. If foreign body does not come out, take patient to a physician.

Nose

1. Stimulate sneezing by having patient sniff pepper or by tickling the opposite nostril. This will usually dislodge a foreign body.
2. If foreign body is not expelled, take patient to a physician.

Skin

1. Only those splinters that protrude from the skin surface should be removed by nonmedical personnel.
2. Grasp firmly and withdraw slowly so as not to break.
3. Apply peroxide or alcohol to area, and cover with sterile bandage.
4. If splinter breaks off beneath the skin, take patient to a physician. Most foreign bodies become infected if permitted to remain in place.
5. Do NOT try to probe deep into the skin for a splinter. You may spread infection or push it deeper!

FRACTURES AND SEVERE SPRAINS

1. If medical aid is available, do NOT move the patient or the injured part. Permit NO weight-bearing!
2. Do NOT try to push back a broken bone if it protrudes from the skin.
3. Do NOT try to straighten a fracture yourself if a physician can be located.
4. Keep the patient warm.
5. If patient must be moved, *splint* the broken bones before moving:

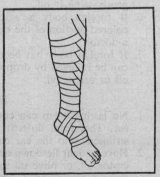

Bandaging

   a. An injured collarbone, shoulder, or arm should be splinted by wrapping the arm securely to the body. Do NOT bend the arm if it is found in a hanging position. If found with elbow bent, then splint it in that position.
   b. Splint fractured leg in a straight position and then tie it to opposite leg, so as to prevent movement.
   c. A cane, umbrella, straight pieces of wood, etc., can be used as a splint. A torn shirt or handkerchiefs can be used as bandage material.
   d. Always pad with something, such as a piece of clothing, between the splint and the injured part of the body.

6. Transport patient in a lying-down position. A blanket or overcoat may be used as a stretcher if several people are available to carry the patient.
7. Give the same first aid to a sprain as you would to a fracture. A layman cannot distinguish between a fracture and sprain.
8. Do NOT apply a tourniquet to limb unless there is uncontrollable bleeding.
9. If the fracture is accompanied by an open wound, cover such wound with a sterile dressing. If this is not available, use a clean handkerchief.
10. Broken neck or back:
    a. Do NOT move patient!
    b. Keep body straight.
    c. Do NOT lift the head or bend it forward!
    d. Keep patient lying down.
    e. If patient *must* be moved, place on stomach and transport on blanket, with head straight for back injury. Transport face up for neck injury.

FROSTBITE

1. Warm the patient gradually (room temperature).
2. Give warm liquids and food.
3. Thaw out frostbitten parts *slowly*.
4. Give medications to relieve pain (aspirin, etc.).
5. Start moving frostbitten part slowly.
6. Do NOT:
    a. Give alcohol to patient.
    b. Immerse frostbitten part in *hot* water.
    c. Rub frostbitten part.
    d. Apply snow.
7. Keep sterile dressing over frostbitten part, as skin may eventually break, leaving an open wound.

GAS POISONING

1. Provide fresh air—open all doors and windows and bring the person to the fresh air. Be careful that there is a minimum of exertion expended.
2. Prevent chilling.
3. Loosen all tight clothing, belts, collars, etc.
4. Keep the person as quiet as possible.
5. Do NOT give alcohol in any form.

6. If the person is unconscious or has stopped breathing, apply artificial respiration.

HEAD INJURIES

1. Have patient lie flat on his back.
2. Keep patient warm.
3. Do not permit patient to get up and walk about.
4. If there has been loss of consciousness, patient should be transported to hospital for further observation.
5. If there is bleeding from an ear, it usually indicates a skull fracture.
6. If there is a cut on the head, apply a sterile dressing or clean handkerchief.
7. Do NOT give alcohol or any medication to relieve headache. This may mask symptoms.
8. Patient must be advised to consult a physician within the few hours after a head injury. Some injuries appear trivial at first but then develop into serious injuries within twenty-four hours.
9. Fractured jaw:
   a. Close the mouth so that the teeth come together as closely as possible.
   b. Tie a handkerchief or scarf so that it circles the head, from beneath the chin to the top of the head.
   c. Permit patient to remain in a sitting position.
   d. Urge patient not to attempt to move the jaw or to talk.

HEART ATTACK

1. Do not move patient!
2. Keep patient in semisitting position.
3. Open collar, loosen tie and belt.
4. Encourage deep breathing.
5. Give patient medication that he may have in his possession (if he has had previous attacks).
6. If heart stops beating, use "closed-chest method" cardiac massage:
   a. Place patient flat on back.
   b. Kneel and straddle patient.
   c. Place heel of palm of right hand on patient's breastbone.
   d. Place left hand over your right hand and push down so that breastbone is depressed about one inch.

    e. Release.

    f. Repeat this every 1-2 seconds for at least 10 minutes or until heartbeat and breathing are resumed.

    g. If someone else is also available, have him render mouth-to-mouth artificial respiration at the same time as you are conducting cardiac massage.

7. Do not permit a patient who has obviously undergone a heart attack to move until he has been examined by a physician. (Pains that have subsided may return with greater intensity if the patient is allowed to exert himself.)

HEAT STROKE AND HEAT EXHAUSTION

1. Get patient out of the sun or out of the hot place.
2. Place him in cold water or, if that is not possible, keep pouring cold water over him.
3. Wrap in cold wet sheets or towels.
4. Give cold water to drink (4-5 glasses).
5. Give ½ teaspoonful of ordinary table salt with water every half hour for 3 or 4 doses.
6. Give an enema with iced water.
7. Keep patient quiet.
8. Call a doctor.

LACERATIONS (CUTS), ABRASIONS, AND CONTUSIONS

1. If you are giving first aid, wash your own hands before touching someone's laceration or abrasion.
2. If possible, place injured part under running, tepid tap water for 5 minutes.
3. With absorbent cotton or sterile gauze, wash out wound for 5 minutes with soapsuds, using any plain soap.
4. If this is done, dirt and pieces of clothing will become dislodged. Wipe away any remaining dirt or clothing.
5. A deep abrasion (scratch or scrape) occurring in dirt or cinders must be scrubbed thoroughly to remove all visible dirt particles. This should be carried out, even if painful, in order to avoid subsequent infection, such as tetanus (lockjaw).
6. Most superficial wounds will stop bleeding spontaneously unless a large blood vessel has been severed. If marked bleeding and spurting continue, apply a tourniquet above the wound. Be sure to release it every 15 minutes.

7. Cover wound with sterile gauze or clean handkerchief. Apply direct, steady pressure to stop bleeding.

8. Do NOT pour alcohol, iodine, or other strong antiseptics on an open wound! Soap-and-water cleansing is much better as a safeguard against infection!

9. If tissues beneath the skin can be seen through the open wound, it is usually an indication that suturing (stitching) will be necessary. Take patient to a surgeon or nearest physician.

10. It is particularly important to get medical care for cuts and abrasions that originate outdoors, in dirty areas. Such wounds are more prone to infection. Wounds incurred in fields where cattle, horses, etc., are present, should be watched for tetanus. Tetanus antitoxin or toxoid is usually given in cases where wounds have resulted from possibly contaminated objects.

11. A severe contusion (bruise) should be treated by the application of steady pressure with the hand over the injured area. Ice or cold water should be applied for 20 minutes at a time, with a similar period of withdrawal of the application. Bruises more than a few hours old can no longer be helped by cold applications. Raise the injured part, such as a leg, to body level so that there will be less tendency for blood to gravitate to the area.

12. Pain, redness, heat, swelling, or pink streaks leading away from a lacerated area are indications that infection has set in. See a doctor!

NOSEBLEED

1. Place patient in a sitting position.

2. Pack the bleeding nostril with a piece of clean absorbent cotton.

3. If there are nosedrops handy, moisten the packing with a few drops, as this may help to contract the bleeding vessel.

4. Exert firm finger pressure against the bleeding nostril for at least 10 minutes.

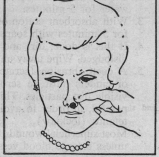

Method for controlling nosebleed

5. Have patient bend head slightly forward during this maneuver. This will prevent blood from trickling down the throat.
6. Leave cotton packing in place for 2-3 hours.
7. If bleeding does not stop, take patient to a doctor, who will cauterize the bleeding point.
8. If bleeding is coming from the back part of the nose (only about 10 percent of cases) the above first aid will not help. Take such people to physicians as soon as possible. Do NOT panic; nosebleeds do not cause healthy people to hemorrhage seriously.

POISONING (Gas)
(See Carbon Monoxide Poisoning above)

POISON IVY OR POISON OAK

1. Wash the skin thoroughly with soap and water immediately after contact.
2. Wash with rubbing alcohol to relieve itching.

RADIATION EXPOSURE

1. Get out of the radiation area as quickly as possible.
2. Cleanse all parts of your body in soap and water. Wash over and over again.
3. Discard all clothing and all other objects that were with you in an exposed area.
4. Contact the local authorities for further instructions.

SHOCK*

1. Place the patient on his back with his feet at a higher level than his head.

*The diagnosis of shock can be made by noting the following symptoms and signs:

1. The skin is gray, cold, and sweaty.
2. There may or may not be loss of consciousness.
3. Pulse is weak and rapid.
4. Breathing is rapid and shallow.
5. Pupils of the eyes are dilated.
6. Patient is excessively thirsty.
7. If conscious, patient is apprehensive and frightened.

2. Loosen any tight clothing.
3. If there is active bleeding contributing to the shock, measures should be taken to stop it (*see* pp. 271–73).
4. Keep patient warm but do not overheat.
5. If there is severe pain (one of the greatest causes of shock), medication should be given as soon as possible to relieve it.
6. If there is a fractured bone (a frequent contribution to shock), it should be splinted and immobilized at once.
7. If it can be ascertained positively that there has been no abdominal injury and that the cause of the shock does not have anything to do with abdominal organs, then warm fluids may be given.
8. Do NOT give alcohol, tea, or coffee!
9. Transport patient in lying-down position to the nearest hospital.

STAB WOUNDS; PUNCTURE WOUNDS

1. Move the patient as little as possible.
2. If the stabbing object (a knife or pick) can be withdrawn easily, do so. This may prevent further injury to tissues when the patient moves.
3. Note carefully the angle and depth of the stabbing object so that you can report it accurately to the attending physician.
4. If the wound is in the chest and air is being sucked into and blown out of the chest, cover the opening tightly. It can be plugged best with a sterile gauze dressing and adhesive tape.
5. Stop active bleeding (*see* pp. 271–73).
6. If any internal organs are protruding through the wound, cover them with a sterile gauze dressing or a clean handkerchief.
7. Stab wounds always require expert care. Take patient to a doctor, who will, in most instances, give tetanus antitoxin or toxoid.
8. Small puncture wounds should have their edges spread so as to promote some bleeding and prevent the sealing in of dirt, rust, etc.

SUFFOCATION OR STRANGULATION

1. Place patient in open air or open all windows.

2. Loosen anything tight around the neck, chest, and abdomen.
3. Lift up the chin to improve airway.
4. Wipe away any secretions that may have collected in the mouth.
5. If foreign body is lodged in the throat, turn patient upside down and strike sharply on the back.
6. Put index finger in mouth and try to sweep out any foreign body that may be stuck in back of throat.
7. Encourage deep breathing and then a forceful cough.
8. Employ mouth-to-mouth breathing (*see* ARTIFICIAL RESPIRATION).
9. Summon police or fire department, who will respond with pulmotor and oxygen.

TOOTHACHE

1. Apply a hot-water bag or ice bag to the side of the face, whichever gives most relief.
2. Take aspirin or other pain-relieving medications.
3. Call your dentist. You *will* be able to reach him at night if you try.

UNCONSCIOUSNESS

1. If patient is not breathing but has a pulse or heartbeat, employ mouth-to-mouth breathing (*see* ARTIFICIAL RESPIRATION).
2. Search the patient's clothing. You may find information that he is a diabetic, epileptic, heart patient, etc.
3. Keep patient lying flat on back with chin up.
4. Loosen tight clothing.
5. Check for possible head injury or bleeding.
6. Summon ambulance by telephoning the police.
7. Give nothing by mouth.
8. Do NOT throw cold water in face.
9. Keep patient warm. Cover with coat or blanket.
10. If patient is convulsing, try to place folded handkerchief between teeth. Be careful that you are not accidentally bitten.

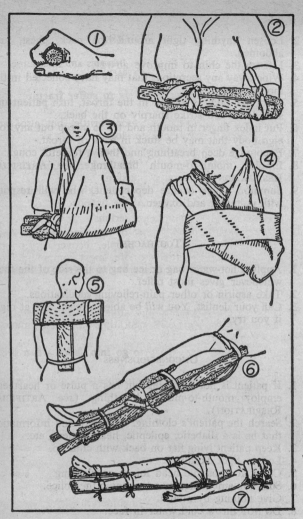

Methods for splinting fractures

Splints
1. Bandage roll in hand for broken fingers or hand bones (metacarpals)
2. Splints of scrap wood padded with towels for broken forearm
3. Broken forearm supported by a sling
4. Sling and band for broken collarbone or dislocated shoulder
5. "T" board for broken collarbone
6. Splint of scrap wood or tree limbs padded with towels and bound with handkerchiefs and belts
7. Splints for severe back injury or high thigh break or broken pelvis

FRACTURES

See BONES AND JOINTS; FIRST AID; INJURIES AND ACCIDENTS;
REHABILITATION AND PHYSICAL THERAPY.

Are people over sixty more likely to suffer fractures than younger ones?

Yes. Not only are their bones more brittle, but also their reactions to impending injury are slower.

What are the two major types of fractures?

1. Simple fractures, in which the broken fragments have not broken or penetrated the skin.
2. Compound fractures, in which the skin is cut and fragments have burst through to the outside.

Are compound fractures more serious?

Yes, because there is great danger of infection with an open wound. Bones, especially in older people, recover very poorly from bacterial infection. Furthermore, most compound fractures require surgery, whereas many simple fractures can be set by manipulation only.

What is the desired goal in the treatment of all fractures?

To get the broken fragments into alignment and to see that solid healing takes place, with restoration of normal function and appearance.

Are older people more likely to go into shock when there is a fracture?

Yes. For this reason, it is essential to give first aid quickly and to get the patient to the nearest doctor or hospital as soon as possible.

Do broken bones heal more slowly in people over sixty?

Yes, because there is usually less calcium in their bones. In addition, the muscles and tendons surrounding the broken bone have less recuperative power.

What extra measures should be taken to promote healing of fractures in older people?

1. If the patient has a vitamin or mineral deficiency, tablets or injections should be given to supplement the usual intake of these chemicals.
2. Calcium tablets may be given if a blood analysis shows the amount of this chemical to be low.
3. If the patient is anemic, iron and other blood-building medications should be given.
4. Many older people will benefit from hormone injections given during the period of bone healing.

5. If the patient is undernourished, every encouragement should be given him to maintain a high-calorie diet.

6. If the patient is diabetic, it is important to see that the disease is well controlled.

7. If there has been a compound fracture, in addition to the usual measures, large doses of antibiotics should be given until it is certain that infection is under control.

If open surgery is necessary to set a fracture, can an older person withstand such an operation?

Yes. Naturally, an older person's reaction will be more severe. Furthermore, greater care must be exercised in placing metal supports to the fractured fragment. Older people often have greater difficulty in encapsulating (covering over with fibrous tissue) foreign bodies, such as metal plates, nails, wires, etc.

Should older people be kept in bed longer after a fracture?

No. The opposite procedure should be followed. It is very important that they get up and about quickly, and that they are hampered as little as possible by heavy casts.

Why is it so important that an older person move about quickly after his fracture has been set (reduced)?

This is essential for the following reasons:

1. Inactivity in bed predisposes one to form blood clots, with the potential danger of embolism (*see* EMBOLUS AND EMBOLISM).

2. Inactivity in bed predisposes one to pneumonia and other lung complications.

3. Older people tend to lose muscle tone more quickly, and inactivity will markedly prolong the period of rehabilitation.

4. The more active the patient, the quicker the healing.

Should older people exercise during the time they are forced to remain in bed with a fracture?

Yes, definitely. Bed exercises are essential to prevent stiffening of the unaffected joints and to maintain muscle tone in the uninjured limbs.

What are some of the bones most susceptible to fracture in older people?

The hip (fracture of the neck of the thighbone is the most

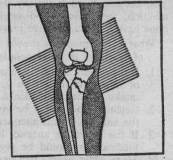

Diagram showing badly shattered tibia

common fracture in people in their seventies, eighties, and nineties); the wrist; skull; spine; ankle; pelvis.

Are fractures of the hip serious?

Yes. First of all, they may be followed by numerous complications, such as pneumonia and embolism. Secondly, they often lead to permanent deformity, with resultant limitation of walking.

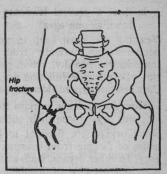

Fractured hip, one of the most common sites of fractures in older people

Are hip fractures treated by long periods of bed rest and immobilization in a cast?

No. A metal pin is hammered through the neck of the fractured bone to hold it in place and the patient gets out of bed in a day or two. Casts are not applied.

What are the usual lengths of time for recovery from fractures in older people?

1. Hip bone—1 year
2. Wrist bone—3 months
3. Skull fracture—2 months
4. Spine fracture—6 months
5. Ankle fracture—6 months
6. Pelvic fracture—4 months

Is it usual for older people to require exercises, baths, heat therapy, and other forms of treatment after the fracture has healed?

Yes. They will usually require extensive physical therapy and rehabilitation. (*See* REHABILITATION AND PHYSICAL THERAPY.)

FUNCTIONAL CHANGES WITH AGING

See ANATOMICAL CHANGES IN ORGANS; DEGENERATIVE CHANGES OF AGING; LONGEVITY; NERVES; PREMATURE AGING.

Does the function of an organ change during one's lifetime?

Generally speaking, no. The organ's function remains the same, but the ability to perform that function may be somewhat modified with aging. For example, the heart's function is to pump blood throughout the body; this function begins before birth and continues throughout life.

Is there a general tendency of all body functions to slow down as one ages?

Yes, but one must keep in mind that the age at which this occurs varies markedly from person to person. There are innumerable healthy, active people in their sixties and seventies whose organs function normally and whose body metabolism has not slowed down appreciably.

How does science explain the different rates at which various organs lose their ability to function normally?

Some organs are thought to lose efficiency of function because of fatigue from overuse. The heart falls into this category. In other organs, such as the brain, function may become impaired because of insufficient blood supply secondary to hardening of the arteries. In this connection it should be pointed out that the brain cells themselves might be perfectly capable of functioning normally if the supply of blood and oxygen were adequate. Other structures may lose their ability to function because of injury, infection, tumor growth, or undernourishment.

Is it true that people who take good care of themselves during their early and middle years have a much better chance for their important organs to maintain normal function during their later years?

Yes. This is absolutely true.

Does a strenuous physical life cause functional decline to take place prematurely?

If one lives a life of excess, in which various parts of the body are abused, these structures will certainly show early decrease in function. However, when one works strenuously but sensibly, the physical exertion will not lead to premature loss of function.

How important is heredity in determining the age at which one shows evidences of functional changes?

It is thought to play an extremely important role. People whose parents retained good vision, hearing, heart action, and other functions well into their seventies or eighties have a very good chance of doing the same. If in addition to a healthy background the individual lives a sane, sensible life, the chances are that his structures will function better and longer than those of his forebears. It should not be forgotten that good hereditary factors can be more than counterbalanced by a life of stress, disease, and indiscretion.

What role does emotional tension play in the onset of functional changes?

It is thought that a life of stress may lead to disturbed body function. When the time comes that an organ can no longer react normally to stress, function failure results. The phenomenon is seen particularly in such vital glands as the pituitary, thyroid, and adrenals. One of the keys to a healthy old age is the ability to handle the strains and stresses of youth and the middle years.

If one knows in his younger years that there is a defect or weakness in a structure or organ, can special care be taken to prevent early impairment of its function?

Yes. For example, the young man or woman who has hepatitis or jaundice with impaired liver function should always avoid diets rich in fat and excessive drinking of alcoholic beverages. Similarly, the person who has had tuberculosis in his youth should never work too strenuously or ignore even the most minor respiratory infection. Extra care can preserve weakened organs so that they will function satisfactorily throughout life.

One often hears that within another century the average life-span will be increased to one hundred years. Does this mean that new methods will be devised to prolong the functional capacity of organs?

Not necessarily. Most organs *in health* are capable of functioning efficiently for one hundred years. The trouble is that undue stress, arteriosclerosis, injuries, and diseases shorten their functional capacity. If a time comes when we can control arteriosclerosis and eliminate certain stresses, injuries, and diseases, then our vital organs may be able to function normally for one hundred years or more.

Can anything be substituted for organs that have stopped functioning?

Fortunately, as one ages the demands made by the body on the organs diminish. Thus, it is no longer necessary for the ovaries or testicles to secrete certain of their hormones; the thyroid is not called on to manufacture such large quantities of its hormone; the muscles are required to do less strenuous work. When there is a need for increased function, artificial means can be found to supply it. Thus, for example, ovarian, testicular, thyroid, and adrenal hormones can be prescribed to make up for the inactive glands; braces and supports can be worn to aid failing muscles.

Can medical treatment improve the function of a failing organ?

Yes, but its efficacy will depend greatly on the cause of functional failure. If an organ is injured or overworked and begins to falter, rest may restore it to normal. If the inability to function is due to inadequate oxygen and blood supply, this condition can be improved by giving specific medications to correct faulty circulation. If the trouble originates from an infection, antibiotics may overcome the difficulty and permit normal function to be restored. If an organ suffers because of malnutrition or vitamin or mineral deficiency, it will be helped by adequate diet and by taking the appropriate vitamins and minerals.

Can surgery help to improve the function of an aging organ?

Yes. Tremendous advances in this field have been made within the past decade. Frequently, when functional loss is secondary to impaired blood supply, blood-vessel surgery may be effective. The brain, liver, kidneys, and lower extremities can all benefit from blood-vessel grafts and transplants.

When the function of an organ is impaired because of an ulcer or tumor, normal function can often be restored by surgical removal of the ulcer or tumor.

FUNGUS INFECTIONS

See DERMATITIS; FEET; FEMALE ORGANS; INFECTIONS; SKIN.

Do fungus infections occur frequently in older people?

Yes, particularly since so many antibiotic drugs are in general use. It has been found that antibiotics, most of which are ineffective against fungi, kill off many of the bacteria that normally inhibit the growth of fungi. For example, when a powerful antibiotic is taken by mouth, many of the bacteria that normally live in the intestinal tract will die, and the fungi will therefore grow and multiply.

Where are the common sites for fungus infections in older people?

In the corners of the mouth, around the genitals, in the vaginal canal, in the intestinal tract, between the toes, in the groin, and between folds of the skin, where perspiration accumulates.

Are any medications helpful in combating fungus infections?

Yes. Great strides have been made in the treatment of these stubborn infections. New substances containing such ingredients as griseofulvin, fulvicin, and mycostatin have been most helpful in eradicating fungal infections. Some of these substances are applied locally; others are given orally.

Is the repeated application of soap and water helpful in treating fungus conditions?

If the patient is unclean the fungus infection will thrive. However, soap and water does very little good once a fungus infection has taken hold.

How are fungus infections in the vaginal tract treated?

By various douches, powders, and suppositories. There are now many effective medications that will clear up these infections (trichomonas), although they do have a tendency to recur.

Are fungus infections between the toes particularly serious in older people?

Yes, because of the poor circulation in the feet that sometimes exists, secondary bacterial infection is more likely to set in. Such infections (e.g., athlete's foot) must be treated promptly by a physician to ward off the possibility of gangrene.

GALLBLADDER AND BILE DUCTS

See Hepatitis; Jaundice; Liver; Pancreas.

Is the gallbladder capable of functioning normally throughout the entire life-span?

Yes. There is no evidence that a healthy gallbladder loses its ability to function merely because of age.

Is there an increase in the incidence of gallbladder disease and gallstones in people over sixty?

Yes.

What causes this increased tendency to develop gallbladder disease in older people?

1. It is thought that an upset in cholesterol metabolism takes place in most people as they age, and that this imbalance is often associated with the formation of gallstones.
2. Other factors that contribute to an increased incidence

of gallstones are alcoholism, obesity, and the sedentary habits people develop in their later years.

What is the incidence of gallstones in people past sixty?

Recent estimates show that approximately one out of three women and one out of eight men have stones in their gallbladder by the time they reach sixty years of age.

Do gallstones form after sixty years of age?

Yes. Many people who have been X-rayed for stones in their late fifties and have shown none will show them when X-rayed several years later.

Can gallstones and gallbladder disease be demonstrated by X ray?

Yes. The procedure is as follows:

1. Pills containing an opaque dye are swallowed the night before the X-ray examination. When the patient is X-rayed, the next morning, the dye will be seen filling up the gallbladder. If stones are present, they will appear as negative shadows in the gallbladder.

2. To see the gallbladder and the bile ducts, the patient's veins are injected with an opaque dye; X rays taken soon after will show this dye in the gallbladder and bile ducts.

3. In certain cases of gallstones, they block the entrance to the gallbladder. The gallbladder will therefore not admit the dye and X rays will not show up the gallbladder. Failure of the gallbladder to be seen on X ray after taking of the dye is proof that it is inflamed and probably contains stones.

Do many older people have gallstones without symptoms?

Yes. It is estimated that approximately 50 percent of persons past sixty who have gallstones will have no symptoms. Knowledge of their presence is gained by a gallbladder X-ray examination.

Are there medications that will dissolve gallstones?

No. Charlatans have made great sums of money selling drugs that supposedly will dissolve stones. No such medication exists.

What are the most common symptoms of gallbladder disease?

1. Severe colicky pain in the upper abdomen, more often on the right side beneath the ribs. This pain may spread to the back or around the right side of the abdomen or to the region of the right shoulder blade. These excruciating episodes of pain come on suddenly and last an hour or two before subsiding.
2. Discomfort in the upper abdomen after eating.
3. Inability to digest fried foods, foods containing large quantities of fat, raw fruits, and raw vegetables (particularly those in the cabbage family).
4. Belching, heartburn, nausea, or vomiting.
5. Chronic constipation.
6. In some cases a gallstone passes out of the gallbladder and enters the main bile duct; jaundice, chills, and fever will then develop.

Is the colic associated with gallbladder disease ever mistaken for a heart attack?

Yes. The pain is sometimes so high up in the abdomen that it is felt beneath the breastbone and a heart attack is suspected.

Is it thought that there is a connection between the symptoms of gallbladder disease and heart symptoms such as angina pectoris?

Yes. Some physicians think that angina pectoris may be associated with gallbladder disease. Although this has not been proved, it has been noted that in certain cases the removal of a diseased gallbladder relieved heart symptoms.

Can people over sixty be X-rayed for gallbladder disease without danger?

Yes.

Is it just as easy to make a diagnosis of gallbladder disease in older people as it is in younger people?

Not always. Occasionally, a patient in his seventies or eighties may have a severe infection of the gallbladder without developing the usual symptoms of fever, abdominal pain, tenderness, and muscle spasm. There are cases on record in which the process has proceeded almost to the point of rupture or gangrene without the doctor's having made the diagnosis.

Is acute inflammation and infection of the gallbladder a common occurrence in older people?

Yes. One of the dangers of permitting gallstones to go untreated in the earlier years is that there will be a serious acute inflammation of the gallbladder in later life, when the patient is less able to overcome it.

What usually causes an acute inflammation of the gall-bladder?

One of the stones gets caught in the narrow cystic duct that leads from the gallbladder to the bile duct. When this happens, circulation to the gallbladder may be shut off and gangrene may result. In other cases, the impaction of a stone in the small cystic duct will cause the gallbladder to become infected and to fill with pus.

Does an acute inflammation of the gallbladder in someone past sixty always produce symptoms as described above?

No. Unfortunately, occasionally older patients may have a gangrenous gallbladder or one that is about to rupture because of an acute inflammation without the development of characteristic symptoms. In some, the temperature remains normal and there is only slight tenderness in the abdomen.

What type of person is most susceptible to gallbladder disease?

One who is stout, drinks large quantities of alcoholic beverages, eats large quantities of fatty and fried foods, and leads a sedentary life.

Do gallstones ever pass into the intestinal tract and obstruct the intestines?

Yes, although this is rare. In these instances the stone must be at least as large as a hen's egg; the walls of the gallbladder and intestines become ulcerated, allowing the stone to break through. Its passage is usually obstructed just before it reaches the large bowel.

Do older people with gallstones ever develop cancer of the gallbladder?

Statistics show that approximately 1 percent of people who have had gallstones for a number of years will develop cancer within the gallbladder. This is a potent argument in favor of removing all gallbladders containing stones.

It is interesting to note that cancer of the gallbladder is rarely found in an organ that does not contain stones.

Is cancer of the gallbladder curable?

This is one of the least curable types of cancer.

Should all people past sixty with gallstones but without symptoms be submitted to surgery?

No. This decision must be made according to the individual circumstances by the physician and surgeon.

1. If the patient is in good health and between the ages of sixty and seventy, it is perhaps best to remove the gall-

bladder even though there are no symptoms. The mortality for this type of operation is less than one-half of 1 percent, and the chances for developing cancer of the gallbladder are about 1 percent.

2. If the patient is beyond seventy years of age and in good health, it is perhaps wisest to treat him medically, rather than submit him to surgery.

When is a gallbladder operation absolutely essential no matter what the age and general condition of the patient?

1. When jaundice is present and does not recede within a period of a week to ten days.
2. When there are evidences of gangrene of the gallbladder.
3. When there is evidence of an acutely inflamed gallbladder with pus in it.
4. When there have been repeated attacks causing great pain and the general condition is thought to be deteriorating because of the recurring attacks.

Can people over sixty tolerate gallbladder surgery as well as younger people?

Not quite. The mortality rate for healthy people in their thirties, forties, and fifties is considerably less than for those over sixty.

Can physicians tell if jaundice is caused by gallstones or by some other condition?

Yes. Many blood and urine tests will distinguish among the various types of jaundice. It should be stated, however, that whatever the cause of the jaundice, if it is caused by an obstruction of the bile ducts, surgery will be necessary.

Is surgery on an older jaundiced patient more serious?

Yes. This is one reason why it is best to operate on all healthy people with gallbladder or bile-duct disease before they have reached sixty.

In an operation for gallbladder disease in older people, is the gallbladder always removed?

The surgeon usually will remove the entire organ. In the occasional case in which the general condition is so precarious that life is in danger, he may elect merely to open the gallbladder, remove the pus and stones, and insert a drain into it. A second operation for removal of the gallbladder may have to be performed at a later date, when the general condition of the patient has improved.

What are the possible complications from not operating on an older patient who has gallstones?

Statistics vary, but most physicians and surgeons agree that considerably more than half of those over sixty who have had gallstones for a long time will eventually develop serious complications if they are not operated on. These complications may be:

1. A stone may become jammed in the cystic duct, at the base of the gallbladder, causing acute infection or gangrene.
2. A stone may pass from the gallbladder into the bile duct and cause jaundice.
3. One out of a hundred untreated gallstones cases will develop cancer of the gallbladder.
4. A large stone may break through the gallbladder into the intestinal tract and cause obstruction.
5. Liver inflammation and damage culminating in cirrhosis may result from untreated gallbladder disease of many years' duration.
6. Malnutrition and anemia may result from inability to eat because of gallbladder disease.
7. Repeated attacks of pain and colic will predispose one to heart attacks, especially older people.

Should people past sixty receive special preoperative care before gallbladder surgery?

Yes. It is important that the internist and the surgeon co-operate to see that the preoperative general health of these patients is as good as possible. Special care should be taken to support the heart; and special tests should be performed prior to surgery to ascertain the state of liver and kidney function. If these organs are not functioning satisfactorily, special measures should be taken to aid them before gall-bladder surgery is undertaken. It is particularly important to support liver function preoperatively by giving large quantities of sugar, protein, and vitamins.

Are complications following gallbladder surgery more fre-quent in people past sixty?

Yes. This is a decisive factor in a physician's or surgeon's decision to remove a diseased gallbladder when the patient is still young.

Can older people return to their normal activities after removal of the gallbladder?

Yes. They must, however, continue to be careful of their diet.

What are good dietary rules for those who have gallbladder disease?

1. Do not eat a large meal at any time. It is much better to eat four or five small meals than three large meals.
2. Avoid foods rich in fat.
3. Avoid fried foods.

4. Avoid raw fruits and raw vegetables, particularly the skins. Vegetables such as radishes, pickles, cabbage, cauliflower, brussels sprouts, turnips, and lettuce may be particularly indigestible.

5. Avoid drinking large quantities of alcoholic beverages.

6. Avoid condiments and spices such as horseradish, pepper, mustard, chili, and hot sauces.

7. Avoid rich pastries and pies.

Is the normal life-span affected by the removal of the gallbladder?

No. One can live a perfectly normal life without the gallbladder.

Once the gallbladder has been removed, do gallstones ever form again?

Rarely do new stones form in the bile ducts after the gallbladder has been removed. In such cases another operation may be required to remove the newly formed stones.

What medical regimen should people follow who have gallbladder disease?

1. A diet low in fat, fried foods, raw fruits and vegetables, spices, and alcoholic beverages is best.

2. If the patient is overweight, he should reduce.

3. Bile salts may be given to promote better bile drainage from the gallbladder.

4. If there is an acute inflammation of the gallbladder but surgery is inadvisable because of poor general health, massive doses of antibiotics should be given to control spread of infection.

5. Antispasmodic medications should be given to relieve attacks of colic due to gallstones. If these medications do not relieve the attack, it may be necessary to give a strong narcotic.

6. If vomiting causes dehydration, the patient should be hospitalized and fed and medicated intravenously.

7. Older people should not be given strong laxatives if they suffer from gallbladder disease. If mild laxatives do not work, an enema should be given.

Can people during their middle years prevent the onset of gallbladder disease when they get older?

The following are effective to a certain extent:

1. If there is disturbance in cholesterol or thyroid metabolism, it should be actively treated. People so afflicted are more likely to develop gallbladder disease.

2. If people are overweight, they should reduce and stay thin.

3. People should continue to avoid foods rich in fats and cholesterol.

GAS AND SMOKE POISONING

See ARTIFICIAL RESPIRATION; FIRST AID.

Are the effects of gas or smoke poisoning more severe in older people than in younger ones?

Yes, because most of these poisons interfere with the oxygen-carrying capacity of the blood. Since older people may require larger quantities of oxygen to keep the heart, lungs, brain cells, and other vital organs functioning smoothly, they will suffer severe damage from oxygen deprivation.

What first-aid measures should be carried out for victims of gas poisoning?

1. The source of the poison gas should be shut off and the patient should be exposed to fresh air.
2. If the gas is indoors, he should be taken outside.
3. If the fumes are outside, he should be brought indoors and the windows closed tightly.
4. The patient should be covered with blankets to keep him warm. (Gas poisoning predisposes one to pneumonia.)
5. If breathing has stopped, artificial respiration should be started immediately. (*See* ARTIFICIAL RESPIRATION.)
6. Loosen tight clothing—collars, belts, etc.
7. Call the police immediately. They will respond with an emergency squad and a pulmotor with oxygen.

If someone has stopped breathing because of gas poisoning, how long should artificial respiration and other first-aid measures be continued?

Until a doctor decides that the patient is dead.

How soon after spontaneous breathing has resumed can artificial respiration be discontinued?

When breathing has become deep and regular, usually 12 to 20 respirations per minute.

How long may unconsciousness last after exposure to gas poisoning?

Anywhere from a few minutes to several hours, depending on the length of time of exposure to the gas and the type of gas that was inhaled.

Is it common for older people who recover from gas poisoning to have mental changes?

Yes. Serious damage to the brain sometimes follows gas poisoning and it may be several days, weeks, or months before full recovery takes place. Some people may never regain their full mental faculties.

If the cause of the poisoning was an attempt at suicide, the person must be watched very carefully, since there is a tendency to repeat the act.

Can smoke, smog, or other fumes created by chemical decomposition in the air seriously affect older people?

Yes. It has been shown that people in their seventies and eighties may suffer severely from breathing smoke or from living in a polluted atmosphere. Every attempt should be made to transfer them to a place where there is clean, fresh air, free of smog or the products of industrial smoke. Smoke poisoning is particularly injurious to the very aged, who already may suffer from marked limitation of lung and respiratory function.

Should those exposed to smoke poisoning, fume poisoning, etc., be given oxygen?

Yes. They should either be placed in an oxygen tent or be given oxygen through a mask.

GASTRITIS

See ALCOHOL AND ALCOHOLISM; STOMACH AND DUODENUM; ULCERS OF STOMACH AND DUODENUM.

What is gastritis?

An inflammation of the lining of the stomach.

What are the various types of gastritis?

1. *Acute gastritis.* This is an acute inflammation with swelling and congestion of the lining membrane of the stomach secondary to dietary indiscretion, eating spoiled or infected food, or drinking excessive amounts of alcoholic beverages. Such a case of gastritis usually lasts for several days and then subsides. Severe cases may be accompanied by weakness and dehydration. Other symptoms of acute gastritis include pain in the upper abdomen, nausea, and vomiting, sometimes with blood.

2. *Chronic gastritis,* which is either *atrophic* or *hypertrophic.*

a. In atrophic gastritis there is thinning of the mucous membrane lining the stomach and degeneration of the cells that secrete gastric juice and hydrochloric acid. This type of gastritis is seen in cases of pernicious anemia. It is thought that the lining of the stomach normally secretes a hormone that is necessary for the development of red blood cells and that this hormone is not produced in a stomach with atrophic gastritis.

b. Hypertrophic gastritis is a chronic condition in which there is swelling and congestion of the mucous membrane lining of the stomach. This may cause recurring pain in the upper abdomen, indigestion, and nausea with vomiting of blood.

Does the stomach tend to secrete less acid as one ages?

Yes. This is characteristic of the later years. It is estimated that more than 25 percent of all people over sixty-five secrete no hydrochloric acid.

Can an older person live a normal life despite the fact that his stomach no longer secretes hydrochloric acid?

Yes. Approximately 10 percent of people of *all* ages have no hydrochloric acid in their gastric juice. The great majority of them lead perfectly normal lives with normal digestive functions. If indigestion appears in individuals who have stopped secreting acid, the necessary amounts of acid can be supplied artificially by taking drops of dilute hydrochloric acid by mouth. The acid is mixed with milk, fruit juice, or any other liquid.

What causes atrophic gastritis?

The cause of this condition is not known. It is recognized, however, that when people have atrophic gastritis they tend to secrete little or no hydrochloric acid. Also, people with chronic atrophic gastritis seem to have a great tendency to develop cancer of the stomach.

What causes hypertrophic gastritis?

Although the exact cause is unknown, it is recognized that chronic alcoholism and chronic abuse of the stomach through repeated dietary indiscretion may lead to chronic hypertrophic gastritis.

Does bleeding or ulcer formation often complicate cases of hypertrophic gastritis?

Yes, vomiting of blood and the formation of ulcers in the stomach are seen in a great number of cases of hypertrophic gastritis.

What is the treatment of gastritis?

1. This depends on the type. Acute gastritis requires relatively little treatment beyond temporary withdrawal of food and taking large quantities of milk and antacid medications. The acute inflammation will subside within a few days if the patient does not eat, and is kept at rest.
2. No treatment will cure chronic atrophic gastritis. If the patient develops pernicious anemia in conjunction with atrophic gastritis, he can be helped by prolonged therapy with liver extract, vitamin B_{12}, and other substances to control the anemia. These patients must be observed carefully over the years, by repeated X-ray examination, to ensure early detection of cancer of the stomach.
3. Many cases of chronic hypertrophic gastritis can be helped by eliminating the irritants that have contributed to its onset. High on the list is the elimination of alcoholic beverages. People suffering from hypertrophic gastritis should eat a bland diet, with no spices or condiments. They should also be given medications to reduce the amount of stomach secretions and medications to reduce and neutralize the secretion of acid.

GLAUCOMA

See BLINDNESS; EYES.

What is glaucoma?

It is a disease in which the pressure within the eyeball is increased. If this increased tension becomes great, it may lead to irreparable damage to the eye and resultant blindness.

How common is glaucoma?

It is estimated that approximately 3 percent of all people over sixty will develop glaucoma. Fortunately, many of those who do will have a mild form of the disease, which can be held in check by use of appropriate eyedrops.

What causes glaucoma?

The underlying cause is unknown. The symptoms occur because of the inability of the fluid within the eyeball to drain out of the eye at a normal rate. Farsighted people are more prone than nearsighted people to develop glaucoma.

What are the symptoms of glaucoma?

Simple glaucoma has very few symptoms. One of the early

symptoms is the appearance of halos around lights. There may also be pain and a sense of fullness in the eyeball.

If there are no symptoms in the early stage of simple glaucoma, how is a diagnosis made?

When people visit their eye doctor, as they should at least once a year, he will test reactions of the pupils and tension within the eyeball and will map out the field of vision to see if there are blind spots. An increase in tension in the eyeball plus a limitation of the visual field indicates that glaucoma is present or is developing.

What is a tonometer?

It is an instrument that measures the pressure of the fluid in the eyeball.

Does glaucoma usually involve both eyes?

Yes, if it goes untreated. As a rule, it develops in one eye first. If the other eye is treated regularly, it may never develop glaucoma.

What is the treatment of glaucoma and how successful is it?

The great majority of glaucoma patients can be treated successfully by medication if they have the simple type of the disease. Pilocarpine drops or drops of a similar drug are placed in the eye to keep the pupil constantly contracted. This will permit excess fluid to exit from the eyeball. Glaucoma patients should try to avoid emotional upset and should limit their fluid intake.

What is the surgical treatment of glaucoma?

When it has been established that medical treatment will no longer restrict the pressure in the eyeball to a safe level, surgery is advisable. The operation consists of cutting a hole in the anterior chamber of the eyeball to permit the fluid to drain out under the conjunctiva (the thin membrane covering the white of the eye).

Is surgery effective in preventing blindness when glaucoma has developed?

Yes, if the surgery is performed before blindness has already occurred. However, if the glaucoma has already resulted in blindness, surgery may not help.

Does acute glaucoma differ from chronic glaucoma?

Yes. In the acute form of the disease there is abrupt onset of pain in the eye, headache, marked reduction in vision, redness of the eye, nausea and vomiting, dilatation of the pupil, and a greenish reflex on shining a light into the eye. Chronic glaucoma, on the other hand, develops over a period of months or years. Many times the patient is unaware that something is wrong until the disease is well advanced.

Does treatment of acute glaucoma differ from that of chronic glaucoma?

Yes. Unless the acute symptoms subside within a few hours, immediate surgery is necessary to save the sight. A piece of iris (the colored portion of the eye) is removed in order to permit fluid to escape from the anterior chamber of the eye. This operation is called an iridectomy.

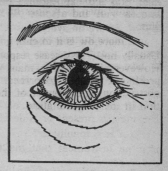

Iridectomy for glaucoma

How successful is surgery for acute glaucoma?

If surgery is performed before loss of vision has persisted for more than a few hours, about 90 percent of the operations are successful.

How successful is surgery for chronic glaucoma?

If performed before extensive damage has been done to the optic nerve and to vision, most operations are successful.

Is it necessary to use eyedrops to keep the pupils dilated even after successful surgery for glaucoma?

Yes.

GONORRHEA

See Cystitis and Interstitial Cystitis; Prostate Gland; Syphilis; Urinary Bladder and Urethra.

Are older people just as susceptible to gonorrhea as younger people?

Yes, if they are exposed to it. There is no such thing as immunity to gonorrhea. Of course, the incidence of this disease in people in their sixties, seventies, and eighties is very low, since sexual contact is reduced.

If a woman past menopause did develop gonorrhea, would it tend to spread to the uterus, fallopian tubes, or ovaries?

No. When the disease is contracted by an older woman, the germ tends to limit its area to the vagina and bladder.

Does gonorrhea produce the same symptoms and signs in older men as it does in younger men?

Yes.

Is it more difficult to cure gonorrhea in an older person?

Usually not. The disease responds well to the antibiotic drugs. However, if an older man who already has an enlarged prostate contracts gonorrhea, it may lead more readily to obstruction of the outlet of the bladder or to abscess formation in the prostate gland.

GOUT

See ARTHRITIS AND RHEUMATISM; BONES AND JOINTS; DIET.

What is gout?

A metabolic disorder in which an excess of urates is produced by the body. These urates are deposited in and around bones, joints, the kidneys, the skin, and other tissues.

Is gout commonly seen in people over sixty?

Yes, although younger people may develop it.

What are some of the symptoms of gout?

Excruciating pain and redness and swelling in the vicinity of a joint. An attack of gout usually comes on suddenly without warning.

What areas are most frequently involved in gout?

The toes (especially the big toe), feet, ankles, hands, wrists, and the sacroiliac joints.

How does the physician make a diagnosis of gout?

He notes the symptoms listed above; in addition, he will have a blood chemistry taken. A person with gout will show an abnormal amount of uric acid circulating in his blood.

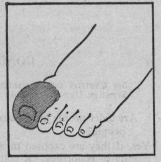

Gout of big toe

What tends to bring on an attack of gout?

1. Overeating, particularly of rich foods and those with a high purine content. (See DIETS.)

2. Drinking large quantities of alcoholic beverages.
3. Emotional upsets.

How long does an acute attack of gout usually last?

From two days to two weeks. It subsides completely, but it may recur several weeks or months later if the patient fails to stay on his diet or if he discontinues his medication.

What is the treatment of gout?

There are many medications that relieve the symptoms of an acute attack and several drugs that will keep the uric acid down to nearly normal levels. However, the long-range treatment of gout involves strict adherence to a prescribed diet and avoidance of alcoholic beverages and foods rich in purine.

HAIR

See DERMATITIS; PREMATURE AGING; SKIN; TRICHIASIS.

Can anything be done to prevent loss of hair as one ages?

In most people, loss of hair is a natural accompaniment of the aging process. However, if a scalp infection is contributing to the loss of hair, clearing up the infection will delay the onset of balding.

Why is it that men lose their hair and women do not?

It is not true that women do not lose their hair as they age. Of course, they lose it in smaller quantities and usually do not become bald. Although there is no exact explanation for the difference, it is thought that hormonal secretions play a major role.

Will giving female hormones to a man prevent balding?

No.

What are the natural changes in hair as one ages?

1. Hair on the head tends to become brittle, falls out readily, and turns gray.
2. Hair in the nostrils, on the eyebrows, and in the ears increases in quantity and becomes bristly.
3. In women, hair on the upper lip and chin grows longer and thicker.
4. There is graying of the hair on the rest of the body, with a tendency toward thinning.
5. The hair loses its sheen and appears dull.

Does graying of the hair indicate that other body structures are also aging?

As one advances in years all body structures grow older. But graying hair does *not* give a clue as to the aging process in vital organs. Many healthy, vigorous men and women have gray hair in their twenties or thirties and show little or no signs of aging.

Does premature graying of the hair indicate that the life-span may be short?

Absolutely not. People who have gray hair early in life have as much chance of living to a ripe old age as anyone else does. Conversely, people with no gray hair may show marked signs of aging in their fifties or sixties.

What causes hair to turn prematurely gray?

This is often a familial characteristic. In certain families every member is gray by the age of thirty. In other families, hair retains its natural color far into the seventies.

Can vitamins prevent the onset of gray hair?

No. It is thought, however, that a marked vitamin B deficiency may lead to premature graying. In such cases, giving large doses of vitamin B may slow down the process.

Are hair dyes harmful?

Not those that contain only vegetable dyes. However, one should consult a skin specialist before using a particular dye in order to make sure that it contains no harmful ingredients. Of course, they are harmful insofar as their repeated use will dry out the hair and make it brittle.

What precautions should one exercise in the use of bleaching agents and dyes?

1. It must be determined that they contain no arsenic or other potentially harmful ingredients.
2. They should be applied with careful attention to instructions, since some of these agents may cause serious burns of the scalp if improperly used.
3. It is always best to have these agents applied by professionals rather than to attempt self-application.

Is there any truth to the expression that someone's hair "turned gray overnight"?

There have been instances reported in which people have supposedly turned gray within a few days. This phenomenon is usually attributed to a great shock or great grief. However, there is no scientific basis for this, and in all probability the change is not nearly as abrupt as one thinks.

Can older people prevent excessive growth of hair on the face and body?

No. These are natural changes that take place as one ages.

What can older women do about excess hair on the face?

1. It should be shaved or plucked out. It is not true that cutting or shaving hair will make it grow in thicker or grow back more rapidly!
2. If the superfluous growth is not too extensive, it can be removed by electrolysis. This procedure should be carried out only by a licensed electrolysist. Removal of hair with an electric needle is an effective and harmless, although sometimes painful, procedure.
3. If the older woman does not wish to have either of the above procedures performed, she can dye the excess hair a light blond so that it will be less noticeable.

Should older women wear wigs or transformations if they have lost a great deal of hair?

Yes, if they are able to afford them. Nothing makes a woman feel quite so old as loss of hair on the head.

Can hormones make hair grow back again?

No. Moreover, it is unwise to take hormones for this purpose.

Will the giving of male sex hormones to women cause hair to grow on their faces and bodies?

Yes. In certain cases of female gland imbalance, breast or ovarian tumors, etc., large, repeated doses of male sex hormones are given. Hair will form only when three or more injections a week are given over a period of several weeks or months. Such hair should be cut or shaved.

When the hormone treatments are discontinued, the hair will disappear.

HEADACHE

See ARTERIOSCLEROSIS; BLOOD PRESSURE; TIC DOULOUREUX; VERTIGO AND DIZZINESS.

Are migraine headaches common in older people?

No. It is a condition afflicting primarily young adults and those in their middle years.

What is the significance of headache in older people?

1. Early-morning headaches, usually in the back of the head, are common in older people with high blood pressure.
2. The development of recurrent headaches in those who have not suffered from them previously is a signal to look for some new, organic disease.

What are some causes of recurrent headaches in older people?

1. Recurrent headache may be a warning that a stroke is imminent.
2. Headache may be due to hardening of the arteries, with insufficient blood reaching the brain.
3. Headache may be caused by an infection in the sinuses, the ears, or the teeth.
4. Headache may be caused by neuralgia or neuritis involving one of the cranial nerves.
5. Headache may be secondary to an allergy or sensitivity to a vapor that has been inhaled or a food that has been eaten.
6. Headache may be brought on by constipation.
7. Headache may be secondary to poor kidney function, with impending uremia.
8. Headache can be caused by emotional upset.
9. Headache may be secondary to overeating or drinking excessive alcoholic beverages.
10. Headache can be the result of eye strain.
11. Headache is an early symptom of brain tumor.
12. Headache may be associated with an infection such as encephalitis, meningitis, or syphilis.

Should people who suffer from recurrent headaches seek medical advice?

Most certainly, yes. The physician will conduct a thorough examination to determine the cause of this distressing symptom. In some cases the source of the trouble can be located readily; in others it may require extensive search, with many tests, such as electroencephalography, spinal puncture, X rays, blood-pressure determination, electrocardiography, blood and urine tests, and others.

Are headache-relieving drugs such as aspirin and codeine just as effective for older people?

Yes. And they can be used without fear of hurting the heart or causing addiction.

If the headaches can be relieved readily with medication, is it still necessary to consult a physician?

Yes, if the episodes recur. It is poor practice to give pain-relieving drugs over and over again without uncovering the underlying cause of the headache.

Do all people with high blood pressure get headaches?

No.

What is the treatment of recurrent headaches?

This will depend entirely on the cause. Naturally, it is of little benefit to give pain-relieving drugs to someone suffering from a serious disorder.

HEALTH INSURANCE AND HOSPITAL INSURANCE

See INSTITUTIONAL CARE; NURSING HOMES; ORGANIZATIONS AND AGENCIES; SOCIAL SECURITY BENEFITS.

Are there nonprofit or commercial health-insurance companies that will insure people over sixty years of age?

Yes. Some policies are now being written specially for those over sixty-five. The policies are limited somewhat in their benefits; therefore the prospective purchaser should read the exclusions very carefully.

Are most health-insurance policies for older people all-inclusive?

No. Many of these policies exclude coverage for preexisting illnesses and conditions. Also, many do not give benefits for some of the chronic diseases so prevalent in older people.

What is the best type of health insurance for older people to buy?

Whenever possible, they should buy the service type insurance. This means that for a single premium all or most medical care is paid for. In these plans (such as HIP in New York and the Kaiser Plans on the West Coast), there is little fee-for-service. The patient pays his premium and is entitled, with few extra charges, to medical care from general practitioners and specialists in the doctor's office, in the home, and in the hospital. At the present time, many insurance companies limit the number of older people they will insure, since older people utilize benefits approximately twice as much as those in their early or middle years.

Should people over sixty-five cancel their present hospital insurance or medical insurance policies?

Not necessarily. It is a good idea for them to discuss the matter thoroughly with the agent or insurance carrier through whom they obtained their coverage. Some hospital insurance policies taken out through commercial or nonprofit carriers may supplement the Social Security hospital insurance, thus obviating all monetary obligations on the part of the beneficiary. Similarly, medical insurance policies currently in force may afford the beneficiary coverage sufficient for all doctor bills.

Will people over sixty-five be forced to use doctors selected by the Federal or State Government?

No. Free choice of physicians will exist.

Will physicians accept the payment schedule of the Social Security medical insurance program as "payment in full" for services rendered?

Not necessarily. The new medical insurance program merely pays a set amount of money to the beneficiary for each type of service rendered by a physician. It is entirely up to the individual doctor whether he wishes to accept this amount as full payment.

Are hospital facilities utilized to a greater extent by people who are sixty-five years of age or older?

Yes. It is estimated that they require approximately three times as much hospitalization as those who are in their middle years. This is one of the reasons why the so-called Medicare hospital insurance program was put into effect.

Are most people over sixty-five able to afford private hospital insurance?

No. Statistics show that the average American over sixty-five has an income less than half that of individuals in their forties and fifties. And their need for hospitalization is approximately three times that of younger people. Thus, the new Medicare hospital insurance program is essential to enable them to afford semi-private accommodations in hospitals.

Will people over sixty-five have to take a physical examination before being accepted for the new federal hospital insurance?

No. All individuals over sixty-five, no matter what their present state of health, will be entitled to this coverage.

Are existing health and hospital insurance benefits under the Kerr-Mills federal law still in effect?

Yes. Some of them will be expanded greatly under new arrangements which are yet to be concluded between the Federal Government and the participating states. (*See* the SOCIAL SECURITY MANUAL.)

Are older people entitled to health and hospital insurance or other medical care under existing federal laws?

To a limited extent, yes. A federal law (Kerr-Mills) provides matching funds in those states that have medical-care programs for the indigent aging over sixty-five. At present, more than thirty states participate in this program to varying degrees. In some states, only hospital benefits are provided; in other states, more extensive medical-care programs have been instituted.

Up-to-date information on the latest legislation and benefits can be obtained by contacting local Social Security offices or by writing:

U.S. Department of Health, Education, and Welfare
Social Security Administration
Baltimore, Maryland 21203

What are the existing laws governing medical benefits for veterans who are over sixty years of age?

Medical care is available to all veterans in Veterans Hospitals, regardless of age. Under special circumstances such benefits might also be accorded to the families of veterans, but this is not the general rule.

For specific information, contact the local Veterans Administration.

HEARING AND DEAFNESS

See INJURIES AND ACCIDENTS; SPEECH.

Does hearing tend to decrease as one gets older?

Yes. Natural changes include a slight progressive decrease in the acuteness of hearing, beginning as early as the thirties.

This loss in hearing progresses slowly with each succeeding decade; it is usually limited to the high tones and does not appreciably interfere with normal hearing.

How can one tell if there has been a slight hearing loss?

An audiometric test will measure the loss. This simple procedure can be carried out in a few minutes by the ear specialist.

How accurate is the audiometer?

It is a very accurate instrument and can measure hearing loss to a very fine degree. Periodic audiometric readings will show if the loss is stable or if it is progressive.

How often should healthy people over sixty have their hearing checked?

Once a year.

Does a collapse, or blockage, of the eustachian tube, which leads from the back of the throat to the ear, often result in hearing loss?

Yes. Air from the throat is transmitted through these tubes to the middle and inner ear. When they are collapsed, or clogged with mucus, loss in hearing results. Many people experience this phenomenon when they have a bad cold or throat infection or when they descend rapidly from a high to a low level.

Can the eustachian tubes be cleared and hearing impairment thereby relieved?

Yes. Patients can often be taught a simple procedure for clearing the eustachian tubes. On the other hand, if the tubes are blocked because of infection, the condition must be treated by an ear specialist.

How can one clear the eustachian tubes?

Take a deep breath, hold the nostrils tightly closed, close the mouth tightly, and then forcefully expel the air from the lungs. This will force some of the expelled air up into the blocked tubes. This procedure should be carried out only on a doctor's advice.

Do most people past sixty retain hearing sufficient to perform the usual daily tasks?

Yes. Despite the natural hearing loss, most people past sixty retain hearing sufficient for normal living.

What is the incidence of deafness in people over sixty?

It is estimated that 10 percent of all people have hearing loss sufficient to interfere with normal living. In people past sixty, it is estimated that approximately *one out of four* has a hearing loss that might be categorized under the general heading of deafness.

Does hearing often improve as people advance in age?

No. Hearing may remain the same throughout life, but it rarely improves spontaneously.

What are some of the common causes of deafness in older people?

1. The most common cause of deafness is degeneration of the auditory nerve (the eighth cranial nerve), which transmits the sound impulse from the inner ear to the brain. A reliable gauge of the aging process is loss of efficiency and deterioration of this nerve.
2. Changes within the cochlea (the sense organ within the inner ear), with replacement of its normal cells by fibrous tissue.
3. Otosclerosis is an extremely common cause of deafness in older age groups. In this process the bones surrounding the middle and inner ear tend to become hardened and overgrown; this will result in interference of the transmission of sound waves.

Does deafness always occur in both ears simultaneously?

No, but conditions that initiate loss of hearing in older people do tend to affect both ears. Usually, hearing loss occurs in each ear at different times and in different degrees.

Can anything be done in the younger years to prevent deafness later on?

Yes. The following care of the ears in youth and in the middle years will help:

1. Ear infections should be treated immediately. A great number of people become deaf because of neglect of an ear infection incurred early in life.
2. The maintenance of a good level of general health is important in the preservation of hearing. If one has been anemic throughout life or has ignored chronic infections of the teeth, tonsils, etc., damage to the ears may result.
3. People who work in factories where there is extremely loud noise or who are exposed to repeated explosions should protect their ears by plugging the external ear canals.
4. It is almost too obvious to state, but people should never pick at their ears or put hairpins, toothpicks, etc., into their ear canals. Often eardrums have been injured and infections have resulted, with permanent hearing damage, from this practice.
5. People who have temporary impairment of hearing should seek medical advice promptly. Many ear conditions can be remedied if discovered during their early stages.

324   Health in the Later Years

What is a fenestration operation?

It is an operation performed to relieve deafness in patients in whom there has been disease and damage to the bones of hearing (the incus, stapes, and malleus). A hole is drilled in the bone within the ear canal, permitting sound waves to bypass the damaged middle ear and to reach the inner ear.

What is a stapes-mobilization operation?

It is an operation to relieve deafness in which the stapes, a small bone of hearing, is freed of adhesions and manipulated so that it will vibrate normally.

When is a fenestration operation or mobilization-of-the-stapes operation beneficial to older people?

When the hearing loss has been caused by a condition in the middle ear. These procedures will not be very helpful if deafness has been caused by degeneration of the auditory nerve, which extends from the inner ear to the brain.

How successful are operations for the restoration of hearing?

If the operation has been performed on a patient whose underlying condition can be helped through surgery, four out of five will result in improvement. Most of the failures occur in operations on people whose deafness is caused by nerve degeneration, and therefore poor candidates for surgery.

Are the beneficial effects of these operations permanent?

In four out of five patients who have been helped, the improvement is permanent. However, some of the remaining 20 percent (in whom deafness returns) can be helped by another operation.

Are operations for deafness safe for older people?

Yes. Recovery from the operation itself always takes place, even when hearing is not improved.

Is hearing impairment ever caused by the accumulation of wax in the ear canals?

Yes. A visit to a physician will reveal such a condition. Removing the wax is a simple procedure, and is often accompanied by immediate restoration of hearing.

People should never attempt to clear their own ear canals of wax, since this may seriously injure the eardrums.

Are ear infections common in older people?

Not nearly as common as in children or young adults. When they do occur, however, they are likely to be of a more serious nature.

Is it safe for older people with ear infections to travel by airplane or to visit places of high altitude?

Such trips should be postponed until the infection has subsided since the infection may spread to the mastoids.

Is ringing in the ears a common symptom in older people?

Yes. This condition, known as tinnitus, may be caused by otosclerosis, collapse of the eustachian tubes, disturbance in the inner ear, upset in salt metabolism, or, occasionally, by a tumor of the auditory nerve.

What is the treatment of ringing in the ears?

This depends entirely on the cause. The important thing to remember is that recurrent ringing in the ears requires medical attention.

Is impairment of the sense of balance (equilibrium) due to disturbance in the inner ear?

Yes, in the great majority of cases. It often indicates that there are degenerative changes in the cochlea and in the nerve that originates in the inner ear and goes to the brain.

Is dizziness or vertigo ever a sign of ear trouble?

Yes. It may be due to a disturbance in the cochlea and inner ear.

What can be done to correct recurrent dizziness or vertigo?

If the condition is associated with the so-called Ménière's disease, in which the salt metabolism is upset, then a salt-free diet may relieve the dizziness. If the dizziness is caused by an ear infection, antibiotics may clear it up. If the dizziness is caused by high blood pressure, medications to lower the pressure may relieve this symptom. If the vertigo is caused by arteriosclerosis of the blood vessels that supply the ear, various medications to dilate these vessels may be helpful. If the vertigo is secondary to anemia, it may be relieved by correction of the anemia.

Should deaf people wear hearing aids?

Yes. Not only will these aids improve hearing of sounds in the great majority of cases, but they will protect the wearer against possible injury or accident. Few people, including some deaf people, realize how dependent they are on their hearing for protection.

Can any type of hearing aid be used?

Yes, but individual tastes will vary. It is characteristic of people with impaired hearing to experiment with different types of

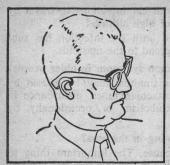 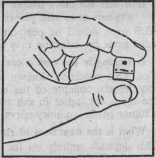

Eyeglasses with attached hearing aid   Small hearing aid that fits into ear
Courtesy of Sonotone Corporation

instruments. What is best for one person may not suit another at all.

Some people get excellent results with the hearing aids that are attached to eyeglasses; others find the type that plugs into the ear and utilizes a small transistor apparatus most satisfactory; the majority of people still prefer the conventional type of instrument, which is attached by a wire to a battery.

Should deaf people consult their ear specialist about their hearing aids?

Yes. It is always wise to have one's ear specialist approve the choice of hearing aid.

Can older people learn lip-reading?

Yes, but it may take them a little longer than it takes young people. It is sensible for those who have progressive hearing loss in their middle years to learn how to read lips early so that they will have the knowledge when they need it later.

Can anyone learn lip-reading?

Yes, if he has a competent instructor and if those who live with him at home will help him to master the rules of lip-reading.

Where can one find out about hearing aids and lip-reading?

Ear specialists will advise one on these matters, as will special agencies set up for this purpose. (*See* ORGANIZATIONS AND AGENCIES.)

Is it important for the family, friends, and coworkers of deaf people to follow certain rules of lip-reading?

Yes. Often those who surround the deaf person are unaware

that they play an essential role in the lip-reading process. Here are some good rules for them to follow if they really want to be helpful:

1. They should not shout. This often interferes with the deaf person's ability to read lips.

2. They should move their lips naturally when addressing a deaf person. Artificial lip movements, although well intentioned, distort things for the lip-reader.

3. They should keep their hands away from their mouths and should look directly at the deaf person when they speak.

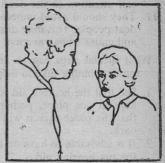

Proper way to address a deaf person

4. They should avoid addressing a deaf person when the sun or a bright light is shining in his eyes. This may make it impossible for him to see the speaker's lips.

5. They should not mumble or whisper.

6. They should not approach the side of the deaf person and shout in his ear.

7. They should address the deaf person only when he has full view of the speaker's face.

8. Those addressing a deaf person should avoid speaking when others are speaking.

9. The radio or television should be turned off when speaking to a deaf person.

10. They should discreetly inform strangers about the deaf person's hearing loss. Many deaf

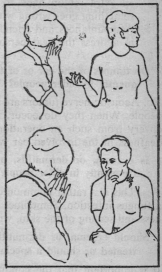

Incorrect way to address a deaf person

people will not let others know of their impairment. On the other hand, if the deaf person has a satisfactory hearing aid, or if he is a good lip-reader, it is better not to call attention to his deafness.

11. They should avoid unnecessary gestures when addressing deaf people. This may draw the attention of other people and cause embarrassment to the deaf person.

What special steps can an attendant, companion, nurse, or family member take to help an older person who is deaf?

1. See that the hearing aid is always available. It should be kept in one place, perhaps by the bedside at night, so that the older person will not have to hunt for it in the dark.

2. It is advisable to have on hand one or two extra batteries for the hearing aid.

3. It is important to see that the older person gets into the habit of taking his hearing aid with him wherever he goes. Also, an extra supply of essential parts should be available.

4. If the older person can afford it, it is a good idea to have an extra set on hand to be used as a substitute when something goes wrong with the hearing aid.

5. Acquaintances and friends should be instructed on how to address the deaf person.

Do tumors of the ear or of the nerves of the ear occur frequently in older people?

No. Acoustic-nerve tumors are usually encountered in younger people. When they do occur, neurosurgery is necessary. Recovery from such an operation is the general rule, although deafness in the involved ear will result.

Is eczema, or dermatitis, of the external ear canal seen frequently in older people?

Yes. This is a rather common condition. Often it is caused by a fungus infection. Sometimes the irritation results from dryness and scaling of the skin, with excessive scratching.

Should eczema, or dermatitis, of the external ear be self-treated or should a specialist be consulted?

It is important that the condition be treated by an ear specialist, in order to avoid a chronic infection that may result in impairment of hearing.

HEART

See ANEMIA; ANGINA PECTORIS; ARTERIOSCLEROSIS; BLOOD
PRESSURE; CHOLESTEROL; CIRCULATION; CORONARY-ARTERY
DISEASE; EMBOLUS AND EMBOLISM; HYPERTENSION; PHYSICAL
ACTIVITY AND EXERCISE; SMOKING; THROMBUS AND THROM-
BOSIS.

What is the potential life-span of a normal heart?

A healthy heart has the capability of functioning satisfactorily
for well over 100 years. This figure, of course, assumes that
the arteries supplying the heart muscle are free from significant
degrees of arteriosclerosis. Laboratory experiments with heart
muscle taken from the body of an individual who has just died
show that it will continue to contract and relax for an almost
indefinite period of time if maintained under proper conditions. Such heart muscle, supplied with oxygen and all the
necessary chemicals, vitamins, and nourishing elements, may
live for many years in a laboratory.

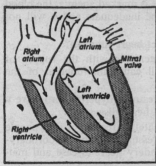

Diagram of the heart chambers

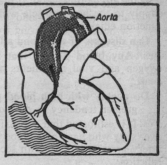

The aorta, the large artery leading
away from the heart

Does a normal heart give out just because it is tired?

Not really. If the person is healthy and has no marked evidences of disease in other vital organs, his heart should continue to function normally for at least 100 years.

If one reaches the age of sixty with a healthy heart, is it likely that he will develop heart disease during his later years?

Not if he maintains good general health. This statement must,
however, be qualified, for a certain amount of hardening of
the arteries will set in and affect the heart as time passes.

329

However, if he has normal heart function at sixty, he will probably not develop rheumatic fever, pericarditis, or other conditions seen so often in younger people.

What is the greatest cause of heart disease after sixty?

Coronary arteriosclerosis and coronary thrombosis. These conditions are actually diseases of the artery supplying the heart, rather than a disease of the heart muscle itself.

Does continued emotional stress affect heart function in older people?

Yes. The heart is greatly influenced by the large network of nerves that supply it. Also, the blood vessels supplying the heart undergo severe spasm and contraction under the influence of emotional strain.

Excess stimuli along the nerves and prolonged contraction of the blood vessels to the heart may interfere seriously with heart function.

Does severe anemia impair heart function?

Yes. The heart depends on the amount of oxygen, chemicals, and nutriments such as protein and sugar that are brought to it by the circulating blood. If there is marked anemia, the blood supply to the heart muscle will be inadequate and it will not function efficiently.

Can diseases of the blood affect heart function?

Yes. Any blood disease that interferes with the supply of oxygen and vital nutriments will cause malfunction of the heart.

Do people with high blood pressure (hypertension) have a greater tendency to develop heart disease?

Yes. It is estimated that approximately three out of four people over sixty who have high blood pressure will develop coronary-artery arteriosclerosis, with secondary heart disease and malfunction.

How does high blood pressure injure the heart?

When someone has chronic high blood pressure it signifies that there is also arteriosclerosis. This means that the heart must exert itself beyond the normal amount in order to pump the blood and oxygen through the narrowed blood vessels to all the parts of the body. This effort will eventually cause permanent heart strain and may eventually lead to heart failure.

Can liver disease impair heart function?

Yes. The liver is the all-important organ in the metabolism of sugars, proteins, fats, and other nutriments. If its function is impaired, the heart may be supplied with insufficient nourishment.

Can kidney disease affect heart function?

Yes. If there is hardening of the arteries to the kidneys, high blood pressure will result. Prolonged high blood pressure forces the heart to do extra work. Also, when the kidneys are damaged by disease or infection, they may fail to eliminate poisons from the system. These poisons will remain in the bloodstream and may interfere with normal nourishment of the heart muscle.

How does overactivity of the thyroid gland affect the heart?

Excessive secretion of the thyroid hormone will cause the heart to assume an abnormally rapid pace and too forceful a beat. If this speed-up is continued over a long period of time, permanent damage will result.

How does underactivity of the thyroid gland affect the heart?

Inadequate secretion of the thyroid hormone will lead to an abnormally low basal metabolic rate. This may spare a damaged heart, although the patient must live in a more or less inactive state.

Is thyroid function ever purposely lowered in order to spare a damaged heart?

Yes. Patients with impending heart failure or who suffer from severe angina pectoris are sometimes given radioactive iodine or antithyroid drugs in order to decrease thyroid secretion. In about half of such instances, the patients are relieved of some of their heart-disease symptoms.

Will excessive sexual activity after sixty in any way damage the heart?

Yes. It may cause blood pressure to rise precipitately; it usually results in a too-rapid heartbeat and may be associated with spasm of the blood vessels supplying the heart muscle. It should be realized, however, that sexual activity does not differ significantly from any other strenuous physical activity that is injurious.

What precautions should people take in their middle years to ensure a healthy heart during their later years?

1. They should stay thin or get thin.
2. They should restrict their salt intake. Large quantities of salt will cause fluid to collect in the body tissues and thus cause extra work for the heart.
3. They should not smoke. Heavy smoking may cause contraction or spasm of the coronary arteries, which supply the heart muscle.
4. They should avoid overindulgence in alcohol.

5. They should avoid self-medication. Many drugs can damage heart muscle if taken in large quantities over long periods of time.

6. They should do their best to minimize emotional strain.

7. Physical exercise should be engaged in regularly, but in moderation.

8. Get adequate sleep, at least 6 hours per night, to allow sufficient time for the tissues to rest and to restore themselves.

9. All infections should be treated promptly and thoroughly.

10. Fluid intake should be maintained at about 8 glasses of liquid per day.

11. A doctor should be consulted about any chest pain or other symptoms that might possibly be related to the heart.

What are the signs when the heart is beginning to age?

1. Shortness of breath when walking at the ordinary pace, or while talking or during periods of excitement.

2. The need to sleep on three or four pillows instead of the usual one pillow.

3. Constriction or pain beneath the breastbone, sometimes radiating to the left arm.

4. Swelling of the feet and ankles toward the end of the day.

5. A sensation of a "bump" or "thump" in the heart region every once in a while.

If one or more of these heart symptoms develop should the patient seek medical advice?

Yes. Older people should have their hearts checked regularly even if they do not develop symptoms.

What is heart strain?

This is a term not often used by physicians. It refers to temporary damage to the heart muscle, rather than the more permanent kind of damage associated with coronary thrombosis. It is a warning that a serious heart attack may be imminent.

How does a physician test the heart to see if it is in good condition?

1. The rate, regularity, and quality of the pulse will be checked.

2. A stethoscope will be placed over various areas of the heart and the beat will be analyzed.

3. The blood pressure will be checked.

4. The size of the heart will be ascertained by percussion with the fingers.

5. The size of the liver will be ascertained.

6. The ankles will be examined for edema (swelling).
7. The heart may be fluoroscoped or X-rayed to note its size and contours.
8. An electrocardiogram will be taken.

Will an electrocardiogram always show whether or not there is heart disease?

No. The machine merely records the electrical impulses that pass through the heart during contraction and relaxation. Although the test often reveals heart disease, people have been known to have serious heart conditions despite normal electrocardiographic findings.

Does the heart tend to enlarge as one gets older?

If older people are in good general health, heart enlargement is of minor significance. On the other hand, if they have marked arteriosclerosis, kidney disease, liver disease, or elevated blood pressure, the heart will become enlarged as they grow older.

Is heredity an important factor in determining how long the heart will continue to function normally?

Yes. One inherits a tendency toward early or late hardening of the arteries. Those who develop arteriosclerosis late in life will tend to maintain normal heart function longer.

If the heart is beginning to function poorly, can it be supported with specific medications?

Yes. There are several medications that will support heart action. Foremost among these, of course, is digitalis.

What is cardiac decompensation?

This is the technical term for heart failure. It means that the heart is not performing fully and is failing to pump adequate amounts of blood to all the body tissues. It does *not* mean that the heart has stopped beating altogether.

What are some of the causes of heart failure?

1. Extensive hardening of the arteries.
2. Kidney disease.
3. Rheumatic heart disease with damage to the heart valves.
4. Heart disease associated with marked hypertension.
5. Extensive disease in the lungs, such as chronic emphysema (*see* EMPHYSEMA), bronchiectasis (*see* BRONCHIECTASIS), or tuberculosis (*see* TUBERCULOSIS).
6. Severe anemia.
7. Bacterial infection in the heart valves.
8. Extensive liver disease.
9. Pericarditis, which is an inflammation of the membrane surrounding the heart.

What are the symptoms of heart failure (cardiac decompensation)?

1. Shortness of breath during ordinary exertion or while at rest.
2. The need to sleep in a sitting or semisitting position.
3. An irregular pulse and heartbeat.
4. A chronic cough, with the bringing up of pink-colored sputum.
5. Swelling of the ankles, especially toward the end of the day.
6. A feeling of anxiety, as if one is in danger.
7. In some cases, a rattling or wheezing noise when breathing.

What is dropsy?

An abnormal accumulation of fluid in the tissues. An example is the swelling of the ankles seen in cases of heart failure. It decreases when one is at rest in bed or when the feet are elevated.

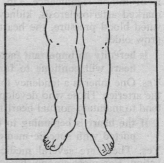

Dropsy, seen often in heart failure

Can heart failure be corrected?

Yes, in the great majority of cases. The treatment varies according to the cause. If, for example, the condition is caused by overactivity of the thyroid gland, medications are given to slow down that gland's activity. If failure is due to marked anemia, attention is directed to correcting the anemia.

What specific measures are carried out for people suffering from acute heart failure?

1. They are placed in a sitting position in bed and kept at rest.
2. Fluid intake is restricted.
3. Diuretics are given to eliminate excess body fluids.
4. The intake of salt is restricted so that the body will not retain fluids.
5. Digitalis or other heart medications are given to support the action of the heart muscle.
6. Sedatives are given to allay anxiety.
7. If shortness of breath is marked, oxygen is given, either by placing in the nose a tube attached to an oxygen tank or by placing the patient in an oxygen tent.

8. If there is an excess of blood volume, bloodletting is sometimes done.

Can most older people with heart failure be helped by the foregoing regimen?

Yes, if treatment is begun promptly.

Is it ever necessary to keep a patient in bed for several weeks because of chronic heart failure?

Yes, if heart-muscle damage is extensive.

Is it important for a patient with heart failure to lose weight?

Yes, if he is at all overweight.

What dietary precautions should people take if they have a tendency to develop heart failure?

1. The diet should be low in fats, particularly in animal fats.
2. The diet should be low in salt and spices.
3. The amount of fluid intake should be limited to 4 or 5 glasses of liquid daily.
4. The diet should contain adequate amounts of protein, sugar, and vitamins.

What is the significance of a heart murmur in older people?

Many heart murmurs are produced by disease of the heart valves or by a deformity of the heart that has been present since birth. Normal, healthy people over sixty do not often develop a heart murmur. Such a symptom coming on late in life would therefore indicate an infection of a heart valve, anatomical changes associated with the aging process, or, perhaps, severe anemia. People who have had a recent coronary thrombosis may also develop a murmur.

Is it possible for people to have heart disease throughout their lives and still live into their seventies and eighties?

Yes, if they follow their physician's instructions carefully. Many of those with rheumatic heart disease, angina pectoris, coronary-artery sclerosis, and other serious heart conditions live well into their seventies—and even eighties—though their hearts have not functioned normally.

Does climate affect heart function?

Yes. Extremes of temperature, both of heat and of cold, tend to affect heart function adversely.

Should older people with heart disease move from a cold to a milder climate?

Yes, if satisfactory arrangements can be made for living in the new environment.

Is the amount of oxygen one breathes important to the maintenance of normal heart function?

Yes. But almost everyone breathes adequate quantities of oxygen. Only people who live at very high altitudes actually lack sufficient oxygen in the inhaled air. This is one of the reasons why cardiac patients are advised not to live at places of high altitude.

Should people with heart disease avoid eating large meals?

Definitely. A large meal may precipitate a heart attack in someone who has a weakened heart.

What effect does being overweight have on heart function?

It is the job of the heart to pump blood, with its life-giving oxygen and nutriments, to every cell in the body. When a person is markedly overweight, the heart must work harder to get blood to each cell. Since excess fat is unnecessary, functionless tissue, it makes unnecessary work for the heart. It is calculated that for every 10 pounds of extra weight, the heart must work 10 percent more.

What is the effect of diabetes on heart function?

The person with uncontrolled diabetes develops premature arteriosclerosis. This causes the heart to work harder to distribute its blood throughout the body. Moreover, if there is generalized arteriosclerosis, it probably involves the coronary artery. This may lead to angina pectoris or coronary thrombosis.

What is the effect of alcohol on the heart?

In moderation, drinking alcoholic beverages does no harm and may even do some good, since it causes blood vessels to dilate and therefore carry more blood. On the other hand, an excessive amount of alcohol acts as a poison to the entire system, and therefore to the heart.

What is the effect of heavy smoking on the heart?

Nicotine causes blood vessels to contract and go into spasm. If people have a tendency to develop heart disease, smoking may cause the blood vessel supplying the heart (the coronary artery) to go into spasm, and angina pectoris may result. Statistics demonstrate that heavy smokers have a greater incidence of coronary thrombosis than nonsmokers.

Should older people with heart disease stop smoking?

Yes, if they can do so without becoming too emotionally upset. On the other hand, if discontinuing smoking causes them great emotional strain and unhappiness, it is perhaps better that they continue to smoke.

What is the relationship between rest and heart function?

A heart that functions inadequately will function better when the patient is at rest. Physical activity causes the heart to work harder. This statement should not be construed as meaning that all people with heart disease should be physically inactive. It has been proved recently that a moderate amount of carefully graded exercise is beneficial, since it maintains a more normal circulation of the blood through the body. It should be mentioned that exercise can be carried out even by people who are forced to remain in bed because of a heart ailment.

What is the normal pulse rate?

Anywhere from 60 to 80 beats per minute. During physical exertion, the rate may rise to 100 to 120 beats per minute, but it will return to normal within a few minutes after the activity ceases. During sleep or complete rest the pulse rate may drop to as low as 50 beats per minute.

What is the significance of a particularly slow pulse rate, for example, 30 to 40 beats per minute?

It usually indicates the presence of heart block.

What is heart block?

It is a condition in which the electrical impulses arising from one of the atria (auricles) of the heart are not transmitted normally to the corresponding ventricle.

Is this condition usually an indication of disease?

Yes, but many of those with heart block live relatively normal lives.

What is the significance of an excessively rapid pulse rate?

A rapid pulse, for example, 100 beats per minute, may indicate an emotionally disturbed state. It also occurs when the heart is under the influence of stimulating drugs. Or it may indicate overactivity of the thyroid gland or the presence of anemia or some debilitating disease. The persistence of an excessively rapid heartbeat should be investigated by a doctor.

What is a skipped beat?

It is an occasional irregularity of the heart accompanied by a thump in the heart region, or a peculiar sensation that the heart has missed a beat. It may be due to fatigue, to the toxic effect of a drug, to excessive smoking, or to some general condition, such as an acute infection. Usually the condition has little or no significance. Although a skipped beat does not usually indicate the presence of true heart disease, a person whose heart skips beats repeatedly should see a doctor.

What is auricular fibrillation?

It is a condition in which the heart beats irregularly, with some of its contractions of insufficient force to be felt in the pulses of the wrists.

What is the significance of auricular fibrillation?

It indicates that the heart is not functioning properly and that heart failure is impending.

What is digitalis?

It is the most powerful and helpful of all heart medications. In many cases of heart failure, digitalis restores normal heart rhythm and function.

Does the condition of the heart often determine the life-span of other organs?

It is usually the other way around. More often, the condition of the other vital organs determines how efficiently and how long the heart will continue to function. If one has had a normal heart throughout life and maintains good health in such organs as the thyroid, the liver, and the kidneys, the chances are that his heart will continue to function normally far into the later decades.

HEART SURGERY

Do people past sixty withstand heart surgery as well as younger people?

No. Fortunately, most heart conditions requiring surgery are apparent during youth or the middle years. If people live beyond sixty with heart malfunction, they are usually able to live their normal life-span without needing heart surgery.

Is heart surgery ever advocated for older people who have had a coronary thrombosis?

Yes, but people over sixty are not very good candidates for this form of treatment.

What is one kind of operation that can help people who have had a coronary thrombosis?

If an older person is a fit subject for heart surgery, an operation known as *poudrage* may be performed. Sterile talcum powder is dusted into the pericardial sac, which surrounds the heart. The powder causes irritation of the membranes covering the outside of the heart, which ultimately results in the formation of small new blood vessels. These new vessels will bring additional blood to the impoverished heart muscle.

The benefits of this operation are limited, and the mortality rate for this type of surgery in people over sixty approaches 5 to 10 percent.

Is heart surgery ever helpful to an older patient who has developed an aneurysm of the heart?

Yes, but the mortality rate in this type of surgery is high.

With aneurysm, the heart is so weakened by a blockage of the coronary artery that a portion of its muscle wall bulges out and threatens to rupture. Unless this is repaired surgically, it *will* rupture, causing almost instantaneous death.

CARDIAC ARREST, OR STANDSTILL

What is cardiac arrest, or standstill?

It is an abrupt stoppage of the heart.

What causes cardiac arrest?

This term is most often used in referring to sudden death during surgery, although it also refers to sudden heart stoppage secondary to a coronary thrombosis. When it occurs during the course of an operation, it is usually the result of a combination of factors, the most important being inadequate oxygen supply.

Can the cardiac arrest that occurs during surgery be remedied?

Yes, if the surgeon opens the chest cavity immediately, takes the heart into his hands, and squeezes it rhythmically at the rate of 60 to 70 times per minute. If this is done within 60 seconds after the heart has stopped, life can be restored in approximately one out of three cases. A recently developed method, closed-chest cardiac massage, employs intermittent pressure and relaxation on the breastbone at the rate of 70 to 80 times per minute. This procedure can be carried out as a first-aid measure by anyone, since opening the chest cavity is not required. (*See* FIRST AID.)

HEPATITIS

See ALCOHOL AND ALCOHOLISM; CIRRHOSIS OF THE LIVER; DIET; GALLBLADDER AND BILE DUCTS; JAUNDICE; LIVER.

What is hepatitis?

It is an inflammation of the liver, usually caused by a virus, a toxic drug, or other agent.

What are some of the causes of hepatitis?

1. Infectious hepatitis can arise spontaneously as a result of a virus entering the body through the digestive or respiratory tract.

2. Hepatitis secondary to an injection given by a nurse or physician. It is thought that the virus causing hepatitis adheres to the needle that was used in injecting a person who had hepatitis.

3. Hepatitis transmitted by a blood transfusion from a patient harboring the virus.

4. Contagion from direct contact with a person who has hepatitis.

5. Hepatitis secondary to an infection in the gallbladder and bile ducts.

6. Hepatitis secondary to drugs or medications that have a harmful effect on the liver.

7. Hepatitis secondary to poisoning.

Can hepatitis develop as a result of eating contaminated food or drinking polluted water?

Yes.

Does infectious hepatitis occur very often in people over sixty?

Although it is essentially a disease of young people, people over sixty may develop it.

How is the diagnosis of hepatitis made?

By noting the symptoms and by laboratory tests on the blood, stool, and urine.

What are the principal symptoms of infectious hepatitis?

1. Loss of appetite and a feeling of listlessness.

2. Swelling of the liver, with a dragging feeling in the upper right portion of the abdomen.

3. Slight to moderate temperature elevation.

4. Jaundice (yellow tint to the skin and mucous membranes).

5. Dark brown urine, denoting the presence of bile.

6. Clay-colored stool, denoting an absence of bile in the intestinal tract.

7. Itching of the skin.

What is the treatment of infectious hepatitis?

1. Absolute bed rest.

2. A diet rich in protein and sugar.

3. Withdrawal of all fats from the diet.

4. Abstinence from alcoholic beverages and any medication or drug that might have a toxic effect on the liver.

5. In cases where infection seems to be a major part of the hepatitis, antibiotics are given.

6. In very severe cases where the outcome is in doubt, the steroid drugs, such as cortisone, are given.

How long does hepatitis usually last?

If it is of the acute infectious variety, it may last from 1 to 4 months. If it is of the chronic type brought on by gallbladder or bile-duct infection or by the toxic effects of drugs or poisons, it may last for many months or until the aggravating factors are eliminated.

Does an older person ever die from hepatitis?

Yes, in about 5 percent of cases. Of course, the chances for recovery are excellent if the diagnosis is made early, the cause promptly eliminated (if possible), and instructions followed closely.

Do coma and failure of kidney function ever accompany hepatitis?

Occasionally. In very severe cases where a fatal outcome seems probable, these complications ensue as terminal events.

Can anything be done to protect a person who has been exposed to a patient with hepatitis?

Yes. If it is given early enough after exposure, a gamma globulin injection has been found to be effective in preventing the infectious type of hepatitis or at least in ensuring a milder case. Follow the same precautions used in avoiding any other contagious disease.

HERNIA

See CYSTOCELE AND RECTOCELE; MUSCLES; PHYSICAL ACTIVITY AND EXERCISE.

What is a hernia?

A defect in one of the body cavities, which permits a structure to leave its usual confines and to extend into a region where it does not belong. For instance, there is a hernia in the groin when some of the small intestines leave the abdominal cavity and descend through the sac of the hernia into the scrotum.

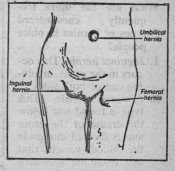

Is a rupture the same thing as a hernia?

Yes.

Are people past sixty more likely to develop hernias than younger people?

They are more likely to get hernias of the acquired type, but less likely to get those of the congenital variety. The latter kind is due to a weakness that is present from birth, but a hernia may not appear clinically until the individual is several years old or until he strains himself severely.

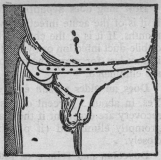

Truss

What are common causes of hernia in older people?

Increase in pressure in the abdominal cavity as a result of marked gain in weight, as a result of severe straining to evacuate the bowels (secondary to chronic constipation), or as a complication of a tumor mass growing in the abdominal cavity. In addition, the muscle and fibrous tissues in older people are weakened and less able to prevent structures within the abdominal cavity from emerging through openings in the abdominal wall. Severe spasms of coughing or sneezing resulting in sudden increase of pressure in the abdominal cavity may also produce a hernia.

Do strains and injuries cause more hernias in older people than in younger people?

Yes. Lifting a heavy object or a sudden twist or strain is more likely to cause a hernia in an older person because of decreased muscle and connective-tissue strength in those structures enveloping the abdominal cavity.

What are the more frequently encountered types of hernias in older people?

1. *Inguinal hernia.* This occurs in the groin, involving one or both sides.
2. *Femoral hernia.* This type is found just below the crease of the groin and is located alongside the blood vessels that exit from the abdomen to enter the thigh.

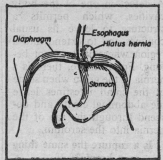

Hernia of the diaphragm, or hiatus hernia

3. *Umbilical hernia.* This is a hernia of the navel. It is seen often in people who have become very fat.

4. *Diaphragmatic, or hiatus, hernia.* This is a common form, particularly in people in their late sixties or seventies. There is an opening (hiatus) in the diaphragm, through which the esophagus (food pipe) passes from the chest into the abdominal cavity. In diaphragmatic hernia, a structure may protrude into this space. It is estimated that somewhere between 5 and 10 percent of all people over sixty-five have a small hernia of the diaphragm.

5. *Epigastric hernia.* This type is located in the midline of the abdomen between the tip of the breastbone and the navel.

6. *Ventral hernia.* This is a hernia in the lower abdomen due to a separation of the two long abdominal muscles, which usually meet in the midline.

7. *Incisional hernia.* This is one that occurs through an opening in a scar of a previous operation. Weakness of an appendectomy, gallbladder, or hysterectomy wound may lead to an incisional hernia.

8. *Recurrent hernia.* This is any hernia that recurs after it has once been repaired.

How is a diagnosis of hernia of the diaphragm (hiatus hernia) made?

By taking X rays of a patient after he has swallowed barium.

What is the treatment of hiatus hernia in people over sixty?

About one out of four of those with this type of hernia have no symptoms at all. No treatment is necessary for them. Another 25 percent have very mild symptoms that require little or no treatment. Still another 25 percent have symptoms that are like those of a stomach ulcer or an inflammation of the gallbladder. A few people have symptoms that are like those of angina pectoris (pain in the heart region). The treatment of all the above-mentioned groups should consist of:

1. Eating only small quantities of food at one time.
2. Walking or standing for about half an hour after each meal.
3. Sleeping propped up on pillows.
4. Eating a diet free of greasy, fried, highly seasoned foods.
5. Taking milk and antacids if symptoms similar to those of an ulcer are present.
6. Reducing, if the patient is overweight.

The last 25 percent have symptoms severe enough to make surgery advisable. These people may develop an ulcer of the

344   **Health in the Later Years**

lower end of the esophagus or the upper end of the stomach at the point of herniation. Such ulcers may be accompanied by severe pain and may hemorrhage dangerously. Others in this group may have a portion of the stomach wedged through the hernial sac into the chest cavity, producing an obstruction of the stomach.

Why does obesity predispose to hernias of all types?

The abdominal cavity is constructed so as to contain the intestines, the liver, the spleen, the pancreas, and other organs. In marked obesity, the space is also occupied by large quantities of fat, thus impinging on the amount of space left to contain the abdominal organs. This overcrowding creates increased pressure on the various weak spots in the abdominal wall.

Is the sudden development of a hernia in an older person sometimes an indication of some more important disease?

Yes. There may be a tumor in the intestinal tract or a growth in some other organ in the abdominal cavity. It also may be associated with enlargement of the prostate gland.

A tumor in the large bowel may necessitate inordinate straining while evacuating the bowels. This repeated straining may lead to the development of a rupture. Similarly, enlargement of the prostate may cause excessive straining while urinating.

Should all hernias in older people be operated on?

The great majority of people in their seventies and eighties who have small hernias will not require surgery or any other form of treatment.

When should surgery be recommended for people over sixty who have hernias?

1. When a structure, such as a segment of intestine, protrudes through the hernia opening and does not readily return to its normal position. This condition is known as *incarceration*. A doctor should be summoned immediately.

2. When *strangulation* of a hernia takes place: when a loop of intestine or large bowel has protruded through the hernia opening and its circulation has been cut off. If surgery is not carried out within a few hours, gangrene of the intestine or bowel will set in and the patient's life will be in danger.

3. When the hernia has become progressively larger, permitting more and more abdominal contents to pass into the sac.

4. When severe pain is a persistent symptom.

5. When a truss or abdominal support cannot hold the hernia in place. In such patients the intestines push through the hernia opening despite the support.

Is it possible to tell whether or not incarceration will be followed by strangulation?

Incarceration means that bowel or other abdominal content is stuck in the hernia sac. This does not necessarily mean that its circulation is cut off or that it will become strangulated. However, one cannot predict whether strangulation will follow incarceration.

What are the symptoms of strangulation?

When bowel is strangulated, the patient will have marked pain and tenderness in the region of the hernia, will develop distention of the abdomen and inability to move his bowels, and will vomit. If the condition goes untreated, he will become markedly toxic and will develop symptoms of peritonitis.

It is imperative that a physician be summoned immediately if such symptoms should appear.

Is it safe to operate on older people for a hernia?

Yes. Almost all hernia operations are well tolerated by older people, even when their general health may not be very robust. Repair of a diaphragmatic hernia is the most serious operation, but even it can be performed safely in the great majority of cases. Inguinal (groin), femoral, umbilical, and incisional hernias are usually minor operations, unless strangulation has taken place.

When should surgery not be performed on older people with hernias?

1. When they are in their late seventies, eighties, or nineties and experience no symptoms.
2. When they are in their late seventies and eighties and a truss holds the hernia in place without causing undue discomfort.
3. When a debilitating condition or organic disease makes the patient a poor operative risk.

Are hernias more likely to recur in older people?

Yes, particularly when the general health is poor.

Can people in their eighties or nineties tolerate surgery for strangulated hernia?

It is remarkable how many people of very advanced age successfully survive this type of surgery. Of course, if too much time has elapsed since onset of strangulation, the outlook for recovery is poor.

What anesthesia is preferred for older people who must undergo surgery for a hernia?

In all probability a general anesthesia will be given. Spinal anesthesia is reserved for healthier, younger individuals in their sixties. Occasionally, a very old patient is operated on under local anesthesia.

Should recurrent hernia in older people be repaired by reoperation?

Repair of recurrent hernias in older people is followed by less rewarding results than in younger people. However, if there is incarceration or if there is danger of strangulation, then reoperation must be undertaken.

Should older people be kept inactive after the repair of a hernia?

No. It has been proved that patients who lie quietly in bed too long after surgery do not heal as well as those who are out of bed and active. Early ambulation seems to stimulate healing and to lessen the incidence of postoperative complications, such as pneumonia and thrombosis of blood vessels.

Is it necessary for older people who have been operated on for hernia to take special postoperative precautions?

Yes. For several months following surgery, they should avoid lifting heavy objects or doing strenuous physical work. It is also advisable that they lose weight if they are obese.

Is it necessary to wear a truss after surgery for hernia?

No.

Should a healthy person past sixty severely restrict his physical activity merely because there is a greater tendency to develop a hernia?

No. If one is healthy and is accustomed to taking physical exercise, he should continue to do so. Normal physical exercise will not cause a hernia. It is sudden, abrupt strain, rapid gain in weight, or the development of an expanding tumor in the abdominal cavity that predisposes one to hernia formation.

HERPES ZOSTER (SHINGLES)

See DERMATITIS; INFECTIONS; NERVES.

What is herpes zoster?

It is an inflammation, thought to be caused by a virus, of endings of nerves that supply sensation to the skin.

At what sites is shingles most likely to develop?

Along the course of the trigeminal nerve (cranial nerve), which supplies sensation to the face; along the course of the nerves that supply the skin of the chest wall; along the course of the nerves that supply the skin of the abdomen.

What are the symptoms of shingles?

1. Excruciating pain along the course of the involved nerve. This may last for several weeks.
2. Blisters, appearing very much like chickenpox blisters, along the course of the nerve. The blisters subside and form crusts.
3. Pain persisting along the nerve pathway for weeks or even months after the crusts have disappeared.

How long does shingles usually take to clear up?

Anywhere from 3 weeks to 3 months.

Is there any satisfactory treatment of shingles?

There is no one specific treatment that will shorten the course of this distressing condition. Various procedures have been tried, including the following:

1. Taking large doses of vitamin B.
2. Applying antibiotic ointments to the blisters.
3. Applying ointments containing anesthetizing ingredients similar to novocaine.
4. Taking antibiotic drugs by mouth.
5. Taking pain-relieving medications to permit sleep.
6. Getting injections of immune serum taken from the blood of a patient who has recently recovered from herpes zoster.
7. Applying ointments containing steroids, such as cortisone.

Does herpes zoster ever involve the nerve that supplies the eye and the cornea?

Yes. This may be the most serious complication of shingles in an older person.

What is the treatment of shingles that affects the eye?

1. Absolute cleanliness must be maintained.
2. The patient should be treated with immune serum from the blood of someone who has recovered from the disease.
3. Medicated drops (antibiotics or solutions containing cortisone) should be placed into the eye in order to avoid infection.
4. Goggles should be worn to protect the eye against flying dust particles.

Do most people with herpes zoster recover?

Yes. However, there may be a great deal of pain for many weeks before total recovery takes place.

Do older people tend to develop shingles more often than younger people?

Yes. Their nerve endings seem to be more susceptible to virus infection and to the effects of vitamin deficiency and the toxic effects of drugs or chemicals.

HOBBIES

See ATTITUDES TOWARD AGING; PHYSICAL ACTIVITY AND EXER-CISE; PSYCHOTHERAPY; REHABILITATION AND PHYSICAL THER-APY; RETIREMENT; SOCIAL BEHAVIOR.

How important are hobbies for older people?

For older people who are still actively engaged in business or professional work or are managing their own homes, hobbies are not very important. They are of greatest value to people who have given up active work.

It is not easy to stimulate interest in a new hobby in people in their sixties or seventies. If they develop an interest in some pastime when they are younger, they may pursue it actively when they retire and have more time to spend on a hobby.

Do older people learn new hobbies easily?

In most instances the ability to learn a hobby is determined by the interest one has in it. It would be difficult, however, to teach a person with a poor educational background a hobby that required knowledge of science, mathematics, or foreign languages. Conversely, people with a good educational background would probably find little interest in a hobby that made few intellectual demands.

How does one go about finding out what kind of hobby an older person might become interested in?

Many community agencies have trained recreation workers who are expert in advising people on finding and developing hobbies. (*See* ORGANIZATIONS AND AGENCIES.)

After talking to an older person and discovering his background and interests, they will suggest several hobbies from which the older person can make a choice. The recreation worker knows from experience that an individual who has been interested in artistic things may want to learn to sculpt or paint; someone who has a plot of ground around his home may want to learn special types of gardening; those who have been mechanically inclined may want to learn how to make furniture, and so on.

Should hobbies be selected in accordance with one's physical as well as mental abilities?

Yes. People who are semiinvalids or must restrict their physical activities should take up hobbies that require little or no physical exertion. Among these are stamp collecting, coin collecting, knitting, sewing, and painting. People who are not so restricted might take up such hobbies as gardening, arts and crafts, or animal breeding.

What are some good hobbies that require little or no physical exercise?

1. Leatherwork, wood carving, ceramics, jewelry making.
2. Painting and sculpting.
3. Stamp collecting.
4. Coin collecting.
5. Collecting semiprecious stones.
6. Becoming a "pen pal" with people who live in distant places.
7. Translating books into foreign languages, if one has the necessary skill; translating and typing books into Braille for the benefit of the blind.
8. Compiling new recipes and experimenting with new methods of cooking.
9. Sewing, knitting, needlepoint.
10. Making and repairing toys.
11. Repairing watches.
12. Repairing radios and television sets.
13. Becoming an amateur radio operator.
14. Writing—memoirs, family history, etc.
15. Learning to play a musical instrument.
16. Learning a new language.

What are some of the better hobbies for older people who are not physically handicapped?

1. Gardening.
2. Animal or fish breeding.
3. Fishing.
4. Carpentry.
5. Bird watching.
6. House painting.
7. Masonry.
8. Repairing broken household equipment.

Should older people try to develop more than one hobby?

Yes, if they are so inclined. It is particularly beneficial when husband and wife develop an interest in each other's hobby.

Where can older people go to learn hobbies?

Many communities have hobby clubs, Golden Age clubs, or similar organizations. There are also community agencies to which people can go for information on this subject.

Is it true that many people who have been retired because of physical disability discover that they can engage in considerable physical activity in pursuing a hobby?

Yes, this is often true. It should be remembered that the pursuit of a hobby usually involves no severe nervous tension, whereas the stress and nervous tension that accompany work often contribute to physical incapacity. Then, too, a hobby can be pursued at the individual's convenience, whereas when he is working he must conform to the demands of his job or position.

Should bedridden patients be stimulated to develop hobbies?

Yes, but bedridden people must develop the kinds of hobbies that will keep them moving about. Hobbies that require a patient to remain in one position in bed for long periods of time are not good.

Will community agencies send representatives to people confined to the house to help them develop hobbies?

Yes. Local church or social agencies should be consulted. Also, some hospitals have developed home-care programs that include recreational benefits. For more information, write to The National Recreation Association.

What is a creative hobby?

It is a hobby that encourages self-expression and the development of latent talents. Frequently an older person will discover for the first time that he can write, paint, or play a musical instrument.

Can the hobbies of retired people sometimes be turned into gainful occupations?

Yes. Many an older woman's home recipes have formed the basis of a successful business enterprise. Similarly, many older men have turned a talent for repairing damaged articles into a successful occupation. It is important that these new occupations not carry with them the tensions that existed in the occupations of their younger days. If they do, the whole purpose of the hobby will be defeated.

Are there agencies that arrange for the sale of items made by older people?

Yes. Agencies in the community should be consulted.

What are some of the psychological benefits derived from hobbies?

A hobby, particularly if it is one that evokes admiration, will restore an older person's ego and will make him feel more vital and alive. It will often uncover latent talent and will stimulate a new interest in living. It can also be a means of making new friends among those who have similar interests.

HODGKIN'S DISEASE

See ANEMIA; BLOOD; LYMPH GLANDS.

What is Hodgkin's disease?

It is a chronic, fatal disease involving the lymph glands. Most pathologists classify it as a tumor or lymphoma. The cause of the disease is unknown.

Who is most likely to get Hodgkin's disease?

Although it is relatively uncommon in all age groups, the greatest incidence is in people in the thirties and forties. It is encountered infrequently in people over sixty.

What are the symptoms of Hodgkin's disease?

Over a period of months or years, the patient will lose weight and appetite, will develop anemia, and will show enlargement of the lymph glands, the liver, and the spleen.

How is the diagnosis of Hodgkin's disease made?

By removal and microscopic examination of one of the enlarged lymph glands.

What is the usual course of Hodgkin's disease?

It terminates in death within three to five years, although many patients who have a slower progressive form of the disease have lived much longer.

Can treatment help Hodgkin's disease?

Yes. Although there is no cure for this disease, life can be prolonged by the use of recently developed chemicals, such as those in the nitrogen mustard group, and by the use of X-ray therapy and some of the newly developed radioactive substances.

HOME-CARE PROGRAMS

See BED CARE; FAMILY RELATIONSHIPS; HEALTH INSURANCE AND HOSPITAL INSURANCE; INSTITUTIONAL CARE; NURSING CARE; ORGANIZATIONS AND AGENCIES; SOCIAL SECURITY BENEFITS.

What is a home-care program?

It is the rendering of assistance to aging people in their own homes rather than in an institution.

What services do home-care programs provide?

These programs differ markedly in the types of services they give, but some of their activities are as follows:

1. They teach older people how to save time and effort in keeping their apartments or homes clean.
2. They arrange for visiting nurses, attendants, companions, domestic help, and cooks to come in to assist people who cannot do all the necessary chores about the house.
3. They show aging, partially disabled people how to wash and dress themselves; how to maintain a clean, neat appearance, and so on.
4. They make suggestions for improving the safety of the home, so that older people will have fewer accidents.
5. They interest them in hobbies, home crafts, and occupational therapy.
6. They bring them books, magazines, and other recreational materials.
7. They send visiting physicians and nurses for those older people who are chronically ill but who would receive little or no benefit from hospitalization.
8. Above all, they teach older people every method for becoming more self-reliant.

Can a home-care program ever act as a substitute for a nursing home or home for the aged?

Yes. In many instances where only partial care is necessary, a home-care program can do a better job than a nursing home or home for the aged. If possible, it is always desirable to preserve the family life of an aging person.

There are experts in this field with great talent for teaching seemingly helpless older people to care for themselves.

Where can one find out about home-care programs?

By contacting one of the following organizations in the community:

1. Church groups.
2. Sectarian charitable and philanthropic organizations.

3. The local medical society.
4. Fraternal organizations.
5. Voluntary or city hospitals in the area.
6. Local health or welfare departments.
7. Federal agencies.

(*See also* ORGANIZATIONS AND AGENCIES.)

HOTELS, APARTMENTS, AND COMMUNITIES FOR THE AGING

See HOBBIES; HOME-CARE PROGRAMS; INSTITUTIONAL CARE; NURSING CARE; NURSING HOMES; ORGANIZATIONS AND AGENCIES.

Are there hotels, apartments, and communities that cater especially to the needs of older people?

Yes. Scattered throughout the country, in rapidly increasing numbers, are hotels, apartment houses, and whole communities built for and run with particular attention to the requirements of older people.

What special programs and arrangements do these hotels offer older people?

1. Most of the hotels limit their guests to people over sixty-five who are able to care for their physical needs. They will not accept those who are bed- or room-confined, those who cannot wash and dress themselves, or those who need constant medical attention.
2. Rooms are usually for single or double occupancy.
3. Rates are on a weekly basis, ranging from as little as $50 to as much as $120, depending on the particular accommodations, the location of the hotel, and other considerations. Monthly rentals can be arranged in most of these establishments. Food, specially prepared to meet the tastes and needs of older people, is included in the cost.
4. Maid service is available.
5. Many of these hotels have a trained nurse on duty.
6. Physicians are on call, should emergency care be required.
7. Many of these hotels have well-developed social programs and facilities, including libraries, reading clubs, lecture series, movies, party rooms, game rooms, workshops, solariums, sun decks, and swimming pools.

What special provisions do the apartments and communities make for the needs of older people?

Many of them have been and are being built in warm climates —for example, in Florida, Arizona, and Southern California— where living is easier for older people. Buildings are often of only one story and ramps often replace steps. Floors are made of nonslip materials; night lights are provided. If furniture is supplied, it is built so that older people can get into and out of it easily. Some of the facilities have meeting rooms, workshops, private garden plots, and so on. Some of the newer ones have built-in markets, movies, laundries, garages, and other facilities.

Is it wise for older people to move out of their own communities to communities in which facilities especially designed for them are available?

Not necessarily. It has been found that the great majority prefer to stay where they are. Their roots are deep in their hometowns and they prefer not to move. However, for those who want to move, the sunnier climates do provide many of these special facilities.

Do any of these communities for the aging have work facilities for their residents?

Yes. Some of the big industries are constructing whole communities for their retired employees. In these communities are plants and factories built for the express purpose of utilizing the skills of the retired or semiretired residents. Many workers forced to retire from a strenuous 40-hour work week because of age or failing health can and want to put in 2 or 3 hours of work a day in a plant located in some sunny climate. Here, with fewer working hours and less arduous conditions, they can enjoy the fruits of their years of labor and at the same time retain their interest in life and earn extra money.

Who should move to these specially constructed hotels, apartments, or communities?

It should be emphasized that only those older people who actually want to live in them should do so. It would be a great mistake to urge that they make the move if they prefer not to. Children of aging parents must remember that their parents' greatest joy may come from their association with younger people—their grandchildren, for example. Moreover, the subject of moving must be approached delicately to avoid making the aging parents feel that they are being "sent away." Many older people want to remain right where they are, no matter how inconvenient and outmoded their living quarters.

Do these specially constructed apartments and community housing projects serve as an adequate substitute for permanent residence in nursing homes or homes for the aged?

No. Most of these communities are designed primarily for *healthy* older people.

Where can one get information about hotels, apartments, and communities for older people?

Contact the local branch of one of the agencies on housing. (*See* ORGANIZATIONS AND AGENCIES.)

HYGIENE

See BED CARE; BED-WETTING; BOWEL FUNCTION; CLOTHING; NURSING CARE; SOCIAL BEHAVIOR; TEETH.

Should people pay more attention to personal hygiene as they grow older?

Yes. Some older people, especially those in their seventies and eighties, tend to forget those things that are necessary for the maintenance of cleanliness. Since their social lives make fewer demands on them and since they appear less often in public, older people may become unkempt. This tendency must be combated by those who live with or who are charged with the care of older people.

Does the body require special personal-hygiene measures as one advances in age?

Yes. The skin often gets dry and scaly, resulting in dandruff and accumulation of skin debris. This condition is often accompanied by unpleasant body odors. Older people should bathe frequently and use skin oils and ointments on the advice of a physician.

Will special attention to personal hygiene throughout earlier life delay the onset of the appearance of old age?

Yes. To prove this point, look at the youthful appearance of many of the aging professional actors and actresses.

What attitude should the family or attendants of older people assume about their personal hygiene?

It is particularly important to compliment them when they are well dressed or when they have purchased a new suit or dress. They must be reminded regularly to have their hair washed, set, or cut. New hairstyles on women should always evoke a

pleasant comment. Older people should be urged and reminded to have their clothes cleaned and pressed.

A positive approach will do much more good than unkind
criticism. (*See* CLOTHING.)

Should older women be encouraged to visit beauty parlors regularly?

Yes, if they can afford it.

Should older women continue to use cosmetics and perfumes?

Yes, but with discretion. It is sometimes helpful for older
women to receive professional advice from a beautician as to
the cosmetics and perfumes that will suit them best.

Is it ever necessary to remind older people to brush their teeth frequently?

Yes. This is quite important, since people tend to neglect
mouth hygiene as they grow older. Unpleasant mouth odors
may become marked as tooth decay and gum infection increase during the later years.

How often should people over sixty bathe?

The usual custom in the United States is to take a daily bath
or shower. This practice can be continued throughout the
later years unless the skin becomes so dry that it cracks or
otherwise rebels against the daily application of soap and
water. If the skin shows signs of irritation, itching, or rash
formation, professional advice from a dermatologist should be
sought. It is well known that the skin of older people reacts
unfavorably to strong soaps and detergents.

What can older people do if their skin is so sensitive that they cannot take regular baths or showers?

See SKIN.

Are there special medications that older people can use to make their skin look more youthful?

If used regularly, many of the skin ointments will give the skin
a more youthful appearance temporarily. (*See* SKIN.)

Can older women douche regularly?

Yes, but only on the advice of a doctor. If there is a vaginal
discharge or an unpleasant odor, douching once or twice a
week is usually quite helpful. However, it is important to
consult one's physician for treatment of the cause of the
discharge, and thus perhaps make douching unnecessary.

Can older women shave under the arms and use underarm deodorants?

Yes. However, discontinue the use of the deodorant if any
rash or allergic reaction takes place.

Are the various hand lotions helpful?

Yes. Most of these products will enhance the appearance of the hands and will prevent chapping.

Can older women dye their hair without doing themselves harm?

See HAIR.

Do older men tend to wet themselves or the floor when they void?

Yes. Men with this condition should be advised to sit on the toilet when they urinate.

What agencies will instruct older people in the methods of hygiene?

Many communities have visiting-nurse associations. These associations send nurses to the homes of older people to instruct them on how to care for themselves. Some hospitals have home-care programs for the same purpose. (*See* HOME-CARE PROGRAMS.)

Do fingernails and toenails tend to become coarse and thickened in the later years?

Yes. For this reason it is important that they be manicured regularly. Older people should also be encouraged to keep their fingernails clean. Nothing gives the appearance of hopelessness and resignation more than dirty, unkempt nails.

Is it ever necessary to encourage aging men to shave regularly?

Yes. Men in their seventies or eighties who stay at home a great deal often abandon the daily shave. This is not good for their morale or for the morale of their wives. They should be stimulated not only to shave daily but also to keep the hairs that grow out of the ears and nose closely cropped. By the same token, they should be reminded whenever they need a haircut.

Do people in their seventies or eighties ever drool saliva when eating?

Yes, if the older person has poorly fitting dentures or has recently recovered from a stroke. If the drooling is due to excess saliva secretion, medications such as belladonna will sometimes control it.

If the drooling is due to poor eating habits and failure to wipe the corners of the mouth with a napkin, then the older person must be reminded to observe better table manners. Scolding should be avoided, however.

Do older people tend to soil themselves or fail to cleanse themselves completely after evacuating the bowels?

This does occur among invalid or semiinvalid people of very advanced age. They must be taught, just like children, how to keep themselves clean. Often it is better for such people to be instructed to wash their anal area with soap and water after each bowel evacuation.

HYPERTENSION

See APOPLEXY, OR STROKE; ARTERIOSCLEROSIS; BLOOD PRESSURE; CIRCULATION; FAINTING; HEADACHE; HEART; KIDNEYS; PHYSICAL ACTIVITY AND EXERCISE; SMOKING; VERTIGO AND DIZZINESS.

What causes hypertension (high blood pressure)?

It is thought that arteriosclerosis (hardening of the arteries) is the greatest single factor in the development of high blood pressure. In arteriosclerosis the arteries become narrower and less elastic, and the heart must pump harder to get blood to circulate through them. It is the more forceful contraction of the heart that is recorded as high blood pressure.

Must arteriosclerosis involve the major arteries for hypertension to develop?

No. If the process involves the tiny arterioles of the kidneys, hypertension will result even when there is no advanced hardening of major arteries.

Is hardening of the small arteries (arterioles) in the kidneys one of the commonest causes of high blood pressure?

Yes.

Can people have elevated blood pressure without hardening of the arteries?

Yes. Spasms of arteries, if widespread, can produce temporary elevation of blood pressure, as can excitement, emotional instability, and

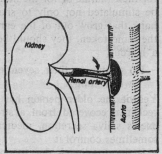

Hardening of the main artery supplying the kidney, a common cause of hypertension

strenuous physical exercise. If one remembers that increased force of heart contractions is reflected in higher blood pressure readings, he will understand how these factors operate to cause hypertension.

Are there people with marked arteriosclerosis who do not have hypertension?

Yes, if the process has not progressed greatly in the small arteries of the kidneys.

Can hypertension be caused by disease in the pituitary or adrenal glands?

Yes. Tumors in these structures may cause an excessive amount of adrenalin to be secreted into the bloodstream. This will result in elevated blood pressure.

Is chronic high blood pressure dangerous?

High blood pressure in itself is not dangerous, but it often indicates that a serious degree of arteriosclerosis is present. Advanced arteriosclerosis can have dangerous complications.

Can people past sixty lead healthy, normal lives even though their blood pressure exceeds 200?

Yes. Many people lead normal lives despite a persistent blood pressure of 200 or more. However, such a condition requires constant medical observation and supervision.

Should people who are in their sixties and seventies receive medications to lower their blood pressure?

Not always. It must be realized that high blood pressure is produced by the necessity for the heart to pump blood harder in order to supply adequate quantities of oxygen and nutriments to all the body tissues. If the blood pressure is lowered artificially, the result may be an inadequate blood supply to the brain, kidneys, or other vital structures.

Does an older person with chronic high blood pressure often develop low blood pressure?

This does not occur very often, except in conditions of disease or shock. A fainting spell may cause an abrupt drop in blood pressure. An acute coronary thrombosis is often associated with a marked fall in blood pressure.

Does high blood pressure in older people ever tend to correct itself spontaneously?

No. If someone over sixty has chronic hypertension, he usually has it for the rest of his life. There are exceptions, of course, as when high blood pressure is caused by an infection of the kidneys. If the kidney infection is cured, the high blood pressure may disappear.

**Does high blood pressure in people over sixty indicate the
need for limiting physical activities?**

Since high blood pressure is often associated with damaged,
brittle blood vessels, strenuous physical exercise should be
avoided. This does not mean, however, that sensible, moderate
physical exercise should be abandoned.

**Can older people with high blood pressure safely undergo
surgery?**

Yes. Surgeons and anesthesiologists know how to control
blood pressure during and after surgery, even when it is
extremely high. It is important that blood pressure not be
dropped too precipitately before or during surgery. Patients
with high blood pressure should *not* take medications preoperatively to lower their blood pressure.

**Is it true that many people can live into their eighties and
nineties even though they have had blood pressure over
200 for many years?**

Yes, the body will frequently be able to compensate for this
elevated blood pressure. Much will depend on the health of
the kidneys.

Does high blood pressure always produce symptoms?

No. Many physicians think that high blood pressure per se
causes very few symptoms; it is believed that most of the
symptoms are produced by the disease underlying the elevated pressure.

**Does an increase in cholesterol in the blood predispose one
to high blood pressure?**

Yes, insofar as a high blood-cholesterol level predisposes
one to hardening of the arteries. It is quite possible that if
people maintain low blood-cholesterol levels in their younger
years, the onset of arteriosclerosis and consequent hypertension will be delayed.

Do people tend to inherit high blood pressure?

People do not inherit high blood pressure itself, but they do
inherit types of structures and tendencies to certain diseases.
Thus, if arteriosclerosis developed early in one's parents, one
will have a tendency to the same condition. And if hardening
of the arteries is extensive, hypertension usually follows.

When is elevated blood pressure a matter of concern?

The doctor can best determine the seriousness of the condition. As stated above, the mere presence of high blood pressure
does not mean that major illness is imminent or that activities
must be curtailed markedly. However, shortness of breath,
severe repeated headaches, chest pain, swelling of the ankles,

or other symptoms of disease should be matters for concern, and a doctor should be consulted if any of them develop.

Are people with high blood pressure more susceptible than others to heart attacks?

Yes, because chronic high blood pressure is associated with hardening of the arteries, including the coronary artery which supplies the heart.

Are older people with high blood pressure more susceptible to apoplexy (stroke)?

Yes, because chronic high blood pressure is usually associated with hardening of the arteries of the brain.

Should older people with high blood pressure not eat red meat?

No. This is an old belief that has no validity.

Should older people with high blood pressure restrict their salt intake?

Yes. It has been found that people with high salt intake tend to retain more fluids. The retention of fluids increases the volume of blood circulating throughout the body, which makes more work for an already overworked heart.

Should older people with high blood pressure take trips in airplanes?

Yes. Modern airplanes are pressurized, so that no matter how high they fly, the pressure within the cabin is safe for hypertensive patients.

Are vacations at high altitudes advisable for older people with high blood pressure?

No. People with high blood pressure will be much more comfortable vacationing near sea level. However, a location one or two thousand feet above sea level is safe and will cause no discomfort.

What can people do in youth and in the middle years to prevent the development of high blood pressure in the later years?

1. Stay thin or become thin.
2. Restrict their intake of animal fats, which contain large quantities of cholesterol.
3. Avoid excessive intake of alcohol.
4. Smoke in moderation or, preferably, not at all.
5. Visit their doctors regularly.
6. All infections, particularly of the kidneys, should be treated early and thoroughly.
7. Try to live moderately and avoid prolonged periods of stress.

What is the recommended treatment of hypertension in older people?

1. A thorough examination is conducted to isolate the underlying cause of the elevated blood pressure. If the cause is a kidney infection, it should be eliminated with intensive antibiotic therapy. If it is an isolated arteriosclerotic blood vessel, it may be replaced by a blood-vessel graft. If it is a tumor in the pituitary or adrenal glands, surgery should be performed. If the thyroid gland is overactive, this condition should be treated.

2. If no disease is found as an underlying cause, and if there are no symptoms, no treatment or medication is necessary.

3. If there are symptoms, such as headache, blurred vision, or intestinal upset, these symptoms should be treated with appropriate medications.

4. All chronic hypertensives should try to get 8 hours of sleep a night; they should restrict salt and fluid intake; they should stay thin but should eat a diet rich in the necessary vitamins and proteins.

5. Medications to bring down the blood pressure should be given only during times of crisis or stress. It is now fairly well agreed that hypotensive drugs may interfere with adequate heart function in elderly patients.

How effective is the "rice diet" treatment for high blood pressure?

Rice, alone, will do little for high blood pressure. However, a rice and fruit diet is good in that it eliminates salt and substances containing large amounts of cholesterol. Also, a person on a rice diet tends to eat fewer calories and will therefore stay thin. Loss of weight will lower blood pressure, especially in the obese.

Are there effective drugs for lowering high blood pressure?

Yes, there are highly effective drugs, but they should be taken only when prescribed by a doctor.

What effect does smoking have on high blood pressure?

The nicotine in tobacco causes constriction of blood vessels. People with chronic hypertension already have constricted blood vessels, and smoking will cause greater constriction. It is wise, therefore, for people with high blood pressure, especially those with marked elevation, to give up smoking. This should be recommended only after consideration is given to the importance of tobacco to the patient, however. There are cases in which the emotional strain of giving up smoking would cause more harm than the good that would follow its abandonment.

Can people with high blood pressure continue to drink a moderate amount of alcoholic beverages?

Yes. Since drinking of alcohol causes dilatation of blood vessels, *moderate* amounts may be safely taken. However, excessive drinking may cause liver and kidney damage, which will offset any benefits that might be derived.

Does diabetes predispose one to high blood pressure?

Yes, since diabetes is often associated with premature hardening of the arteries.

Is it necessary for people over sixty to give up physical exercise because of high blood pressure?

This will depend largely on the severity of the hypertension and the symptoms produced by physical exercise. If the patient does not have marked hypertension, has no major underlying disease, and has few symptoms, he can engage in ordinary physical exercise. In severe cases, associated with advanced disease, complete inactivity may be essential. There are, of course, many gradations between these two extremes. The hypertensive patient should seek the advice of his physician, who will outline precisely the activities that are permitted and those that are not.

ILEITIS

See DIARRHEA; INTESTINES.

What is ileitis (regional enteritis)?

It is a serious, nonspecific inflammation of that portion of the small intestine known as the ileum. The ileum is the last few feet of small intestine before the beginning of the large bowel.

Ileitis is characterized by abdominal pain, fever, ulceration of the intestinal lining, abscess formation, and inflammatory adhesions between loops of small intestine.

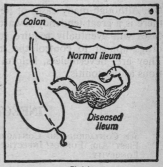

Ileitis

In advanced cases, intestinal obstruction and peritonitis may result.

Do older people get ileitis as frequently as younger people?
No. It is primarily a disease of young adulthood; however, it does sometimes affect those over sixty.

Is ileitis an acute or chronic condition?
Its onset is often acute and simulates the symptoms of appendicitis, but the inflammatory process goes on for several weeks or months to become a subacute or chronic condition.

What is the treatment of ileitis?
Ileitis can be helped greatly by surgery. The small intestine is cut across in a healthy area above that involved in the inflammation and is stitched to the large bowel beyond the area of inflammation. This is known as a bypass operative procedure, or ileotransverse colostomy.

In some cases, the entire diseased area of small intestine, along with the right side of the large intestine, is removed. When this is done, the healthy ileum above the inflamed area is sutured to the healthy transverse colon.

Is an ileostomy or colostomy (opening of the intestine or bowel through the abdominal wall) necessary in cases of ileitis?
No. The continuity of the intestinal tract is restored by surgery.

Is recovery usual after surgery for ileitis in older people?
Yes. The great majority will recover, unless the condition has been neglected and severe intestinal obstruction and advanced peritonitis have set in.

Is there any satisfactory method of treating ileitis without surgery?
No. Although many cases of ileitis will subside by themselves, there is a great tendency toward recurrent acute attacks. Such cases will eventually require surgery. None of the antibiotic drugs appear to control the inflammation caused by ileitis. They are, nevertheless, helpful in combating such complications as peritonitis.

INFECTIONS

See CONTAGION AND CONTAGIOUS DISEASES; COUGHS; FEET; FIRST AID; FUNGUS INFECTIONS; INJURIES AND ACCIDENTS; LONGEVITY.

Are healthy older people able to combat infections as well as younger people can?
Yes. The body's ability to overcome bacterial or viral infec-

tions does not diminish greatly if general health is maintained. This is especially true today because of the new antibacterial drugs.

Are aging people more susceptible to the development of such infections as abscesses, boils, and other pus-forming conditions?

Yes. Certain structures, such as the feet, are more likely to become infected because of decreased blood supply, resulting from hardening of the arteries. The entire skin surface, too, becomes more susceptible with age because some of the protective skin oils diminish. Dried-out skin is more readily invaded by bacteria.

What are the general effects of arteriosclerosis on the incidence of infection and in the ability of older people to fight off infections?

Having arteriosclerosis implies that less blood is supplied to the organ or structure invaded by bacteria. With decrease in blood supply, fewer antibodies and white blood cells are carried to the area to combat the infection. Thus, people afflicted with extensive arteriosclerosis are less able to combat infection.

Do diabetes and arteriosclerosis play major roles in making older people more susceptible to infection?

Yes.

Can people over sixty develop immunity to infections to which younger people are not immune?

Yes, to some of the viruses that cause the contagious diseases of childhood. But they develop no added immunity to the streptococci, staphylococci, pneumonia germs, etc.

If an older person is exposed to a venereal infection, can he develop it as readily as a younger individual?

Yes, but, owing to decreased sexual contact, this happens infrequently.

What factors determine the ability of older people to combat an infection?

1. The general state of health. If an individual is undernourished, that is, lacks sufficient body proteins, vitamins, or essential minerals, he will be poorly equipped to combat an infection.
2. The extent of arteriosclerosis is often vitally important in determining ability to withstand infection.
3. The presence or absence of degenerative diseases, such as arthritis, cirrhosis of the liver, or diabetes, will play an important role in determining how well one can fight off infection.

4. Anemia will interfere with the body's ability to overcome an infection.

Are older people more susceptible to lung infections, such as pneumonia, influenza, bronchitis, and lung abscess?

(*See* under specific conditions.)

Are people past sixty more likely than younger people to develop viral infections?

Not necessarily. As a matter of fact, many of the viruses—infantile paralysis, the contagious diseases, and viral pneumonias, for example—most often affect young people. However, there is no natural immunity to viral infections in those who are in their sixties or seventies.

Do people past sixty produce antibodies to combat infections as readily as they did when they were younger?

This essential body function may be somewhat diminished as time passes, but not enough to interfere with ability to combat the usual infections. When there is decreased natural ability to overcome infections, the antibiotic drugs prove most helpful.

Are older people susceptible to development of boils and carbuncles?

Yes. The skin is one of the first structures to show signs of aging. Consequently, skin resistance to such bacteria as staphylococci or streptococci decreases.

When an older person has an infection, does the fever usually run as high as it does in younger people?

No. Temperatures as high as 105°F. or 106°F. are quite rare in older people but are frequent in children and young adults. When high temperature does occur in older people, it usually signifies an overwhelming infection and septicemia (blood poisoning).

What should be done when an older person develops an abscess, carbuncle, or other infection?

1. Such infections should never be self-treated. A physician should be consulted promptly.
   a. A pimple, boil, or other pus-containing infection should never be squeezed. This will only spread the infection and may lead to blood poisoning.
   b. A needle should never be inserted into a boil or abscess by anyone other than a doctor. This may spread the infection and blood poisoning.
   c. Black ointments or other medications should not be applied. They will not affect the pus-bearing area and may do more harm than good.

    d. Patients should not medicate themselves, not even with antibiotics.
2. Temperature should be taken regularly whenever there is an infection. If the temperature is high, the patient should stay in bed until the doctor arrives. If a physician is not available, the patient should be taken to the emergency room of the nearest hospital.
3. Warm salt, epsom salts, or boric acid soaks and compresses benefit most infections. Care should be taken not to apply solutions that are too hot, for this might superimpose a burn upon the infection. It is *not* necessary to buy special medications for warm soaks.
4. The infected part should be kept at rest. If a hand or arm is infected, it should not be used. Bed rest is essential if the infection involves the toes or feet.
5. It is best not to use hot-water bags, electric pads, and other heating devices on infected areas. This may result in a burn, which will aggravate the infection.
6. If an infection, no matter how minor, does not disappear within twenty-four hours, a physician should be consulted.

Do people over sixty tend to develop infections of the feet?

Yes. *See* DIABETES for explicit instructions on the care of the feet.

Are kidney infections more frequent in people past sixty?

Yes. This is due mainly to two factors:
1. With advanced age there is usually a certain amount of hardening of the arteries that supply the kidneys.
2. There is often obstruction to the free drainage of urine from the kidneys because of enlargement of the prostate gland in men or cystitis in women.

Are bladder infections very common in older people?

Yes. In older women there is often increased laxity in the ligaments and muscles that support the bladder. This condition may prevent the bladder's emptying completely on voiding. As a result, urine stagnates and the bladder becomes infected. In older men, enlargement of the prostate gland often interferes with complete bladder emptying and will result in infection.

Is pneumonia very common in older people?

Yes. There is increased susceptibility to lung infection as one ages.

Is there a tendency for people past sixty to develop gallbladder infections?

Yes, especially if stones are present. It is estimated that 25 to

30 percent of all women past sixty and approximately 10 to 15 percent of all men have gallstones. The stones often cause obstruction to outflow of bile or interference with circulation of blood to the wall of the bladder. Either of these conditions may result in gallbladder infection.

Is hepatitis (inflammation of the liver) very common in people past sixty?

No. It is essentially a disease of younger people. Recently, however, there has been an increase in the number of older people who have suffered from hepatitis. Hepatitis in older people may be due to toxic effects of some poisons rather than to bacterial or viral invasion.

Are people past sixty more susceptible to nose, throat, or sinus infections?

No. On the contrary, people past sixty rarely develop acute tonsillitis or streptococcal throat infections. Most sinus infections in older people are chronic and have been present since the middle years.

Are such intestinal infections as colitis, ileitis, and dysentery encountered frequently during the later years?

No. Ileitis and colitis are more common in younger people. Of course, if an older person is exposed to the bacteria or parasites that cause dysentery, he will develop the disease as readily as anyone else.

Does septicemia (blood poisoning) ever affect older people?

Yes. Because older people sometimes have diminished local resistance to infection, deadly bacteria may enter the bloodstream. The possibility of septicemia should be kept in mind when a minor infection is present in an older person.

Is acute rheumatic fever common in people past sixty?

No, although older people are more likely than younger ones to develop rheumatoid arthritis and other joint diseases. Acute rheumatic fever, with its high temperature and painful swollen joints, is not very frequently encountered, however. Formerly it was thought that older people *never* developed acute rheumatic fever; recently, investigations have shown that they do occasionally.

Do people in their later years ever develop appendicitis?

Yes. *See* APPENDICITIS.

Are fungus infections common in older people?

Yes, if they are exposed to such infections. However, resistance does tend to increase with the passing of years. This is particularly true for vaginal fungal infections.

Do older people respond as well as others do to the anti-biotic and chemical drugs used in combating infections?

Most of the antibiotic drugs and chemicals are effective in combating infections in older people. However, special care should be taken to make sure that no sensitivity or allergic reaction to these drugs has developed over the years. For example, no older person should be given penicillin without certainty that no allergy exists.

Is the treatment of infection usually the same for older people as for others?

Yes, with emphasis on more strenuous methods.

What measures should be taken to prevent infections in the aged?

1. Efforts should be directed toward maintenance of good general health. It is essential that a well-rounded diet, with adequate amounts of protein, carbohydrates, vitamins, and minerals, be maintained.

2. Bed rest and prompt treatment of minor infections, such as head colds or other upper respiratory infections, will often prevent the onset of a more serious infection, such as pneumonia. Minor infections in older people should be treated from the onset as if they were major infections.

3. Older people should be especially instructed in the need for cleanliness and general care of their skin, since this is often the point of entry for invading bacteria.

4. Meticulous care of the feet is essential for all older persons, particularly those who show signs of hardening of the arteries. One of the most serious infections afflicting older people is infection of the toes or feet, since it may lead to gangrene.

5. The diabetic patient should receive special instructions on how to ward off and treat infections. If an infection does occur in a diabetic, it is often necessary to increase his insulin dosage. Diabetics should be instructed to consult a doctor for every infection—no matter where it is or how minor it may appear.

6. Surgery is often indicated to prevent an overwhelming infection in older people. For example, someone with a markedly enlarged prostate gland should have it operated on in order to avoid major kidney and bladder infections. Similarly, people with gallstones should have their gall-bladders removed in order to avoid the possible development of gangrene of the gallbladder or overwhelming infection of the bile ducts and liver.

7. Sedentary people should be encouraged to perform as much physical exercise as can be safely done. Nothing is more conducive to the development of pneumonia or other infections than physical inactivity.

INFLUENZA AND GRIPPE

See BRONCHITIS; COMMON COLD; COUGHS; PNEUMONIA; RESPIRATORY TRACT.

Is influenza the same as grippe?

Yes. Both are thought to be caused by various forms of the same virus. Grippe is classified by most doctors as a mild form of influenza. It usually shows less lung involvement.

Are there many types of influenza and grippe?

Yes. Each type is caused by a different strain of virus. In 1918, a virus produced an epidemic of influenza that spread throughout the world.

Do people past sixty often get grippe or influenza?

Yes. It is seen frequently in the older age groups. When it does affect them, it is usually much more serious than the same disease in younger people.

What are the symptoms of grippe or influenza?

1. Running nose with discharge of mucus.
2. Sore throat.
3. Fever, ranging from 100°F. to 104°F.
4. Malaise (general feeling of weakness and discomfort).
5. Severe pains in the muscles and joints throughout the body.
6. Headache.
7. Diarrhea (in some cases).
8. Coughing, with the bringing up of large amounts of yellow-green sputum.

Will vaccination for influenza help older people to make a speedier recovery from grippe or influenza?

No. Influenza vaccination is prophylactic; it must be given several weeks to months before the time of year when the disease usually strikes.

At what time of year are grippe and influenza most common?

During December, January, February, and March in the north temperate zone.

Are grippe and influenza highly contagious?

Yes. The infection is air-borne; it is often spread, through coughing and sneezing, to all the members of a family or to the entire staff of an office.

Does the treatment of grippe and influenza differ for older people?

Yes. They should stay in bed for several days longer than younger people with that disease. Since influenza tends to be more serious in older people, prophylactic antibiotic drugs are sometimes prescribed to prevent such complications as pneumonia. This is particularly true for those in their late seventies or eighties.

Are the antibiotic drugs effective in curing the average case of grippe or influenza?

No. These medications have little or no effect on the viruses causing grippe or influenza; they should be used only when a physician deems it wise from a prophylactic point of view.

What are some of the common complications of grippe and influenza?

1. Bronchitis.
2. Pneumonia.
3. Inflammation of the sinuses.
4. Heart malfunction, especially if there is a preexisting heart condition.
5. Invasion of the bloodstream by bacteria that have invaded the body secondary to the weakened condition.

What can older people do to avoid contracting grippe and influenza?

1. Take influenza vaccine injections several weeks before winter, or when an epidemic is imminent.
2. Maintain good nutrition with ample intake of protein, minerals, and vitamins.
3. Avoid exposure to drafts, damp, wet, and cold, making especially sure to change wet or damp clothing when coming indoors.
4. Avoid contact with people who have colds, coughs, or sore throats.
5. Go to bed and call a doctor at the first sign of a cold.
6. If possible, people who are particularly susceptible to upper respiratory infections should be in warm climates during the winter months.

What is the treatment of grippe and influenza?

1. Bed rest, until 48 hours after fever has subsided and until most of the symptoms have disappeared.

2. Large quantities of water, fruit juices, and other liquids should be taken, unless there are restrictions because of a heart condition.

3. The room should be kept warm and moist, but a window should remain open to allow for free circulation of air.

4. The patient is usually most comfortable if he is propped up on several pillows.

5. If coughing is severe and distressing, a cough medicine may be prescribed.

6. Analgesics such as aspirin or aspirinlike products are often prescribed if aches and pains are severe.

7. If the patient is very old and has shortness of breath or marked difficulty in breathing, an oxygen mask or tent may be necessary.

8. If the heart shows impairment of function, cardiac stimulants should be given.

9. If complications such as pneumonia set in, antibiotic drugs will be prescribed.

INJURIES AND ACCIDENTS

See ARTIFICIAL RESPIRATION; BURNS AND FROSTBITE; DRIVING; FAINTING; FIRST AID; FRACTURES; GAS AND SMOKE POISONING; REHABILITATION AND PHYSICAL THERAPY; SHOCK; TRAVEL.

Are injuries from accidents common among older people?
Yes. Although people over sixty make up only 15 to 20 percent of the population, between 35 and 40 percent of all pedestrian fatalities occur in this age group. Also, four out of five fatalities resulting from accidental falls are among people over sixty years of age. Accidents constitute the fourth leading cause of death for persons over sixty-five in the United States.

Why do older people suffer more accidents than younger people?
Older people have a slower reaction time than younger people. Furthermore, they often suffer impairment of various senses, such as vision, hearing, and balance. Thus, an older person with impaired hearing fails to hear an approaching automobile and so is more likely to be injured. Similarly, because of visual impairment, an older person may not see the curled-up edge of a rug or a jagged area in the pavement.

Should healthy, vigorous older people limit their activities because of the increased chances for accidental injury?

No. If they are in possession of all their senses and in good physical health, their chances for accidental injury are insignificantly greater than those for younger people.

What is the most common type of accident affecting people past sixty?

A fall that results in a fracture.

What measures can be taken to prevent accidents in a home where elderly people live?

1. Furniture should be kept in its usual place. Most people assume that a particular piece of furniture always remains in the same place; when it is moved, they may stumble over it. This is important because older people frequently get up and walk about at night.

2. Footstools, though they may be useful, are frequent causes of accidents. They are much too easy to move. It is perhaps best to discard them when old folk are about.

3. Scatter rugs should be taken up because they may cause slipping. Rugs should be firmly attached to the floor.

4. Ashtrays with stands should be replaced by table ashtrays.

5. If the floors are bare or if they are covered with linoleum or asphalt tile, they should not be highly polished or waxed. If they are waxed, a nonskid variety of wax should be used.

6. Chandeliers should be raised above head level.

7. Household articles that are frequently used should be kept in closets at knee-to-shoulder heights. It should not be necessary for older people to get down on their hands and knees to reach frequently used items, nor should they be forced to climb onto chairs or up ladders. Head injuries, especially, may be sustained while getting up from a kneeling position or falling off a chair or ladder.

8. When children live with older people, it is important that their toys and playthings be put away each night so that they are not tripped over.

9. Frail or damaged chairs should not be used. Older people find it especially difficult to regain their balance once a chair tips.

10. Staircases should have bannisters. Wooden stairs should not be highly polished. If stairs are covered by runners or carpets, it is important that the edges are not frayed.

11. Every room should have adequate provisions for ventilation. This will reduce the possibility of suffocation from the fumes of gas heaters and stoves.

12. If a bedroom is far from the front door, a doorbell extension should be installed, so that older people with diminished hearing can hear it.

What are some special precautions for prevention of bathroom accidents?

1. A rubber mat should be placed in the bottom of the bathtub.

2. A handrail should be available to enable older people to lift themselves out of the tub without the need to grab a faucet handle.

3. Enamel faucet handles should be replaced by steel ones because they may break and cause serious lacerations of the hand.

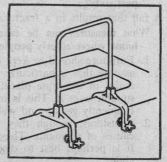

Handrail to aid people in getting into and out of bathtub

4. If eyeglasses are worn, they should always be kept at the bedside, so that when an older person gets up at night he can put them on.

5. A small, low-watt night light should be kept on, so that older people are not forced to move about in complete darkness.

6. Medicines in the bathroom medicine cabinet should be clearly labeled with large letters. This can be done by applying adhesive tape to the front of the bottle and then printing the name of the drug in large block letters.

7. Older people should be advised not to lock bathroom doors. In certain instances, it is wise to remove locks.

8. Older people should not take hot baths or showers with the windows and doors tightly closed. This may cause a fainting spell, resulting in an injury or burn. Someone should always be within earshot when an older person takes a hot bath or shower.

9. Older people should be cautioned not to enter a tub or shower without first carefully testing water temperature.

What are special precautions for prevention of kitchen accidents?

1. A stove or burner should never be lighted by a person

wearing a kimono, nightgown, bathrobe, or other garment with large loose-fitting sleeves or sashes. The material might catch fire.

2. If someone customarily wears eyeglasses, they should be put on before striking a match or lighting a stove.

3. Old-fashioned kettles with the handle near the top are safer than the modern containers, which have tricky handles placed near the bottom of the vessel.

4. Hot liquids should not be poured out of shallow pots or pans. Such vessels are difficult to balance and may cause burns on tipping.

5. When carving, the strokes should be *away* from, not toward, the body.

6. Bent or broken can openers should not be used.

7. Since the sense of smell may not be as acute in older people, it is particularly important to make certain that all gas jets are closed tightly and that the pilot light is burning. A kitchen window should always be left open a crack, but care should be taken not to permit a draft, which could blow out the pilot light.

8. China and kitchen utensils should be stored at comfortable levels, so that it is not necessary to use chairs or ladders to reach them.

What are special precautions for prevention of accidents in bed?

Although beds are supposedly the safest places in the home, this is not always the case. The following precautions should be observed:

1. People should never smoke in bed. This is one of the greatest causes of accidental death.

2. Electric pads and hot-water bottles should be removed before one goes to sleep. Their potential danger far outweighs their possible beneficial effects.

3. Older people should be taught to get out of bed slowly. They should sit up in bed for a few minutes before standing. This will help them to reestablish their sense of balance.

4. One side of the bed should be placed against a wall or another bed if the individual is very old or if there is a chance that he may fall out of bed.

5. It is sometimes wise to place the back of a straight chair against the bed in the region of the individual's head. This also will prevent the person from falling out of bed.

6. Older people who have been given sleeping tablets or sedatives require special treatment. They should be protected by rails along the sides of the bed.

What special precautions will help older people to avoid accidents when they are out-of-doors?

1. If there is impairment of vision, glasses should be worn.
2. When the sun is strong, sunglasses should be worn.
3. Those who have hearing loss should use hearing aids.
4. Older women should wear sensible shoes with substantial "stack" heels. Spike heels give insufficient support.
5. People who tend to lose their balance or who have arthritic joints should carry a cane.

What precautions can people take as passengers in automobiles?

1. They should sit back in their seats, so that they are not thrown forward when the car stops suddenly.
2. Seat belts should be used at all times.
3. A window should always be left open for ventilation, even if the weather is bad.
4. In getting out of a car, the curb side should always be used. Car doors should be opened wide and the entire body rotated so that both feet are planted solidly on the ground before an attempt is made to step out.

What special measures are necessary for older people who take airplane trips?

Usually none if the older person is healthy. Modern airplanes are pressurized, so that comfort is maintained even when the plane flies at great heights. Moreover, oxygen is available for passengers who may experience shortness of breath. Heavy meals and heavy drinking are best avoided during a plane trip.

INSTITUTIONAL CARE

See ATTITUDES TOWARD AGING; FAMILY RELATIONSHIPS; HOME-CARE PROGRAMS; HOTELS, APARTMENTS, AND COMMUNITIES FOR THE AGING; MENTAL CHANGES; NURSING HOMES; ORGANIZATIONS AND AGENCIES; SOCIAL BEHAVIOR.

What is meant by the term "institutional care for the aged"?
It refers to a home or hospital that specializes in the physical and mental care of those incapable of caring for themselves. Some institutions limit admission to those who are mentally competent; others care for people with mental difficulties.

Who is eligible for admission to institutions for the aged?
Formerly, people as young as sixty were eligible for admission. Today, with improved health of older people, it is rare for persons under sixty-five to enter such institutions. Most admissions are now of people over seventy.

When is it advisable to institutionalize an older person?

Only when the person's physical or mental faculties have diminished to a point where he can no longer care for himself. Most social workers agree that aging people, even if they are in their late seventies or eighties, should not be admitted to a home for the aged if they are capable of caring for themselves physically and if their mental capacities are relatively unimpaired. In the majority of cases, it is best to get their voluntary acceptance of the idea before arranging admission.

Are home-care programs a good supplement to institutional care of the aging?

Yes. Recent advances in the care of the aging include the creation of home-care programs. Workers are provided who visit aging people in their own homes and give them assistance. (*See* HOME-CARE PROGRAMS and SOCIAL SECURITY MANUAL.)

Social workers who do home-care work are usually affiliated with institutions for care of the aging. When the workers conclude that home care is no longer feasible, they recommend institutionalization. The knowledge that there is an affiliated institution that will care for him if it becomes necessary often relieves the aging person and his family of a great deal of anxiety. Relief from fear of abandonment is often a substantial factor in keeping the aging individual in his home and community for many additional years.

What agencies should be consulted about institutionalizing an aging person?

1. Many cities have sectarian institutions for the aged. It is therefore advisable for the family of an aging person to discuss the matter first with a minister, priest, or rabbi.
2. The local welfare department should be consulted. Welfare departments almost always have special sections with personnel trained to handle problems of this kind.
3. Each state has a department of social welfare, which should be consulted if local agencies cannot supply sufficient help.
4. At the federal level, the Department of Health, Education and Welfare can be consulted. This agency has a large, efficient section that devotes itself to the assistance of the aging. (*See* ORGANIZATIONS AND AGENCIES.)

Can financial assistance be obtained from federal sources when institutionalizing an individual of sixty-five years?

(*See* SOCIAL SECURITY MANUAL.)

What is the best procedure to follow when one member of an aging couple requires institutionalization and the other member does not?

1. If financial circumstances permit, the healthy individual should employ an attendant to care for his or her spouse. If this is feasible, it will permit the couple to remain together for a longer period of time.

2. If the symptoms of aging have advanced to the point where an attendant will not solve the problem or if there is insufficient money to employ an attendant, it then becomes necessary to admit the individual to an institution. A nearby institution should be chosen, preferably one that has a liberal policy concerning visitors.

Does separating an aging couple often cause family conflict and unhappiness?

Yes. Often both husband and wife resist the idea of institutionalization. In order to forestall such a situation, an expert social worker should be consulted early—several months *before* the actual need for institutional care. This will give the social worker time to adjust the couple to the idea. Visits to nearby institutions may allay much of the fear that naturally exists.

Are there hotels and boarding houses that specialize in permanent residence for the aged?

Yes. *See* HOTELS, APARTMENTS, AND COMMUNITIES FOR THE AGING.

Is it natural for older people to become depressed when they first enter a home for the aged?

Yes. Many of them take two to three months to adjust. This group is composed mainly of those people who were depressed before they entered the institution.

Modern, up-to-date institutions are prepared for the treatment of maladjusted new residents. They have special programs to bolster their morale. In addition, many of the larger institutions have full-time psychiatrists who are trained in the care of the emotional problems of the aging.

Is psychiatric consultation available in most homes for the aged?

Yes. The larger ones usually have a staff psychiatrist. Smaller institutions that cannot afford full-time psychiatrists usually offer courses to the staff in the handling of psychological problems of the aging. Also, well-trained psychiatric social workers are on the staffs of most of these institutions.

Do homes for the aged tend to specialize in the type of aged person they admit?

Yes. Some will take as residents only people who are able to care for themselves physically; others will admit people who require a considerable amount of medical care; still others specialize in the care of those showing mental changes.

Some of the larger institutions care for all types of residents, with separate buildings and staffs for the various special needs.

Can the average family afford the rates of a home for the aged?

Many different types of institutions are devoted to the care of the aging. Some are private organizations run for profit and may charge for a year's care from $3,000 to $15,000. However, there are a large number of nonprofit, voluntary institutions, which cost much less. In these institutions a certain number of patients are admitted free; others will be accepted if checks received from old-age assistance or if social security benefits are turned over as payment. Nonprofit institutions frequently have private pavilions too and may charge from $10,000 to $15,000 a year for those who can afford it.

In addition to private, profit-making institutions and voluntary nonprofit institutions, there are city and state institutions, which take monies received from social security benefits and old-age assistance as full payment for their residents.

What information should be sought before selecting a home for the aged?

1. One should look into the sponsorship of the institution. It should be ascertained if the organization or people that run the home appreciate the need for maintaining the dignity of the residents and will help the aging to continue as worthwhile members of the community. It must also be determined that the attitudes of the sponsors are acceptable to the aging person and his family.
2. The standard of care should be studied thoroughly and the following questions answered:
   a. Is the institution well staffed?
   b. Are the living quarters adequate?
   c. Are the meals adequate in content and variety?
   d. Are there provisions for maintenance of good hygienic standards?
3. The available medical and nursing services should be investigated, with particular attention to whether or not there are staff nurses and physicians always on duty.
4. It should be determined whether there are professional social service workers on the staff. The training and

attitudes of the social service department should be investigated to see if they satisfy the requirements of the aging resident and his family.

5. The availability of recreational and occupational facilities—library, assembly hall, game room, theater, etc.—should be inspected.

6. Facilities for the maintenance of privacy should be considered. Many aging people will insist on privacy in their living quarters. If this is lacking, an otherwise excellent institution may not appeal to a prospective resident.

7. The composition of the group of residents should be noted. It is possible to have an excellent home for the aged that does not suit the particular intellectual or social needs of a prospective resident.

8. The location of a home for the aged is important. If a home is located in a place difficult for the family to reach, it may cause unhappiness to the new resident.

9. The visiting hours and policies pertaining to visiting must be determined before a member of the family enters a home for the aged. Many new residents will insist on liberal visiting policies.

10. The cost of continued residence must be carefully calculated. Great unhappiness may result if money gives out after a year and a well-adjusted resident must be taken out of a pleasant environment.

11. The physical appearance of a home—the grounds surrounding it, the cheerfulness of the decor, etc.—are often extremely important to the happiness of a new resident. These must be carefully considered before selecting a particular home.

How should one go about convincing an individual to enter a home for the aged?

This is often a difficult task that requires the combined efforts of many people. The family should be advised by trained workers in this field before introducing the subject to an aged person.

Many who should be in institutions have resisted the idea indefinitely because the original approach by the family lacked understanding. Skilled social workers can often convince the most reluctant potential resident by selecting an appropriate and attractive institution and by painting a picture of the happy life he would live as a resident in such a place. And, of course, the family physician and clergyman can be most helpful by supporting the plans proposed by the family and social worker.

Since it is often difficult for the aging individual to make up his mind to enter a home, advance preparation should be made. Visits to some of the better homes for the aged, before the time that institutionalization is actually required, will often do away with false notions about such homes and will facilitate eventual acceptance.

Who should make the decision about whether or not institutionalization should be advised for an aging person?

This decision should be made by the entire immediate family, in consultation with the aging person's physician and representatives from a home for the aged.

Can a family force institutionalization on an aging individual?

No, unless there is accompanying mental illness. In such instances there must be proof, beyond doubt, that the mental illness is of such proportions that institutionalization is essential.

Do most homes for the aged have facilities for recreational and occupational programs for their residents?

Yes.

What types of recreational programs do homes for the aged often provide?

1. Movies.
2. Music programs, often with resident participation. Many homes for the aged have excellent choirs and small orchestras made up entirely of residents.
3. Dramatic programs, often with resident theater groups.
4. Literary societies and reading circles.
5. Birthday-party groups.
6. Festivities for important holidays.
7. Publication of an institution newspaper.
8. Sewing circles.
9. Arts and crafts facilities.
10. Games such as shuffleboard and darts.
11. Card and other parlor games.
12. Discussion groups on social and political matters.
13. A visiting-celebrity program. These are available to most large nonprofit institutions.

Are residents of homes for the aged allowed to visit their families and to go on weekend trips?

Yes. Most institutions encourage this practice for residents who are physically and mentally able to take care of themselves on visits.

Do most institutions permit unlimited visits from the family of residents?

No. They usually have regular visiting days and hours. This procedure is necessary so that they can regulate their programs.

Is the average nursing home as satisfactory as a larger institution especially designed to care for the aged?

Usually not. Most nursing homes have limited facilities and it has been found that a large institution is necessary for a well-rounded program. As an example, the average nursing home for the aged cannot afford to employ full-time social service workers, full-time physicians and psychiatrists, or full-time recreational and occupational therapists, all of whom contribute so much to the well-being of the residents. Finally, many nursing homes are maintained primarily as profit-making institutions, which by their nature are forced to limit their facilities; whereas most of the larger homes for the aged are either voluntary nonprofit institutions or publicly owned and can therefore maintain more costly programs.

How should one select a nursing home for the aged?

Apply the same criteria as those for selecting a home for the aged. If a nursing home is found to be deficient in too many of the essentials for a good home for the aged, then it should not be selected.

The family physician will be most helpful in choosing the most suitable nursing home.

Should the members of an aging person's family keep close watch on the care rendered in a nursing home?

Yes. Many of these institutions are not well equipped, and local communities have not as yet set minimal standards for operation. On the other hand, there are many excellent nursing homes, which render fine service to their patients.

The outward appearance of a nursing home is not always a good measure of its worth.

Do homes for the aged try to rehabilitate aging residents so that they may return to their families?

Yes. Rehabilitation techniques have been tremendously developed in the past twenty years, and a large number of aging people have been taught to care for themselves again. It is not, however, the prime purpose of a home for the aged to rehabilitate older people so that they can return to their homes. Their activities are devoted more toward improving the state of well-being of the residents, so that they can care for themselves in whatever environment they live.

It has been the experience in many homes that people who

are admitted in a bedridden condition can be rehabilitated so as to become ambulatory and self-sufficient.

How do most residents of homes for the aged feel about visitors?

Most residents anxiously look forward to having visitors. Among other things, it makes them feel less detached from their former environment; it gives them status with their fellow residents; and it provides material for extended conversations with fellow residents long after the visitor is gone.

Are there any homes for the aged that also have hospital facilities?

Yes. Some of the larger public-sponsored institutions have complete hospital facilities to care for the physical ailments of their residents. Many of these institutions are fully accredited by the American Hospital Association.

How should one select a mental institution for the aged?
See MENTAL CHANGES.

Should the presence of children in a home where old people also live influence the decision to send an older person to a home for the aged?

Yes. Not only is it bad for the children to see an old person deteriorate but also the presence of small children often irritates and aggravates the condition of an aging individual. It is essential that children be brought up in a happy, healthy home environment, and the presence of an ill, aging grandparent can often create much strife in an otherwise tranquil home.

What steps should be taken to confine a mentally incompetent older person to a mental institution?
See MENTAL CHANGES.

Do most homes for the aged separate the mentally alert and well from the mentally infirm?

Modern concepts advocate that persons who show signs of senility be permitted to live with those who are mentally alert until they create a disturbing influence on the community in the institution. It is only then that they are segregated.

What steps should the family take if an older person who has been in a home for the aged wants to leave and return home?

Consultations should be held with the director, the social service worker, the physician, the psychiatrist in charge of the institution, and the patient's own family physician. The prime consideration in making a decision should be the welfare of the whole family unit rather than just the welfare of the aged individual. If the family can see its way clear to receiving the individual, it should do so. Otherwise, the patient should be persuaded to remain in the home or to transfer to one more to his liking.

INTESTINES

See APPENDICITIS; BOWEL FUNCTION; CONSTIPATION; DIARRHEA; DIVERTICULOSIS AND DIVERTICULITIS; ILEITIS; LAXATIVES; POLYPS OF THE LARGE BOWEL; RECTUM AND ANUS; STOMACH.

Does the intestinal tract lose much of its ability to absorb and digest foods as people grow older?

Usually not. Healthy older people retain normal intestinal function. There are not many consequences of the aging process in the intestinal tracts of healthy people, even in the eighties and nineties. The glands lining the intestines will continue to secrete normal amounts of enzymes and other substances necessary for the digestion of food and the elimination of waste.

Can the intestinal tracts of healthy older people readily handle large quantities of food?

Not as easily as during the younger years. As people advance in age they should eat smaller quantities of food. As people grow older their need for large quantities of food diminishes.

Do older people's stomachs usually secrete a sufficient quantity of gastric juice to digest food?

Yes, although there may be a marked diminution in the quantity of hydrochloric acid that the stomach secretes. Contrary to popular belief, most of the important digestive processes take place in the small intestine, not in the stomach. But even at advanced ages, the stomach normally continues to churn the food and to start the processes of digestion. The absence of acid seems to interfere very little with stomach function.

When problems of digestion do develop in older people, what forms do they usually take?

Even healthy older people often complain about their digestion. Belching, the passage of large quantities of gas by rectum, distention of the abdomen, diarrhea, constipation, intestinal rumbling, and a general feeling of abdominal discomfort are the most frequent complaints.

What are some common causes of digestive disturbance in older people?

1. Eating too much carbohydrate (starches and sugars).
2. Eating too much fat, grease, and fried foods.
3. Eating too quickly and chewing food inadequately. This will cause large chunks of food to enter the stomach, thus placing an extra load of work on that organ.
4. Allergies to certain foods. This may cause swelling of the mucous membrane of the intestinal tract, with consequent failure of the food to be properly absorbed.
5. Emotional disturbance, particularly around mealtime.
6. Anemia, so common in older people, may interfere with proper digestion and utilization of ingested food.
7. Vitamin and mineral deficiencies of various types may interfere with proper digestion and absorption of food.
8. The pancreas sometimes shows evidences of the aging process and may secrete an insufficient quantity of digestive juices.

What can be done to combat faulty digestion and absorption of food in older people?

1. The general health of the person must be carefully examined, and any underlying general disease must be eliminated.
2. If anemia is present, medications must be given to remedy it. Liver extract is sometimes necessary to correct this condition.
3. If there is insufficient hydrochloric acid in the gastric juice, digestion can often be helped by giving small quantities of dilute hydrochloric acid with the meals.
4. If a vitamin deficiency exists, appropriate vitamins should be given.
5. If pancreatic function is inadequate, pancreatic extracts should be prescribed.

Should older people cut down on the amount of carbohydrate and fat in their diets even if they are in good health?

Yes. The older one gets, the less carbohydrate and fat and the more protein should be ingested.

Is it wise for people past sixty to undergo a routine X-ray examination of the intestinal tract?

Yes. Ideally, all people past forty should have an X-ray examination of the intestinal tract once every year, even if they are in good health. It is *not* dangerous for older people to have X rays taken.

Do older people often develop colitis?

Inflammation of the large bowel (colitis) does occur in older people, but it is not usually the serious, ulcerative form of the disease.

How can people tell if they have colitis?

Anyone with recurrent diarrhea or one who passes mucus and blood through the rectum should see his physician for a thorough examination. This will include inspection of the anal area, manual examination of the anal canal, passage of an instrument known as a sigmoidoscope into the rectum, and taking of special (barium enema) X rays.

Do people tend to develop colitis more often as they grow older?

On the contrary; colitis is a disease that more often affects younger people.

What is sigmoidoscopy?

It is the passage of a metal hollow tube, measuring approximately ten inches in length, into the anal-rectal canal. The tube is lighted, and through it, the examining physician can inspect the last twelve inches of the large intestine. He will be able to see any inflammation or tumor growth that may be present.

Should people past sixty be sigmoidoscoped regularly?

Yes. Since benign tumors and cancers of the rectum and lower bowel are common conditions, it is wise for all older people to be sigmoidoscoped yearly, or at any time they develop rectal bleeding or other bowel symptoms.

What is a barium enema X ray?

It is an X ray taken after barium, an opaque substance, is instilled into the rectum by an enema syringe. This procedure will make the entire large intestine visible on X ray, and will outline any obstruction or tumor growths.

Are sigmoidoscopy and barium enema X rays painful?

No. Although they do cause some discomfort, these tests can be made without pain.

Are people in their later years more likely than younger ones to develop hemorrhoids?

Yes. (*See* HEMORRHOIDS.)

Are people past sixty likely to develop appendicitis?

See APPENDICITIS.

Is constipation more common in people past sixty?

Yes. (*See* CONSTIPATION.)

Is itching of the anus very common in older people?

Yes. (*See* RECTUM AND ANUS.)

Are fissures and fistulas of the anus very common in people past sixty?

See RECTUM AND ANUS.

What intestinal symptoms should lead an older person to consult his physician?

1. Unexplained loss of appetite.
2. Unexplained loss of weight.
3. Repeated episodes of nausea or vomiting.
4. Repeated belching, heartburn, or a feeling that food is not being adequately digested.
5. Difficulty in swallowing, with the feeling that the food is not readily passing down the foodpipe into the stomach.
6. Distention of the abdomen and excessive passage of gas.
7. Repeated episodes of abdominal pain.
8. A change in one's usual bowel habits, with the onset of diarrhea or constipation.
9. Change in the appearance and character of the stool, especially the appearance of blood.
10. Repeated episodes of bleeding from the rectum.
11. The appearance of undigested food in the stool.
12. Repeated appearance of a tarry, jet-black stool.
13. Inability to pass gas through the rectum.

INTESTINAL OBSTRUCTION

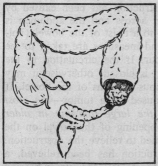

Intestinal obstruction due to a malignant tumor of the bowel

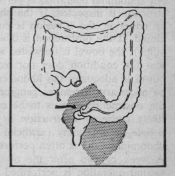

Volvulus, or twist of the bowel

Do older people develop intestinal obstruction very often?
Yes. Since tumors of the bowel occur more frequently as one advances in age, intestinal obstruction is seen more often in the aging. Moreover, other conditions such as adhesions or volvulus (a twist of the bowel) tend to affect older people more than those in their younger years.

What are the major symptoms of intestinal obstruction?
1. Increasing difficulty in moving the bowels.
2. Complete inability to move the bowels.
3. Inability to pass gas by rectum.
4. Colicky, sharp abdominal pains.
5. Distention of the abdomen.
6. Nausea and vomiting, eventually consisting of fecal contents originating from the small or large intestines.
7. Overwhelming toxemia.

What is the treatment of intestinal obstruction?
1. A rubber tube is passed through the nose into the stomach and on into the small intestine. This will drain off gas and fluids that have accumulated above the point of obstruction.
2. The patient is fed intravenously, replacing the chemicals that have become depleted by vomiting.
3. X rays of the abdomen are taken to determine the exact site of the obstruction.
4. Surgery is performed after the site of the obstruction has been determined and the general condition of the patient has been improved by removing excess gas and fluids and by giving appropriate intravenous medication.

What are the surgical procedures for intestinal obstruction?
An abdominal operation is performed and the site of the obstruction is inspected. If the obstruction has been caused by an adhesion, the adhesion is cut across and the abdomen is closed. If the obstruction is due to a twist of the bowel (volvulus), the bowel is untwisted and measures are taken to see that the condition does not recur. If the circulation to the bowel is adequate, the abdomen is closed; otherwise it may be necessary to remove gangrenous portions of the bowel. If the obstruction proves to be caused by a tumor—*the most likely cause of obstruction of the large intestine in older people*—a colostomy (artificial opening of the bowel on the abdominal wall) is often performed to relieve the obstruction. A week or two after the obstruction has been relieved, a second operation is performed to remove the tumor-bearing segment of the bowel. In certain cases where the obstruction

is not very severe, the tumor-bearing segment of the bowel is removed without a preliminary colostomy.

Does intestinal obstruction ever cure itself without the necessity for surgery?

Yes, in a small percentage of cases when the obstruction is due to an adhesion, to a twist, or to a kink in the bowel. In such instances, the obstruction can sometimes be relieved by passing a rubber tube into the intestinal tract and deflating the obstructed bowel. The patient, however, must be told that the chances for recurrent obstruction are great, and that if it does recur, surgery will be necessary.

What are the chances for older people to recover from surgery for intestinal obstruction?

In a modern hospital and with a competent surgeon, most patients will recover from this type of surgery. Much will depend on how soon treatment is instituted after obstruction has developed. By far the greatest chances for recovery are when treatment is begun within 24 hours of the onset of the obstruction.

TUMORS OF THE LARGE INTESTINE

Is cancer of the large bowel a common disease in people past sixty?

It is one of the most frequently encountered forms of cancer in the older age group.

What are the symptoms of cancer of the large bowel?

1. A change in bowel habits, such as the onset of episodes of diarrhea and constipation.
2. A change in the appearance of the stool.
3. Blood in the stool or bleeding when evacuating the bowels.
4. Such evidence of intestinal obstruction as distention of the abdomen, difficulty in passing gas, and difficulty in moving the bowels.
5. Complete inability to pass gas or move the bowels.
6. Colicky abdominal pains.
7. Anemia.
8. Loss of appetite.
9. Loss of weight.
10. The feeling of heaviness or a lump in the abdomen.

How does the physician make a diagnosis of cancer of the bowel?

If the characteristic symptoms are present, the doctor will

order a barium enema X ray. This will, in almost all instances, reveal the presence or absence of a tumor.

The examining physician will also perform a sigmoidoscopic examination; if the tumor is located in the last ten to eleven inches of the bowel, he will be able to see it directly. He will also be able to cut off a small piece of tissue (biopsy) and send it to a laboratory for microscopic examination.

What is the surgical treatment of cancer of the bowel?

1. If the cancer is on the right side of the large bowel, the entire right side of the colon (large bowel) is removed and the small intestine is stitched to the transverse portion of the large bowel in the midabdomen. In this procedure, no artificial opening of the bowel (colostomy) is performed, and the patient will continue to evacuate his bowels through his rectum.

2. If the tumor is in the transverse portion of the large bowel, that entire segment is removed. In this instance, too, there will be no colostomy, and the patient will continue to move his bowels in the normal way.

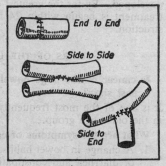

3. If the cancer is in the left side of the colon, that entire segment is removed and the transverse colon is stitched to the upper portion of the rectum. In this instance, too, the patient will continue to move his bowels through the normal rectal route.

Methods of joining one portion of intestine to another

4. If the cancer is in the last few inches of the rectum, then the entire rectum and part of the descending colon on the left side are removed. When this type of operation is performed, the patient will evacuate his bowels through a colostomy, an opening of the colon onto the abdominal wall.

Is cancer of the bowel curable?

Yes, in more than 50 percent of cases, cancer of the large intestine can be cured. If the cancer is discovered in the early stages of its development, approximately three out of four cases can be permanently cured.

Can older people return to normal living after surgery for cancer of the bowel?

Yes, even those patients who must have a colostomy can learn to live a fairly normal life.

Are all tumors of the large intestine cancerous (malignant)?

No. Many older people have benign tumors, known as polyps or adenomas. These are wartlike growths and should be removed surgically. (*See* POLYPS OF THE LARGE BOWEL.)

Where in the large bowel are benign polyps most likely to occur?

In the rectum, or descending colon, although they occasionally occur in the right side of the colon or in the transverse colon.

How can one tell if he has a polyp in the large intestine?

The outstanding symptom of polyps is painless bleeding through the rectum. Occasionally, a polyp of the bowel will grow sufficiently large to cause intestinal obstruction.

How does the physician make the diagnosis of a large bowel polyp?

1. By noting the symptoms, such as painless rectal bleeding.
2. If the polyp is within the last 10 to 12 inches of the intestinal tract—a common site of a polyp—it can be seen directly through a sigmoidoscope.
3. Polyps higher up in the bowel are usually diagnosed by barium enema X-ray examination.

How can a physician distinguish between a benign polyp and a cancer of the bowel?

For positive identification, a biopsy and microscopic examination must be carried out.

What is the treatment of polyps of the large bowel or rectum?

1. If the polyp is in the right side of the colon, the transverse colon, or the descending colon, surgery must be performed. This will involve an abdominal incision, opening of the large bowel at the site of the polyp, and removal of the polyp from the lining wall of the colon.
2. If the polyp is located low down, within the last 10 inches of the bowel, it can usually be removed through a sigmoidoscope. In such cases, a snare is placed around the base of the polyp and it is burned away from the bowel wall.

Do benign polyps ever turn into cancer?

Certain types do; others do not. For this reason it is important that *all* polyps be removed.

How large are polyps of the large intestine?

They vary from the size of a pea to that of a golf ball. The majority are about the size of a lima bean and contain stalks about ¼ to 1 inch in length. Some, however, are flat and have no stalks.

Do all polyps cause rectal bleeding?

The majority do, but some do not. The latter group may not be diagnosed until they grow to a large size or become malignant. This is another reason why people over sixty should undergo periodic barium enema X-ray examinations.

JAUNDICE

See CIRRHOSIS OF THE LIVER; GALLBLADDER AND BILE DUCTS; HEPATITIS; LIVER.

What is jaundice?

It is a yellowish discoloration of the skin and eyes, resulting from bile pigments in the blood. There are many causes of jaundice, but most fall into one of two categories:

1. Jaundice secondary to obstruction of the flow of bile from the liver to the intestines.
2. Jaundice secondary to disease in the liver.

What are some of the common causes of the obstructive type of jaundice?

1. Stones in the bile ducts.
2. Cancer of the head of the pancreas, obstructing the outlet of the bile duct into the intestines.
3. A tumor of the bile duct.
4. Inflammation of the bile duct, especially in the region where it empties into the intestinal tract.

What are some of the common causes of jaundice secondary to diseases in the liver?

1. Infectious hepatitis (*see* HEPATITIS) secondary to a virus infection.
2. Cirrhosis of the liver. (*See* LIVER.)
3. Homologous serum jaundice, secondary to a blood transfusion.
4. Toxic hepatitis, secondary to poisoning by a drug or poison.
5. Infection of the liver, with abscess formation, secondary either to a germ or a parasite, such as that found in amebic dysentery.

6. Blood diseases, with inability of the liver to secrete bile.
7. Cancer of the liver.

Does jaundice often affect those over sixty?

Yes. It is frequently encountered in older people.

What types of jaundice are most likely to affect older people?

They have no immunity to any type, although jaundice precipitated by virus infections and/or associated with blood diseases are more common in younger age groups.

Can a physician diagnose which of many causative agents has produced the jaundice?

Yes. Laboratory tests, as well as X rays, will aid him in making a precise diagnosis.

What is the treatment of jaundice?

This depends on the cause of the jaundice. If the cause lies outside of the liver (obstructive jaundice), such as a stone blocking the bile duct or a tumor of the bile duct or of the head of the pancreas, then surgery will be necessary to relieve the obstruction. If the jaundice is caused by cirrhosis of the liver, surgery to shunt the blood from the portal vein should be considered. (*See* CIRRHOSIS.) If the jaundice is the result of a blood disease or disease in the liver substance, then medical management of the disease must be undertaken.

Can there be a full recovery from an attack of jaundice in a person over sixty?

Yes, if the underlying cause has been eradicated. However, when jaundice persists for several weeks it often results in permanent damage to the liver.

What regimen should older people follow who have recovered from jaundice?

1. They must not overwork or subject themselves to physical strain for 6 months to a year.
2. They should avoid all fatty, greasy, or fried foods for at least one year.
3. They should eat large amounts of protein and sugar for at least one year.
4. They should not drink alcoholic beverages.
5. They should take no medications or drugs without the explicit approval of their physician.
6. They should take supplemental vitamins.
7. They should be checked by a doctor each month for a year after an attack of jaundice.

KIDNEYS

See ARTERIOSCLEROSIS; BLOOD PRESSURE; CYSTITIS AND INTERSTITIAL CYSTITIS; HYPERTENSION; PROSTATE GLAND; TESTS; URINARY BLADDER AND URETHRA.

Where are the kidneys located and what is their structure?

The kidneys lie on either side of the back region of the abdomen, high up in the abdominal cavity beneath the diaphragm. Each kidney measures approximately four by two inches in diameter. They are made up of hundreds of thousands of tiny units called *nephrons,* which connect with little ducts known as *tubules.* Each nephron forms urine from the plasma of the blood passing through it. The urine from the tubules drains out of the kidneys and passes down the ureters leading to the bladder.

What is the function of the kidneys?

To extract waste, poisons, and excess minerals and water from the blood. It is also the function of the kidneys not to remove certain chemicals and substances needed to maintain normal body chemistry and metabolism.

Is adequate kidney function necessary to the maintenance of good health?

Yes. One cannot live long if the kidneys fail to function adequately.

What happens when kidney function does fail?

There is loss of essential chemicals from the bloodstream and accumulation of chemical poisons in the body. When kidney failure assumes too great a proportion, other organs and body tissues will be unable to function because of the consequent chemical upset.

Is there a normal tendency for the kidneys to show signs of aging as one enters the later decades?

Yes. But the body is endowed with a great deal of kidney reserve; that is, there is a surplus of kidney tissue to perform the necessary functions to maintain chemical balance. As a result, even though the kidneys may show marked signs of aging, there may be enough functioning kidney tissue to maintain normal health.

How much healthy kidney tissue is required to maintain normal function?

About one-fourth of the total amount. Thus, when it is necessary to remove a damaged or diseased kidney, normal life can continue if the remaining kidney is normal or near normal.

How is kidney function determined?

By chemical tests of the urine and blood. There are dozens of such tests, each of which demonstrates the adequacy or inadequacy of some aspect of kidney function.

Will eating large quantities of red meats throughout life cause ultimate kidney damage?

No. If kidney function has been normal, this will do no harm.

What are some of the more common laboratory tests for determining kidney function?

Urine Tests:

1. Albumin concentration.
2. Examination for the presence or absence of casts (a mass of plastic matter, which indicates organic damage).
3. Determination of the quantity of chloride, sodium, potassium, and other chemicals in the urine.
4. The specific gravity of the urine, and its power to dilute and concentrate.
5. The quantity of urine excreted during a 24-hour period.
6. Examination for the presence of white blood cells, red blood cells, and pus.

Blood Tests:

1. The urea nitrogen quantity.
2. The quantity of nonprotein nitrogen.
3. The quantity of uric acid.
4. The quantity of creatinine.
5. Various dye tests to determine ability of the kidneys to excrete.
6. Intravenous pyelogram. An X-ray examination to determine the ability of the kidneys to excrete an opaque dye that has been injected into the bloodstream.

Will impaired kidney function accelerate the aging process?

Yes. People with diseased kidneys will soon develop other conditions that will lead to rapid aging. Some of these conditions are high blood pressure, heart disease, uremia, anemia, and malnutrition.

Do healthy people in their sixties and seventies normally show impaired kidney function?

No. In healthy people, the kidneys continue to perform satisfactorily throughout life.

Will arteriosclerosis ultimately damage kidney function?

Yes. Hardening of the renal arteries, which supply the kidneys, will cause marked impairment of kidney function. When these blood vessels become narrowed, insufficient blood and oxygen will be supplied to the kidneys, and their function will be impaired. The kidneys require large quantities of blood rich in oxygen.

What are some of the common causes of decreased kidney function in people past sixty?

1. Hardening of the arteries going to the kidneys and of the small arteries (arterioles) in the kidneys.

2. Degeneration of the small nephrons (units of the urine-secreting function) and replacement of functioning tissue by fibrous tissue. This is part of the aging process, which ultimately takes place in all organs.

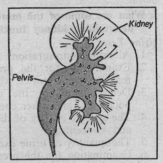

Pyelitis, an infection of the pelvis of the kidney

3. Kidney infections of bacterial origin, such as pyelitis.

4. Blockage of the kidney exit by the presence of kidney stones.

5. In the male, blockage of free drainage of urine because of an enlarged prostate gland.

6. Damage to kidney structure from drug poisoning or toxins that circulate in the bloodstream.

7. Marked anemia, with inadequate quantities of blood and oxygen reaching the kidneys.

8. Undernourishment, with inadequate maintenance of protein levels in the body.

9. Replacement of kidney tissue by tumor cells, as in cancer of a kidney.

Can the extent of kidney damage be evaluated from the results of the various blood and urine tests?

Yes.

Can older people maintain a relatively normal existence even though they have kidney damage?

Yes, provided the damage is not so great that it results in the retention of large amounts of urea and other poisons in the bloodstream. Post-mortem examination of people who have lived into their eighties and nineties frequently reveals extensive kidney damage although there had been no symptoms of active disease.

Can people live a normal life with only one functioning kidney?

Yes. The body has extra kidney tissue so that adequate function can be maintained with one normal kidney.

Is the life-span shortened when a kidney has been removed?

Not if the remaining kidney is normal.

Can impaired kidney function cause anemia?

Yes, but the reverse is more likely.

Can impaired kidney function cause diabetes?

No. Sugar in the urine of diabetics is not due to kidney disease. Diabetes is primarily a disease of the pancreas.

Can kidney function be improved by eliminating an anemic condition?

Yes.

Will successful treatment of malnutrition and vitamin deficiency help to improve kidney function?

Yes.

What medications or drugs may lead to kidney damage?

1. Poisons that have been taken accidentally, particularly those containing mercury, lead, arsenic, or other heavy metals.
2. Overdose of an otherwise beneficial medication or drug.
3. Certain medications prescribed to increase the output of urine. Many of these drugs contain mercury.
4. Occasionally, one of the antibiotics used in the treatment of infections.
5. Occasionally, certain of the newer chemicals (such as nitrogen mustard) used in the treatment of tumors.

Is dropsy (swelling of the ankles and legs) evidence of impaired kidney function?

Dropsy is more often caused by impaired heart function. Ankle swelling caused by kidney disease is usually associated with swelling of the thighs and legs, and puffiness under the eyes.

How common is hardening of the arteries of the kidneys?

This is very common in aging people. Almost everyone past sixty with high blood pressure has some hardening of the arteries in the kidneys.

Is arteriosclerosis of the vessels in the kidneys usually part of a generalized process occurring throughout the body?

Yes, but in some people it may be by far the most serious evidence of the aging process.

Can kidney infections or infections elsewhere in the urinary tract cause permanent damage to kidney tissue?

Yes, especially if the infections are chronic.

Can kidney infections in youth or during the middle years lead to premature impairment of kidney function in later life?

Yes, if the infection was a serious one.

If kidney tissue has once been destroyed, does it regenerate?

No, but the body has an excess of kidney substance, so that it can withstand considerable damage of kidney tissue.

Should older people have their urine examined at regular intervals?

Yes. Everyone over sixty should have a urine examination at least twice a year. This will often uncover malfunction of the kidneys at a time when it can be remedied. It may also reveal diabetes, bladder infection, the presence of stones, or other conditions.

Do female kidneys differ from male kidneys?

No. It should be mentioned, however, that older men's kidneys are somewhat more susceptible to damage because of the high incidence of prostate-gland enlargement in the later years.

Does acute nephritis (inflammation of the kidney) occur frequently in people past sixty?

No. It is much more common in youth and early adulthood.

What is uremia?

It is a serious condition caused by failure of kidney function. Urea and other substances normally excreted by the kidneys remain in the blood and poison the entire system.

What are the symptoms and signs of uremia?

1. There may be drowsiness and lethargy during the early stages of the condition.
2. The breath may have a urinelike odor.
3. Urine analysis will reveal the presence of albumin, casts, and other substances not found in normal urine.
4. Blood analysis will show an accumulation of urea nitrogen, creatinine, nonprotein nitrogen, and other waste products.
5. There may be twitching of muscles in the arms and legs.
6. In the final stages, the patient lapses into coma.

Is uremia more common in older people than in younger ones?

Yes, because diminished kidney function is more common in older people.

Is uremia ever curable?

Yes, if the cause can be determined and eliminated. For instance, uremia caused by blockage of urinary outflow due to an enlargement of the prostate gland can be relieved by the surgical treatment of the enlarged prostate. Uremia caused by acute poisoning sometimes clears up when the poison is eliminated from the system. Uremia brought on by an acute kidney infection can sometimes be relieved by curing the infection.

If, on the other hand, the uremia is the terminal phase of a long-standing disease of the kidneys, then in all probability it will not be cured and will lead to the patient's death.

How does an artificial kidney function?

The patient's blood flows through the artificial kidney and various poisons are filtered out, thus relieving uremia. The artificial kidney has saved many lives by tiding a patient over a period of acute kidney failure, when poisons are accumulating in the bloodstream. Occasionally, a patient with urea nitrogen values of ten to twenty times the normal value has been saved by this device.

Is the artificial kidney of value when someone has taken an overdose of poison?

Yes, particularly for an overdose of the barbiturates or the heavier metals, such as mercury or arsenic.

What is kidney failure?

The inability of the kidneys to excrete those wastes and toxins that would normally be eliminated from the body. Also, it is the inability to retain in the bloodstream certain essential chemicals.

Does kidney failure mean that the kidney has completely failed and cannot function at all?

No. Kidney failure is a term that denotes either partial or complete inadequacy of kidney function.

Will severe kidney failure lead to the development of uremia?

Yes.

What is kidney "shutdown"?

The kidneys are excreting no urine or an insignificant amount of urine.

How much urine should normal kidneys excrete during a 24-hour period?

Anywhere between three and five pints of urine, depending largely on fluid intake.

What is anuria?

A condition in which there is no output of urine—in other words, a kidney "shutdown."

Is renal failure the same as kidney failure?

Yes.

Are operations sometimes complicated by postoperative renal failure, kidney shutdown, anuria, and other kidney malfunctions?

Yes. This is one of the most serious complications of major surgery.

How can one guard against the development of renal shutdown after surgery?

The internist and the surgeon must discover before surgery whether or not the body chemistries are adequate to withstand the contemplated surgery. This is determined by examining the blood and urine and by performing other tests to determine the adequacy of vital organs, such as the liver, heart, and kidneys. If the operation is not absolutely essential, it should not be carried out if the patient shows marked impairment of kidney function.

Is failure of liver function often associated with kidney failure?

Yes, especially after a major operation. This is called hepatorenal failure or the hepatorenal syndrome.

If impairment of liver and kidney function has been discovered preoperatively, is there any way to improve it so that surgery can be performed safely?

To a limited extent. The liver should be supported by feeding large quantities of sugar and by withholding fats from the diet. The kidneys should be supported by attempts to bring the various blood chemicals into more normal balance. This is a complicated procedure and should be supervised by the internist. Of course, people with advanced kidney damage cannot be helped greatly, but sufficient temporary improvement may be obtained to permit essential surgery.

If kidney failure or kidney shutdown does take place after surgery, what can be done about it?

1. Measures will be taken to maintain in the patient as normal a balance of electrolytes (chemicals such as sodium, chloride, and potassium) as possible.
2. Fluid intake and output will be carefully watched and attempts will be made to bring them into proper balance.

3. If poisons, such as urea nitrogen, accumulate in large quantities in the blood, the artificial kidney may be used.
4. If kidney failure is associated with blood loss, blood transfusions will be given.

Do older people ever recover from kidney failure?

Yes, but not very often.

Is there a tendency for older people to form kidney stones?

The development of kidney stones occurs most often during the early and middle years, although people past sixty can develop them. Kidney stones often remain quiescent during most of life, but may cause trouble when the patient enters his seventies or eighties.

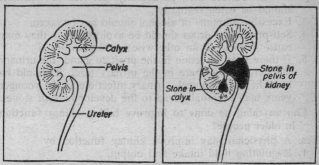

Normal kidney and kidney with stones

What are some of the symptoms caused by stones in the kidney?

1. Excruciating pain in the loins.
2. Marked tenderness over the area of the involved kidney.
3. Painful urination.
4. Blood in the urine.

Do kidney stones often impair the function of a kidney?

Yes, if they cause obstruction of the urinary outflow or if they are associated with infection.

Is infection often associated with kidney stones?

Yes. Since stones frequently obstruct the urinary outflow, the urine stagnates and becomes infected.

What is hydronephrosis?

It is a condition caused by obstruction of the outflow of urine from the kidney. The kidney becomes dilated and distended with urine, leading eventually to destruction of the organ.

Can an enlarged prostate gland lead to kidney damage?

Yes. In such cases, the obstruction of urine outflow causes a backflow of the urine from the bladder all the way to the ureter and into the kidney.

If one takes precautions during the middle years, can he prevent the formation of kidney stones in later life?

There is no sure way to prevent the formation of kidney stones. However, certain precautions should be taken if there is a tendency to develop stones:

1. At least eight to ten glasses of fluid should be taken every day, unless there is some medical reason for limiting liquid intake.
2. A well-rounded diet, particularly one rich in vitamins, should be eaten regularly.
3. Excessive amounts of alcohol should not be taken.
4. Self-prescribed drugs should be avoided, since they may cause damage to an otherwise healthy kidney.
5. If there is an infection in the prostate gland, the urinary bladder, or elsewhere in the urinary tract, it should be brought under control. Urinary infections in the younger years may eventually lead to the development of stones.

Can anything be done to improve failing kidney function in older people?

Yes. A physician may improve kidney function by
1. Regulating fluid intake and output.
2. Regulating the amount of minerals in the diet.
3. Clearing up a kidney or bladder infection.
4. Eliminating an obstruction of the outflow of urine from the kidneys and bladder.
5. Correcting dietary insufficiencies.
6. Correcting anemia.
7. Eliminating kidney irritants such as alcohol or harmful drugs.
8. Attempting to improve the circulation and to lower high blood pressure.

Will the drinking of excessive amounts of alcohol over a long period of time lead to premature impairment of kidney function?

Yes.

Does tuberculosis ever affect the kidneys?

Yes, but it usually shows up during the younger years. Whereas kidney removal used to be necessary for tuberculous infections, today, antibiotics and other drugs cure many such cases.

CYSTS

Do cysts of the kidney occur in older people?

Occasionally, but they usually develop early in life.

Should a cyst of the kidney in an older person be operated on?

Only if it produces symptoms or causes extensive kidney damage. In many cases, the cyst causes no symptoms and does not interfere with kidney function.

CANCER OF THE KIDNEY

Is cancer of the kidney common in older people?

Malignant tumor of the kidney comprises about one-half of 1 percent of all cancers. It occurs in people past sixty in about that proportion.

What are the signs and symptoms of cancer of the kidney?

1. A lump (tumor mass) may be felt in the flank area.
2. There is pain in the flank.
3. Blood appears in the urine.

Is it difficult to establish a diagnosis of malignant tumor of the kidney?

No. Special X rays will show a distortion of the outline of the kidney. Such a distorted picture will indicate the presence of a tumor.

Are most tumors of the kidney malignant?

Yes.

What is the treatment of cancer of the kidney?

Removal of the kidney.

Can older people tolerate kidney removal?

Yes; if they are in satisfactory general health.

What are the chances of cure in cancer of the kidney?

If the organ is removed early enough, cure can be obtained in approximately half of the cases.

What can people do in their earlier years to avoid kidney trouble later in life?

1. They should try to forestall the onset of premature hardening of the arteries. This will include leading a life of moderation and eating a diet low in fats.
2. They should obtain prompt treatment for any infection of the urinary tract.

3. They should drink large quantities of fluids.
4. Kidney stones should be removed as soon as it is apparent that they will not pass spontaneously.
5. They should drink alcoholic beverages only in moderation.
6. They should avoid drugs that might cause kidney damage.
7. Any tendency to high blood pressure should be treated energetically, and all efforts should be made during earlier years to control it.

LAXATIVES

See BOWEL FUNCTION; CONSTIPATION; DIARRHEA; DRUGS AND MEDICINES; INTESTINES; RECTUM AND ANUS.

Do people require laxatives more often as they grow older?
Yes. Bowel function does tend to become sluggish during the later years. This is caused by laxity of the muscles in the abdominal wall and surrounding the rectum. The lack of muscle tone makes it more difficult to expel feces from the rectum. Moreover, older people engage in less physical exercise, thus making it harder for them to maintain good muscle control.

What are some good general rules for older people to follow when taking laxatives?
1. They should always use the mildest laxative that will produce a result.
2. If a bland lubricant such as mineral oil will regulate the bowels, it should be used instead of a laxative.
3. If the taking of substances such as prunes and bran will produce satisfactory bowel evacuation, they are preferable to laxatives.
4. The smallest possible dose of a laxative should be used.
5. As many days as possible should be skipped between doses of laxatives.
6. When a laxative that has previously been effective begins to lose its effect, another laxative should be substituted.
7. Those laxatives that produce the least dehydration should be used. In other words, if a laxative causes diarrhea with the loss of large quantities of fluid, older people should not use it.

Are laxatives habit-forming?

In the sense that people become dependent on them. People do not, however, develop a true addiction to laxatives.

Do most laxatives tend to irritate the lining of the intestinal tract?

Yes, and for this reason they should be avoided whenever possible.

Are bulk-forming medications a good substitute for laxatives?

Yes, when they produce satisfactory evacuation. It must be understood, however, that they may occasionally cause stagnation of feces in the lower intestinal tract.

These medications should not be used by older people unless prescribed by a physician.

What are the best foods to take to avoid constipation and the need for laxatives?

1. Stewed fruit and fruit juices.
2. Fresh fruit.
3. Fresh vegetables.
4. Bran products.
5. Foods containing a large amount of roughage.

Diets containing such foods cannot always be tolerated well by elderly people. A doctor should be consulted in cases of chronic constipation.

LEUKEMIA

See BLOOD; CANCER AND OTHER MALIGNANT GROWTHS; HODGKIN'S DISEASE; LYMPH GLANDS; SPLEEN.

What is leukemia?

It is a disease of the blood-forming organs, characterized by excessively large numbers of white blood cells in the bloodstream. Many of these cells are abnormal in size and shape; others are immature and are released into the bloodstream by the bone marrow before they have fully formed.

Is leukemia considered to be "cancer of the blood"?

Yes.

Is leukemia seen often in elderly people?

Yes. It affects people in all age groups, although it is somewhat more common in the young. The chronic form of the disease is seen more often in older people; the acute form is seen most frequently in children and young adults. The greatest incidence of leukemia of the chronic type is in people between the ages of sixty and eighty.

How can someone tell if he has leukemia?

There are very few early symptoms. The disease is often discovered unexpectedly when taking the blood count of a patient who complains of loss of appetite and decrease in energy.

Is leukemia ever curable?

No, but there are drugs that can often retard the progress of the disease and cause it to remain static for years.

Is leukemia always fatal when it affects older people?

No. The chronic form may extend over a period of ten to twenty years. Thus, an older individual may live out his normal life-span and succumb to some totally unrelated condition.

What is the treatment of leukemia?

1. Drugs to destroy white blood cells are given.
2. X-ray treatment of the bone marrow is sometimes given.
3. Certain new radioactive isotopes to destroy excess white blood cells are given.
4. Blood transfusions are given to counteract the anemia that almost always accompanies leukemia.
5. Bone-marrow transfusions have been used recently on an experimental basis and have occasionally proved helpful in delaying the progress of the disease.
6. Antibiotics are prescribed whenever infection sets in. People with leukemia are particularly susceptible to infection.

LEUKOPLAKIA

See CANCER AND OTHER MALIGNANT GROWTHS; FEMALE ORGANS; MOUTH, LIPS, AND TONGUE; SMOKING; VITAMINS.

What is leukoplakia?

Thickened white patches of epithelium appear on the mucous membranes, most often of the mouth, the gums, the inner lining of the cheeks, the palate, and the tongue. It may also affect the mucous membranes of the female genitals. Leukoplakia of the female genitals is characterized by thickening, dryness, and itching of the membranes at the entrance to the vagina.

Is "smoker's tongue" the same as leukoplakia of the tongue?

Yes.

Does leukoplakia frequently affect older people?

Yes, although middle-aged people may also develop this condition.

What causes leukoplakia of the mouth?

Although the exact cause is not known, it is thought that

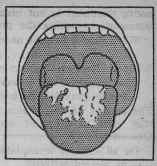

Leukoplakia of tongue

tobacco smoking and poorly fitting dentures are the most important contributing factors. Chewing tobacco and snuff, used extensively some years ago, were also thought to cause leukoplakia.

Does leukoplakia usually develop into cancer?

In the great majority of cases, it does not. However, measures must be taken to check it, or cancer may result. It is commonly considered to be a precancerous condition.

What measures should be taken to prevent leukoplakia of the mouth from developing into cancer?

1. Smoking should be discontinued.
2. Chewing tobacco and snuff should not be used.
3. Drinking alcoholic beverages should be stopped, except for an occasional drink.
4. All possible sources of local irritation, such as rough edges of teeth, infected decayed teeth, and badly fitting artificial teeth, should be remedied.
5. General health should be checked regularly to make certain that there is no underlying vitamin deficiency or disease such as syphilis.
6. Patches of leukoplakia that seem to be growing or developing into ulcerations should be removed. This can be done either by burning the plaques away with an electric needle or by surgical excision.

Should older people with leukoplakia of the mouth visit a doctor frequently?

Yes, it is wise to visit the doctor every three to four months so that he may note whether any changes have taken place in the appearance of the patches of leukoplakia.

Must leukoplakia of the mouth always be treated actively?

No. In the great majority of cases, the process is so slow that active treatment is not necessary. Most cases can be held stationary by taking the precautions listed above.

When does it become necessary to treat leukoplakia actively?

When it ulcerates or shows marked growth.

What measures can be taken to prevent leukoplakia of the female genitals from becoming cancerous?

The patches of leukoplakia should be removed surgically if they start to grow or become ulcerated. (*See* FEMALE ORGANS.)

Do all cases of leukoplakia of the female genitals have to be treated actively?

Not unless areas of ulceration appear, or if the spread of the disease is extensive.

LIVER

See ALCOHOL AND ALCOHOLISM; CIRRHOSIS OF THE LIVER; DIET; DRUGS AND MEDICINES; GALLBLADDER AND BILE DUCTS; HEPATITIS; JAUNDICE; TESTS; WEIGHT.

Where is the liver located?

The liver, the largest organ in the body, is located in the upper right portion of the abdomen beneath the diaphragm. It measures approximately eight inches by seven inches in diameter.

What are its functions?

The liver is one of the most important structures in the body and is essential in regulating chemical reactions. It has many functions. Some of the most important are:

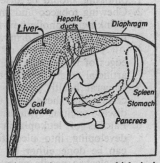

Liver and organs to which it is attached

1. The storage of sugar (in the form of glycogen).
2. The production and storage of proteins and the regulation of the many byproducts of protein metabolism.
3. The storage and utilization of fats.
4. The production of substances important for blood coagulation.

5. The production of bile acids and bile salts, which are secreted through the ducts leading from the liver to the intestinal tract.
6. The elimination of poisons and toxins that circulate throughout the body.
7. The production and storage of substances important to the manufacture of blood and blood cells.

Is adequate liver function essential to the maintenance of life?

Yes.

Is the liver capable of maintaining normal function throughout all of life?

Yes. In healthy people, the liver can function adequately into the eighties and nineties. Even if there is considerable cirrhosis (fibrous replacement of liver tissue), a sufficient amount of functioning liver substance often remains to sustain life.

What are the effects of the aging process on the liver and on liver function?

Aging brings about destruction of liver cells and their replacement by fibrous (scar) tissue. This process is known as cirrhosis of the liver. Also, during the process of aging there may be a replacement of the liver tissue by fat cells. This is called fatty degeneration of the liver.

But the body has such an excess of liver tissue that marked loss of some of it can occur without endangering function too greatly.

What are some of the common causes of impairment of liver function in older people?

1. The normal aging process.
2. Infection of the liver, usually caused by a spread through the bile ducts, the lymph channels, or the blood vessels of the liver.
3. Liver poisoning due to toxic drugs, poisons, or other substances.
4. Obstruction of the outflow of bile from the liver.
5. Inadequate sugar in the diet.
6. Interference with blood supply to the liver.
7. Failure of the kidneys to eliminate poisons from the body. These poisons will eventually cause liver damage.
8. Cirrhosis of the liver, with replacement of its functioning cells by fibrous tissue.
9. Cancer of the liver.

How can one tell if the liver is failing?

Any of the following conditions may point to impaired function:

1. Marked enlargement of the liver. This condition may be felt as a heavy, dragging sensation in the upper right portion of the abdomen. An examining physician will be able to tell if the liver is enlarged merely by feeling the abdomen.
2. Jaundice (yellowness of the skin, eyeballs, and mucous membranes).
3. Extreme fatigue, loss of appetite, and a generally sluggish feeling.

Are there tests for determining the adequacy of liver function?

Yes. Dozens of tests, performed on blood and urine, will permit the doctor to gauge quite accurately the adequacy or inadequacy of liver function.

Should older people have liver-function tests performed?

Yes, if any of the above symptoms appear. Also, a blood-chemistry analysis, which should be done once a year, will show any abnormality in liver function.

Is it true that alcoholics tend to develop liver disease?

Yes. Chronic alcoholics have a greater incidence of cirrhosis and other liver diseases.

What effect does being overweight have on liver function?

It is generally agreed that those who are obese place added strain on their livers. Fatty infiltration of the liver definitely interferes with adequate function.

Can liver function in overweight people be improved if they reduce?

Yes.

Is an adequate supply of sugar and other carbohydrates in the diet important in maintaining normal liver function?

Yes.

Is an adequate intake of protein necessary to maintain normal liver function?

Yes.

Is it particularly important to test liver function in older people who are about to undergo surgery?

Yes, this is essential. Postoperative liver failure is one of the commonest causes of death among older surgical patients.

How can a surgeon tell if the liver is functioning properly before he operates?

1. Liver-function tests are performed, especially those to determine the liver's ability to regulate sugar and protein metabolism.

2. Tests will be made to determine the liver's capacity to maintain normal blood coagulation.

3. Tests for jaundice will be conducted.

4. The amount of protein circulating in the bloodstream will be noted.

Does the liver tend to enlarge when circulation is inadequate or when the heart is failing?

Yes, because the liver becomes filled with blood that is slow in passing through its veins. When heart function is restored by use of digitalis and other medications, the liver tends to return to normal size.

Does liver poisoning, with extensive destruction of liver tissue, ever take place as a result of taking toxic drugs or medications?

Yes. It is especially likely to happen when people medicate themselves.

Does an elderly individual have to follow a special routine in order to maintain normal liver function?

No. The liver will perform its duties if the general health remains satisfactory.

What can one do to ensure the continuation of normal liver function?

1. Avoid excessive alcohol and drugs that may cause liver damage.

2. Stay thin, so that excess fat is not deposited in the liver.

3. If the gallbladder is infected or contains stones, have it removed.

4. Maintain a diet rich in proteins, sugar, and vitamins.

What is a fatty liver?

It is a liver that contains more than the normal quantity of fatty substances.

Does a fatty liver interfere with adequate liver function?

Yes, since the fat cells replace functioning liver cells.

What are some of the causes of fatty liver?

1. Alcoholism.

2. Diabetes.

3. Marked obesity.

4. Marked anemia.

5. Marked undernourishment.

6. Chemical poisoning of the liver by drugs or poisons.

What is the treatment of fatty liver?

1. Elimination of the above precipitating causes.

2. A diet containing large amounts of protein and sugar, and adequate quantities of minerals and vitamins.
3. Limiting the amount of fats eaten.
4. Medication for anemia.
5. If the heart is not functioning properly, appropriate medication for that condition.
6. Bed rest, if there is acute liver failure.

What is the treatment of jaundice?
See JAUNDICE.

What is cirrhosis, and what is the treatment of it?
See CIRRHOSIS OF THE LIVER.

Does cancer of the liver occur frequently in older people?
Cancer *originating* in the liver is a rather rare disease in older people, but it does occur occasionally. However, cancer of the liver that had its origin elsewhere in the body is extremely common. Since all of the body's blood will eventually pass through the liver, it will carry cancer cells with it. The liver filters out these circulating cells and thus becomes involved in a secondary cancer growth.

Cancers of the breast, the stomach, the intestines, the prostate, the rectum, and the pancreas have a tendency to spread and deposit cells in liver substance.

Is it ever possible to cure cancer of the liver?
Yes, in an occasional case it is possible to remove an involved section of the liver. But in the vast majority of cases, cancer spreads to so many areas in the liver that surgery cannot bring relief.

Is it possible to live without a liver?
No.

LONGEVITY

See ALCOHOL AND ALCOHOLISM; ANATOMICAL CHANGES IN ORGANS; ARTERIOSCLEROSIS; ATTITUDES TOWARD AGING; CLIMATE; DEGENERATIVE CHANGES OF AGING; ENDOCRINE GLANDS AND HORMONES; PREMATURE AGING; WEIGHT.

What is meant by the term "full life-span"?
It is the number of years that people are capable of living under ideal circumstances. This does not necessarily mean that there is a set length of time for all individuals. As we know, people sometimes live for more than 100 years. Also, the length of the full life-span is different for various races

and in various climates. Generally speaking, the full life-span means that after a certain specific number of years, vital organs will deteriorate to such an extent that life can no longer be sustained.

Is it likely that the average life-span will be significantly lengthened in years to come?

Yes. As medical science discovers more and more about the causes and origins of the aging process, new methods for delaying its onset will undoubtedly be found. Even now, great progress is being made in discovering the underlying causes of arteriosclerosis (hardening of the arteries).

What predictions can be made concerning the number of added years one can expect to live within the foreseeable future?

Most scientists feel that another five to ten years will be added to the average life-span by the end of the twentieth century.

Do diseases of childhood and youth decrease the life-span of an individual?

Yes. In this area, too, we can anticipate much progress. When medicine discovers how to eradicate some of the more serious bacterial and viral infections of the earlier years, the aging process will be retarded considerably.

In looking back over the past hundred years, we can see how the life-span in many parts of the world has been prolonged enormously by the eradication of such diseases as typhoid fever, cholera, hookworm disease, tuberculosis, and many other killers that plagued man for centuries.

How does elimination of childhood infections increase longevity?

Repeated infections in childhood, youth, and early adulthood often lead to permanent damage to organs that are vital to longevity. Such organs as the liver, heart, and kidneys, when damaged by infection in youth, will show deterioration earlier in one's adulthood. As one example, rheumatic fever can now be controlled with the antibiotic drugs, thereby saving hundreds of thousands of children from developing valve disease of the heart. People with diseased heart valves have a much shorter life expectancy than those with healthy heart valves.

Will increased knowledge concerning chemical and physical factors involved in the aging process tend to lengthen man's life expectancy?

Yes. For instance, great strides have been made in understanding the arteriosclerotic process. The entire subject of cholesterol metabolism and its possible relationship to premature hardening of the arteries may ultimately lead to the retardation of this degenerative process.

Toward what goal is the medical profession directing its attention, insofar as life expectancy is concerned?

Efforts are being made today to see that more and more people attain their *full* life expectancy. By the elimination of some of the causes of premature aging and, consequently, of premature death, we have been able to extend the *average* life-span from the forty years of a century ago to approximately seventy years today.

What are some of the major factors that have contributed to longer life expectancy?

1. The control of infection and sepsis during childbirth has led to a tremendous decrease in newborn and maternal mortality.

2. Elimination of infant diarrhea (dysentery) and other infections during the first year of life has greatly lowered infant mortality.

3. The control of the more serious childhood contagious diseases, such as diphtheria, typhoid fever, and infantile paralysis, has lowered child mortality to such an extent that deaths from these causes are now rare in the United States.

4. The control and elimination of such epidemic diseases as plague, cholera, smallpox, and typhus fever in the more scientifically advanced parts of the world have lowered the mortality rates of both children and adults.

5. The control of such diseases as pneumonia and tuberculosis, through the introduction of antibiotics and other new drugs, has produced a sudden drop in mortality rates.

6. Vast improvements in surgery and anesthesiology have lowered surgical mortality rates tremendously.

7. Improved hygienic standards and measures to eliminate dietary-deficiency diseases have lowered mortality among poor peoples.

8. Greatly improved diagnostic techniques have aided medicine in reaching correct diagnoses, so that serious illnesses can be treated more accurately.

9. Distribution of medical care has been improved, so that more and more people are able to receive expert help for serious illness.

10. Society's realization that the health of its people is a vital social responsibility has led to the development

of medical-care programs and the assumption by voluntary and public agencies of responsibility for the health of their communities.

Is life expectancy now greater for healthy people who are over sixty?

Yes, but the increased expectancy is not as great as that for a child who is in good health. In other words, man's increased longevity is due more to the decrease in infant and child mortality. Of course, some of the factors mentioned before are responsible for a longer life expectancy for older people too, but this increase can be measured in terms of a few years, not in terms of decades.

Is heredity an important factor in longevity?

Yes. Certain families tend to age early, whereas others show the signs of aging much later in life. Everyone is familiar with families in which the parents and most of the children have lived for more than seventy or eighty years. In such families, arteriosclerosis and other evidences of aging occur exceptionally late in life.

It is the consensus of science that we inherit only a *tendency* toward longevity. There is a tendency in families to inherit good blood vessels or bad blood vessels. Further, there is a tendency in families to inherit conditions that predispose one to early or late deterioration of vital structures.

It should be noted that heredity is only one factor in the process of aging, and that it may be modified greatly by environmental factors. Thus, an individual with an inherited tendency toward late development of arteriosclerosis may counteract this tendency by living a dissolute life. If he eats and drinks too much or if he is not emotionally stable, he may develop arteriosclerosis at an early age.

Many men in their forties or early fifties suffer fatal heart attacks even though they come from families in which the parents and grandparents had lived far into their seventies and eighties. It cannot be emphasized too strongly that the emotional factors of life may modify or nullify hereditary factors.

If one has a history of longevity in his family, can he, too, expect to live a long life?

Not necessarily, but he has a potentially long life-span.

If one has a family history of short life-span, does this necessarily mean that he, too, will have a relatively short life-span?

Absolutely not. The awareness of poor heredity often is beneficial, in that an individual can take steps to offset those factors that caused the early death of his parents and grandparents. For instance, if a young man knows that his parents developed diabetes and high blood pressure at an early age, he can take preventive measures. Such an individual can follow a dietary regimen that is the least conducive to diabetes and hypertension, and he can lead a life as free from stress as possible.

If a young person knows that there is a tendency toward cancer in his family, he can have frequent periodic examinations so that if he does develop cancer, it will be discovered in its early stages. A medically conscious individual with a poor family history of longevity has a much better chance for long life than one with an excellent family history of longevity who neglects his health.

Does the average woman have a greater life expectancy than the average man?

Yes. In the United States the female life-span is approximately five years longer.

Is life expectancy increasing more rapidly for women than for men?

Yes. According to Metropolitan Life Insurance statistics, between 1900 and 1950 the expectation of life increased by 17.6 years for men and 20.3 years for women. These statistics are reflected in the fact that women outnumber men in the later years, even though there are about 105 males born for every 100 females.

Why do women have a greater life expectancy than men?

1. The average woman, particularly in the United States, leads a life of less stress.
2. The average woman is exposed to fewer physical hardships and hazards.
3. The average woman gets more rest and sleep.
4. Those conditions that formerly produced the greatest number of deaths in young women, namely, deaths due to complications arising from childbearing, have been largely eliminated.
5. Chemical factors involved in cholesterol and estrogen metabolism lead to much later onset of arteriosclerosis in women. It is estimated that arteriosclerosis sets in about seven to ten years later in women than in men.
6. Accidents, a rapidly increasing cause of death among young people, kill fewer women than men.

Is it true that glandular factors in women make it possible for them to live longer?

A definite answer cannot be given to this question. A great many investigators in this field believe that steroid metabolism (including cholesterol and female sex hormone metabolism) greatly influences the onset of arteriosclerosis, and it is well known that there is considerable difference between the metabolic processes in the two sexes.

Does the age at which a woman undergoes change of life (menopause) influence the length of her life-span?

No.

Does the age at which a man loses his potency influence the length of his life-span?

No. Loss of potency is more often a psychological phenomenon than a physical one.

Can a doctor make an accurate prediction as to how long an individual is likely to live?

Yes, by noting the state of health of organs that are important to long life.

What organs are most important in judging the potential life-span of an individual?

The heart, arteries, kidneys, liver, adrenal glands, pancreas, lungs, and brain.

Do hormones play an important role in determining longevity?

Yes. Many investigators feel that an upset in hormone secretion and chemical reactions is largely responsible for the onset of the aging process. One whose hormone metabolism continues to function normally late in life has a much better chance of a long life-span.

Is it true that if one inherits good blood vessels he can live a long life?

The ability of the blood vessels to remain free from arteriosclerosis is certainly an extremely important factor in the aging process, but so many other factors may alter the situation that this statement is not invariably true.

What is the relationship between obesity and longevity?

Statistics indicate that thin people live longer than fat people. This is not because obesity in itself terminates life at an early age, but because obese people are much more likely to develop diseases and infections.

What effect does multiple childbirth have on longevity?

There is no evidence that bearing an average number of children shortens the life-span. On the contrary, women who have never borne children have a shorter life-span.

Does diet affect longevity?

Yes. Those who have chronic dietary deficiencies are more

likely to develop diseases that shorten life. In underdeveloped countries, where food shortage is great, the life expectancy is much lower than in the United States, for example.

Do vegetarians tend to live longer than people who eat meat?

No.

Does climate influence longevity?

Yes. People who live in the extremes of temperature tend to have shorter lives than those who live in a temperate climate. This is to be expected, since those who are exposed to the heat of the tropics and uncivilized conditions in the jungles are more likely to develop diseases that can terminate life. Similarly, those who live in frigid areas are prone to develop diseases associated with their rigorous existence.

Do people who have suffered repeated serious illness in youth tend to live shorter lives?

Yes, because repeated serious illness may permanently damage those organs that are essential to long life.

Does the rapid pace of modern living tend to shorten the life-span?

Yes, because excess stress is associated with an increased incidence of disease in vital organs.

What influence does an occupation demanding strenuous physical exertion have on longevity?

If people become accustomed to hard physical labor, their life-spans will not be shortened by it. On the other hand, people who are not accustomed to strenuous physical work and who engage in it sporadically may do themselves irreparable harm. For example, a banker who sits behind his desk all day for twenty to thirty years may suffer a fatal heart attack while playing a set of tennis. On the other hand, a man who labors in the construction business year in and year out can tolerate other physical exertion without undue danger.

Will people who have led an "overactive" sex life tend to have a shorter life-span?

No, unless their activities are associated with insufficient rest, excessive drinking, etc.

Will abstinence from sexual activity prolong the life-span?

No.

Does chronic alcoholism shorten the life-span?

Yes. Damage to vital organs, such as the brain, the heart, the liver, and the kidneys, often occurs among alcoholics.

Does excessive smoking shorten the life-span?

This has not been proved, although it is known that smoking is bad for people who have hardening of the arteries. If they continue to smoke, the smoking may precipitate a heart attack or cause further damage to the blood vessels.

Will taking vitamins throughout the middle years tend to prolong the life-span?

Only if a major dietary deficiency has necessitated the continued use of supplementary vitamins.

Does one's attitude toward living affect one's longevity?

Yes. The will to live is of inestimable importance. Almost all physicians agree that people who lack a desire to live tend to die at earlier ages. There are, however, many events that occur over the years that can alter this situation. In other words, an intense desire to live will go unrewarded if one develops an incurable malignancy or if the blood vessels are markedly sclerotic.

Do married people tend to live longer than single people?

Statistics show that married people do tend to live longer. Medical investigators believe that this is due to the care that one spouse will take of another. When a husband is ill, the wife will urge him to seek medical attention early in the course of an illness. A single person tends to neglect his health until disease is far advanced.

Can any drugs prolong the life-span?

No. There are specific medications for specific illnesses, but there is no special "longevity drug."

Are there differences in the life-spans of various occupational groups?

Yes, but these differences are based on statistics for the group, rather than for the individual.

Does poverty influence longevity?

Yes. Poor people have diets deficient in essential ingredients. Furthermore, poor people seek medical attention less often and later in the course of an illness than those who have adequate financial means. Also, the poor are less able to observe hygienic practices, which increases the incidence of infection and disease among them.

Does worry adversely affect longevity?

Yes. Recent investigations have demonstrated that organic disease can result from excessive emotional stress.

Can older people expect to live longer today?

Yes. According to statisticians of the Metropolitan Life Insurance Company,* senior citizens share substantially in the marked reductions in mortality during recent decades.

Spectacular reductions in mortality among children and young adults have tended to obscure the progress in lengthened lifespan for older people. However, mortality rates at ages sixty and over for 1958 show marked reduction over those for the 1929–31 period.

Among men, a mortality-rate reduction was recorded at each age from sixty to eighty, the decrease averaging about 13 percent. For example, at age sixty, the death rate fell from 26.4 per 1,000 in 1929–31 to 22.6 in 1958; at age seventy-five, the death rate dropped from 85.3 to 73.3 per 1,000 in the same period. Women have made considerably greater gains than men, the reductions ranging from as much as 47 percent at age sixty to more than 30 percent through age eighty.

Reductions in mortality have been accompanied by increases in longevity for older persons. In 1958 women at age sixty had an expectation of remaining life of 19.2 years, a gain of 3.1 years since 1929–31. At age eighty, the remaining lifetime averaged 6.4 years in 1958, a gain of 0.8 years. For men, the age sixty figure was 15.7 years in 1958, a gain of one year; at age eighty, life expectancy was 5.8 years, a gain of half a year.

A reflection of the improvement in decreased mortality and increased longevity is seen in older people's increased chances of surviving an additional ten years. For those currently reaching age sixty-five, the chances of living at least another ten years are almost 3 in 5 for men and 3 in 4 for women. Even at age seventy-five, the chances of survival for ten years are almost 1 in 3 for men and more than 2 in 5 for women.

What are the statistics for life expectancy of women between the ages of sixty and seventy?*

FEMALES

Age	Years of Life to Live
60	19.2
61	18.4
62	17.6
63	16.9
64	16.1
65	15.4
66	14.7

*Statistics in this section furnished by Metropolitan Life Insurance Information Service.

67	14.0
68	13.3
69	12.7

What are the statistics for life expectancy of men between the ages of sixty and seventy?*

MALES

Age	Years of Life to Live
60	15.7
61	15.0
62	14.4
63	13.8
64	13.2
65	12.7
66	12.1
67	11.6
68	11.1
69	10.6

LUNG TUMORS

See CANCER AND OTHER MALIGNANT GROWTHS; RESPIRATORY TRACT; SMOKING.

Do tumors of the bronchial tubes develop very often in older people?
Yes. They are among the most common tumors in people past sixty, especially in men.

Do benign (noncancerous) tumors ever affect the lungs?
Yes, although they are not as common as the malignant type. These tumors may be adenomas, fibromas, neurofibromas, lipomas, or papillomas. When they do occur, they usually produce symptoms similar to those of malignant tumors.

What are the symptoms of lung tumor?
1. Chronic (often hacking) cough.
2. Coughing up blood.
3. Pain in the chest on the affected side.
4. Shortness of breath and a consequent desire to sleep in a semisitting position.
5. Loss of appetite, weakness, fatigue, anemia.

*Metropolitan Life Insurance Company.

Do people with lung tumor develop symptoms early in the course of the disease?

No. For this reason it is important that older people undergo periodic physical examinations, including X ray of the lungs.

Why are men more likely than women to develop cancer of the bronchial tubes and lungs?

The exact reason is not known, but some investigators feel that cigarette smoking, formerly more common among men, has something to do with it. This theory is supported by the fact that the incidence of this form of cancer in women is now increasing, paralleling their increased use of tobacco in recent years.

Is cancer of the lungs and bronchial tubes increasing?

Yes.

Is tobacco smoking thought to be an important factor in the development of cancer of the lung?

Yes. Statistics demonstrate a much greater incidence of lung cancer among those who smoke. This is especially true in men.

Does the type of smoking make any difference?

It seems to. The greatest incidence of cancer is among those who smoke cigarettes. Cigars and pipes seem to be much less influential in development of cancer.

Does lung cancer ever develop in nonsmokers?

Certainly, although the incidence is much less than among those who are heavy smokers.

Will a chest X ray always allow diagnosis of lung cancer?

No. It may suggest the presence of a lung cancer, but many other conditions give a somewhat similar picture on X ray.

How is a definite diagnosis of lung cancer made?

In addition to taking chest X rays, the doctor usually makes a bronchoscopic examination. This entails passing a metal tube from the mouth down the throat and into the trachea (windpipe). In the majority of cases, the bronchoscopist will be able to see an obstruction of the bronchial tube in the tumor area. Often a piece of tumor tissue is removed (a procedure called *biopsy*) and then submitted for microscopic examination.

What is a scalenus node biopsy?

This is a procedure in which an incision is made in the base of the neck, and lymph glands that lie above the dome of the lungs are removed and sent to the laboratory for examination. If these glands are cancerous, removal of the lung will in all likelihood be of little help to the patient. If, on the other hand, the biopsy is negative, the surgeon will operate for removal of the lung.

Does a negative finding from bronchoscopic examination always mean that no cancer is present?

No. In many cases the final diagnosis will depend on surgical exploration of the chest.

When is surgical exploration usually recommended?

When symptoms persist for more than several weeks.

What is the surgical procedure when lung cancer is suspected?

A long incision is made between the ribs on the affected side of the chest. The chest cavity is opened and the lung thoroughly inspected. If a tumor is present, it is not difficult for the surgeon to detect it.

What is the surgical procedure for a tumor of the lung?

In the great majority of cases, the involved lobe is removed. If the tumor has extended to more than one lobe or to the root of the lung, then the entire lung on that side will be removed.

How dangerous is surgery for lung cancer?

Today there is little more risk in lung surgery than in abdominal surgery. For this reason, whenever doubt exists as to the presence of a lung tumor, surgery is advocated, even for the aged.

What is a lobectomy?

It is the removal of a lobe. The left lung is composed of two lobes; the right has three lobes.

What is pneumonectomy?

The removal of an entire lung; that is, the three lobes of the right lung or the two lobes of the left.

Do older people usually recover from lobectomy or pneumonectomy?

Yes, in over 85 percent of cases. This does not necessarily mean, however, that a total cure has been effected.

Is there any treatment other than surgery for cancer of the lung?

Yes. Patients who cannot undergo surgery because of poor general health may be given X-ray or cobalt therapy. Such treatment may bring about substantial prolongation of life.

What percentage of patients are seen early enough to permit surgical removal of lung tumor?

It is estimated that because of improved diagnostic techniques and greater realization by the public that early treatment of chest symptoms is important, nearly half of those with lung tumor are now reaching the surgeon in time for surgical removal of the growth.

Is cancer of the lung curable?

Yes, in many cases in which the tumor has not spread beyond the confines of the lung. But often people go for a medical examination too late in the course of the disease.

What is the treatment of benign lung tumor?

The involved lobe of the lung is removed in the same way that a malignant growth is.

Are benign lung tumors curable?

Yes, in almost all cases, provided the patient is able to withstand the operation.

Is surgery for benign lung tumors very serious?

Yes, but recovery is the rule in almost all instances.

LYMPH GLANDS

See HODGKIN'S DISEASE; INFECTIONS; LEUKEMIA.

What are lymph glands and where are they located?

Lymph glands, or, more accurately, lymph nodes, are oval structures about one-quarter to one-half inch in length and about one-eighth to one-quarter inch in diameter. They are made up mainly of white blood cells and connective tissue.

They are present in every part of the body. Some lie deep within the tissues; others are superficial, lying beneath the skin. The lymph glands congregate in the areas where they drain major lymph channels. Normally, one can feel lymph glands beneath the skin in the neck, under the armpits, and in the groin.

What is lymph?

The fluid that is derived from connective tissue and tissue between organs. Lymph travels through special lymph channels.

What are the functions of the lymph glands?

They filter the lymph and block the spread of infection and

disease. For instance, an infection in the tonsils or throat will cause swelling of the lymph glands in the neck. The infectious process will often be halted in the lymph glands, thus preventing spread of the infection to the circulation. Similarly, cancer of the breast often spreads to the lymph nodes in the armpits, where an attempt will be made to prevent the spread of the cancer to the rest of the body.

How do the lymph glands stop the spread of infection?

The various cells in the lymph glands fight the bacteria or viruses and often destroy them. Most infections are halted or controlled by this mechanism.

Are the lymph glands as effective in halting the spread of cancer or infection in older people as in younger ones?

Most observers believe that lymph glands continue to function normally throughout life, although there may be some replacement of the white cells by fibrous tissue. There may also be some tendency for tumor cells to pass through the lymph glands more readily in older people, but this is not certain.

What happens when the lymph glands are overwhelmed by a powerful infection?

They break down and form abscesses. It then becomes necessary to make a surgical incision into the area and permit the pus to drain out.

How can one tell if there is an infection in the lymph channels or in the lymph glands?

If the lymphatics (lymph channels) are infected, a red streak will appear, originating near the site of the primary infection. An infected lymph gland will become swollen, hot, and tender to the touch.

Are lymph glands removed when cancer has spread to them?

Yes. A thorough operation for cancer will include the removal of as many involved lymph glands as possible. Thus, in breast removal for cancer, those lymph glands that normally drain the breast area are removed. Similarly, in operations for cancer of the bowel, the lymph glands in the vicinity of the involved bowel are removed. Extensive removal of nearby lymph glands often results in eradication of all tumor cells.

Will surgical removal of the lymph glands in the armpit or in the groin ever lead to swelling of the arm or leg?

Yes. Permanent swelling of a limb frequently does follow such an operation. This is because lymph collects in the limb when the channels for exit have been removed. Such a condition is called *lymphedema.*

Do the lymph glands become enlarged in leukemia?

Yes. *See* LEUKEMIA.

How can one tell if the swelling in lymph glands is due to an infection, to a tumor, or to some other condition, such as leukemia?

1. Infected glands are almost always painful, hot, and tender. Furthermore, there will be an accompanying infection nearby.
2. If the glands are swollen because of a tumor, the primary growth will be found somewhere in the region.
3. If the gland swelling is due to leukemia or to some other blood disease, a blood count and blood-chemistry analysis will reveal the underlying disease.

LYMPHOMA

What is lymphoma?

This is a general term denoting a malignant disease of the lymph glands. The term is used for many different types of malignancy; for example, lymphosarcoma, Hodgkin's disease, and even leukemia.

Do lymphomas ever affect older people?

Yes.

Is lymphoma always associated with the presence of leukemia, Hodgkin's disease, or lymphosarcoma?

No. Many odd types of tumors of lymph glands do not fall precisely into any one category. Occasionally, only one gland is involved; in such a case, the removal of the involved gland may bring about a complete cure. In other instances, lymphoma is part of a generalized process in which all glands—in the abdomen, in the chest cavity, or in some other area—are involved.

How is the diagnosis of lymphoma made?

By surgical removal and microscopic examination of the involved gland.

LYMPHOSARCOMA

What is lymphosarcoma?

It is a form of malignancy of the lymph glands.

How common is it in people past sixty?

It is found infrequently in older people, although it does sometimes occur.

Is lymphosarcoma ever limited to one gland or to one set of glands?

Occasionally. It is more likely to involve all or most of the lymph glands in the body.

How is lymphosarcoma treated?

If it is limited to one gland or to one set of glands, these glands are removed surgically. In the majority of cases, however, lymphosarcoma does not lend itself to surgery. Some of the newer chemicals, such as nitrogen mustard, can inhibit the growth of lymphosarcoma for months or years. Other cases can be helped tremendously by X-ray or cobalt treatments or by the use of radioactive substances.

Can people past sixty live very long with lymphosarcoma?

Yes. Some of these tumors, especially in very old people, grow at an extremely slow pace. If the general health of the patient is maintained at a satisfactory level and if treatment is carried out vigorously, he may live for many years.

Is there a close relationship between leukemia and lymphosarcoma?

Yes, but they are not the same disease. (Leukemia is a disease of the blood-forming organs.)

MARRIAGE AFTER SIXTY

See FAMILY RELATIONSHIPS; HEART; LONGEVITY; SEX AFTER SIXTY; WIDOWHOOD.

Is it wise for older single people to marry?

In the introduction to this book a proposal is made that age should be calculated not only by counting the number of years since birth but also by attempting to estimate the number of years that lie ahead. The thought was propounded that many people in their sixties are both mentally and physically young, whereas others in their thirties and forties are in actuality old. If this idea is valid, then one should not determine the advisability of marriage merely on the basis of chronological age. In general, it can be said that people who have remained single for, say, sixty years will find adjustment to married life more difficult than they would have at an earlier age. It is perhaps easier for the single male to marry after he is sixty because sexual experience will probably not be new to him. On the other hand, some women who have remained single for sixty years may find these adjustments quite complicated.

What special factors should be considered carefully when older people contemplate marriage?

1. The age of the intended spouse: A man in his sixties, seventies, or eighties should weigh seriously the advisability of marrying a woman in her twenties or thirties. He should make sure that the relationship is truly one of love, that he is not being married for his money or his reputation, and that he is not substituting for a father. Similarly, a woman in her sixties or seventies should think twice before marrying a very young man. In many instances, such a marriage is based on finances rather than on true physical and spiritual affection.

2. The mental competence of the older persons contemplating marriage: It should be determined whether or not the older man or woman is mentally capable of deciding to marry. Furthermore, the family should investigate to make sure that coercion plays no part in the marriage. They should also keep in mind the fact that, all too often, older men and women are "taken in" by the false protestations of love offered by self-seeking younger people.

3. The physical condition of the person contemplating marriage: There are very real physical hazards for an older man who marries a young woman. It should be determined beforehand that the male is physically capable of performing all the duties of a husband.

4. The length of time that the couple have known each other: Older people should be cautioned to go slowly and not to marry after a short courtship. Capricious, compulsive acts are sometimes evidence of the onset of senility. It should be remembered that it is rather easy to marry, but to get an annulment or divorce is much more difficult.

5. The intellectual compatibility of the couple: Nothing destroys a marriage of older people more quickly than widely divergent intellectual interests.

Do older widows or widowers find remarriage more difficult than older people who are marrying for the first time?

No. On the contrary, people who have been married previously have a greater knowledge of how to make a marriage work. They know more about the responsibilities of a marital relationship, and they have already proved their ability to demonstrate affection. (Incidentally, it has been determined statistically that people who remarry in their later years extend their life-span considerably.)

Is sexual incompatibility a serious problem when people over sixty marry younger mates?

This need not be true, although of course it is sometimes true. A great many older men and women retain their physical competence and are often capable of continuing an active sexual life well into their seventies. This does not mean, however, that sexual incompatibility is a minor issue. Naturally, when a man in his late seventies marries a girl in her twenties, the basis for sexual incompatibility is already present. This may also be true when an older woman marries a young man, but it is less likely.

What is the main physical danger when an older man marries a young woman?

Sexual intercourse sometimes places a strain on the heart and blood vessels. Coronary-artery spasm or thrombosis or cerebral-artery spasm or a stroke all too often follow sexual exertion.

A thorough physical examination, with medical clearance, should be obtained before an older man marries a young woman.

Is the incidence of emotional incompatibility greater when people past sixty marry?

Statistics show that the chances of emotional incompatibility are greater among older newlyweds. This happens because the ability to adjust and make changes in their pattern of living diminishes as people advance in age.

Is the incidence of infidelity greater when older people marry younger people?

Yes. The reasons for this are quite obvious. This is another strong argument for caution before marrying a person who is much younger.

What role should the family of an older person play when they learn of an "unwise" contemplated remarriage?

It is not advisable for the children to attempt to impose their wishes on a parent or to take too positive a position before consulting the family physician, a clergyman, or a marriage counselor. Many good relationships between children and parents have been disrupted by premature or unwarranted opposition to remarriage.

Are there legal factors to be considered when an older person remarries?

Yes. It should be made clear to an older person that his or her legal and financial situation may be completely changed by remarriage. This will also affect the position of his or her children and grandchildren. Those who contemplate remarrying should consult their attorney first.

MENTAL CHANGES

See ATTITUDES TOWARD AGING; DEATH AND FEAR OF DEATH; DEGENERATIVE CHANGES OF AGING; FAMILY RELATIONSHIPS; INSTITUTIONAL CARE; PSYCHOTHERAPY; RETIREMENT; SOCIAL BEHAVIOR.

When does the average person begin to show mental signs of aging?

There is so much individual variation that a precise answer to this question cannot be given. If the question refers to evidence of actual mental deterioration, it can be stated that this rarely occurs among normal older people before the eighties. If it refers to the little variations, such as forgetfulness, slowed reaction time, loss of memory for unimportant recent events, etc., these changes frequently have their onset in the forties and early fifties.

How common is mental illness in older people?

It is estimated that one-third of all patients in mental hospitals are sixty-five years of age or older. Since the sixty-five-and-older age group represents only about one-tenth of the total population, it can be seen that mental illness is three times more common in the aged. Most of this illness—more than 80 percent—can be attributed to varying degrees of arteriosclerosis.

Does the average individual between sixty and seventy years of age show signs of mental deterioration?

Not if he is in good health!

Are brain cells capable of maintaining normal function even into the eighties and nineties?

Yes, if the blood supply to the brain remains adequate and if there is no physical brain disease.

Do brain cells, once destroyed, ever regenerate?

No.

What is cerebral arteriosclerosis?

Hardening of the arteries that supply the brain. Most people show some slight cerebral arteriosclerosis as they grow older, but they do not necessarily develop mental changes as a result. Only when the arteriosclerosis becomes advanced will mental deterioration become evident.

When hardening of the arteries to the brain does take place, does it affect all parts of the brain in the same way?

On the contrary, certain mental functions may be completely normal, whereas others may be seriously impaired because of sclerosis.

Does cerebral arteriosclerosis occur in men more often than in women?

Yes, slightly more often. Moreover, it generally afflicts women later in life.

Is heredity an important factor in cerebral arteriosclerosis?

Yes. There is a tendency to inherit the same strength or weakness of the blood vessels that one's parents had.

What are some of the symptoms of cerebral arteriosclerosis?

1. Increased irritability.
2. Forgetting of recent events, but remembrance of past events.
3. Inattentiveness.
4. Lessened capacity for work.
5. Periods of depression.
6. Occasionally, headaches and dizziness.
7. Occasionally, slurring of speech and groping for words.
8. Carelessness about personal appearance.
9. Personality changes.
10. Temper tantrums.
11. Obstinacy and stubbornness.
12. Regression to childish habits.
13. Crying spells.

Do people with hardening of the arteries show their symptoms all the time?

No. There are often long periods of complete normalcy, sometimes extending for weeks, which are followed by recurrence of symptoms.

To what can one attribute the periodic disappearance of symptoms in people who have cerebral arteriosclerosis?

Physicians think that psychological factors play a very important role in the condition. If one's emotional state is good, symptoms may abate; conversely, if one is depressed and if the people who surround him fail to show affection, symptoms may become exaggerated.

Can medications help people who have hardening of the arteries to the brain?

Yes, particularly if the symptoms are caused by high blood pressure or by spasm of the blood vessels to the brain. Further, if the general condition of the patient is poor, medications to improve the health will also retard the progress of cerebral arteriosclerosis.

What are some of the common physical and emotional causes of mental changes in older people?

1. By far the most common physical cause is hardening of the arteries to the brain. Arteriosclerosis deprives the brain cells of an adequate supply of oxygen, sugar, and other substances that are essential to efficient function.
2. Physical disease, especially of a chronic nature, often results in mental changes. Everyone is familiar with the aging individual whose alertness and interest in his surroundings are blunted by his constant attention to a physical ailment.
3. Changes in the interpersonal relationships of older people often bring on evidences of mental decline. Thus, an older person who has lost a spouse or close friends or whose family has moved away may begin to lose interest in living and become dull and mentally deficient.
4. Perhaps one of the most important factors leading to premature mental deterioration is the lack of interest demonstrated by those who surround aging people. When an aging person feels unwanted or unloved, he may resign himself to his old age and will lose interest in things about him.

Does shock, such as that caused by the loss of a spouse, ever precipitate mental changes?

Yes. This is one of the most frequent causes of withdrawal from active living. It is important that the children of aging parents sponsor new interests and activities soon after the mourning period has ended.

Does severe illness ever trigger the onset of mental deterioration?

Yes. It is not at all uncommon to see people suddenly show marked mental changes after having passed through a serious illness. Such patients require special attention to encourage them to resume active participation in the activities of their family and community.

What is senility?

As a general term, it applies to the entire period of old age. More specifically, it refers to the mental changes of old age.

What are some of the early signs of senility?

It should be realized that the great majority of people in their sixties and early seventies show only slight evidence of senility. However, some of these signs are:

1. Inattentiveness to things going on about them—loss of interest in current events and in family affairs, for example.
2. Forgetfulness, including the names of people they know very well, telephone numbers, addresses, birthdays, anniversaries, etc.
3. A tendency to repeat things that they have said once or twice before, and a tendency to stress inordinately the importance of trivial matters.
4. Increasing forgetfulness of recent events, with remembrance of things that took place in youth or early adulthood.
5. Increasing irritability over unimportant matters.
6. An accentuation of peculiarities and eccentricities that existed, but were repressed, during the younger years.
7. Rigidity in pattern of living and ways of doing things.
8. Dulling of the sense of time and place. As a consequence, older people who were formerly prompt are late for appointments or may lose their way.
9. Sometimes, a decreasing interest in physical appearance.

Are symptoms of senility continuous, or do they tend to appear and disappear?

If the symptoms have been precipitated by a transient emotional problem, they often disappear completely when the problem is solved. It is well known that widows or widowers who find a new love act, think, and feel many years younger. Also, people whose symptoms of senility were caused by a debilitating illness may make a complete recovery when the illness has subsided.

Why is it that people in their seventies and eighties sometimes forget recent events but remember events that occurred fifty or sixty years earlier?

This peculiar psychological quirk is not fully understood by psychiatrists. One often encounters an aged person who will remember innumerable little things that took place when he was a small child but who cannot recall the name of the street on which he presently lives.

What can be done to aid aging people who are forgetful?

1. They should be supplied regularly with written instructions to guide their activities. For example, if an older person is to meet a member of his family at a certain time and place, this information should be jotted down on a piece of paper and given to him. Telephone numbers, too, should be written down and should be kept

handy for reference. This routine will relieve a great deal of anxiety all around.

2. Older people should be supplied with accurate watches. Those with alarm attachments are often quite useful.

3. They should be instructed to perform specific tasks at specific times each day. If they are in the habit of contacting members of their family every day, they should be taught to do it at the same hour. Regularity of routine is most helpful to older people.

4. Writing out a daily schedule often helps older people tremendously.

5. Relatives of older people should develop regularity in their contacts. A visit or phone call on the same day each week will give them something to look forward to. During such calls or visits, reminders can be tactfully made concerning the following of routines.

6. Calendars should be supplied, so that engagements and special dates can be recorded.

7. Date books, appointment books, etc., should be older people's constant companions.

8. Important telephone numbers, such as those of the physician, the pharmacist, and members of the family, should be posted in well-lighted places, for example, on the backs of bathroom doors, kitchen cupboards, and other places throughout the house.

Are people over sixty susceptible to such mental illnesses as melancholia and manic-depressive states?

Yes. The later years are accompanied by a considerable increase in the incidence of mental disease.

Are there medications that can help mentally disturbed older people?

Yes. Recently discovered drugs, including some of the tranquilizers, can relieve many of the disturbing symptoms of mental illness.

Is there a tendency toward suicide in older people?

Yes. The largest number of suicides occur after sixty.

Is paranoia (the idea that people are conspiring against one) encountered often in older people?

Yes, although the condition occurs in younger people too.

Do people tend to become more jealous as they grow older?
Yes. This can be readily appreciated, since it stems from the mounting fear that they will lose the love of their family and friends. The best remedy for jealousy is love and attention.

Are older people inclined to be overly possessive?

Yes, because they fear the loss of those they love.

Is there such a thing as "second childhood"?

Only if advanced senility has set in. Under such circumstances, some older people will perform childish acts. Regression to infantile habits, such as bed-wetting and soiling, incomplete attire, or silly talk are occasionally encountered. So-called second childhood is almost always associated with marked cerebral arteriosclerosis.

Do older people tend to become more neurotic and hypo- condriacal?

Yes. This is thought by most psychiatrists to be a display of the need for affection. The fear of loss of love may cause older people to conjure up imaginary symptoms in order to enlist the sympathy and attention of those who surround them. Also, as people age they frequently develop an increasing fear of death. This may be accompanied by neurotic symptoms.

How should one handle the neurotic symptoms of older people?

By displaying more affection and attention. Also, excessive fear of impending death should be dealt with through consultation with a psychiatrist.

Are older people often hysterical?

Yes, it is a common neurotic manifestation. Hysteria represents *fear*. It is important that those who are charged with the care of older people realize this and make every attempt to relieve the fear.

What is "senile dementia"?

The loss of mental faculties and the emotional distortions that accompany cerebral arteriosclerosis and consequent degeneration of brain cells.

Do mental traits and peculiarities that have existed through- out life tend to become exaggerated during the later years?

Yes. A person who is finicky and fussy may become unbearably exacting in later life. One who is inordinately possessive and jealous during the early years may show abnormal tendencies in this direction when he gets older.

Do people undergo changes in their basic personality as they advance in age?

Not unless they become senile. Normally, if they were stingy throughout life, the tendency becomes greater later on. If they were outgoing and warm as young people, they tend to be so during their later years.

How can one tell if an older person is mentally incompetent?

This should not be a one-man decision. It is much wiser to hold a family conference and consultation with experts in the field of mental health. Judging an older person to be mentally incompetent is a serious matter and should not be undertaken unless expert advice has been obtained. Such advice should emanate from the family physician, a psychiatrist, and the family attorney. In most states it is necessary for a court order to be obtained in order for someone to be judged mentally incompetent.

Is it advisable for older people who are beginning to show evidence of mental decline to live in the same house with their grandchildren?

Whenever possible, such a situation should be avoided. Nothing is quite so damaging to a young person as being forced to watch a grandparent, whom he may love and revere, become irritable, foolish, and mentally irresponsible. Children of aging parents should anticipate such situations and should make plans well in advance for the care of their aging parents. Too often, children wait until marked mental changes have taken place and an acute crisis develops. They should be informed that it is very difficult to find a good institution for the care of the mentally ill.

When should an older person be institutionalized because of mental deterioration?

See INSTITUTIONAL CARE.

Is surgery ever helpful in treating older people who show signs of mental deterioration?

In recent years it has been discovered that certain people with cerebral arteriosclerosis can be benefited by graft replacement of a sclerotic carotid artery in the neck. The new artery may restore circulation to the brain sufficiently to relieve some of the symptoms caused by the cerebral arteriosclerosis. But the number of cases in which this procedure is applicable is very limited.

Prefrontal lobotomy, an operation in which some of the nerve fibers in the front of the brain are severed, has been performed to relieve some of the symptoms created by senile brain changes. This operation is not used very often today, but in certain cases it has been helpful.

Is there any way for younger people to protect themselves against the emotional problems of later life?

To a limited extent. Some suggestions that may be of help are as follows:

1. Since psychological factors play such an important part in determining how early or late mental changes take place, people in their middle years should do all they can to build a healthy emotional atmosphere for their later years. First, they should maintain good family relations. They should pay great attention to their relationships with their children, so that when they do reach old age they will have their children as *friends*, not merely as relatives.

2. During their middle years they should get into the habit of doing things for others. This will redound to their benefit when they are older and need things to be done for them.

3. Psychiatric treatment during the middle years will often resolve neurotic tendencies, thus placing them in a better position to withstand the shocks and grave problems of the later years. Psychological treatment is not nearly so effective after sixty.

4. Excesses of any kind should be avoided during the middle years. Such excesses may become addictions or major abnormalities in old age.

5. Infections should be treated vigorously during the middle years so that they will not cause damage later on.

6. Since arteriosclerosis is one of the main underlying factors in the development of early mental changes, one should do everything possible to prevent its onset during early and middle life. Staying thin, avoiding a diet rich in cholesterol, cutting down on smoking and drinking, getting adequate sleep, etc., will all tend to slow down the onset of arteriosclerosis with its subsequent mental deterioration.

Are neuroses and psychoneuroses seen very often in older people?

Yes. It is safe to state that those who had neurotic tendencies in their youth and middle years will continue to show them in later years. Conversely, those who were able to control their fears and anxieties during the earlier years will demonstrate the same ability to maintain equilibrium in old age.

Do suppressed neurotic tendencies ever crop up during the later years?

Yes. Often people are able to cope with emotional problems when they are young, but when the anxieties and fears of old age are superimposed on these neurotic tendencies, they may manifest themselves openly.

A simple example of this would be someone who has had

inordinate fear of poverty during his younger days but who
was able to earn a satisfactory living and therefore could suppress the fear. In later life, that same person may not be
capable of maintaining financial stability, and, as a consequence, he may suffer an emotional breakdown. In fact, then,
it is not a new neurosis, but an overt manifestation of an older,
suppressed neurotic tendency.

**Can psychotherapy or psychoanalysis help older people to
deal with their neuroses?**

Psychiatric care is not nearly as effective for older people.
However, relatives, the family doctor, and the psychiatrist can
do much to alleviate anxieties and to help older people live
with their neuroses. (*See* PSYCHOTHERAPY.)

MOLES AND MELANOMAS

See PLASTIC SURGERY; SKIN; XANTHELASMA.

Are moles common in older people?

Yes. Although most of these growths originate in earlier years,
they tend to increase in number and size as one ages.

Is a nevus a mole?

Yes.

Are all moles colored?

No. Some are skin-colored; others are light or dark brown;
still others are blue-black.

What is the difference between a mole and a melanoma?

A melanoma is a malignant mole. Its cells often spread
throughout the body if it is not removed during an early stage
of its development.

How can one distinguish between a mole and a melanoma?

A physician can usually tell the difference. Characteristically,
a melanoma grows and darkens in color as it grows. Benign
moles frequently remain stationary in size and color.

Does the ordinary mole ever turn into a melanoma?

Most investigators believe that this does occasionally happen,
although it should not be assumed that every mole that grows
or changes color is becoming a melanoma. To be on the safe
side, one should have every mole that grows, or changes color,
or is subject to repeated irritation removed by a surgeon.

When is a mole most likely to be irritated?

If it is rubbed by a brassiere, a belt, or a shoe, or if it is on the face or neck, where it will be shaved over repeatedly.

How often do benign moles turn into malignant melanomas?

Infrequently. However, when they do, the process endangers life. When in doubt, have the mole removed.

Should blue-black moles that have been present for many years be removed?

Yes, particularly if they grow larger.

Why are melanomas so dangerous?

Because the cells tend to spread through the bloodstream to other parts of the body.

What is the treatment of melanoma?

It should be removed surgically with a wide surgical incision. Any glands in the area should also be removed. In recent years, certain medications have been found helpful in delaying the growth and spread of melanomas. These chemotherapeutic agents are injected into arteries near the area of the melanoma in order to kill off any cells that may remain after the melanoma has been excised.

If a malignant melanoma is removed surgically, can the patient look forward to a cure?

Yes, if it is removed before cells have spread to other parts of the body. On the other hand, if the melanoma has already spread to other parts of the body, local excision will not usually result in a permanent cure.

Where are the common sites of moles and melanomas?

They may form on any of the body surfaces. Those that occur on the palms of the hands or the soles of the feet are particularly likely to grow because they are subject to constant irritation.

Is it safe to have a mole removed by an electric needle in a doctor's office?

This is usually not a wise practice unless the surgeon has already had a piece of the mole examined microscopically. If such examination reveals that the mole is benign and shows no tendencies toward developing into a melanoma, then it can be removed safely with an electric needle.

To be totally safe, it is wiser to have moles removed surgically with an ellipitical incision through the surrounding skin. This procedure can be performed readily under local anesthesia.

Is the surgical removal of a melanoma a serious operation?

It may be serious if the operation is accompanied by the

removal of the lymph glands that drain the area to which a
melanoma might spread. The simple removal of the local
lesion is not serious.

MOUTH, LIPS, AND TONGUE

See LEUKOPLAKIA; SALIVARY GLANDS; SMOKING; SPEECH;
TEETH; VITAMINS.

**What changes may occur in the mouth and tongue as one
ages?**

1. There is a thinning out of the mucous membrane, often
   accompanied by a decrease in sensitivity to taste, heat,
   and cold.
2. Cracks in the lip membranes and sores at the corners of
   the mouth may develop.
3. There may be a burning sensation on the tip of the
   tongue.
4. Alignment of the teeth may become faulty because of
   loss of teeth or changes in the jawbone.
5. Pain in the joint connecting the lower jaw to the skull
   may develop as a result of poor alignment of the teeth.
6. Leukoplakia of the mucous membranes of the mouth or
   tongue may develop. (*See* LEUKOPLAKIA.)
7. Pyorrhea (infection of the gums around the teeth) may
   develop if the teeth begin to decay.
8. Cancer of the lip, tongue, or mucous membrane of the
   mouth occasionally develops.
9. "Dry mouth," secondary to a decrease in the amount of
   saliva secreted, may occur.
10. Stomatitis (ulceration in the mouth) may occur in de-
    bilitated, sick older people.
11. Loss of teeth, cavities, tooth abscesses, etc., are encoun-
    tered much more often in people in their seventies or
    eighties.

**Do the above changes take place very often in healthy older
people?**
Not if people maintain good health and are regularly checked
by their doctors and dentists. The lips, mucous membrane of
the mouth, and the tongue are all capable of adequate function
throughout life.

Do people naturally develop bad breath as they get older?
Not unless there is infection or disease in the mouth.

Can bad breath usually be corrected?

Yes, by eliminating infection in the mouth and by correcting tooth defects.

What are the pinhead-sized yellow spots seen on the inner surfaces of the lips and inside of the cheeks in some older people?

These are enlargements of the little glands located in the mucous membranes, a condition called Fordyce disease. It has no clinical significance and requires no treatment. Many older people are frightened by it because they think it a sign of cancer.

Do vitamin deficiencies cause alterations in the appearance of the lips and mouth?

Yes.

What changes can vitamin A deficiency produce?

An overgrowth of the mucous membranes of the gums and lips.

What changes can vitamin B deficiency produce?

1. Irritation and ulceration at the corners of the mouth.
2. Inflammation of the tongue.
3. Ulceration of the gums.
4. A swollen, beefy-looking tongue.

What changes may accompany marked vitamin C deficiency?

The gums become red and bleed readily. If the condition goes untreated, scurvy, with ulcerations of the gums, may develop.

Is it common for people in their seventies and eighties to drool from the corners of the mouth?

Not if the person is healthy. However, if dentures do not fit properly or if teeth are out of alignment, the corners of the mouth may not join as they should. This, in some cases, may be accompanied by drooling. Other people may have palsy (parkinsonism), which is frequently associated with drooling of saliva.

Do people of advanced age ever secrete excessive amounts of saliva?

Occasionally, if they have degenerative changes in their nerves or nervous system. It is much more common, however, for older people to secrete less than normal amounts of saliva.

What can be done for excessive salivation?

Several drugs in the belladonna group can be given to lessen the amount of salivary secretion.

Do older people tend to be more sensitive to hot foods and liquids?

They are not usually more sensitive, but their ability to perceive heat may be somewhat diminished. For this reason, burns of the lips, tongue, and gums occur more often.

Should older people pay particular attention to the care of their lips?

Yes.

1. If alignment of the teeth is thrown off by the loss of teeth, it should be corrected. Malocclusion may lead to leakage of saliva from the corners of the mouth and eventual irritation of the lip membranes.
2. Pipe smokers and cigar smokers should consult a physician immediately if they note a nonhealing ulceration or lump on the lip. The constant irritation of a hot pipestem is thought to be an important factor contributing to cancer of the lip.
3. Overexposure to the heat of the sun should be avoided, since it may cause a burn or heat sore on the lips.
4. Vitamin deficiencies and fungus infections should be corrected; they may lead to ulcerations, cracks, and fissures in the lips.
5. Women should not use any lipstick that causes an allergic reaction.

What special care should be given to the gums?

1. If the gums bleed, both the doctor and the dentist should be seen. Bleeding gums may indicate anemia, blood disease, or there may be a collection of debris and tartar beneath the gums near the tooth margin.
2. In brushing the teeth, care should be taken not to scrub them so hard that the gums are torn or lacerated.
3. If there is infection or discharge about the gums, the dentist should be consulted promptly.
4. People with leukoplakia of the gums should stop smoking. (*See* LEUKOPLAKIA.)
5. Ulceration of the gums may indicate an acute infection. It should be treated promptly by a physician.

Do the gums tend to recede from the teeth as people age?

Yes. This condition can often be corrected if it is treated early by the dentist.

What special care should be taken to safeguard the mucous membranes of the cheeks?

1. The most important consideration is that the membranes not be irritated or scratched by sharp edges of broken

teeth or by poorly fitting dentures. Constant irritation over a period of years may cause a cancer to develop.
2. Any lump or ulceration on the inside of the cheek should be treated promptly.

Should older people get into the habit of rinsing their mouths regularly?

Yes. It is best to use a mouthwash prescribed by a doctor or dentist rather than one advertised to the public.

What special care of the tongue should be observed?

1. If white leukoplakia patches develop, smoking and drinking of alcoholic beverages should be discontinued and a physician consulted.
2. Sharp edges of teeth or dentures should be removed. Repeated irritation or scratching of the tongue may produce ulceration or stimulate cancer growth.
3. Burning or tingling and numbness of the tongue is an indication for medical examination. It may signify the presence of anemia or a vitamin-deficiency disease.

What can be done about a burning or tingling sensation of the tongue?

If the symptoms are due to anemia, liver extract and vitamin B injections or capsules may bring relief. However, if the sensation is caused by degeneration of the nerve that supplies the tongue, little can be done to help it.

Can anything be done about the loss of sense of taste, which sometimes occurs as people grow older?

Yes, if it is caused by a vitamin deficiency or anemia. However, if nerve degeneration is the underlying factor, nothing will restore it.

"DRY MOUTH"

What is "dry mouth"?

It is a condition in which insufficient saliva is secreted. This condition may be the result of taking drugs that inhibit the secretion of saliva, or it may be due to a depressed mental state with diminished secretion of saliva as a symptom.

Does "dry mouth" often affect older people?

Yes, particularly in the late seventies or eighties.

What is the treatment of "dry mouth"?

1. Drugs that decrease the amount of salivary secretion should be discontinued.

2. Tranquilizers or sedatives should be given to calm the nerves if it is suspected that emotional upset is the cause of the condition.

3. Vitamin A, neostigmine, potassium iodide, and other medications are sometimes helpful in increasing the amount of salivary secretion.

PERLÈCHE

What is perlèche?

It is an inflammation, with crust formation at the corners of the mouth, thought to be brought on by leakage of saliva, lack of cleanliness, the collection of food particles, and the growth of a yeastlike fungus. Formerly, many doctors believed the condition to be due mainly to a vitamin deficiency.

Do older people get perlèche frequently?

It is seen most often among those who are invalids and who are unable to keep themselves clean.

What is the treatment of perlèche?

1. Dental deformities and malalignment of teeth must be corrected in order to stop drooling of saliva.

2. The corners of the mouth should be cleaned daily to prevent collection of food particles.

3. Fungicidal ointments, such as mycostatin, should be applied regularly.

CANCER OF THE LIP

Is cancer of the lip encountered often in those past sixty?

Yes.

Is cancer of the lip more common in men?

Yes, in a ratio of about four to one.

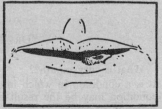

Cancer of lower lip

Is cancer of the lip always caused by smoking?

No. Nonsmokers may develop this disease, too.

Are all lip tumors cancerous?

No. Many lip tumors are benign, for example, blood-vessel tumors, known as hemangiomas. Also, warty growths and patches of leukoplakia are not cancerous.

Is cancer of the lip curable?

Yes, in the great majority of cases, if it is surgically excised in its early stages.

How is cancer of the lip treated?

A wedge-shaped segment of the lip surrounding the tumor is cut away. If lymph glands in the neck are involved, an extensive dissection is carried out to remove the tissues to which tumor cells might have spread. After excision of the cancer, the lip is so sutured that the resulting deformity and scar are minimal.

Do people recover from operations for cancer of the lip?

Yes, and most such cases today are diagnosed and treated during the early stages, when cure is easier to effect.

Does the removal of a large segment of the lip often result in marked deformity?

No. Excellent techniques for the repair of the lip have been developed, so that usually only minor disfigurement results. Furthermore, the lip is composed of elastic tissue, which tends to stretch back into place even when a large section has been removed.

Do cigar and cigarette smoking have the same tendency as pipe smoking to promote lip cancer?

No. It is believed that the hot stem of a pipe, with its constant irritation and burning of the superficial layers of the lip membrane, is mainly responsible for the ultimate development of lip cancer.

CANCER OF THE TONGUE

Is cancer of the tongue common in people past sixty?

Yes.

Is cancer of the tongue more common in men?

Yes. It occurs about four times more often.

What is thought to bring about cancer of the tongue?

1. Leukoplakia that has persisted for many years and has gone untreated.

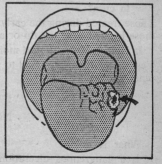

Cancer of tongue

2. Chronic irritation of the tongue, owing to poorly fitting dentures or to repeated abrasion from the sharp edges of broken teeth.

3. Other contributory factors such as chronic infection or debilitating disease.

Does heavy smoking predispose one to the development of tongue cancer?

Yes, inasmuch as it predisposes one to leukoplakia. Since leukoplakia is often a forerunner of cancer, smoking must be considered a major causative factor.

How can one tell if he is developing a tumor of the tongue or mouth?

The diagnosis is simple. During the course of a routine physical examination the physician will undoubtedly examine the oral cavity. When he does, a tumor of the lips, cheeks, or tongue will become apparent at a glance. A suspicious lesion will be biopsied and an exact diagnosis can be made in a few days.

What is the treatment of cancer of the tongue?

A lesion at the tip of the tongue or along its front edges is treated by surgical removal of the tumor-bearing section. Even if half of the tongue is removed, speech remains unaffected.

When a cancer is located toward the base of the tongue, it is often better treated by X-ray radiation rather than by surgical excision.

Are surgery and X-ray therapy ever combined in the treatment of cancer of the tongue?

Yes. Sometimes the combination of surgery and X-ray therapy will afford the best chance for cure.

What types of cancer of the tongue best lend themselves to cure?

Those treated during the early stages of their development and those located near the tip or along the sides of the tongue.

Is cancer of the mouth more easily cured in older patients?

Yes, since all cancers tend to grow and spread more slowly in older people.

NOMA

What is noma?

It is a gangrenous ulceration of the mouth often found in older people who have a generalized debilitating disease such as leukemia or advanced cancer. When noma occurs, it is usually a sign that death is imminent. Local treatment of the ulcerated area is usually of little use.

MUSCLES

See ARTHRITIS AND RHEUMATISM; BACKACHE; BONES AND JOINTS; BURSITIS; CLAUDICATION; FRACTURES; HERNIA; IN-JURIES AND ACCIDENTS; PARKINSON'S DISEASE AND PALSY; PHYSICAL ACTIVITY AND EXERCISE; REHABILITATION AND PHYS-ICAL THERAPY.

Do muscles tend to function less efficiently as people enter their later years?

Yes, although the changes may be imperceptible at first. When people are in their late seventies and eighties, muscle function and coordination undergo the most marked changes.

Do muscles tend to lose some of their strength and tone after sixty?

It is estimated that people over sixty normally retain only about 50 percent of the muscle strength and tone they had at thirty-five to forty years of age. But older people do not suffer greatly from this loss, since their activities require less muscle competence.

Do muscle reflexes become less efficient as one advances in age?

Yes. This loss may be due not to actual muscle degeneration but to changes in the nerves, so that they bring impulses to the muscles more slowly. Also, there is a decrease in agility and sense of balance, which may explain inefficient muscle reflex responses.

Do the tiny muscles surrounding the blood vessels and in-testines tend to lose their strength, too, as one ages?

No. These muscles (the so-called smooth muscles), the actions of which are not controlled voluntarily, show very little signs of aging, even among very old people. This is fortunate, since the smooth muscles control the expansion and contraction of blood vessels and are responsible for the propulsion of food along the intestinal tract.

Do muscles tend to degenerate if they are not used?

Yes. It is essential that older people exercise, even when they are bedridden. In this way, blood circulation to the muscles

will be preserved and there will be a minimum of loss in
muscle tone and strength.

Does muscle bulk usually diminish as one grows older?

Yes. This is a natural phenomenon and will not interfere with
continued muscle function.

Are muscle cramps common in older people?

Yes. Severe muscle cramps often attack the calf muscles, the
tendons and muscles in the feet, and other muscles. Cramps
are brought on by spasm of the blood vessels supplying the
muscles. A muscle cramp may be an extremely painful experience, often coming on without warning during sleep. When
pain and cramps in the calf muscles come on from walking,
the phenomenon is called claudication. (*See* CLAUDICATION.)

**Is calcium sometimes deposited in muscle tendons, especially
    where muscle joins bone?**

Yes, this frequently occurs in older people and leads to decreased muscle efficiency. It may also cause severe pain in the
area.

**Is it natural for older people to have more aches and pains
    in their muscles and joints?**

Yes. The muscles are more susceptible to strain following
physical exertion, and pain in muscles and joints frequently
accompanies old age.

What can be done to relieve muscular aches and pains?

1. Exposure to cold should be avoided and room temperatures should be kept at or near 70°F.
2. Exposure to excessive heat should be avoided, and an
   adequate salt intake should be maintained on very hot
   days.
3. Analgesic medications such as aspirin will usually afford
   great relief.
4. Muscle-relaxing medications can be taken, but only on
   prescription by a doctor.
5. Hot baths often relax muscles and will relieve a great
   deal of pain.
6. Applications of moist or dry heat is often beneficial.
7. If it has been determined that the aches and pains are
   due to hardening of the arteries, medications to relieve
   spasm of blood vessels should be prescribed.
8. Whirlpool baths, diathermy treatments, baking lamps, and
   other forms of physical therapy are often helpful if the
   pains are due to an acute muscle sprain or injury.
9. When the pains and aches in the muscles are chronic,
   physical aids such as braces, splints, and bandages should
   be utilized.

10. A cane or crutches should be used if the muscle and joint pain causes marked disability in walking.
11. A thorough physical examination should be carried out to determine whether or not the muscular aches and pains are caused by some generalized condition. Occasionally, an infection in the nose or throat, the sinuses, the urinary bladder, or the prostate gland will cause toxins to circulate throughout the body. These infections often affect the muscular system. Elimination of such a focus of infection may eventually lead to the disappearance of the muscle aches and pains.
12. Muscles often become painful and function poorly because of arthritis in nearby joints. It will do little good to treat the muscles if the arthritis is permitted to go untreated.

What happens when muscle fibers are injured by a strain?
Muscle fibers are often torn, and hemorrhage into the muscle tissue results. It is followed by tenderness, swelling, and marked pain in the region. There is also inability to contract and relax the muscles normally. A popular name for this condition is charley horse.

How can older people safeguard themselves against muscle strains?
1. By learning their physical limitations. This is a slow and sometimes painful process, often learned only after several episodes of muscle injury. They will have to learn to avoid strenuous labor or physical exertion, such as changing an automobile tire, lifting heavy objects, or attempting a maneuver that will place undue strain on the muscles.
2. By getting into the habit of making deliberate movements and avoiding sudden, unplanned motions.
3. By engaging in a program of regular daily exercises. These exercises should be conducted sensibly, with the physical limitations of advanced age in mind.
4. By avoiding strenuous physical exercise in very hot or very cold weather.

What is the best way for older people to maintain muscle strength and tone?
1. By taking regular physical exercise.
2. By staying at a proper weight.
3. By eating a high-protein, low-fat diet.
4. By maintaining an adequate intake of vitamins and minerals.
5. By avoiding overexertion and undue strain on muscles.

Do muscle tremors, palsy, and twitching indicate muscle disease?

Usually not. These symptoms do occur in many older people, but they are evidence of a nerve disorder rather than of a primary muscular condition. Treatment must therefore be directed toward the former condition.

Are elderly people subject to muscular diseases, for example, muscular dystrophy or myasthenia?

Most of the muscle-wasting diseases afflict people during youth or the middle years. It is most unusual to find a person in his sixties or seventies developing these conditions for the first time.

Do once-paralyzed muscles show a tendency to regain function?

Yes, if the paralyzed nerves that supply the muscles recover. In most instances, loss of muscle function is secondary to nerve damage, as in paralysis from a stroke. If the nerve recovers, as sometimes happens, then the muscle will regain its ability to expand and contract.

After suffering partial paralysis from a stroke, is it possible to regain use of paralyzed muscles?

Yes. Great advances have been made in recent years in the field of rehabilitation. Muscles that were apparently useless have, with the aid of new rehabilitation techniques, been regained. Moreover, unaffected healthy muscles can be trained to take over functions of paralyzed muscles. (*See* REHABILITATION AND PHYSICAL THERAPY.)

Does failure of muscle coordination occur frequently in older people?

Healthy adults in their sixties and seventies do not often show lack of muscle coordination sufficient to lead to abnormal function. However, as one ages there is some lessening of muscle coordination. As a consequence, older people do tend to falter and fall more frequently.

What are some of the causes of muscular incoordination?

1. Decrease in the efficiency of nerve reflexes—a natural phenomenon of aging.
2. Development of palsy or tremor as the result of degeneration of nerve cells within the brain.
3. Brain tumors, which may lead to muscular incoordination or severe, uncontrolled muscle contractions.
4. Degeneration in the inner ear, or disease of the auditory nerve, may lead to loss of equilibrium and balance and to muscular incoordination.

5. Excessive intake of alcohol.
6. Advanced syphilis, which affects the nervous system.

What is chorea?

Involuntary, jerky muscle movements. Although chorea usually affects people while they are awake, it sometimes occurs during sleep.

Does chorea occur often in older people?

Occasionally. When it does, it denotes degeneration of certain nerve cells in the brain.

Can anything be done to relieve chorea?

Not usually, although brain operations that are still in the experimental stage may prove helpful in the near future.

What is ataxia?

A general term for lack of coordination of muscles.

What is locomotor ataxia?

An abnormal gait resulting from syphilis that has affected the spinal cord. (*See* SYPHILIS.)

NERVES

See ANEMIA; APOPLEXY, OR STROKE; BELL'S PALSY; BRAIN TUMOR; COMA; CONVULSIONS; DRIVING; EPILEPSY; FAINTING; HEADACHE; MENTAL CHANGES; OPTIC-NERVE ATROPHY; PAIN; PARKINSON'S DISEASE AND PALSY; PSYCHOTHERAPY; SCIATICA; TIC DOULOUREUX; VERTIGO AND DIZZINESS.

Does nerve tissue tend to degenerate as people grow older?

Yes. A gradual process of replacement of nerve tissue by inactive fibrous tissue takes place. This may be responsible for the decreased muscle tone and slowed reaction time and reflexes so common in old people.

Do nerve reflexes tend to change as people age?

Yes. Although the changes may not become apparent or

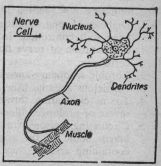

Nerve cell and fiber

significant until well into the seventies or eighties, the reflexes do slow down after sixty. Several instruments can gauge the extent of these changes quite accurately.

Do older people tend to experience loss in skin sensitivity because of changes in the nerves supplying the skin?

To a limited extent. Most healthy older people do not suffer from this loss in sensitivity, but the lessened sensitivity to touch, heat, and cold is responsible for an increased incidence of burns and lacerations in people of advanced age.

Do the senses, smell, hearing, taste, sight, and touch, tend to become less acute as people grow older?

Yes. However, the healthy older individual may show only minor decreases in these sensations. It should be emphasized that these changes do not begin abruptly after one has reached sixty but take place slowly from the thirties and forties onward. (*See* EYES; EARS; etc.)

Do brain cells grow older too?

Yes. Although microscopic examination of the brain of a healthy person in his eighties or nineties may show replacement of brain cells by inert fibrous tissue, mental faculties may continue relatively unimpaired. Only after extensive anatomical brain change does mental deterioration become evident.

Is it natural for older people to develop numbness and tingling in their hands and feet?

Sometimes. It may be a sign of the aging of the nerve fibers. In other instances, it is a symptom of disease.

What conditions may damage nerve fibers, with resulting numbness and tingling in the hands or feet?

1. Diabetes of long standing, especially cases that have not been well controlled. In such instances, there may be degeneration of nerve fibers that originate in the spinal cord.
2. Chronic secondary anemia. (*See* ANEMIA.)
3. Pernicious anemia. (*See* ANEMIA.)
4. Toxins circulating through the body as a result of a severe or prolonged illness or infection.
5. Circulating poisons from drugs the patient may have taken. Some of the popular tonics, particularly those containing arsenic, may have harmful effects on nerve tissue.
6. Vitamin deficiencies, especially vitamin B deficiency.
7. Chronic alcoholism.
8. Direct pressure on the nerves as they exit from the spinal

column or further along in their course. This is seen in cases of herniated disk, spinal-cord tumor, arthritis of the spine, or a tumor anywhere along the nerve.

What is the treatment of numbness or tingling in the hands or feet?

1. If it is caused by diabetes, the diabetes should be brought under control.
2. If it is caused by anemia, the type of anemia must be determined and specific treatment begun.
3. If it has been caused by circulating toxins secondary to prolonged illness, the symptoms will probably clear up spontaneously after the disease has subsided.
4. If it has been caused by a drug, the drug should be discontinued immediately.
5. If it is caused by a vitamin or nutritional deficiency, the deficiency can be remedied.
6. If it is caused by nerve irritation secondary to alcoholism, it will frequently subside after the patient gives up drinking.
7. If it is caused by direct pressure on nerves, surgical correction (as with a herniated disk) will usually bring relief.

Is there a greater tendency for older people to develop inflammation and pain along nerve pathways?

Yes.

Do older people feel pain less than younger people?

There is thought to be little or no decrease in perception of pain with aging. However, people past sixty are subject to more conditions causing pain.

Do pain-relieving drugs act as efficiently in older people?

On the whole, it can be said that older patients' response is as good as that of younger people. However, the dosage may have to be altered for older patients. For example, people in their seventies and eighties require smaller doses of narcotics to relieve pain.

Are neuritis and neuralgia more common during the later years?

Yes. Nerves become progressively more susceptible to inflammatory processes and irritation as one ages.

Is anemia a common cause of neuritis?

Yes, particularly in undernourished older people.

Is vitamin deficiency a common cause of neuritis in older people?

Yes.

What are some of the usual symptons of neuritis?

Severe pain along the course of the nerve, numbness and tingling in the skin area supplied by the nerve, loss of reflexes of the muscles supplied by the nerve, and possible loss of sensation in the skin area supplied by the involved nerve.

Which nerves tend to be most susceptible to neuritis?

Any nerve in the body may become involved, but the ones most often affected are:

1. The sciatic nerve, which arises in the lower back and extends down the back of the thigh and leg into the foot.
2. The brachial plexus, the group of nerves that originates in the neck and supplies the arms, forearms, and hands.
3. The trigeminal nerve, or fifth cranial nerve, in the face. This nerve originates in the brain and supplies the area surrounding the eyes, the nose, the cheeks, the mouth, and the chin. Neuritis of this nerve is known as tic douloureux.

Can neuritis be cured by treatment?

Usually, if the underlying cause can be found. It must be remembered, however, that neuritis is frequently associated with degeneration of nerve fibers. This process cannot be reversed.

Does neuritis ever affect more than one set of nerves at a time?

Yes. This condition is called polyneuritis.

What are the most common causes of polyneuritis?

1. Chronic alcoholism.
2. The aftereffects of a severe illness.
3. Marked anemia.
4. Marked vitamin deficiency.
5. Drug poisoning.

Are the symptoms of polyneuritis different from those of other types of neuritis?

No, except that they occur in more than one area at the same time.

Are the effects of neuritis ever permanent?

In some cases, especially in very old people. Occasionally, the symptoms will persist even after the causative factor has been eliminated. This is due to permanent nerve damage.

Do nerve cells or nerve fibers ever grow back again once they have been destroyed?

If the nerve cell is destroyed, it will not grow back. If the nerve cell is intact and the fiber leading from it is damaged, the fiber may regenerate. However, the process is very slow, often requiring many months.

Is there a natural decrease in sphincter control as one ages?

Yes. Sphincters are circular muscles surrounding various structures, such as the lower end of the esophagus (food pipe), the outlet of the stomach, the anus, and the outlet of the urinary bladder. Diminished sphincter control in the intestinal tract may disturb digestion or cause such symptoms as nausea, vomiting, and diarrhea. Diminished urinary-sphincter control may lead to incontinence. As one ages, the delicate nerve reflexes that govern sphincter action may get out of alignment.

Do healthy older people usually maintain adequate sphincter control?

Yes, even though efficiency may be somewhat decreased.

NURSING CARE

See BED CARE; BED-WETTING; BOWEL FUNCTION; HOME-CARE PROGRAMS; HOTELS, APARTMENTS, AND COMMUNITIES FOR THE AGING; NURSING HOMES.

What special nursing care do many older sick people require?

1. Particular attention should be paid to bodily cleanliness; they may neglect it if left to themselves.

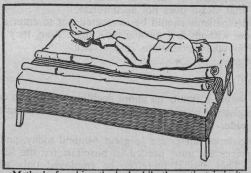

Method of making the bed while the patient is in it

2. Urinary and bowel function must be watched, since older patients may develop urinary retention or fecal impactions.
3. Older patients tend to stay for long periods in one position in bed. They should be moved frequently in order to keep the circulation active and to ensure good aeration of the lungs.
4. Older patients should be watched for bedsores. Frequent changes in position will help. (*See* BED CARE.)
5. Regular muscle exercises, even for bed patients, help prevent stiffness and muscle wasting.
6. Special attention should be paid to mouth hygiene, since gum or tooth infection may spread to other organs of the body.

Is it important that nurses supervise an older patient's personal hygiene?

Yes. This is often quite a delicate task, since many older people strongly resent questions about washing, bathing, brushing the teeth or hair, etc.

What special precautions are necessary when older people take showers or baths?

1. The bathroom door should never be locked.
2. The bathroom door should be left partially open, so that a nurse or attendant can know what is going on.
3. The bathroom window should be left open a crack, so that the room does not become too hot or humid. (This may cause dizziness or fainting.)
4. Older people should be assisted into and out of a tub or shower. (Debilitated patients are particularly susceptible to falls and fractures.)
5. In stall showers, the door should be left partially open so that steam does not accumulate.
6. Older patients should be instructed not to enter a bathroom without first turning on a light. Also, they should never take medications in the dark.

What are bedsores?

See BED CARE.

How should a family go about deciding whether to employ a registered nurse, a practical nurse, or a companion for an older sick person?

1. Registered nurses are in great demand today, and their services are most needed in hospitals for the seriously ill. They should therefore be employed only when a serious illness is present.

2. Practical nurses are usually well trained and are especially suited to home-nursing care. Most states require licensing examinations and that practical nurses be able to perform many of the duties of registered nurses.
3. Companions should not be engaged for sick patients. All too often they are called on to fill the roll of nurse when they are totally untrained for the task.

What are the limitations of duties and responsibilities of a practical nurse as compared to a registered nurse?

It should be recognized that registered nurses have undergone three years of intensive hospital training and therefore can carry out many procedures that the practical nurse is unable to perform. For example, registered nurses can give intravenous medications; they know how to care for drainage tubes and tracheotomy tubes; they can care for oxygen equipment; they can change surgical dressings, and many other things. A practical nurse should not be asked to carry out tasks for which she is not trained.

What special attributes should a family look for in choosing a practical nurse or a companion?

1. It is important that the nurse or companion be in good health. Many a patient has been done a great disservice by the employment of an ailing nurse or companion.
2. It is advisable to inquire into the personal tastes and interests of the nurse or companion, especially if a long association is anticipated. Nothing is more irritating to an older patient than to be in constant contact with someone whose intellect and interests are incompatible with his own.
3. The recreational interests and hobbies of a nurse or companion should be ascertained.
4. The reading capabilities of the nurse or companion should be ascertained before employment.
5. The personal appearance of the nurse or companion is of great importance, since she will come in contact with the friends and associates of the patient.
6. References should always be checked carefully, since it is often necessary to give a nurse or companion considerable freedom in the handling of the patient's financial affairs. (The use of a reputable nurses' registry will minimize the chances of hiring someone who is dishonest.)
7. Salary should be discussed thoroughly prior to employment. For patients who will require prolonged nursing care, it is best to make arrangements for a monthly, rather than an hourly or weekly, salary.

8. The question of duty hours should be thoroughly discussed before employment. Many a good relationship has been spoiled because of misunderstandings about time off.

What special precautions should be observed in employing a nurse or companion for an elderly man?

Many older men are still active and capable sexually. If they are emotionally disturbed as a result of their illness, they may develop peculiar notions concerning their relationship with a female nurse or companion. This must be guarded against, and any untoward advance must be reported immediately by the nurse or companion to the family and to the physician in attendance.

In choosing a companion, is it best to select one of the same sex?

Yes, especially for very old people. Many potentially embarrassing situations can be avoided in this way.

Is it good practice to employ a companion of approximately the same age as the patient?

This is not always a good idea. In many instances elderly patients have had to serve as nurses to ailing companions.

Can one usually make monthly salary arrangements with registered nurses?

No. Most registered nurses now work on an hourly-rate basis. Moreover, very few registered nurses wish to work more than eight, or at the most twelve, hours a day. It is rare to find a registered nurse who will agree to sleep in or work on a twenty-hour basis.

Do older people tend to resist the idea of a permanent nurse or companion?

Yes, especially if they consider themselves to be in a fair state of health. For this reason, it is always wiser to discuss the matter first and to obtain the consent and cooperation of the older person. To many older people, engaging a nurse or companion signifies that they are nearing the end of their days. The family should state the need positively and should attempt to convince the patient that a good companion or nurse will enable him to develop new interests and will make it possible for him to participate more fully in various activities. Renewed interest in one's surroundings often can be stimulated by an alert, energetic companion or nurse.

Are special precautions necessary when choosing a nurse or companion for an older person who has suicidal tendencies?

Yes. Seemingly casual suicide threats often turn out to be

serious. It is therefore essential that a nurse or companion be thoroughly familiar with this aspect of the care of older patients. Whenever possible, an individual who has had previous experience with this type of case should be employed.

What are good sleeping arrangements for an older person and his nurse or companion?

1. Many older patients respond well to the knowledge that there is someone else sleeping in the same room. If this is feasible, it should be permitted.

2. As a general rule, it is better that a female nurse or companion not sleep in the same room with a male patient.

3. If the patient is not sleeping in the same room with the nurse or companion, a good communications system should be arranged. A buzzer, a bell, or an intercom system should be installed.

Should older people be encouraged to go out socially with their nurses or companions?

Yes. For this reason it is important to select a nurse or companion who is presentable and who can mix well with the patient's friends and associates.

To what agencies should one apply to obtain nursing care for a chronically invalided older person?

(For specific agencies, *see* ORGANIZATIONS AND AGENCIES.)

1. The old-age-assistance bureau in the local community.
2. The social service department of a large nearby hospital.
3. The community visiting-nurse association.
4. Public-health nursing agencies.
5. Church, fraternal, and social organizations.
6. The department of welfare or department of social welfare in one's community.
7. Nurses' registries, either private or associated with nearby hospitals.
8. The county medical society in one's vicinity.

NURSING HOMES

See HOME-CARE PROGRAMS; INSTITUTIONAL CARE; ORGANIZATIONS AND AGENCIES.

What are nursing homes?

They are institutions designed especially to care for convalescent patients, chronically ill patients, semi-invalided people who need constant nursing attention, or bedridden invalids.

Are most of the patients in nursing homes over sixty years of age?

Yes, although younger people are also admitted.

Is the need for nursing-home beds increasing?

Yes, tremendously. More and more people are living into the later decades, in which the incidence of chronic and incurable disease is greatly increased. Nursing-home facilities are essential for their care.

Are there enough nursing-home beds available today?

Definitely not, and many that are available are in institutions that have inadequate facilities.

Can institutions for the aged and hospitals for the care of the chronically ill do the work of nursing homes?

No, since the need for beds is so great that such institutions can admit only a small percentage of those requiring care. Furthermore, many of the functions of the nursing homes differ from those of hospitals and homes for the aged.

Who administers the medical care in nursing homes?

Some of the better nursing homes have resident physicians who perform duties similar to those of interns in a general hospital. However, patients in nursing homes must retain their own personal physicians, who will visit them at the home.

Who supervises the day-to-day care of patients in nursing homes?

These institutions have medical directors, who are in charge of the overall management of the home, and a chief nurse, who supervises the nursing care.

What type of older patient is most suitable for admission to a nursing home?

One who can eventually be returned to his own home. Those who cannot look forward to going home and who, in all probability, will live for several years are much better off in a large home for the aged, where social and recreational activities are better developed.

What steps should be taken before one chooses a nursing home?

1. The family physician should be consulted, and the contemplated selection should meet with his approval.
2. Before admission of the patient, all costs should be discussed with those running the nursing home.
3. Advice from the county medical society, the social service departments of neighboring hospitals, and other community agencies (*see* ORGANIZATIONS AND AGENCIES) should be sought before the patient is admitted to a nursing home.

Is there any agency that approves or accredits nursing homes?

Yes. They are under the jurisdiction of the local health department. Those that fail to meet its standards are subject to being closed. Furthermore, a national organization is being set up to establish standards for nursing homes. In the near future, there will be "accredited" nursing homes, just as there are now "accredited" or "nonaccredited" hospitals.

The new Social Security Amendments providing for extended care facilities will undoubtedly lead to the establishment, in the near future, of federal standards for nursing homes. (*See* SOCIAL SECURITY MANUAL.)

OPTIC-NERVE ATROPHY

See ALCOHOL AND ALCOHOLISM; BLINDNESS; DRUGS AND MEDICINES; EYES; PITUITARY GLAND.

What is optic-nerve atrophy?

It is degeneration of the main nerve to the eye. As degeneration progresses it causes increasing loss of vision.

Is optic-nerve atrophy a common cause of blindness in older people?

Yes, but it is encountered less frequently than glaucoma, cataract, and some other eye diseases.

What can cause optic-nerve atrophy?

1. Progressive arteriosclerosis, including changes in the small blood vessels that supply the nerve.
2. Increasing pressure in the skull, as in brain tumor.
3. Pressure on the nerve, as with a tumor of the pituitary gland, which lies in close proximity to the optic nerves.
4. Glaucoma.
5. Chronic, severe diabetes.
6. Chronic alcoholism.
7. Syphilis affecting the nervous system.
8. Drug poisoning, as from arsenic or lead.
9. Direct pressure on the nerve, as in the case of a tumor growing in the eyeball or in the orbit of the skull.

How is the diagnosis of optic-nerve atrophy made?

By direct examination of the nerve through an ophthalmoscope. That portion can be seen that enters the retina in the back of the eyeball. When it has undergone atrophy, a nerve is characteristically depressed and whitish in appearance.

Is there any cure of optic-nerve atrophy?

If the cause can be eliminated before too much degeneration

has set in, the condition may clear considerably. But in most instances, once atrophy has taken place and sight has been impaired or lost, there is no way to remedy the situation.

ORGANIZATIONS AND AGENCIES

Alcoholism
> Alcoholics Anonymous, 133 E. 39th St., New York, N.Y.
> National Council on Alcoholism, 2 E. 103rd St., New York, N.Y.

Arthritic Conditions
> Arthritis and Rheumatism Foundation, 10 Columbus Circle, New York, N.Y.

Cancer
> American Cancer Society, Inc., 521 W. 57th St., New York, N.Y.

Dental Care
> American Association of Public Health Dentists, 1330 West Michigan St., Indianapolis, Ind.

Diabetes
> American Diabetes Association, Inc., 1 E. 45th St., New York 17, N.Y.

Drug Addiction
> National Family Council on Drug Addiction, Inc., 401 West End Ave., New York, N.Y.

Education
> Adult Education Association of U.S.A., 743 N. Wabash Ave., Chicago, Ill.
> American Association for Health, Physical Education, and Recreation, 1201 16th St. N.W., Washington 6, D.C.
> National Home Study Council, 2000 K St. N.W., Washington 6, D.C.

Employment
> American Personnel and Guidance Association, 1605 New Hampshire Ave. N.W., Washington 9, D.C.

Eyes and Blindness
> American Association of Workers for the Blind, Inc., 838 Investment Building, Washington 5, D.C.
> American Foundation for the Blind, Inc., 15 W. 16th St., New York, N.Y.
> Associated Blind, Inc., 147 W. 23rd St., New York, N.Y.

National Council to Combat Blindness, Inc., 41 W. 57th St., New York, N.Y.

National Medical Foundation for Eye Care, 250 W. 57th St., New York 19, N.Y.

National Society for the Prevention of Blindness, 1790 Broadway, New York 19, N.Y.

Health

American Medical Association, 535 N. Dearborn St., Chicago 10, Ill.

American National Red Cross, National Headquarters, Washington, D.C.

American Public Health Association, Inc., 1790 Broadway, New York 19, N.Y.

Health Information Foundation, University of Chicago, Chicago, Ill.

Medical and Surgical Relief Commission, Inc., 420 Lexington Ave., New York, N.Y.

Muscular Dystrophy Association of America, 1790 Broadway, New York 19, N.Y.

National Health Council, 1790 Broadway, New York 19, N.Y.

National Tuberculosis Association, 1790 Broadway, New York 19, N. Y.

(*See also* American Veterans Association; local public health organizations.)

Hearing and Deafness

Alexander Graham Bell Association for the Deaf, Inc., 1537 35th St. N.W., Washington 7, D.C.

American Speech and Hearing Association, 1001 Connecticut Ave. N.W., Washington 6, D.C.

Deafness Research Foundation, 310 Lexington Ave., New York, N.Y.

National Association of the Deaf, 2495 Shattuck Ave., Berkeley 4, Calif.

Heart

American Heart Association, Inc., 44 E. 23rd St., New York 10, N.Y.

Homes for the Aged

American Association of Nonprofit Homes for the Aged, 325 S. Boyle Ave., Los Angeles 33, Calif.

American Society for the Aged, Raymond Commerce Building, Newark 2, N.J.

National Council on the Aging, 49 W. 45th St., New York, N.Y.

Housing

American Society of Planning Officials, 1313 E. 60th St., Chicago 37, Ill.

National Association of Housing and Redevelopment Officials, 1313 E. 60th St., Chicago 37, Ill.

Kidney Disease

Kidney Disease Foundation of New York, Inc., 327 Lexington Ave., New York 17, N.Y.

Medical Care

See Health.

Mental Health

American Psychiatric Association, 1700 18th St. N.W., Washington, D.C.

Mental Health Foundation, 2 E. 86th St., New York, N.Y.

National Association for Mental Health, Inc., 10 Columbus Circle, New York 19, N.Y.

Nursing Homes

American Association of Nonprofit Homes for the Aged, 325 South Boyle Ave., Los Angeles 33, Calif.

American Nursing Home Association, 1346 Connecticut Ave., N.W., Washington 6, D.C.

Nutrition

American College of Nutrition, American Nutrition Society, 10651 W. Pico Boulevard, Los Angeles 64, Calif.

Occupational Therapy

American Occupational Therapy Association, 250 W. 57th St., New York 19, N.Y.

Recreation and Social Activities

American Association for Health, Physical Education, and Recreation, 1201 16th St. N.W., Washington 6, D.C.

American Camping Association, Inc., Bradford Woods, Martinsville, Ind.

American Recreation Society, 1420 New York Ave. N.W., Washington, D.C.

American Social Health Association, 1790 Broadway, New York 19, N.Y.

Council of the Golden Ring Clubs, 25 E. 78th St., New York 21, N.Y.

Golden Age and Senior Citizens Clubs of the United States, R.F.D. 1, Box 275, St. Louis 41, Mo.

National Association of Recreational Therapists, Inc., Athens State Hospital, Athens, Ohio

National League of Senior Citizens, Inc., 1031 S. Grand Ave., Los Angeles 15, Calif.

National Recreation Association, 8 W. 8th St., New York 11, N.Y.

Rotary International, 1600 Ridge Ave., Evanston, Ill.

Senior Citizens of America, 1129 Vermont Ave. N.W., Washington 5, D.C.

Seniors International, Inc., Post Office Box 2391, Lakeland, Fla.

Seniors in Philanthropic Service, Inc., 704 S. Spring St., Los Angeles 14, Calif.

Rehabilitation and Physical Therapy

American Association for Rehabilitation Therapy, 12020 Joan Drive, Pittsburgh 34, Pa.

American Congress of Physical Medicine and Rehabilitation, 30 N. Michigan Ave., Chicago 2, Ill.

American Physical Therapy Association, 1790 Broadway, New York 19, N.Y.

American Rehabilitation Commission, 28 E. 21st St., New York, N.Y.

Federation of the Handicapped, 211 W. 14th St., New York 11, N.Y.

Goodwill Industries of America, Inc., 1913 N Street N.W., Washington 6, D.C.

National Association of Recreational Therapists, Inc., Athens State Hospital, Athens, Ohio

National Association of Sheltered Workshops and Homebound Programs, Inc., 3600 Troost St., Kansas City, Mo.

Religious Agencies

American Baptist Home Mission Societies, 475 Riverside Drive, New York, N.Y.

American Council of Christian Churches, 15 Park Row, New York, N.Y.

American Council for Judaism, 201 E. 57th St., New York, N.Y.

Catholic Social Service, 919 Fairfield Ave., Fort Wayne, Ind.

Central Bureau for the Jewish Aged, 31 Union Square West, New York 3, N.Y.

Evangelical and Reformed Church (United Church of Christ), 1505 Race St., Philadelphia, Pa.

Methodist Church, 740 Rush St., Chicago 11, Ill.

National Benevolent Association of the Christian Churches (Disciples of Christ), Landreth Building, Fourth and Locust, St. Louis 2, Mo.

National Catholic Welfare Conference, Family Life Bureau, 1312 Massachusetts Ave. N.W., Washington 5, D.C.

National Council of Catholic Men, Federation of Catholic Men's Organizations, 1312 Massachusetts Ave. N.W., Washington 5, D.C.

National Council of Catholic Women, Department of Lay Organizations, N.C.W.C., 1312 Massachusetts Ave. N.W., Washington 5, D.C.

National Council of Churches, Department of Social Welfare, 475 Riverside Drive, New York 27, N.Y.

National Council of the Churches of Christ in the U.S.A., 475 Riverside Drive, New York 27, N.Y.

National Council of the Protestant Episcopal Church, Ministry to the Aging, 815 Second Ave., New York, N.Y.

Religious Society of Friends (Friends General Conference), 1515 Cherry St., Philadelphia 2, Pa.

Research and Training

American Society for the Aged, Raymond Commerce Building, Newark 2, N.J.

Gerontological Research Foundation, 5600 Arsenal St., St. Louis 9, Mo.

Retirement

American Association of Retired Persons, Dupont Circle Building, Washington 6, D.C.

Social Security Administration, U.S. Department of Health, Education and Welfare, Washington 25, D.C. (*See also* local community offices.)

Sunset Clubs, Volunteers of America, 340 W. 85th St., New York 24, N.Y.

(*See also* Golden Age clubs, which are often listed in the telephone directory.)

Social Welfare

American National Red Cross, National Headquarters, Washington, D.C.

American Public Welfare Association, Public Welfare Project on Aging, 6006 South Stony Island Ave., Chicago 37, Ill.

Council of Jewish Federations and Welfare Funds, Inc., 729 Seventh Ave., New York 19, N.Y.

Evangelical and Reformed Church (United Church of Christ), Commission on Health and Welfare Services, 1505 Race St., Philadelphia, Pa.

Family Service Association of America, 44 East 23rd St., New York 10, N. Y.

Federation of Protestant Welfare Agencies, Inc., 251 Park Ave. South, New York, N.Y.

Foundation for Voluntary Welfare, Box 72, Burlingame, Calif.

Jewish Family Service, 33 W. 60th St., New York 23, N.Y.

Kiwanis International, 101 E. Erie St., Chicago 11, Ill.

Masonic Foundation for Medical Research and Human Welfare, 71 W. 23rd St., New York 10, N.Y.

Masonic Service Association of the United States, 700 10th St. N.W., Washington 1, D.C.

Methodist Church (Board of Hospitals and Homes), 740 Rush St., Chicago 11, Ill.

National Association of Colored Women's Clubs, Inc., 1601 R St. N.W., Washington 9, D.C.

National Association of Social Workers, Inc., 2 Park Ave., New York, N.Y.

National Association of Voluntary Jewish Institutions for Care of the Aged, 2525 Centerville Road, Dallas, Tex.

National Benevolent Association of the Christian Churches (Disciples of Christ), Landreth Building, Fourth and Locust, St. Louis 2, Mo.

National Catholic Welfare Conference, Family Life Bureau, 1312 Massachusetts Ave. N.W., Washington 5, D.C.

National Committee on the Aging, The National Social Welfare Assembly, 345 E. 46th St., New York 17, N.Y.

National Council of Catholic Men, Federation of Catholic Men's Organizations, 1312 Massachusetts Ave. N.W., Washington 5, D.C.

National Council of Catholic Women, Department of Lay Organizations, N.C.W.C., 1312 Massachusetts Ave. N.W., Washington 5, D.C.

National Council of Churches, Department of Social Welfare, 475 Riverside Drive, New York 27, N.Y.

National Council of the Churches of Christ in the U.S.A., 475 Riverside Drive, New York 27, N.Y.

National Council of Jewish Women, 1 W. 47th St., New York 36, N.Y.

National Council of Senior Citizens, 200 C St. S.E., Washington, D.C.

National Federation of Settlements and Neighborhood Centers, 226 W. 47th St., New York 36, N.Y.

National Jewish Welfare Board, 145 East 32nd St., New York, N.Y.

National Council of the Protestant Episcopal Church, Ministry to the Aging, 815 Second Ave., New York 10, N.Y.

Religious Society of Friends (Friends General Conference), 1515 Cherry St., Philadelphia 2, Pa.

U. S. Department of Health, Education and Welfare, Washington 25, D.C.

(*See also* community family agencies and social welfare agencies, which offer counseling and information, and which are listed in the local telephone directory.)

Speech

American Speech and Hearing Association, 1001 Connecticut Ave. N.W., Washington 6, D.C.

Sunset Clubs

Volunteers of America, 340 W. 85th St., New York 24, N.Y.

Tuberculosis

National Tuberculosis Association, 1790 Broadway, New York 19, N.Y.

Veterans

American Legion, 1608 K Street N.W., Washington 6, D.C.

American Veterans Committee, 1830 Jefferson Place N.W., Washington 6, D.C.

Veterans of Foreign Wars of the United States (Ladies Auxiliary), 406 W. 34th St., Kansas City 11, Mo.

OVARIES

See ADRENAL GLANDS; ENDOCRINE GLANDS AND HORMONES; FEMALE ORGANS; PITUITARY GLAND; SEX HORMONES; THYROID GLAND.

How long do the ovaries continue to secrete hormones?

It is thought that very small amounts of hormone are secreted into the bloodstream even after menopause (change of life).

Does surgical removal of the ovaries shorten the life-span of a woman?

Not at all.

Does any other organ take over the secretion of female hormones after the ovaries have been removed?

It is thought that the adrenal glands secrete substances very similar to the ovarian hormones throughout the life of the female.

What are the symptoms or signs of ovarian undersecretion in women past sixty?

No symptoms have been *proved* to be the result of lack of

ovarian secretion in women past sixty. However, it is thought that obesity, listlessness, arthritis, increased growth of body hair, and other symptoms may be associated with absence of ovarian-hormone secretion.

Should women past sixty be given ovarian-hormone extracts in order to combat the above-mentioned symptoms?

No. It is thought that if a dormant ovarian tumor is present, ovarian-hormone therapy may stimulate it to become active and grow.

Is it possible for a woman past sixty to become pregnant?

There are a few cases on record in which women have continued to menstruate and ovulate into their sixties and have thus been capable of becoming pregnant. However, these cases are extremely rare and constitute medical oddities. Moreover, one would have to examine such reports very closely to make sure that a mistake had not been made in calculating age.

How long after menstruation has stopped can a woman be certain that she has no chance of becoming pregnant?

If a woman has had no natural menstrual periods for one year, it can be assumed that the possibility of pregnancy is almost nonexistent.

Do the ovaries ever become enlarged in older women who have passed the menopause?

Yes, from the development of either a cyst or a tumor.

How does the physician make a diagnosis of an ovarian cyst?

By a pelvic examination. Because such cysts can occur in older women, they should have a pelvic examination every year.

Do benign ovarian cysts ever become cancerous?

Yes, especially in women past menopause.

What is the treatment of an ovarian cyst in older women?

It should be removed surgically through an abdominal incision. In all probability, the gynecologist will also remove the uterus and the other ovary.

Is the removal of an ovary a dangerous operation?

Not at all, unless the general health of the patient is extremely poor.

How does a physician make the diagnosis of an ovarian tumor?

By noting the enlargement of one or both ovaries. In some instances, an ovarian tumor will cause resumption of vaginal bleeding in a woman who has passed the menopause.

Are all ovarian tumors cancerous?

No, but the majority found in women past sixty *are* malignant.

What is the treatment of an ovarian tumor?

Surgical removal of both ovaries and the uterus.

How is a benign ovarian tumor distinguished from a malignant one?

During the operation, the gynecologist may be able to make the distinction visually; for absolute certainty, he will have a biopsy done (a piece of the tumor is examined under a microscope)—even while the operation is in progress.

Is recovery the general rule after this type of operation?

Yes. The operation itself is not dangerous. The important thing is to operate at a stage early in the development of the tumor, before it has become malignant or has spread to other organs in the abdominal cavity.

What are the chances for cure of ovarian cancer?

If it is operated on before it has spread throughout the abdominal cavity, the likelihood of cure is excellent. If, on the other hand, the disease has already spread throughout the abdomen, only a small percentage of cases will be cured.

Are there treatments for ovarian cancer other than surgical removal of the ovary?

Yes. X-ray or cobalt therapy, instilling radioactive gold into the abdominal cavity, giving cancer-inhibiting chemicals, and other treatments have been of help in delaying the growth of malignant tumors. With these newer methods of treatment, life can often be prolonged for many years.

PAGET'S DISEASE

See BONES AND JOINTS.

What is Paget's disease of the bones?

It is a chronic disease of the long bones and the skull, which begins very slowly and, over a period of many years, may cause progressive deformity.

At what age is Paget's disease most likely to manifest itself?

Although it starts during the middle years, it usually does not become apparent until the sixties or later.

Are all the bones of the body affected by Paget's disease?
No, but it does tend to involve many of them.

Is Paget's disease a common condition?
Yes, but in many instances the changes are mild and the process remains almost stationary for years.

How is Paget's disease diagnosed?
X rays will show bone changes typical of the disease, for example, a characteristic thickening of the skull bones and thickening and bowing of the bones of the legs.

What causes Paget's disease?
The cause is as yet unknown.

What is the course of Paget's disease?
Bone deformity advances over the years, occasionally resulting in spontaneous fractures in the long bones.

Does Paget's disease shorten the life-span?
No, but it may cause severe crippling.

Is there any treatment of Paget's disease?
No.

What is Paget's disease of the nipple?
It is cancer of the nipple that has spread outward from a malignant growth in the breast. It is totally unrelated to Paget's disease of the bones.

PAIN

See ANESTHESIA; ANGINA PECTORIS; BACKACHE; CLAUDICATION; HEADACHE; NERVES; SCIATICA; TIC DOULOUREUX.

Does the ability to perceive pain continue throughout life with the same degree of intensity?
It is thought that the threshold of pain for one individual remains almost constant from the time of birth until the end of life. Stated in another way, this means that the body's physical ability to perceive the sensation of pain changes very little with the passage of time.

Do older people feel pain as intensely as young people?
In all probability, although the older person's reaction to it may change as he gets older. Some people become more stoical as the result of years of experience with pain and ill-

ness; others, either consciously or unconsciously, overreact to pain in an attempt to obtain more attention and sympathy from those who surround them.

Are people past sixty more subject to conditions that cause pain?

Yes, especially pain in the muscles and joints secondary to arthritic changes.

Should more emphasis be placed on relieving the pain suffered by older people?

Yes. Many older people, because of impaired heart function, can physically tolerate less pain. Others are emotionally less able to tolerate pain.

Can a heart attack be precipitated by extreme pain?

Many physicians believe that the suffering of intense pain in an area other than the heart may bring on an attack of angina pectoris, or even coronary thrombosis. The exact mechanism that causes this is not known, but it is thought that extreme pain causes excessive stimuli to travel along the nerve pathways to the heart. This overstimulation of the nerves may cause the coronary artery to go into prolonged spasm, with resultant clotting of the blood in its passage.

Can prolonged, excruciating pain cause a stroke?

If a person has high blood pressure and marked arteriosclerosis, it is entirely possible that the anguish and emotional stress created by intense pain could produce a stroke.

Are people past sixty more susceptible to the development of pain along nerve pathways, for example, neuralgia and neuritis?

Yes. Changes in the nerves as one ages make them more susceptible to irritation and inflammation.

How should one treat older people who exaggerate their pain?

Sympathy, attention, and kindness are essential in handling people who exaggerate their pain. Scolding or giving them the impression that they are imagining the pain is a very poor way of handling the problem. It challenges their honesty and will cause them to exaggerate their pain even more.

Is the treatment of organic pain (that resulting from actual disease) more difficult to relieve when it affects older people?

Yes, because the underlying disease is more likely to be chronic in nature. For instance, pain in the legs caused by hardening of the arteries is much more difficult to relieve than a similar pain caused by a muscle tear or sprain.

Do the reactions of older people to the pain-relieving drugs differ from those of younger people?

Essentially, their reactions are the same, although very thin older people often require less than the average dose of these medications.

Should medications be withheld from older people because of their habit-forming or addictive properties?

Not if the patient is very old and the condition for which the drug is being prescribed is chronic or incurable. Often it is better to have the patient depend on the drug than to allow him to suffer continued or repeated pain.

Are ice bags helpful in relieving localized pain?

Yes, if the pain has been caused by an injury resulting in hemorrhage into the tissues. However, it should not be forgotten that burns or frostbite may result from too prolonged an application of an ice bag.

Are hot-water bags, baking lamps, and electric pads helpful in relieving pain?

To a limited extent. Here, too, it is essential that burns be guarded against by regulating the heat and the length of its application.

Are injections of novocaine or similar substances helpful in relieving pain in localized areas?

Yes. In many instances even pain of long duration can be relieved by one or two such injections.

Is surgery ever helpful in relieving the chronic pain caused by a spreading malignant tumor?

Yes. In cases in which the cancer has spread and cannot be removed, the nerve pathways carrying the pain impulses can be cut. This procedure will often give great relief from suffering.

PANCREAS

See ALCOHOL AND ALCOHOLISM; DIABETES MELLITUS; ENDO-CRINE GLANDS AND HORMONES; GALLBLADDER AND BILE DUCTS.

What is the pancreas and where is it located?

It is a yellowish, long, flat organ lying across the upper part of the abdomen behind the stomach and transverse colon. It measures about five to six inches on its longest axis.

What are the functions of the pancreas?

Its main function is to produce chemical substances known as enzymes, which digest the food in the intestinal tract. These secretions reach the small intestine through a tube known as the pancreatic duct.

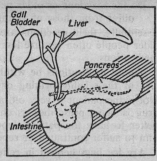

Its other important function is to produce insulin and secrete it into the bloodstream. Insulin regulates the utilization of sugar by the

The pancreas and organs to which it is attached

body and is essential for the transformation of sugar (glucose) into energy.

Is disease of the pancreas common in older people?

Yes. Older people are very susceptible to the development of the following pancreatic diseases:

1. Diabetes.
2. Pancreatitis (inflammation of the pancreas).
3. Cancer of the pancreas.

Does the pancreas wear out as one gets older, or is it capable of functioning satisfactorily throughout life?

In healthy older people the pancreas will continue to manufacture and secrete enzymes sufficient for food digestion and will produce enough insulin to regulate sugar metabolism. Of course, the organ will be subject to the same changes of aging as other structures. Thus, arteriosclerosis of its vessels may eventually lead to inadequate secretion of insulin and enzymes.

Does inflammation of the pancreas (pancreatitis) ever occur in people past sixty?

Yes, especially in those who have gallstones and disease of the gallbladder and bile ducts. Since biliary infection and stones often affect older people, it is not unexpected that the incidence of pancreatitis is high.

What are the symptoms of acute pancreatitis?

Upper abdominal pain, nausea, vomiting, elevation of temperature, distention of the abdomen, a reddish-blue hue to the cheeks, and the characteristic finding of a marked increase in the amount of amylase (an enzyme) in the blood.

In severe cases, a state of shock may be caused by chemical

peritonitis. In other cases, there may be a severe hemorrhage into the abdominal cavity. Pancreatitis can be a very serious disease, especially in people of advanced age. Death from shock or hemorrhage is not unusual if treatment is delayed.

Can acute alcoholism precipitate an attack of pancreatitis?

Yes.

Does cancer of the pancreas occur more frequently in older people?

Yes. The outstanding symptoms of this disease are as follows:
1. Slowly progressive and deepening jaundice (yellowness of the skin).
2. Vague midabdominal pain, often radiating to the back on the left side.
3. Characteristic blood-chemistry findings indicating an obstruction of the passage of bile from the liver to the intestines.
4. Loss of appetite and weight.
5. In some cases, a characteristic X-ray finding on examination of the first portion of the duodenum.

What is the treatment of cancer of the pancreas?

Surgery. But the great majority of patients cannot be saved through surgery because they seek help too late. Nevertheless, some people can be saved by removal of the pancreas. This is a most formidable procedure, accompanied by considerable risk.

What is hyperinsulinism?

It is a condition caused by overactivity of the insulin-producing cells (the islets of Langerhans) of the pancreas. The overactivity may be due to a tumor of these cells or merely to oversecretion of normal cells.

Does hyperinsulinism frequently affect older people?

It is rare in people past sixty, but it does occur occasionally.

What are the symptoms of hyperinsulinism?

When an excessive amount of insulin is secreted into the blood, the patient becomes nervous, tense, and, occasionally, mentally confused. Symptoms include tremor of the hands; spots before the eyes; intense, ravenous hunger; and, in severe cases, convulsions with loss of consciousness.

If the blood were to be analyzed at the time of an acute episode of hyperinsulinism, it would reveal an extremely low quantity of sugar.

Are the symptoms the same as those brought on by an overdose of insulin?

Yes. (*See* DIABETES.)

What is the treatment of hyperinsulinism?

When it occurs in a patient over sixty years of age, it is most likely due to a tumor of the pancreas. Surgery for removal of the tumor is necessary. Such operations can be done with relative safety and the condition can be cured in a large number of instances.

If no tumor is found, the hyperinsulinism must be attributed to an overgrowth of the insulin-producing cells. This will necessitate removal of the major portion of the pancreas in order to cut down on insulin production. Such an operation, although of major proportions, can be carried out with a fair prospect of success.

Is there any way to guard against developing disease of the pancreas in later life?

Yes. Pancreatitis can be avoided in most instances by staying thin, by eating meals low in fat, and by using alcohol in moderation.

If there are stones or infection in the gallbladder or bile ducts, the condition should be corrected surgically. Nothing can prevent the development of a tumor of the pancreas.

PARATHYROID GLANDS

See BONES AND JOINTS; ENDOCRINE GLANDS AND HORMONES; THYROID GLAND.

Where are the parathyroid glands and what are their functions?

They are four small, pea-sized endocrine glands located just behind, and embedded in, the capsule of the thyroid gland in the neck. They manufacture and secrete parathormone, the hormone that controls calcium and phosphorus metabolism.

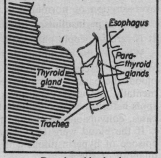

Parathyroid glands

Do the parathyroid glands ever become overactive?

Yes, although not often. The condition is know as hyperparathyroidism.

What are the results of overactivity of the parathyroid glands?

Large amounts of calcium are withdrawn from the bones, and appear in the bloodstream. There is also an abnormally large quantity of calcium excreted by the kidneys. This process leads to thinning out of the bones, bone deformity, bone cysts, and formation of kidney stones. Serious damage to kidney function may also ensue.

How is parathyroid overactivity diagnosed?

There are characteristic changes in the blood chemistry, X rays show changes in bone structure, and kidney stones are present.

Does the withdrawal of large amounts of calcium from the bones lead to marked deformity?

Yes. A characteristic bone condition, known as *osteitis fibrosa cystica,* results. Marked bowing of the long bones, cyst formation, and spontaneous fractures are the main results of this disease.

What are the common causes of overactivity of the parathyroid glands?

1. A tumor in one or more of the glands. The tumors are usually benign; cancer of the parathyroid glands is rare.
2. Overactivity of all of the glands without tumor formation.

What is the treatment of hyperparathyroidism?

Surgical removal of the enlarged gland or glands, whether the enlargement is caused by tumor formation or by gland overactivity. This operation is safe, even for people of advanced age.

Will the bones heal after removal of a tumor of the parathyroid?

Yes. Improvement is usually remarkable. However, if the bones have already become bent and twisted, the deformities will not straighten out.

Are the parathyroid glands ever underactive?

Yes, although this condition is less common than overactivity.

What causes underactivity of the parathyroid glands (hypoparathyroidism)?

Since these glands adhere to the thyroid gland, they may be injured or accidentally removed during surgery for removal of the thyroid.

What are the symptoms of underactivity of the parathyroid glands?

Two conditions may result:

1. Repeated convulsions whenever the blood-calcium level becomes too low.
2. Severe cramps and spasm in the muscles (tetany).

How is the diagnosis of underactivity of these glands made?

By noting the symptoms and by discovering an extremely low blood-calcium level.

What is the treatment of underactivity of the parathyroid glands?

Large amounts of calcium and vitamin D will bring relief from symptoms, but this treatment must continue for as long as the underactivity persists. Injections of parathormone will also control symptoms temporarily. In some cases, a graft of a normal parathyroid gland may prove beneficial.

PARKINSON'S DISEASE AND PALSY

See ARTERIOSCLEROSIS; BELL'S PALSY; MUSCLES; NERVES; RE-HABILITATION AND PHYSICAL THERAPY.

What is Parkinson's disease, or paralysis agitans?

An organic disease of the brain associated with tremors and muscle rigidity. The muscle rigidity slows up all body movements and causes the face to have a blank expression. The shaking tremor is slow, rhythmic, and even, and is most visible in the neck and hands. The fingers particularly are involved in the tremor, especially the thumb and index and middle fingers. The movements of the fingers are similar to those of pill rolling.

Is there actual paralysis in parkinsonism?

No, despite the fact that the condition is often referred to as paralysis agitans.

What are the main causes of Parkinson's disease?

1. Arteriosclerosis of blood vessels in the brain, resulting in degeneration of those nerve centers (ganglia) that control muscle actions.
2. Encephalitis ("sleeping sickness"), a virus inflammation of the brain, which, years later, leads to degeneration of the same nerve centers.

Is parkinsonism a disease of old age?

No, although the type associated with hardening of the arteries is much more common in the seventies and eighties than in earlier life. When the disease follows encephalitis, it usually occurs during the thirties, forties, or fifties.

Are the symptoms of Parkinson's disease the same whether it is caused by hardening of the arteries or by encephalitis?

Yes.

Is Parkinson's disease more common in men than women?

Yes, inasmuch as arteriosclerosis of the arteries in the brain affects men more often than women.

Is mental function impaired in Parkinson's disease?

No, except that mental function might be naturally impaired in patients of advanced age. The masklike appearance of the face is not indicative of stupidity, but is part of the disease process.

Does the shaking palsy continue throughout the night and day?

No. During sleep, the shaking tremors disappear. Also, the shaking disappears or is markedly diminished in intensity while voluntary muscle movements are being performed.

What is palsy?

It is any type of rhythmic tremor (shaking movement), involving the arms, hands, legs, head, or neck.

Is Parkinson's disease usually progressive?

Yes. If untreated, it will get worse as the months or years pass; eventually, it may render the patient helpless.

Is chronic constipation associated with Parkinson's disease?

Yes, and this may be a very troublesome complication. (*See* CONSTIPATION.)

What is the treatment of Parkinson's disease?

1. A rather large group of drugs are helpful in reducing the muscle rigidity and tremors. These drugs must be taken regularly and for long periods of time.
2. Psychotherapy is very helpful in aiding the patient to adjust to his condition.
3. Within recent years, brain operations have been devised that sever those nerves responsible for the tremors and muscle rigidity. With modern surgical techniques good results can be anticipated in the majority of cases.

Does paralysis of the arms and legs follow surgery for parkinsonism?

No.

Are operations for Parkinson's disease safe?

Yes, provided the general health of the patient is satisfactory.

PHYSICAL ACTIVITY AND EXERCISE

See ANGINA PECTORIS; APOPLEXY, OR STROKE; ARTHRITIS AND RHEUMATISM; CLAUDICATION; CORONARY-ARTERY DISEASE; HEART; HERNIA; LONGEVITY; REHABILITATION AND PHYSICAL THERAPY; RETIREMENT; SEX AFTER SIXTY; TRAVEL; WEIGHT.

Should older people engage in active physical exercise?

By all means, provided they are in good health. The exact type of exercise and its extent will differ for different people. The family physician should be consulted, so that he may outline precisely what activities can be undertaken.

What are some of the factors governing the type and amount of exercise that can be taken?

1. Those who have exercised regularly during their earlier years should continue the same type of activity, so long as no untoward symptoms develop.
2. As people enter their late sixties and seventies they should modify the amount of physical exercise they take, even if no symptoms arise. For example, a habitual golfer should use a golf cart no matter how hearty he may feel; a fisherman should cut down on the amount of time he is exposed to the sun.
3. Those who were never very active physically should be especially cautious about taking up new forms of exercise.
4. If symptoms such as pain in the chest, shortness of breath, palpitation of the heart, or headache should appear during exercise, it should be discontinued immediately.
5. People who have been under medical treatment should not exercise without specific permission from the doctor.
6. Activities that are accompanied by emotional excitement or intense competition, such as a golf match, bowling contest, or boat race, should be stopped when people reach their later years or have been through a major illness. Physical exercise in the later years should be a form of relaxation, not a competitive struggle.

Is it safe for people over sixty to begin physical exercise for the first time?

Yes, but they must proceed cautiously and only after consultation with a doctor. It is much easier on the body to continue a form of exercise that has been engaged in for years than it is to start some new activity for the first time.

Does the appearance of muscle and joint pain indicate that the exercise must be given up?

Not necessarily. It usually is a sign that too much exercise has been performed or that the individual failed to pace himself properly.

Is it important for older people to avoid overexposure to the sun during exercise?

Yes. Activities that require long periods in the sun should be modified so that sunstroke and heat exhaustion are avoided. Golfing, fishing, and sailing, for example, are particularly likely to be associated with overexposure to the sun.

When should people over sixty cancel plans to exercise?

1. On extremely hot or humid days.
2. On extremely cold or windy days.
3. After eating a heavy meal.
4. If they do not feel completely well or anxious to exercise.
5. If they suspect that the activity will create too much tension.

How should older people taper off after having engaged in physical activity?

1. They should take a short nap or sit quietly in a lounging chair for half an hour or more.
2. After resting for a half hour or more, they may take a cool shower or a swim.
3. If the exercise has caused a great deal of perspiring, salt tablets and water should be taken.
4. A large meal should not be eaten until at least one hour after completion of the exercise.

Must certain forms of exercise be discontinued merely because one has advanced in age?

No, but the *manner* in which one exercises should be modified. Many healthy people in their seventies can continue to golf, play tennis, fish, sail, ski, ride horseback, etc., provided they are less strenuous in their pursuit of these sports. "Doubles" should take the place of "singles," trotting should replace cantering or galloping, golf carts should replace walking, etc.

What symptoms indicate the need for more physical activity?

1. Low blood pressure, with a chronic feeling of lassitude in an otherwise active individual.
2. A slow pulse in someone who is generally healthy.
3. A sense of air hunger in an otherwise healthy person.
4. Muscle and joint stiffness in a person who shows minimal signs of arthritis.
5. Coldness of the hands and feet in those who have adequate circulation.

What symptoms indicate that too much physical exercise is being taken?

1. Shortness of breath, palpitation of the heart, or headache.
2. A rapid, bounding pulse.
3. Pain in the chest, possibly radiating to the left shoulder and arm.
4. Excess perspiration and flushing of the skin at a time when the humidity is low.

Is walking a good form of exercise for older people?

Yes. It is one of the best forms of exercise for all people. A mile or two a day is not excessive for healthy older people, provided they walk on level ground and pace themselves carefully. Walking up steep grades, rapid walking, and walking against a heavy wind are not advisable. Also, it is perhaps best not to walk immediately after eating a large meal.

Are calisthenics a good form of exercise for older people?

Yes, especially for those who have been in the habit of doing them for years. People who have never engaged in calisthenics before should be more moderate in practicing them.

Is swimming good for older people?

Yes, but very cold or rough water should be avoided.

Can older people continue to hunt?

Yes, but they must realize that their senses are not as keen as they once were. When hearing and sight are not as good as they were and reaction time is slower, accidents are more likely to occur. Also, it is important that older people be familiar with the terrain in which they will hunt, so that they will not be forced to climb steep grades.

Is dancing a good form of exercise for older people?

Yes, in moderation.

Should older people continue to tend their gardens?

Yes, but many garden chores will require help from younger

people. Lifting heavy loads, trimming treetops, or digging deep ditches, for example, should be left to younger people.

Can people who have recovered from heart attacks resume physical activity?

Yes, but the time and the amount of exercise they can perform must be spelled out carefully by their physician. It is now recognized that a certain amount of physical exercise is good for people who have had heart attacks and have made satisfactory recovery.

Should people past sixty take rest periods or naps during the day?

Yes. This is an excellent habit even for those in robust health. The best time is after the noonday meal. Rest should be from one half to one hour, for longer periods may interfere with sleep at night.

PITUITARY GLAND

See ADRENAL GLANDS; ENDOCRINE GLANDS AND HORMONES; THYROID GLAND.

What is the pituitary gland and where is it located?

It is a small endocrine gland that measures about one-half inch in diameter, and is located in the base of the skull beneath the brain. It is divided into an anterior and a posterior portion, each of which secretes different hormones into the bloodstream.

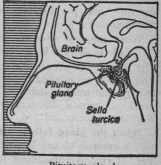

Pituitary gland

What are the main functions of the pituitary?

1. To secrete hormones that influence the activities of other glands such as the thyroid, the adrenals, the mammary glands, the pancreas, the ovaries, and the testicles. Hormones from the anterior portion of the pituitary at times stimulate and at other times inhibit the secretions of these glands. For example, if the thy-

roid is secreting too little of its hormone into the bloodstream, the anterior pituitary will often stimulate it to
greater activity.

2. The posterior portion of the pituitary gland secretes a
hormone that controls the excretion and retention of
water by the kidneys.

3. In childhood and youth, the pituitary secretes a hormone that is responsible for growth. Oversecretion of
this hormone may lead to gigantism; undersecretion, to
dwarfism.

**Will the pituitary continue to function satisfactorily after
sixty?**

Yes, provided the individual is in a normal state of health.

**Does the pituitary gland ever become overactive in older
people?**

Occasionally, when it is the site of a tumor.

**What happens when the pituitary secretes an excessive
amount of hormone into the bloodstream?**

A condition known as acromegaly may develop. This will
produce a distorted, grotesque enlargement of the bones of
the face, hands, and feet.

When other cells in the anterior portion of the pituitary
become too active, the adrenal glands will be overstimulated,
resulting in a condition known as Cushing's syndrome. The
characteristics of this disease are marked obesity, high blood
pressure, and purplish-blue streaks across the skin of the
abdomen.

**What happens when the anterior portion of the pituitary
fails to secrete its hormones?**

The function of all other endocrine glands will be depressed.
The person so affected suffers weakness, weight loss, loss of
energy, and marked debility. The skin becomes wrinkled and
dried out, mental deterioration sets in, and the aging process
is greatly accelerated.

**When the gland fails to function adequately, are pituitary
hormones of any benefit?**

Yes. Hormone-replacement therapy can sometimes maintain
the health of patients with pituitary-gland deficiency for a
long time.

**What happens when the posterior portion of the pituitary
gland fails to function properly?**

A disease known as diabetes insipidus results. This is a serious condition in which the kidneys can no longer control

the amount of water they excrete. People with diabetes insipidus must drink huge quantities of water in order to prevent dehydration.

Is diabetes insipidus related to diabetes mellitus?

No.

Can diabetes insipidus be helped by treatment?

Yes. Hormones will greatly alleviate the symptoms. However, the patient may have to take these medications for the rest of his life.

Can people in their sixties and seventies safely take pituitary hormones, or pituitarylike hormones, such as ACTH?

Yes, but such drugs should be taken only under the strictest surveillance by the physician. Their actions are so potent and the reactions to their effects so intense that great care must be exercised in their use.

How is the diagnosis of a pituitary tumor made?

If the tumor is large, it will press on the optic nerves going to the eyes, and there will be visual disturbance. If the tumor is in the anterior part of the gland, the features of the face become distorted with overgrowth of the bony prominences. The hands and feet, too, will show bone growth. Speech may become slurred as the contours of the mouth change.

Other symptoms such as weakness, debility, and loss of appetite and weight also indicate the possibility of a pituitary tumor.

A tumor in the posterior portion of the pituitary will usually cause the typical Cushing's syndrome, mentioned above.

Evidences of tumor growth may be seen on X ray of the base of the skull. An erosion (eating away) of that portion of the skull in which the pituitary gland lies (the sella turcica) may appear.

Can pituitary tumors be treated successfully in older people?

Yes, in the great majority of instances.

1. The gland may be removed by a neurosurgeon. Most older people can successfully withstand this type of surgery, and the chances of recovery are excellent.
2. The gland may be treated by intensive X-ray therapy. New radiation techniques and super-voltage X-ray machines can pinpoint the rays on the pituitary gland and destroy the tumor cells almost as efficiently as surgery.

PLASTIC SURGERY

See ANESTHESIA; BELL'S PALSY; BREASTS; PREMATURE AGING; SKIN; SURGERY; WEIGHT.

What is plastic surgery?

That branch of surgery devoted to the correction, repair, and restoration of malformed tissues. It is concerned not only with return to normal appearance but also with restoration of normal function.

What is cosmetic surgery?

It is the branch of plastic surgery primarily concerned with restoration of tissues to normal *appearance*.

Do older people ever need cosmetic surgery?

Yes. Contrary to common belief, there are perhaps more indications for this type of surgery in older people than in younger ones.

A good many older people, particularly those in professions in which physical appearance is important, suffer both economically and emotionally because of the onset of the aging process. If cosmetic surgery can help them to appear young longer, there is little point in withholding it from them.

What are some of the cosmetic operations that can benefit older people?

1. The so-called face-lift-ing procedure to obliterate wrinkles.

   a. Operations to remove "crows' feet" about the eyes.

   b. Operations to remove "pouches" beneath the eyes and wrinkles in the upper eyelids.

   c. Operations to remove "double chins" and wrinkles in the neck.

2. Breast plastic operations.

   a. For pendulous breasts.

   b. To trim down excessively large breasts.

   c. To remove excessively large, pendulous male breasts.

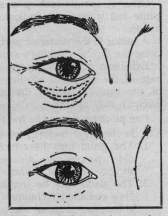

Before and after plastic operation for removal of "bags" under the eyes

3. Operations to remove skin blemishes, such as moles, "brown spots," hemangiomas (red spots), and areas of wartlike growth (hyperkeratoses).

With age, skin growths tend to appear in large numbers for the first time. For some unknown reason, those that have been in existence for many years grow larger as one advances in age.

4. Operations to remove excessive fat on the abdomen (lipectomy).

5. Plastic operations on the nose (usually applicable to younger people, but there is no reason to deny this type of surgery to older people who want it badly).

Are the results of the above-mentioned cosmetic operations usually permanent?

Many of them are not. However, nasal plastic surgery and surgery to make the breasts smaller do have permanent results. Older people should know in advance that wrinkles will eventually return, no matter how effective the cosmetic operation. Similarly, if an older person overeats, he will grow new fat tissue on his abdomen. Moreover, cosmetic surgery cannot prevent the formation of new skin blemishes.

Is plastic surgery dangerous for people of advanced age?

Not if they are in good general health. Skin healing should take place almost as quickly and with as little scarring as it does in younger patients. The surgery itself is not dangerous, although in certain cases special care must be exercised to make sure that the patient can safely undergo prolonged general anesthesia. Postoperative medical observation is essential.

PNEUMONIA

See BRONCHIECTASIS; BRONCHITIS; COMMON COLD; COUGHS; EMPHYSEMA; INFLUENZA AND GRIPPE; RESPIRATORY TRACT.

What is pneumonia?

An acute infection of the air spaces of the lungs.

Are there many different types of pneumonia?

Yes. Pneumonia may be caused by virus or bacterial infections, and even by fungal infections.

What is lobar pneumonia?

It is a type of pneumonia involving one or more lobes of a lung. It is often caused by the pneumococcus germ. The onset

488					Health in the Later Years

is sudden, with chills, fever, cough, and pain in the chest. It lasts several days if untreated, and terminates with a sudden drop in temperature and symptoms. The abrupt change is called a crisis. Today, however, the antibiotics have so modified the course of the condition that it rarely lasts more than a day or two and true crisis does not occur.

What is bronchopneumonia?

It is an inflammation of the lungs involving many small, patchy areas, rather than an entire lobe. It can be caused by several different bacteria, such as the streptococcus and staphylococcus.

What is virus pneumonia?

This is a specific type of pneumonia caused by a virus, rather than by bacteria. It is characterized by low-grade temperature and a rather slow, subacute course lasting up to several weeks.

**Do older people tend to get pneumonia more often than
    younger people?**

Yes. The lungs have less resistance to infection as one gets older. Emphysema (*see* EMPHYSEMA) and fibrous replacement of elastic tissue decrease aeration and blood supply to the lungs, thus causing them to be more susceptible to infection.

What are the symptoms of the various forms of pneumonia?

Although each type may have a somewhat different set of symptoms, the following are common to all:

1. Fever. In the severe types of lobar pneumonia and bronchopneumonia, fever often stays at 105° or 106° F., until it breaks abruptly during the crisis.
2. Chills. They are most common in lobar pneumonia, but people with viral or bronchopneumonia may also have chills.
3. Pain in the chest. If the pneumonia is limited to one lung, the pain will be localized in that area. In bronchopneumonia, pain may be distributed throughout the chest.
4. Cough, often associated with rust-colored or blood-tinged sputum.
5. Rapid, shallow breathing.
6. Malaise (feeling of being sick).

How is the diagnosis of pneumonia made?

1. By listening to the chest with a stethoscope and noting the characteristic sounds.
2. By tapping (percussing) the chest and noting areas of dullness.
3. By noting the characteristic symptoms (listed above).
4. By taking an X ray of the chest.

What is the treatment of pneumonia?

1. Bed rest until the temperature becomes normal.
2. Large quantities of fluids, unless there is an associated heart condition.
3. Antibiotic drugs.
4. Oxygen, when breathing is difficult.
5. Heart stimulants if heart function is adversely affected.

Is pneumonia more serious when it affects older people?

Yes, but recovery takes place in the great majority of cases if treatment is adequate and is begun early.

Should people in their seventies or eighties be hospitalized when they have pneumonia?

Only when it is not feasible to give nursing care at home.

What are the chances for recovery from pneumonia?

Formerly, pneumonia was one of the greatest causes of death in people past sixty. Today, with the antibiotics, the great majority of older people recover from this disease. Naturally, the incidence of complications is greater in the older age groups.

What measures can be taken to prevent pneumonia in older people?

1. Sudden changes in temperature should be avoided.
2. Precautions should be taken against exposure to dampness and wetness.
3. Contact with people who have upper-respiratory infections should be avoided.
4. A good state of nutrition should be maintained.
5. Fatigue and strenuous physical exertion should be guarded against.
6. During an epidemic of grippe or influenza, influenza vaccine should be given.
7. When a minor respiratory infection, such as a cold, comes on, older people should go to bed and be treated as if they had a more serious illness.

POLYCYTHEMIA

See ANEMIA; BLOOD; CIRCULATION; CORONARY-ARTERY DISEASE; THROMBUS AND THROMBOSIS.

What is polycythemia?

A chronic, slowly progressive condition characterized by an excess of circulating red blood cells, an increase in blood volume, and an increase in the viscosity (thickness) of the blood.

Is polycythemia seen very often in later life?

It occurs most often in older people.

Does polycythemia occur more often in men than women?

Yes, it is twice as common in men.

What causes polycythemia?

The cause is unknown.

What are the symptoms of this condition?

1. The skin is a reddish-purple.
2. Weakness, headache, dizziness, and vague aches and pains are present in the more serious cases.
3. Examination of the blood shows an increased number of red blood cells, anywhere from 7 million to 13 million per cubic millimeter. (Normal is 5 million per cubic millimeter.)
4. Clots in veins and inflammation of a vein (phlebitis) are seen in advanced cases.
5. Evidences of heart failure may develop.
6. Hemorrhages from the nose, intestinal tract, and other areas are common.
7. The spleen is usually enlarged.

What are the dangers of polycythemia?

1. Heart failure may result from the extra load placed on the heart by the increased blood volume.
2. Cerebral thrombosis or thrombosis of other important veins may result from the thickened state of the blood and the slowed circulation.
3. Severe, sometimes fatal, hemorrhages may occur in severe cases.

How long does polycythemia last?

It is a chronic disease, usually lasting ten to twenty years. Thus, if someone over sixty develops it, it may not shorten his life-span to any appreciable degree.

Can treatment keep polycythemia under control?

To a certain extent.

What is the treatment of polycythemia?

1. Repeated bloodletting reduces blood volume and often relieves the symptoms for a month or two.
2. Radioactive phosphorus will often arrest the disease for several months or even years.
3. Nitrogen mustard and other chemical agents are also helpful in bringing about prolonged remissions.

POLYPS OF THE LARGE BOWEL

See INTESTINES; RECTUM AND ANUS.

What is a polyp?

It is a benign, wartlike growth of a mucous membrane. Some polyps have long stalks; others look like a small sprig of cauliflower. Polyps range in size from that of a pea to that of a golf ball or plum.

In what part of the intestinal tract do polyps occur?

Although polyps do occasionally occur in the stomach, the usual site is the large bowel, especially the rectum and the left side of the descending colon.

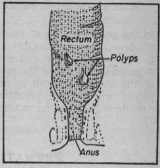

Polyps of large bowel

Are polyps of the large bowel very common in older people?

Yes.

What are the symptoms of a polyp of the rectum or bowel?

The characteristic symptom is painless bleeding on defecation. A slight amount of blood may be passed, or the entire toilet bowl may appear to be filled with bright red blood.

Can polyps of the rectum be removed in a doctor's office?

In many instances. Since a great many of these polyps are in the last ten inches of the intestinal canal, they can be easily reached through a sigmoidoscope. A rectal specialist (proctologist) can easily remove them. However, some polyps are so large or so high up that hospitalization will be required for their removal.

Can polyps of the descending colon, or the area higher up in the large bowel, be removed through the rectum?

No. These tumors will require removal through an abdominal incision in which the bowel is opened, the polyp removed, and the bowel stitched together.

Do rectal polyps of the large bowel ever turn into cancer?

Yes, a certain number will become cancerous if not removed. This is the main reason why *all* polyps of the bowel should be removed.

How can a surgeon distinguish between a benign polyp and one that has undergone cancerous changes?

When a polyp is removed, it is sent to the pathology laboratory for microscopic examination. Such examination will determine whether or not the tumor has become cancerous.

What procedure is carried out if a polyp is found to be cancerous?

In the great majority of cases, the cancer-bearing segment of the bowel is removed. Only when the patient is very advanced in age or when the cancerous changes are limited to the superficial portions of the polyp is the tumor-bearing segment of the bowel permitted to remain. If it is not removed, the patient must return periodically for examination to make sure there has been no recurrence of the tumor.

PREMATURE AGING

See ARTERIOSCLEROSIS; ATTITUDES TOWARD AGING; DEGENERATIVE CHANGES OF AGING; HAIR; INTRODUCTORY REMARKS ON AGING; LONGEVITY.

What is premature aging?

Premature aging is the onset of degenerative changes in organs or within the entire body earlier than one would ordinarily expect. The concept of *premature* aging presupposes that each organ, as well as the whole individual, has a definite limit to its life. This is probably true, and from this point of view, any organ that deteriorates before its limit is reached is actually showing evidence of premature aging. So, even though life usually lasts for seventy years (in America and Europe), the *potential span* is nearer to one hundred years. Even people who show signs of aging in their seventies or eighties are, in reality, growing old prematurely. However, according to most physicians, premature aging consists of major evidences of degeneration during the forties, fifties, or early sixties.

Do most organs tend to age at the same time or at the same rate of speed?

No. (*See* DEGENERATIVE CHANGES OF AGING.)

What role does heredity play in premature aging?

Most investigators feel that people inherit *tendencies* toward certain conditions. These tendencies can be modified greatly by the life one leads and the diseases one has. Thus, an individual may inherit the *tendency* toward early arteriosclerosis, but if he has lived a healthy, sensible life, he may so delay the onset of arteriosclerosis that the tendency is completely nullified. Similarly, one who inherits a tendency toward diabetes may overcome this tendency by following special precautions in youth and middle age.

What effect does climate have on premature aging?

Extremes of climate may expose people to hardships that the body must strain to overcome. Many years in such areas undoubtedly lead to premature aging, as we have learned from study of peoples who live in the Arctic or in the Tropics.

Will malnutrition and vitamin deficiency lead to premature aging?

Yes, if they have existed for many years.

Will chronic alcoholism lead to premature aging?

Yes. (*See* Alcohol and Alcoholism.)

Does repeated serious illness in early life tend to cause premature aging?

Yes, if any of these illnesses have damaged vital structures. For example, rheumatic fever may leave, as an aftermath, damage to heart valves. An individual who has recovered from rheumatic fever may show premature aging because his heart will not function normally later in life.

On the other hand, if one makes a recovery from a serious illness without associated damage to important structures, he will not, in all probability, age prematurely.

Can excessive smoking throughout life cause one to age prematurely?

Medical investigators are not agreed on this subject. For someone who is sensitive to the effects of nicotine, smoking will most definitely cause premature changes in the blood vessels and heart. Many people, however, are not at all sensitive to the effects of nicotine, and they may live well into their eighties or nineties in spite of the fact that they have always been very heavy smokers.

There is little doubt about the connection between excessive smoking over a long period of time and the development of lung cancer in men. Although premature aging may or may not result from smoking, life can certainly be brought to an end prematurely by the development of lung cancer.

Will chronic lack of sleep and rest cause premature aging?

Yes. It is agreed by most investigators that adequate rest and sleep are essential to the maintenance of normal metabolism.

Do one's emotional makeup and attitude toward living play an important role in the aging process?

Yes. People with an optimistic, zestful attitude toward life have a much better chance of delaying the onset of aging.

Can a great unhappiness, such as the loss of a loved one, cause premature aging?

Although organic changes do not often directly follow emotional upsets, it is true that people who make poor adjustments do become old before their time. This may be *psychological* aging rather than *physical* aging. Nevertheless, it is just as real as if it were caused by hardening of the arteries.

One hears that people "turn gray" overnight. Is this true?

Not really, although they may appear to turn gray suddenly. Moreover, those who have suffered a great shock may neglect their appearance to such an extent that their gray hair becomes more noticeable than it ever was before.

Can chronic worry lead to premature aging?

Yes. Recent studies have revealed a very intimate connection between stress and the development of organic disease. Continued stress may result in the degeneration of such vital organs as the adrenal glands and other hormone-producing structures in the body.

Does one's outward appearance necessarily reflect the state of health of his internal organs?

No. Perfectly healthy people with little deterioration in their vital structures may have markedly wrinkled skin and gray hair.

Will people who have undergone repeated surgery tend to age prematurely?

Not if recovery from each operation is complete and there is no residual damage to important organs. For example, many women have undergone surgery for benign breast tumors, benign goiters, gallstones, fibroid tumors of the uterus, and other operations, and have recovered fully from each. They will not have a shortened life-span.

Do people who lead sedentary lives tend to age later than those who lead a strenuous life?

Not necessarily. For example, the middle-aged laborer may show such signs of aging as wrinkling of the skin and a stoop, whereas the middle-aged banker may have smooth skin and may stand erect. However, the banker may have arteriosclerosis and a liver infiltrated with fat. These latter changes are much more significant evidences of premature aging than the superficial signs shown by the healthy laborer.

Will excessive sexual activity in youth and the middle years cause one to grow old prematurely?

It is difficult to define "excessive" sexual activity. If it is accompanied by insufficient sleep and high consumption of alcohol, then sexual activity may be said to influence the aging process. These accompanying factors are more important than the amount of sexual activity. There is no scientific proof that sexual activity alone can cause premature aging.

What are some significant signs of premature aging?

1. A loss of interest in one's family and friends and in the community and world events.
2. Hardening of the arteries, as evidenced by elevated blood pressure, and impairment of various body functions.
3. Deficient kidney function, as evidenced by abnormalities discovered by urine analysis.
4. Cirrhosis of the liver, as shown by blood-chemistry analysis.
5. Heart disease, as shown by electrocardiographic findings and by the development of shortness of breath, swelling of the ankles, chest pain, and other symptoms.

Can hormones help to prevent premature aging?

Not to any appreciable degree. It is true that giving female sex hormones may delay the onset of the symptoms of menopause, and the giving of male sex hormone may delay loss of potency in a man. However, their action lasts only so long as the medication is continued. In addition, there is considerable danger in taking hormones over a long period of time. (*See* OVARIES; PROSTATE GLAND.)

Whom should one consult about fears of premature aging?

A consultation with the family doctor, preferably in young adulthood, should be very helpful. If such fears are discussed with him, he will inquire into the patient's medical history and that of his family; then he will perform a complete physical examination. With the information thus gathered, he will be able to lay out a regimen for the patient to follow.

What specific steps should a young person follow in order to avoid premature aging?

1. It has been definitely shown that fat people tend to age more quickly than thin people. Those who have a tendency toward obesity should follow a reducing diet.
2. One who eats insufficient quantities of food or an unbalanced diet should start eating more sensibly.
3. An adequate intake of vitamins and minerals should always be maintained.

4. Ample rest should be had, in order to allow tissues to restore themselves.

5. Adequate physical exercise should be taken, to keep metabolic processes functioning smoothly.

6. Emotional problems should be resolved, whenever possible, and excessive stress should be avoided.

7. Heavy drinking and smoking should be discontinued.

8. A thorough physical examination should be carried out each year.

PROSTATE GLAND

See CYSTITIS AND INTERSTITIAL CYSTITIS; GONORRHEA; KIDNEYS; SEX AFTER SIXTY; SURGERY; URINARY BLADDER AND URETHRA.

What is the prostate gland?

It is a gland in the male, normally the size of a large horse chestnut, surrounding the outlet of the urinary bladder. Through its center passes the urethra, the duct leading from the bladder to the outside.

What is the main function of the prostate?

To secrete the seminal fluid, which transports sperm from the ejaculatory ducts through the penis to the outside.

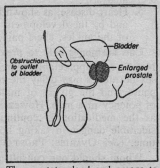

The prostate gland and organs to which it is attached

How is the prostate gland examined?

1. By inserting a finger into the rectum. The gland's size and contour can be readily determined by this method of examination.

2. By examination through a cystoscope inserted through the penis into the bladder. By this method, enlargement of that portion of the gland surrounding the bladder outlet can be discovered.

What are the main diseases affecting the prostate gland in older men?

1. Benign enlargement of the prostate (benign hyperplasia, or prostatism).

2. Stones in the prostate gland (calculi).
3. Cancer of the prostate.
4. Acute inflammation (acute prostatitis).
5. Chronic inflammation (chronic prostatitis).

Is inflammation of the prostate gland very common in men over sixty?

No. It is more common in younger men.

What is the usual cause of acute inflammation of the prostate in older people?

An infection that has reached it through lymph channels or through the bloodstream. In a small number of cases in older men, it is secondary to a gonorrheal infection.

What are the symptoms of acute prostatitis?

1. Pain between the scrotum and the rectum (the perineum).
2. Temperature rise to 101°–103° F.
3. Pus in the urine.
4. Frequent urination accompanied by a burning sensation.
5. Blood in the urine.

How is acute prostatitis diagnosed?

1. By examining the prostate gland by inserting a finger into the rectum, swelling and tenderness will be noted.
2. By urine analysis.
3. By noting the characteristic symptoms and signs.

What is the treatment of acute prostatitis?

1. Bed rest.
2. Large quantities of fluids to flush out the bladder and to keep the urine dilute.
3. Administration of antibiotic or sulfa drugs.
4. Frequent hot baths.

Do most cases of acute prostatitis subside completely?

Yes, if treated properly and promptly. If they are neglected, chronic inflammation may set in. Also, the inflammatory process may spread upward and involve the kidneys.

Does chronic inflammation of the prostate occur very often?

Yes. It is a common condition, often associated with enlargement of the gland (prostatism).

Can chronic inflammation of the prostate take place without a history of acute inflammation of the gland?

Yes.

Does chronic inflammation of the prostate always have symptoms?

No. A certain amount of inflammation is almost always associated with benign enlargement of the gland, and this may be present without any symptoms.

What are the symptoms of chronic prostatitis?

1. Frequent urination accompanied by a burning sensation.
2. Pain in the bladder region or lower part of the back.
3. Loss of potency or premature ejaculations.

What is the treatment of chronic prostatitis?

The standard treatment is periodic massage of the gland. This is best performed by a physician who specializes in disease of the genital organs (urologist). Antibiotic drugs are of little use in chronic prostatitis.

What is prostatism?

It is the enlargement of the prostate gland, which takes place in almost all men as they enter their sixties or seventies. The enlargement often causes an obstruction to the free flow of urine from the bladder out through the urethra.

Is prostatism a benign or a cancerous condition?

The typical, slowly progressive, enlargement is benign.

How can one know whether or not he is suffering from prostatism?

1. It takes longer to start to urinate.
2. There is a decrease in the force of the urinary stream.
3. There is a tendency to urinate more frequently.
4. It is necessary to get up from sleep to urinate.
5. There is dribbling of urine at the end of urination.
6. The bladder is not emptied completely on voiding. This may lead to infection of the retained urine, cystitis, and, possibly, kidney infection.
7. When prostatism is advanced, inability to void may be complete.

Is examination through a cystoscope usually necessary for a diagnosis of prostatism?

No. In a great majority of cases the diagnosis can be made by digital examination through the rectum.

What causes benign enlargement of the prostate gland?

It is thought to be initiated by hormone imbalance secondary to decreased male sex hormone secretion by the testicles. It may also be influenced by alteration in the amount of adrenal and pituitary hormones being secreted.

How does a doctor determine whether or not there is obstruction to the outflow of urine from the bladder?

1. By feeling the lower abdomen, the rounded distention caused by the full bladder will be noted.

2. He will pass a rubber tube called a catheter through the urethra into the bladder after the patient has voided as much as he can. If urine remains in the bladder, it is proof that some obstruction prevents complete emptying.

Do cystitis and urinary infection usually take place when there is obstruction to bladder emptying?

Yes, if obstruction lasts for several weeks.

Does kidney infection eventually result from obstruction to the outlet of the bladder?

Yes.

Do all men who show enlargement of the prostate have to undergo treatment?

No. In many cases the enlargement takes place so slowly, over a period of years, that the symptoms are minimal. In such cases, although there may be some increased difficulty in voiding and some retention of urine in the bladder, no treatment is required.

How does a physician determine which cases require treatment?

If the patient is able to void and can empty most of the urine from the bladder, treatment is not necessary. It will, however, probably take him longer to pass urine and the act must be performed at more frequent intervals. If, on the other hand, the bladder retains large amounts of urine or if there is total obstruction to the passage of urine, treatment is necessary.

Is there any way to halt enlargement of the prostate gland once it has begun?

No. Formerly, some physicians advocated administration of male sex hormone to retard the process, but this method of treatment has not proved efficient. Moreover, there is the possible danger that large doses of male hormone in older men may stimulate the growth of a dormant tumor in the prostate gland.

What medical treatment will help people with enlarged prostate glands?

1. Ample quantities of water should be taken to stimulate bladder emptying and to prevent stagnation of urine.
2. Antibiotic medications and urinary antiseptic drugs should be given to prevent cystitis or kidney infection.
3. Alcoholic beverages and highly seasoned foods should be avoided.
4. Sedatives and relaxant drugs may be given to aid in urination.
5. Exposure to very cold climate should be avoided.

How does the urologist decide which case of prostatism requires surgery?

If there is a large amount of residual urine, marked difficulty in emptying the bladder, and bladder infection with decreased kidney function, surgery will be advocated.

What surgery is performed in prostatism?

1. *Transurethral resection.* This entails the removal of the enlarged portion of the prostate that obstructs the outflow of urine. A cystoscope is inserted into the bladder, and the obstructing portion of the gland is removed by electric current.
2. *Prostatectomy.* The gland is removed surgically through an incision in the abdomen or through the perineum (the region between the base of the scrotum and the anus).

What percentage of cases can be treated by transurethral resection through a cystoscope, and what percentage will require surgical incision?

Approximately 70 percent of cases can be treated by transurethral resection; the other 30 percent will require prostatectomy.

Is a transurethral resection as effective as prostatectomy?

No. However, if transurethral resection fails to relieve the symptoms, the surgeon can, at a later date, remove the entire gland.

Are operations on the prostate gland dangerous?

No. Even a man of greatly advanced age will recover from this type of surgery, unless his general condition is exceptionally poor.

Is there such a thing as a man's being too old to have his prostate removed?

If the gland is to be removed because it is cancerous, there is probably no age limit for prostatectomy. A more important consideration is the ability of his heart, kidneys, and other vital structures to withstand this type of surgery.

If the surgery is to be carried out for benign enlargement with urinary obstruction, there is no alternative to surgery.

Is the removal of the prostate a one-stage or a two-stage procedure?

1. If the patient is very old, has complete urine retention, and suffers marked kidney damage, the surgeon may elect to do the operation in two stages. In such instances, he will first make an abdominal incision into the bladder to relieve the urinary obstruction (cystostomy). If the general condition of the patient permits, several days

to several weeks later the surgeon will complete the operation by removing the prostate through the opening he has previously made into the bladder.

2. If the general condition of the patient permits, the surgeon may perform the entire procedure in one stage. The gland may be removed through an incision into the bladder or through an abdominal incision that avoids opening into the bladder (retropubic prostatectomy).

The gland may also be removed through an incision in the perineum.

How does the surgeon determine whether to perform a prostatectomy or a transurethral resection?

If, through cystoscopic examination, the urologist determines that burning away small segments of the gland will suffice to relieve symptoms, he will follow that procedure. If he believes transurethral resection will prove insufficient to relieve symptoms, he will perform a prostatectomy.

Will surgery relieve the symptoms of prostatism?

Yes. Eventual return to normal voiding is the rule.

Does benign enlargement of the prostate gland tend to recur after it has been corrected surgically?

Not after a surgical prostatectomy. In some instances, it will recur after transurethral resection.

What is a median-bar obstruction?

This means that the segment of the prostate surrounding the bladder outlet is enlarged and is causing obstruction.

Does enlargement of the prostate gland interfere with sexual relations?

Not unless there is urinary retention and bladder infection.

Does transurethral resection often cause loss of potency?

No.

Does the ordinary prostatectomy cause inability to perform the sexual act?

Not in the majority of cases, although it does sometimes. Since most men who have these operations are in their seventies, eighties, or nineties, loss of potency presents relatively little hardship.

Does radical, or total, removal of the prostate interfere with potency?

Yes, although this procedure is done only in cases of cancer of the prostate gland.

Do most men regain urinary control after prostatectomy?

Yes.

Do stones ever form in the prostate gland?

Yes. The presence of stones will often be revealed by X-ray examination of this region.

Are stones most often found in association with prostatism?

Yes.

Can stones in the prostate gland be felt on rectal examination?

Occasionally, but the more precise method of diagnosis is by X-ray examination.

Do prostate stones often cause symptoms?

No, but when they cause obstruction to the outflow of urine or when they are associated with infection, they will cause symptoms and necessitate removal of the prostate gland.

How frequent is cancer of the prostate gland?

Although this may be a shocking statistic, it is estimated that approximately *one out of four* men will develop cancer of the prostate before they reach their seventies or eighties. Cancer of the prostate is the most common malignancy in the male.

What causes cancer of the prostate?

The cause is not known.

How is cancer of the prostate diagnosed?

In most cases, it can be diagnosed by rectal examination. Small, stony, hard nodules can be felt through the rectal wall.

Is cancer of the prostate gland slow in developing, or is its progress rapid?

This type of malignancy grows very slowly, and it may not shorten the life-span very much. Cancerous nodules may grow slowly and may not spread outside the gland for three to five years. Once the cancer has spread outside the prostate, it grows more rapidly.

What are the symptoms of early cancer of the prostate?

There are none. Only when the cancer has spread beyond the prostate and has caused an obstruction to the outflow of urine do symptoms develop. Thus, nearly nine out of ten cases go unrecognized until late in their course.

What can be done to make an earlier diagnosis of cancer of the prostate?

Every adult male, especially one over sixty, should have a rectal digital examination at least once a year. Change in urinary habit—frequency of urination, inability to empty the bladder, burning on urination, and so on—should be investigated promptly.

Does benign enlargement of the prostate (prostatism) lead to cancer of the prostate?

No. The two conditions, although both characterized by prostatic enlargement, are unrelated.

What is the treatment of cancer of the prostate?

In about 50 percent of those cases in which the cancer is confined to the gland, cure can be obtained by the surgical removal of the gland. However, the great majority of patients consult the urologist *after* the cancer has already spread beyond the gland, and these people are not helped greatly by surgery.

Does the prostate always have to be removed when cancer is discovered in it?

No. In many men in their seventies or eighties the cancer will grow so slowly that it will not interfere with the natural life-span. These people can be maintained in a fair state of health with medical management or by another form of surgical treatment.

What is another form of surgical treatment of cancer of the prostate?

It has been discovered that removal of both testicles will slow down the rate of growth of the cancer. This is a safe operation and can be carried out in men in their late seventies or eighties without adverse effects.

What is the medical treatment of cancer of the prostate that has already spread beyond the gland?

The administration of large doses of female sex hormone. This is a most effective method of slowing down its rate of growth. The treatment is particularly effective in older men who have already had both testicles removed.

PSYCHOTHERAPY

See ATTITUDES TOWARD AGING; DEATH AND FEAR OF DEATH; INSTITUTIONAL CARE; MENTAL CHANGES; PREMATURE AGING; REHABILITATION AND PHYSICAL THERAPY; RETIREMENT; SOCIAL BEHAVIOR.

What are some of the conditions of older people that require psychiatric treatment?

1. Obvious mental deterioration, with loss of ability to understand and perceive. This is usually associated with arteriosclerosis of the blood vessels supplying the brain.
2. Acute psychosis—with loss of the sense of reality and lack of orientation to surroundings.

Health in the Later Years

3. Organic brain infection with mental changes; paresis, caused by syphilis, is an example.

4. Acute or chronic mental depressions (melancholia). Such states are extremely common in aging people.

5. Involutional changes associated with sleeplessness and self-depreciation.

6. Paranoid reactions. These are states in which one feels that his family, neighbors, or the entire community is conspiring against him.

7. Psychoneurosis. Psychoneurotics are not psychotic, but they do show extraordinary anxieties and fears relating to various body activities and functions.

8. Suicidal tendencies. It is estimated that suicidal tendencies are more common after sixty than at any other period in life.

Many other mental conditions require psychiatric treatment, but they cannot be classified readily.

What is psychotherapy?

Any form of treatment for emotionally disturbed or mentally ill patients.

Do older people respond as well to psychotherapy as younger people?

No. As people age their ideas become more fixed, and they tend to resist changes in their thought patterns. Psychotherapy will thus be less effective. However, in many areas psychotherapy can be very helpful to the aging.

Do older people respond well to psychoanalysis?

No, although some psychoanalytic techniques are being adapted to the treatment of older neurotic patients. It seems that the psychoanalytic approach delves too deeply into the past life and may, thereby, create too great an upset in established patterns of thinking and behaving.

What are some of the effective methods of treating emotionally and mentally disturbed older patients?

1. Recently, many fine new drugs have been used to relieve anxiety and depressed states. Although these medications are not in themselves curative, they often relieve symptoms to a point where the psychiatrist can begin psychotherapy.

2. Electric-shock therapy is sometimes helpful in the treatment of acute depression. The electric shock causes a temporary period of convulsion and unconsciousness. Shock treatment is rarely used as the sole form of therapy but is usually combined with other psychotherapeutic approaches.

3. Hormone therapy is helpful in an occasional case in which it has been found that the underlying cause of the disturbance is glandular malfunction. It must be emphasized, however, that hormone treatment is limited to a very small group of cases. Certainly, it should not be the only form of treatment but should be given only in conjunction with psychotherapy.

4. Where arteriosclerosis appears to be the main cause of mental changes, medical treatment often brings about good results. In an occasional case in which sclerosis of the carotid artery in the neck is responsible for mental changes, surgical replacement of the artery with a graft has proved beneficial.

5. By far the greatest number of mentally ill patients are treated by psychiatrists using the standard psychiatric measures. It should not be forgotten that psychiatrists can often bring about strikingly good results. All too often, psychiatric care is withheld because of the erroneous belief that "Nothing can be done to help someone whose ills are imaginary."

6. Prefrontal lobotomy, an operation in which certain nerve fibers in the brain are severed, is occasionally helpful in cases in which there are advanced, irreversible mental changes. Today, however, lobotomies are rarely done.

Can psychotherapy help people who have paranoid reactions?

People with paranoid delusions respond poorly to treatment. Since they believe that people are conspiring to harm them, it is important to try to relieve their fears and to alert those who live with them to their abnormal thoughts. Paranoids should be treated with kindness and sympathetic understanding. This will do them almost as much good as the ministrations of the psychiatrist.

Should people who threaten suicide be treated psychiatrically?

By all means. At the first indication that suicidal ideas exist, the patient should be placed in the hands of a psychiatrist. Also, it is often necessary to place a person with suicidal tendencies under constant surveillance.

Is psychotherapy of much value in the treatment of hardening of the arteries in the brain?

No, except that the psychiatrist can be helpful in advising the family how to handle the patient's various problems.

Is electric-shock therapy dangerous for older patients?

Yes, unless it is performed under ideal conditions. Fractures, dislocations, and damage to the heart may ensue. It is therefore wisest to perform shock therapy in a hospital, where all emergency facilities are readily at hand.

How effective are the tranquilizer drugs in the treatment of the depressed older patient?

Although they can be somewhat helpful in certain cases, their usefulness is limited. Certainly, they cannot serve as a substitute for psychiatric care.

Is it possible to prevent emotional and mental disturbance in the later years by undergoing psychotherapy while one is still young?

Yes, if treatment is instituted early enough, that is, in the twenties, thirties, or forties. Much good can be accomplished by alerting young people to coming events. They should think out how they are going to handle the death of close relatives and friends; they should plan how they will spend their years of retirement; they should project themselves into a time when they will be forced to spend most of their days alone and on their own. Society is just beginning to recognize the great need for better mental adjustment in older people. Our planning must take into account the elongated life-span and the new problems it will create.

What are some of the symptoms that should lead a family to consider placing an older person in a mental institution?

1. Repeated threats of suicide or an actual attempt at suicide.
2. Inability of the patient to dress, feed, and care for himself.
3. Threats by the patient against members of the family or neighbors.
4. Paranoid delusions, such as the feeling that others are trying to harm him.
5. Behavior of such an unsocial nature that it repeatedly embarrasses those with whom the patient lives.
6. Emotional upset of children or others who live with the older individual.
7. Melancholia of such intensity that it depresses the healthy members of the family.
8. A home situation in which the patient has little opportunity for social contacts that might improve his mental attitude. Mental institutions provide programs and contacts that often lift the patient out of himself, thus improving his condition.
9. The desire of the patient himself to go to an institution where he feels he will receive more expert care.

How should a family go about making the decision to institutionalize a mentally disturbed relative?

This is a most difficult decision to make and should never be attempted by a single member of the family, unless absolutely necessary. A family conference should always precede such a decision. Also, it is advisable to plan far in advance for this eventuality rather than to wait until a crisis arises. Those who live closest to an aging person should be in contact with the family physician, a psychiatrist, and a psychiatric social worker for many months before institutional care becomes necessary.

Do mental institutions provide psychotherapy as well as custodial care?

Yes. Most mental institutions today provide excellent psychotherapy, and many of the most recent advances in psychiatry have originated in these institutions.

Do mentally ill older patients often improve sufficiently to return home from a mental hospital?

Sometimes. However, it must be remembered that most mental illness in older people is due to irreversible anatomical changes, such as hardening of the arteries and degeneration of brain cells. Moreover, as stated above, psychotherapy is not as effective for older people as it is for younger people.

PTERYGIUM

See CONJUNCTIVITIS; EYES.

What is pterygium?

A marked thickening and growth of mucous membrane extending from the inner corner of an eye toward the colored portion. It is usually triangular in shape, with the apex pointing away from the pupil.

Is pterygium seen in people past sixty?

Yes. This condition represents a degenerative change in the covering membrane of the eye.

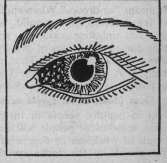

Pterygium

Does pterygium interfere with vision?

In the majority of cases the tissue does not grow so far that it covers the pupil. Therefore, vision is usually not disturbed.

What is the treatment of pterygium?

If it is not extensive and has not grown near to the colored portion of the eye, it is left alone. On the other hand, if it has grown large and endangers the colored portion of the eyeball, it should be removed surgically.

How successful is surgery for pterygium?

Most cases can be cured through surgery. However, the condition tends to recur, and a second operation may occasionally have to be performed.

Is it ever necessary to use a graft in performing an operation for pterygium?

Yes. In some cases where large patches of tissue covering the eyeball have been removed, a patch of mucous membrane from the inside of the mouth will be used as a graft to cover the raw area.

Is X-ray treatment ever helpful in treating pterygium?

Recent reports state that some cases can be helped by certain types of X-ray therapy. However, this does not apply to the great majority of cases.

PTOSIS OF THE EYELID

See BELL'S PALSY; EYES.

What does ptosis mean?

It means "to droop." When applied to the eye region, it refers to the drooping of an eyelid. When used in speaking of the stomach, intestines, kidneys, and other structures, it means that due to the forces of gravity, these organs have dropped down to lower positions. Thus, a "floating kidney" is a *ptosed* kidney. A ptosed stomach ("dropped stomach") occupies a position in the lower abdomen.

Does ptosis of an eyelid occur frequently in older people?

Not in healthy people in their sixties and seventies. However, some older people will develop a drooping eyelid as a result of weakness or degeneration of the nerves that supply the muscle of the upper eyelid. Also, in some people who have recently had a stroke (cerebral hemorrhage or thrombosis), paralysis of the nerve supplying the upper eyelid will result.

What is the treatment of ptosis of an eyelid?

If the drooping is only partial, treatment is not necessary. On the other hand, the lid may be so paralyzed that vision is completely shut off. In such cases, plastic surgery is indicated to refashion the lid so that vision is possible.

Are special protective measures necessary for someone who has ptosis or paralysis of an upper eyelid?

Yes. The blinking mechanism helps to spread tears over the surface of the eyeball, thereby working out dust particles. If this ability is lost, dust and dirt may remain in the eye and cause inflammation or ulceration. It is therefore essential that the eyes of people with ptosis of the eyelid be washed out every few hours and that they be shielded by special glasses when out of doors.

RECTUM AND ANUS

See BOWEL FUNCTION; CONSTIPATION; CYSTOCELE AND RECTOCELE; DIARRHEA; DIVERTICULOSIS AND DIVERTICULITIS; INTESTINES; LAXATIVES; POLYPS OF THE LARGE BOWEL.

What are some anatomical changes of aging that take place around the anus and rectum?

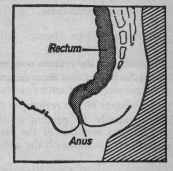

The normal rectum and anus

1. The muscles supporting the anus and rectum may weaken. This may eventually lead to constipation or to prolapse, a protrusion of the mucous membrane through the anal opening.

2. The blood vessels surrounding the anus may dilate and form varicosities, thus producing hemorrhoids.

3. The skin of the anus frequently becomes dry and scaly, resulting in intense itching (pruritus ani).

Does the skin around the anus require special attention in older people?

Yes. The following routine should be observed:

1. Since the skin becomes dry and scaly, it should be kept lubricated with vaseline or some other soothing ointment.
2. The anus should never be wiped strenuously, as this may injure the already delicate skin. It is good practice to cleanse the anus after a bowel movement with cotton moistened in warm water, rather than using toilet tissue.
3. Medicated ointments can be used to relieve irritation and itching. (Such medications should not be used unless a doctor has prescribed them.)
4. Occasionally, it is found that nylon, rubber, or synthetic undergarments irritate the anal area. If so, cotton underwear should be worn.
5. Excessive scrubbing with soaps or detergents should be avoided, as it may injure the delicate tissues of the anal outlet.

Does bleeding from the rectum usually denote cancer of the rectum?

No. Although bleeding does occur with cancer, it also occurs in many other conditions. Among the more common of these conditions are the following:

1. Hemorrhoids (piles).
2. Fissure (a crack or tear in the mucous membrane of the anal outlet).
3. Pruritus ani. In this condition the bleeding is caused by intensive scratching.
4. Colitis.
5. Rectal polyps (benign tumors). (*See* POLYPS OF THE LARGE BOWEL.)

Is cancer of the rectum common in people past sixty?

Yes. It is one of the most frequently encountered cancers in older people. (*See* CANCER; INTESTINES.)

Can cancer of the rectum be cured by surgery?

Approximately 50 percent of those operated upon will be cured. After removal of the diseased rectum, a false orifice (colostomy) is made on the abdominal wall for exit of feces.

HEMORRHOIDS

What are hemorrhoids?

They are dilated varicose veins in the anus and rectum. When these veins are on the outside of the anus, they are called external hemorrhoids; when they are inside the anal canal, they are called internal hemorrhoids.

Are piles the same as hemorrhoids?

Yes.

Do people tend to develop hemorrhoids as they grow older?

Yes. Constipation and straining to evacuate the bowels predispose toward formation of hemorrhoids.

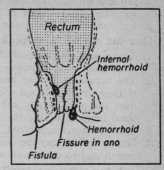

Hemorrhoids and fissure and fistula in ano

What is meant by the term "prolapsed hemorrhoids"?

Prolapsed hemorrhoids, which originate in the rectal canal, are hemorrhoids that are forced out during evacuation. In many cases the sphincter muscle of the anus contracts after the bowels have been evacuated, and the hemorrhoids are left on the outside.

What can older people do to prevent hemorrhoids?

1. Attempts to move the bowels should be made at the same time each morning. Right after breakfast is the most desirable time.
2. No more than 15 minutes should be spent in attempting to have a movement. Excessive straining predisposes toward hemorrhoids.
3. If there is constipation, fresh fruits, raw vegetables, and bran products should be eaten regularly and a lubricant such as mineral oil should be taken daily.
4. If attempts to move the bowels fail, a small enema should be taken. This is much better than excessive straining.

What are the most common causes of hemorrhoids in older people?

1. A natural tendency toward varicose-vein formation.
2. Chronic constipation.
3. Poor bowel habits.
4. Excessive straining at the stool secondary to poor muscle tone.
5. An obstruction, often caused by a tumor, in the bowel.
6. Cirrhosis of the liver resulting in increased back pressure on the veins originating in the rectal area.

7. An abdominal tumor that creates pressure on the rectum, for example, a tumor of the uterus.
8. Inflammation or infection in the anal canal.

How can one tell if he has hemorrhoids?

1. There may be grape-sized lumps on the outside of the anal canal after a bowel movement.
2. The hemorrhoids may become very painful and swollen if they develop blood clots within them. After a few days the pain usually subsides, leaving a hard, marble-sized lump alongside the anal opening.
3. Some hemorrhoids bleed.
4. Hemorrhoids may be associated with a discharge of mucus and blood, which will stain the undergarments.

Are all hemorrhoids painful?

No. The most painful are external hemorrhoids in which clots develop (thrombosed hemorrhoids) and internal hemorrhoids that protrude outside the anal orifice and, because of spasm of the sphincter muscle, cannot be pushed back inside. These latter are called strangulated hemorrhoids.

Are hemorrhoids ever an indication that something else is wrong with the intestinal tract?

Yes. A tumor higher up in the large bowel may cause hemorrhoids to appear.

How does the physician rule out the possibility of a tumor as the cause of hemorrhoids?

By examining the rectum with a finger; by inserting a sigmoidoscope, which will permit inspection of the last 10 to 12 inches of the bowel; and by performing a barium enema X ray of the entire large bowel.

What is a barium enema X ray?

Barium is an opaque substance that, when injected into the rectal canal, will fill the entire large bowel. X rays are then taken, and the contours and outline of the bowel can be seen. Departure from the normal contours, obstruction to the passage of the barium, and other distortions usually demonstrate the existence of a bowel tumor.

Is bleeding from the rectum a sign that hemorrhoids are present?

Yes, in some cases. In others, the bleeding may originate from a polyp, a tumor, or an inflammatory condition.

What is the treatment of hemorrhoids?

1. The mere presence of hemorrhoids does not always indicate the need for surgery. Many older people have

hemorrhoids that do not bleed or cause pain or constipation. Such hemorrhoids require no treatment.

2. Other types will respond to medical management. Treatment will consist of taking lubricants such as mineral oil to keep the stool soft, avoiding alcohol and spices, which irritate the anal outlet, local treatment (including sitz baths), the application of soothing ointments, and the insertion of specially medicated suppositories.

3. If bleeding from the hemorrhoids persists, if the hemorrhoids continue to be painful, if they become strangulated or thrombosed, and if the above medical measures fail, then surgery will be necessary.

Is removal of hemorrhoids a serious operation for older people?

Not unless their general condition is extremely poor. Even then, measures can be taken so that they can safely undergo hemorrhoidectomy.

Is the "injection" treatment of hemorrhoids effective?

Yes, but only for certain cases of *internal* hemorrhoids. Since most people have the combined form of internal and external hemorrhoids, injection treatment will often not solve the problem.

Will repeated rectal bleeding from hemorrhoids produce anemia?

Yes, even of small amounts of blood, if bleeding continues for several months. This is a very common cause of secondary anemia in the aging.

Will high blood pressure cause hemorrhoids to bleed more often?

Yes.

Are hemorrhoids in older people likely to recur after surgical treatment?

No. However, if they happen to be associated with a bowel tumor that has not been removed, recurrence is quite possible.

Do hemorrhoids ever lead to the development of cancer?

It is thought that they do not.

What measures should be taken to avoid recurrence of hemorrhoids?

1. Keep bowel movements regular by using lubricants and eating a proper diet.

2. Avoid straining at the stool or sitting too long on the toilet.

3. Avoid excessive use of alcoholic beverages or highly seasoned foods.

FISSURE IN ANO

What is a fissure in ano?

It is a tear, split, or ulceration of the skin and mucous membrane at the anal outlet.

Are fissures very common in people over sixty?

Yes. Since constipation is one of the primary causes of fissure in ano, a high incidence in older age groups is to be expected.

What are the symptoms of anal fissure?

Severe, sharp pain in the anal region, especially on attempting to move the bowels. The fissure becomes exceptionally painful when the anal outlet is dilated. Constipation and bleeding from the base of the ulcer are also frequent symptoms.

What is the treatment of fissure in ano?

1. If the fissure is superficial and of recent origin, the treatment is the same as medical care for hemorrhoids. Most cases of this type heal within a few weeks.
2. If the fissure is a little deeper, it may respond to medical management, plus repeated cauterization with silver nitrate.
3. If the fissure is deep and has been present for several months, surgery will be necessary.

What surgery is carried out for a fissure?

All the tissue on both sides of and beneath the ulcer is removed, and the underlying sphincter muscle is cut. This will permit the sphincter muscle to remain in a relaxed state so that the overlying membranes will heal. Healing usually takes place within a few weeks and normal bowel function is restored.

Is surgery for anal fissure serious?

No. It can be safely carried out on people of all ages, provided their general health is satisfactory.

Does fissure tend to recur in older people if they fail to follow good bowel-movement habits?

Yes.

FISTULA IN ANO

What is a fistula in ano?

It is a false tract or tunnel leading from the mucous membrane in the anal canal out onto the external surface of the skin at the site of the anus.

What causes fistula in ano?

It is the result of an infection that originated in the lining membrane of the anus and extended outward to empty on the skin. An abscess alongside the anal orifice (a perirectal abscess) frequently precedes the formation of a fistula.

Do older people develop fistulas?

Occasionally. They are much more common in young adults, however.

What causes abscesses to form in the area surrounding the anus?

1. An infection in one of the little pouches of the mucous membrane (crypt of Morgagni) in the anal canal.
2. Lack of cleanliness.
3. Ulceration and infection of a hemorrhoid.
4. Rarely, a foreign body may puncture or scratch the mucous membrane and lead to infection.
5. An undernourished or anemic condition may make it easier for bacteria to invade the tissue in this region.
6. Diabetics are especially likely to develop abscess in the anal area.

What is the treatment of an abscess that has formed in the anal region?

1. Hot baths should be taken, to bring the abscess to a head.
2. Mineral oil or a mild laxative should be given to keep the bowels moving.
3. Since these infections are usually very painful, the patient should be kept in bed most of the time.
4. Antibiotics should be given only when the infection appears to be spreading rapidly and affecting the general health of the patient.
5. When the abscess has come to a head, it should be opened surgically. Often the patient must go to the hospital for this operation, which will be carried out under general anesthesia.

Do abscesses alongside the rectum or anus frequently lead to formation of a fistula?

Yes, about half the time. The fistula will open and close, discharging a few drops of pus, for a period of several weeks after the original incision into the abscess.

What is the treatment of a fistula in ano?

It must be excised (removed) surgically. This is done by cutting out the entire tract from the skin level into the anal canal. In this operation, the sphincter muscle is cut.

How long does it take the wound to heal after surgery for fistula?

Several weeks, but the patient is confined to the hospital for only 4 to 7 days, and is out of bed most of the time.

Is the removal of a fistula (fistulectomy) serious?

No.

Do fistulas tend to recur in older people who fail to follow good bowel-movement habits?

Occasionally.

PROLAPSE OF THE RECTUM

What is a prolapse of the rectum?

An abnormal descent of the mucous membrane of the rectum to the outside of the anal canal.

Are older people susceptible to the development of this condition?

Yes. The basic cause is weakness and loss of tone of the muscles that hold the rectum in place. Chronic constipation, with repeated straining at the stool, is also conducive to the development of prolapse.

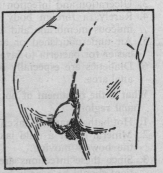

Rectal prolapse

When does the prolapse become most evident?

After moving of the bowels.

Does the prolapsed mucous membrane go back inside after bowel evacuation?

Sometimes it goes back spontaneously. More often, it must be pushed back inside the anal opening.

What is the treatment of prolapse of the rectum?

Many attempts have been made to treat this condition medically, but most attempts are unsuccessful. Some of the medical measures that have been recommended are as follows:

1. If the patient is undernourished and underweight, as many people with prolapse are, they should be brought up to normal weight. Muscle and sphincter tone will be improved if the patient gains weight.

2. If the patient lacks vitamins or minerals in his diet, they should be given.

3. If the patient is chronically constipated, lubricants, mild laxatives, or small enemas should be given to bring about evacuation without muscle strain.

4. The patient should be shown how to replace the prolapsed mucous membrane in the anal canal. This should be done immediately after bowel evacuation, in order to prevent strangulation of the prolapse.

5. A rectal specialist (proctologist) should be consulted. He may, in mild cases, try to cure the prolapse by injecting various sclerosing substances alongside the anal canal. These may cause fibrous tissue to form in the region between the mucous membrane and the muscle wall of the bowel. If sufficient fibrous tissue does form, it may hold the mucous membrane in place.

If medical measures fail to cure a prolapse, is surgery recommended?

Yes, provided the general health of the patient will permit it. There are a dozen or more operative procedures designed to cure prolapse. Few of these operations are totally successful, but a substantial measure of improvement can be gained from some of them.

What percentage of patients can be cured of prolapse?

Perhaps two out of three patients can be helped appreciably, but not all of them will be entirely rid of their prolapse. However, if good medical management (as described above) is carried out in combination with surgical repair, the ultimate result will usually be satisfactory.

PRURITUS ANI

What is pruritus ani?

Chronic itching of the anus, with irritation of the skin in the entire anal area.

Does pruritus ani affect people past sixty?

Yes. There is a greater incidence of this condition in older people because the skin in this region tends to be thinned out, sensitive, dry, and scaly.

What are some of the conditions that predispose to itching around the anus?

1. Fungus infections, such as those involving the vagina.
2. Emotional disturbance, often in neurotic people.

3. Diabetes; pruritis ani is sometimes a secondary condition in this disease.
4. Allergies, either to foods or to nylon, rubber, or other types of undergarments.
5. Drinking excessive quantities of alcohol or eating highly seasoned foods.
6. Hemorrhoids, fissures, or fistulas sometimes lead to development of pruritus ani.
7. Excessive perspiration due to heavy underwear and clothing sometimes precipitates itching about the anus.

What is the treatment of pruritus ani?

1. If the patient is allergic, elimination of the offending irritant will often relieve the pruritus.
2. If the patient is an uncontrolled diabetic, measures to bring his diabetes under control may stop the itching.
3. Excessive drinking of alcohol and eating of spicy foods should be stopped.
4. If the origin appears to be emotional, psychiatric care may prove helpful.
5. If the condition originates from hemorrhoids, fistula, or fissure, correction of these conditions will often eliminate the pruritus.
6. People with pruritus ani should cut their fingernails very short, so that they will not damage the area by scratching in their sleep. Often, scratching by sharp nails will cause secondary infection.
7. People with pruritus should dress lightly and should avoid tight undergarments, which will cause excessive perspiration. If the patient tends to perspire excessively, talcum powder should be dusted onto the area. At night, as few blankets as possible should be used.
8. Various ointments containing anesthetic agents and cortisonelike ingredients should be applied regularly, but only on prescription by the physician.
9. Various antihistamine tablets may be taken to relieve the itching.
10. People with pruritus often have the habit of scrubbing the area with soap and water. This should not be done. Scrubbing with soap and water will only serve to *increase* the itching. If soap is used it should be a very mild one.
11. If there is swelling and redness in the area, warm baths or local applications of witch hazel will often bring temporary relief from the itching.
12. An occasional case of pruritus can be helped by a surgical procedure known as "tattooing." Other operations,

for example, undermining the skin of the region in order to separate it from the underlying nerves, have proved helpful in an occasional case, but no operation can be recommended as a routine procedure.

13. The patient must be instructed that the less he scratches, the quicker the pruritus will heal. Although it is extremely difficult not to scratch, self-control is essential. A few days of complete abstinence from scratching may cause the pruritus to disappear completely.

Does pruritus ani usually interfere with sleep?

Yes. Many people with this condition complain bitterly that they are unable to sleep because of the intense itch. These people may require sedatives and sleeping pills.

REHABILITATION AND PHYSICAL THERAPY

See AMPUTATION; APOPLEXY, OR STROKE; ARTHRITIS AND RHEUMATISM; BED CARE; BLINDNESS; BURSITIS; FRACTURES; HEARING AND DEAFNESS; HOBBIES; INJURIES AND ACCIDENTS; MUSCLES; NERVES; PARKINSON'S DISEASE AND PALSY; PHYSICAL ACTIVITY AND EXERCISE; SPEECH.

What is rehabilitation?

It is a form of treatment employing physical therapy, together with attempts at social and psychological readjustment of those people who are handicapped.

Is rehabilitation for older people worthwhile?

Yes. Great advances have been made in recent years toward reeducation and rehabilitation of older people who have been handicapped as a result of injury or disease. Specialists in physical medicine have discovered ways of increasing the physical capacity of handicapped older people and of restoring many of their lost abilities.

What are some of the general areas in which rehabilitation is most helpful?

1. People who have been partially paralyzed by a stroke can often be taught to walk again and to get the most use possible out of their damaged limbs.

2. Those who have lost their ability to speak can, in some instances, benefit greatly from speech therapy. Others, who are unable to have their speech restored, are taught

methods of expressing themselves so that they can be understood by people who come in contact with them.

3. Those who are deformed or crippled by arthritis are taught exercises to limber their stiff joints, to preserve those joints that are unaffected, and to get the maximum use out of their hands and feet.

4. People with permanent joint, bone, nerve, or muscle infirmities are supplied with appliances to support their bodies, to maintain as near-normal posture as possible, and to get the most use possible out of partially damaged structures.

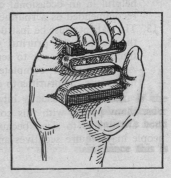

A grip exerciser, used to limber up stiff fingers and to improve the strength of the hand

5. Special ways to walk, to get up and down curbs or stairs, to sit and stand, have been devised for people who are crippled.

6. People who have undergone amputation of a limb are taught how to use artificial limbs and appliances.

7. Those afflicted with Parkinson's disease are given special treatment and training for rigid muscles; they are given speech therapy and occupational training that will help them to work with their tremor and palsy.

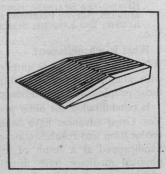

A ramp for people who are unable to step up

8. Occupational retraining is given to fit in with existing deformities.

9. Psychotherapy is given to aid those who are depressed and to better adjust the handicapped person to the world in which he lives.

Can people who have been invalids for many years ever be helped through rehabilitation techniques?

Yes. Some who have not used their arms or walked for years can be taught how to do so again. Of course, the sooner the rehabilitation is started after an injury, the better the final results will be.

Should older people go to physicians who specialize in rehabilitation?

Yes. Rehabilitation techniques are highly specialized, and only doctors who confine their practice to this field will be able to give expert care.

Do most communities have rehabilitation centers?

No. However, the larger voluntary and municipal or county hospitals do have departments to give this type of service. The nearest county medical society will provide the required information.

Should patients who have had a stroke be referred to rehabilitation clinics?

Yes. If such an installation is not available, they should be referred to a physician who specializes in rehabilitation.

How soon after a stroke can rehabilitation measures be started?

Within a day or two. One of the first procedures is to control the patient's position in bed so that unnecessary contractures will not set in. Also, exercises of a *passive* type will be instituted, so that muscles and joints do not become stiff. As soon as the patient has regained consciousness, he will be shown how to assist himself.

How are psychological factors used in aiding rehabilitation?

Seeing others improve as a result of treatment has an uplifting effect on patients who are depressed by their misfortune. Group therapy and classroom techniques may prove especially beneficial. Also, patients will often form stimulating new relationships with others who have similar difficulties.

What is physical therapy?

It is a branch of medicine that concerns itself with the restoration of function to damaged structures and aims toward helping the convalescent patient to recover.

What methods does physical therapy employ?

1. *Heat therapy*
   a. Baking lamps. Such lamps do not have great powers of penetration, but they will aid superficial circulation and will relax muscle spasm.

b. Infrared rays. These rays have some power of penetration, but they do not reach the deeper tissues.
c. Hot compresses.
d. Diathermy. These heat waves have the power to penetrate the muscles, tendons, and bones.
e. Paraffin baths.
f. Steam baths.
g. Ultraviolet rays.
h. Natural sunlight.

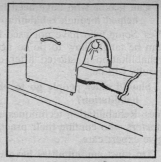

Baking lamp

2. *Hydrotherapy*
   a. Wet compresses.
   b. Whirlpool baths.
   c. Swimming tanks and pools.
   d. Tub baths.

3. *Electrical stimulation*
   a. Galvanic current.
   b. Faradic current.

4. *Massage*

5. *Exercises*
   a. Passive exercises. These are muscular movements carried out by the physical therapist, not by the patient himself. Passive exercise is most applicable to those who have been paralyzed and cannot move by themselves.

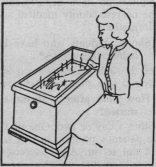

A paraffin bath to aid those with arthritis

   b. Active exercises. These are prescribed by the physician but carried out by the patient.

6. *Manipulation.* This is carried out by physical therapists, nurses, or the

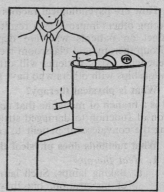

Arm and foot bath used in heat treatment

physician in charge of the case in order to restore motion to a stiff or "frozen joint." Some of these procedures can be performed without anesthesia; others require anesthesia in order to overcome pain and spasm.

7. *X-ray therapy.* These treatments are sometimes helpful in loosening up a "frozen joint," especially when it is caused by bursitis, or inflammation of the fibrous tissues surrounding a joint.

8. The application and teaching of proper use of braces, plaster casts, artificial appliances and limbs, crutches, canes, walking aids, supports, etc.

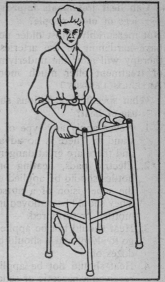

A walker, which aids convalescent patients

Is it safe for people in their sixties, seventies, or eighties to take physical-therapy treatments such as ultraviolet rays, heat treatments, baths, or diathermy?

Yes, but physical therapy should be under the supervision of a specialist in this field of medicine. There are real dangers in permitting older patients to treat themselves or to be treated by commercial laboratories. Older patients require special care because they are more sensitive to the effects of physical therapy.

Why are older people more sensitive to the effects of physical therapy?

Because their skin is more easily damaged by excessive heat or cold. Also, aging muscles and joints are easily injured by inept massage, manipulation, or use of diathermy.

Should special care be taken in massaging older people?

Yes, although healthy people in their sixties and seventies usually require no special handling. Sick or bedridden patients must be massaged very gently so as not to rupture muscle fibers or damage brittle blood vessels. Overzealous massage may do more harm than good to some older patients.

Can heat treatments improve the deep circulation in the legs of older people?

Not measurably. Most older people with impaired circulation have hardening of the arteries, and no amount of physical therapy will alter the underlying condition. Surgical methods of treatment offer much more hope in this regard. (*See* ARTERIOSCLEROSIS.)

What specific precautions should older people take in the use of heat?

1. Never apply any type of heat as hot as the patient can stand it. There is no advantage in making it so intense, and there are great dangers of serious burns.
2. Electric pads, heating or baking lamps, or hot-water bottles should be applied only on the order of and under the supervision of a nurse or other qualified attendant. They should be removed immediately if the skin becomes mottled or turns red.
3. Heat should not be applied when the patient is about to go to sleep, and it should be removed as soon as a patient dozes off.
4. Heat should not be applied to a patient who has just received a narcotic or sedative. The medication may dull his sensibilities to such an extent that he will be unaware of the heat's intensity.
5. Cold applications should not be left in place for more than a half hour at a time. Damage to circulation or frostbite may result.

Is it safe for older people to take hot cabinet baths or Turkish baths?

Healthy, active older people can tolerate these baths well, but it is unwise to "sweat out" someone who is ill or underweight. The loss of large quantities of body fluids and salt can be dangerous.

Are whirlpool baths, hot tub baths, and swimming tanks safe for older people?

Yes, but the temperature of the water must be watched carefully so as not to cause a burn. Also, if older people have a tendency to faint or are unable to communicate easily, they must be watched very carefully while they are in the water.

Do older people tolerate exposure to ultraviolet or sun rays?

Yes. Here, too, precautions must be taken to avoid overexposure and burns.

Does massaging take off weight?

No. It is an erroneous notion that appreciable amounts of

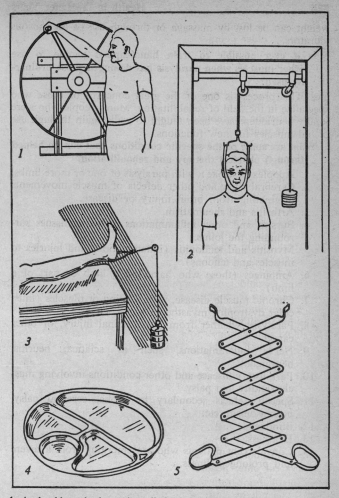

1. A shoulder wheel, used to limber up stiff shoulder joints
2. Head and neck in traction apparatus for people with neck pain, slipped disks, etc.
3. Traction, often used in cases of sciatica, slipped disk, or fractures of the leg
4. A divider dish, used to prevent spilling of food
5. A reacher, to aid a bedridden patient to grasp a distant object

weight can be lost by massage or through use of the various vibrators.

Is it ever possible to train handicapped people to use other muscles when paralysis has damaged those ordinarily used?

Yes. This process is one of the great concerns of those who specialize in the field of rehabilitation. Many people who were totally bedridden have been taught to walk again through use of old muscles for new functions.

What are some of the specific conditions that can be helped through physical therapy and rehabilitation?

1. Apoplexy (stroke), with paralysis of one or more limbs.
2. Cerebral palsy and other defects of muscle movements originating from brain injury or disease.
3. Arthritis and rheumatism.
4. Bursitis and other inflammations involving tissues surrounding the joints.
5. Myositis and tendonitis (inflammations and injuries to muscles and tendons).
6. Amputees (those who have lost a limb or part of a limb).
7. Chronic muscle disease, with wasting of muscles (muscular dystrophy, myasthenia gravis, etc.).
8. Paralysis, whether from polio, spinal injury, or other causes.
9. Nerve inflammations, such as sciatica, neuritis, neuralgia.
10. Parkinson's disease and other conditions involving muscle rigidity and palsy.
11. Speech defects secondary to stroke, cerebral palsy, parkinsonism, etc.
12. Blindness.
13. Deafness.
14. Convalescent patients who are emerging from a severe and prolonged illness.

RESPIRATORY TRACT

See ALLERGY; ASTHMA; BRONCHIECTASIS; BRONCHITIS; COMMON COLD; COUGHS; EMPHYSEMA; GAS AND SMOKE POISONING; INFLUENZA AND GRIPPE; LUNG TUMORS; PNEUMONIA; SMOKING; TUBERCULOSIS.

What structures make up the respiratory tract?

The nose, sinuses, throat, pharynx, larynx, trachea, bronchial tubes, and lungs.

Does the respiratory tract become less subject to infection as people get older?

Some people may develop a certain amount of immunity to respiratory infections as they get older, but the majority do not. It is important to note that when respiratory infections do develop in the older age groups, they tend to be more serious.

What effect does climate have on the respiratory tracts of older people?

Most people past sixty, especially those in their seventies and eighties, are much more sensitive to abrupt changes in climate and to extremes of climate. Sudden changes in temperature or humidity often bring on the common cold, sinus infection, bronchitis, and other respiratory ailments.

What influence does the aging process have on susceptibility to respiratory infections?

The mucous membrane lining the respiratory tract tends to become less capable of secreting protective mucus. As a result, bacteria and viruses can more readily invade the system. Moreover, the mucus that is secreted tends to stagnate in the lungs and bronchial tubes because of the older person's decreased ability to expel it through coughing.

What is the best climate for older people who are especially susceptible to respiratory infections?

A dry temperate climate. Extreme humidity, smog, and extremes of temperature should be avoided if possible.

Why is it especially harmful for older people to breathe soot and smog?

Soot and smog contain chemicals that lodge in the bronchial tubes and air sacs of the lungs and must eventually be expelled in the sputum by coughing. Since people of advanced age often are unable to cough up sputum lodged deep in the lungs, the chemical irritants may result in impairment of respiration. Moreover, stagnation of mucus in the bases of the lungs predisposes to the development of pneumonia.

Is air conditioning harmful for older people?

No. As a matter of fact, well-regulated air conditioning is ideal for older people. It rids the air of dirt and dust particles and regulates temperature and humidity.

Are older people normally short of breath?

Not during the performance of ordinary activities, such as walking on level ground or around the house. It is natural for people in their seventies and eighties to become short of breath while walking up hills, climbing stairs, or during physical exertion.

When should shortness of breath be considered abnormal?

1. When it occurs while the person is at rest.
2. When it comes on from walking about the house.
3. When it takes place as a result of talking.
4. When it is accompanied by a sense of suffocation.
5. When it is associated with other symptoms such as irregular heartbeat, swelling of the ankles, pain in the chest, or severe coughing.

Is it difficult for a doctor to distinguish between natural shortness of breath and that brought on by disease?

No.

What is the significance of blood in the sputum?

It may be caused by one or more of the following conditions:

1. An inflammation or small ulceration in the mucous membrane of the nose or throat, with a dripping down of the blood into the bronchial tubes. The blood is later coughed up with the sputum.
2. An inflammation in the throat, larynx, or bronchial tubes.
3. An inflammation in the lungs, such as bronchitis or pneumonia.
4. Tuberculosis.
5. A tumor of the bronchial tubes or lungs.

How often should older people have their chests X-rayed?

Once a year.

Is there any danger of overexposure to X rays if the chest is X-rayed once a year?

No.

Is there a close relationship between the respiratory tract and heart function?

Yes. In order for the heart to function properly, its muscle tissue must be supplied with large quantities of oxygen. A normally functioning respiratory tract extracts this oxygen from the inhaled air and transports it through the bloodstream to the heart. If insufficient oxygen is extracted from the inhaled air, the heart will not function normally. Conversely, if the heart does not pump a sufficient amount of blood to the lungs, inadequate amounts of oxygen will be extracted from the inhaled air. In other words, normal function of one is essential to normal function of the other.

Will the position in which one sleeps influence respiratory efficiency?

Not if an individual is in good health. However, older people with heart or lung impairment can breathe more easily when they sleep in a semirecumbent or sitting position.

TUMORS OF THE RESPIRATORY TRACT

(*See* LUNG TUMORS.)

What areas of the respiratory tract are the most common sites of tumors, both malignant and benign?

The larynx, bronchial tubes, and lungs.

Are tumors of the larynx common in people past sixty?

Yes, particularly in men. The incidence of tumors of the larynx is seven times greater in men than in women.

Is cancer of the larynx thought to be associated with excessive smoking?

This is a very difficult question to answer unequivocally, but, more and more, scientists are gaining evidence of the injurious effects that tobacco has on the respiratory tract.

What are the main symptoms of a tumor of the larynx?

Hoarseness that persists for several weeks. It is often associated with coughing, difficulty in breathing, and pain in the throat.

Are all tumors of the larynx malignant?

No. There are benign conditions, such as fibromas and polyps. But the majority of laryngeal tumors in older people are malignant.

Is cancer of the bronchial tubes or lungs common in older people?

Yes. This is one of the most common types of cancer in aging people. (*See* CANCER.)

Are men more susceptible to the development of cancer of the bronchial tubes and lungs?

Yes, it is much more common in men than in women, although recent statistics point to an increase in this type of cancer in women.

Is cancer of the bronchial tubes or lungs increasing?

Yes.

Is there such a thing as a nonmalignant tumor of the bronchial tubes or lungs?

Yes. But most tumors of the bronchial tubes and lungs in older people are malignant.

Is excessive smoking thought to be an important factor in the development of lung cancer?

Yes. (*See* LUNG TUMORS.)

RETINAL DETACHMENT

See BLINDNESS; EYES.

What is the retina?

It is the structure in the back of the eye that receives light rays and transmits their impulses to the brain, where they are interpreted as "sight."

What is retinal detachment?

It is a separation, usually partial, of the retina from its underlying layer, the choroid.

What are the symptoms of retinal detachment?

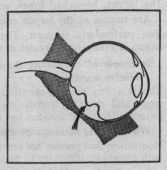

Detachment of retina

1. The abrupt appearance of a dark veil before one eye. Usually the dark area is located at the outer rim of the field of vision, but it gradually spreads toward the center of the eye.
2. There is loss of sight over part of the field of vision that may spread, over a period of days, weeks, or months.
3. A diffuse fog before one eye may develop.
4. Prior to development of blindness, there is often a period of seeing distorted shapes, flashes of lights, and spots before the eyes.

Does retinal detachment often affect people over sixty?

Yes, but it is not especially prevalent in this age group.

What causes retinal detachment?

1. Extreme nearsightedness predisposes one to detachment of the retina, though it is not a direct cause.
2. A severe blow to the head, causing a hemorrhage in the choroid layer beneath the retina.
3. A tumor in the choroid, which will push away the overlying retinal layer.
4. Inflammatory adhesions that pull the retina away from the choroid.

Is it difficult to diagnose detachment of the retina?

No. It can be readily diagnosed by examination with an ophthalmoscope, which allows the physician to see directly into the back of the eye.

What is the treatment of retinal detachment?

1. Diathermy coagulation (electric-needle application) to the sclera (the white of the eye). The coagulation is applied directly over the area of detachment and the resulting inflammatory reaction will pull the retina back to its underlying attachments.
2. If the detachment has been caused by a tumor of the choroid, the eyeball must be removed.

How successful is treatment of retinal detachment?

In more than half the cases, one or more treatments with electric coagulation will bring about a cure, with restoration of vision. If the underlying cause is a tumor, cure can come about only through early removal of the eye.

Does retinal detachment ever recur?

Yes, in about one out of four cases. The same treatment is repeated.

RETINAL THROMBOSIS

See BLINDNESS; EMBOLUS AND EMBOLISM; EYES; THROMBUS AND THROMBOSIS.

What is retinal thrombosis?

The blockage of either the retinal artery or the retinal vein in the eye.

Does retinal thrombosis occur often in people past sixty?

Yes. It is a condition closely associated with the aging process.

What causes retinal thrombosis?

1. A blood clot in an arteriosclerotic retinal artery.
2. An embolus, a blood clot arising in the heart and passing through the bloodstream to the central retinal artery.
3. Severe spasm of the retinal artery, followed by clot formation.
4. A blood clot in the main retinal vein of the eye.

What are the main symptoms of retinal thrombosis?

Sudden, painless loss of sight in one eye. The blindness may come on instantaneously if the artery is involved but may take an hour or so if the retinal vein is involved.

How is retinal thrombosis diagnosed?

By examination of the retina with an ophthalmoscope. There is a marked difference in the appearance in retinal-artery thrombosis and retinal-vein thrombosis.

What is the treatment of retinal thrombosis?

1. Reduction of the pressure in the eyeball in an attempt to dislodge the blood clot. This is done by removing some of the fluid in the eye chamber.
2. Administration of medications, such as the nitrites, in an attempt to relieve possible spasm of the retinal artery.
3. Administration of anticoagulant drugs, such as heparin, in order to prevent further clot formation.

Is treatment of retinal thrombosis usually successful?

Only in an occasional case, in which the above measures are carried out within an hour or two of the onset of symptoms.

RETIREMENT

See ATTITUDES TOWARD AGING; FAMILY RELATIONSHIPS; HOBBIES; INTRODUCTORY REMARKS ON AGING; HOTELS, APARTMENTS, AND COMMUNITIES FOR THE AGING; LONGEVITY; ORGANIZATIONS AND AGENCIES; PHYSICAL ACTIVITY AND EXERCISE; SOCIAL SECURITY BENEFITS; TRAVEL.

Should healthy people retire from their business or profession merely because they have attained the age of sixty or sixty-five?

No. As stated in the beginning of this book, chronological age is often a poor indicator of physiological or psychological age. Many people in their sixties and seventies retain such healthy bodies and minds that they should give little or no consideration to retirement.

What is modern thinking about compulsory retirement at a predetermined age?

The tendency is to get away from mandatory retirement and to let specific factors, such as the physical and mental well-being of the particular individual, determine whether or not retirement is necessary.

What are some of the factors that operate in modern retirement policies?

1. The occupation in which the individual is engaged. If one is forced to do strenuous physical work, he will, of course, be governed by an entirely different set of retirement rules than if he were a clerk or office worker.
2. The ability to replace the aging person by someone just as competent. If the individual is engaged in a highly

specialized job, and if he has skills that are difficult to replace, mandatory retirement is often waived, provided the worker is in good health.

3. If there are available younger men who can do the job as well, most businesses will insist on retirement of older employees.

4. The ability of the worker to support himself in permanent retirement. Fortunately, the government has helped private industry to provide for this time of life by establishing social security benefits and old-age assistance programs. These apply to men who have reached the age of sixty-five and to women who have reached the age of sixty-two. Those who can see their way clear to supporting themselves will be much better candidates for retirement than those who will become a burden to their families or the community.

5. Perhaps the most important factor to be considered is the personal desire of the worker himself. Rules should be much more liberal for those who do not wish to retire and who demonstrate continued competence.

Should there be fixed ages for retirement?

Wherever possible, there should not be. Of course, it must be recognized that in large industries rules must be made to apply to hundreds or thousands of workers. In such organizations it is almost impossible to have anything but a fixed retirement age. In smaller businesses, retirement rules are often constructed so that workers can continue beyond the retirement age but are reevaluated each year.

Is it wise for people in their middle years to plan for their retirement?

This is an essential component of modern living in our society. Many businesses and industries are beginning to realize that they must construct elaborate programs, far in advance, for the eventual complete retirement of their employees and officers. With the provision of rewards, benefits, travel opportunities, recreational facilities, etc., many aging officers and workers are converted from opponents to advocates of retirement.

Whom should one consult about planning for retirement?

1. An attorney.
2. An insurance broker.
3. An investment adviser.
4. Adult children should consult their parents and parents should consult their adult children. Together, they should talk over their financial status.
5. Agencies such as the Social Security Agency, the Vet-

eran's Bureau, the regional office of the Department of Health, Education and Welfare, etc., should be consulted to ascertain the specific benefits that will accrue at retirement age.

6. The supervisor or personnel director of the business in which one is employed should be consulted, in order to learn the benefits that will be received on retirement.

7. If one belongs to a union, he should consult the union's social security or welfare department.

What are some of the good things about retirement?

One of its greatest advantages is the freedom from the stresses of competition. In addition, it will permit more time to be spent with one's spouse, children, and grandchildren.

More and more, retired people are realizing the significant role they can play in their community. They often participate actively in social work, community fund raising, church programs, etc.

Retirement offers the opportunity to spend more time doing things one enjoys. It allows the exploitation of hobbies and other recreational pursuits.

If one has been financially successful, the retirement years offer remarkable opportunities for travel and furtherance of educational desires that had been neglected during the more active years.

What are some of the disadvantages of retirement?

Enforced retirement often results in loss of self-esteem and in feelings that one is no longer needed. This can have a serious, damaging effect on the psyche of an aging individual. It is a well-known medical fact that when one stops work and disengages himself from active participation in the struggle of life, he may deteriorate mentally and physically.

Is it true that retired people do not live as long as those who continue to work?

This is difficult to answer statistically, but many authorities think that mandatory retirement of a healthy individual is not conducive to longevity.

Can it harm a healthy person to discontinue physical work abruptly?

Yes. Most bodies become geared to a certain pattern of activity. As they get older they depend more and more on the continuation of their established pattern. Thus, sudden inactivity may upset one's physiological balance. Digestion may suffer; sleeping habits may change; depression may set in. Healthy older people who retire should engage in substitute physical activity.

How important is the spouse in plans for retirement?

It is important for husbands to discuss with their wives the details of retirement long before it actually goes into effect. Differences of opinion concerning specific plans for retirement often occur between husband and wife and are a source of great unhappiness during the later years. Prior to retirement, there should be agreement between husband and wife on how they are going to live later on. It should not be forgotten that a wife may have to assume an entirely new role toward a retired husband, and this requirement comes at an age when *she* is least able to make radical changes in her own pattern of living.

Should retirement mean inactivity?

Absolutely not. Those who plan to sit around the house after they stop working should do everything possible not to retire. Retirement represents a challenge. It is the *beginning* of a new period in life, not the end of all living.

What specific steps should people take before retiring?

1. They should come to an agreement with their spouse as to the kind of life they both want to lead.
2. They should mutually agree on where they want to live.
3. They should plan to do those things they have both wanted to do in their earlier years.
4. They should consult experts in the retirement field, such as social agencies in the community, church organizations, community agencies, and old-age clubs.
5. They should plan to develop hobbies. (*See* HOBBIES.)
6. Whenever possible, they should outline the specific activities in which they will engage; and they should keep a calendar so that they will be aware of their daily activities far in advance.

Should retired people move to communities or housing projects where other older people live?

Yes, if *both* the husband and wife wish to do so. A good rule to follow, however, is to make no commitment from which they cannot withdraw.

Are old-age clubs of value to retired people?

Yes, for older people who feel the need for added companionship. Retired people should try these communal organizations if they want to, but they should be in a position to withdraw if the organizations fail to suit their particular needs.

Is it wise for retired people to give up retirement and return to work?

Many people who have voluntarily retired at the age of sixty or sixty-five return to work on discovering that inactivity is distasteful to them. It is a wise move for them, provided they are in good physical and mental health. Naturally, special precautions should be taken not to overexert oneself when first resuming physical tasks.

Is it wise for retired people to embark upon a new occupation?

Yes, provided the new activity does not create the same stresses as the old one. Many hobbies of older people accidentally turn into profitable money-making businesses. This can give a new lease on life to people who thought their accomplishments finished. It is interesting to note that occasionally people who have been engaged in nonimaginative, humdrum physical labors throughout most of their lives develop surprising proficiency in imaginative and creative fields, such as painting, sculpting, or woodworking. The sixties and seventies are wonderful years for the exposure and development of hidden talents.

Is it important for people who have retired to consult their family physician?

Yes. Eating habits, sleeping habits, physical and mental activities, etc., undergo changes during retirement. It is important that the family physician know about these changes and that he be asked for advice concerning them. For instance, someone who has been accustomed to strenuous physical labor should cut down on his food intake after retirement. Someone who has sat at a desk throughout most of his working life should avoid hobbies or recreations that necessitate great physical exertion.

SALIVARY GLANDS

See MOUTH, LIPS, AND TONGUE.

Where are the salivary glands and what is their function?

There are three salivary glands on each side of the head. The *parotid glands* are located in front of and below each ear. The *submaxillary glands* are located about an inch in front of and below the angle of the lower jaws. The *sublingual glands* lie on the floor of the mouth beneath the tongue.

The salivary glands manufacture and secrete saliva, which reaches the mouth through tubes (ducts) leading from the glands to the mouth.

Do the ducts leading from the salivary glands ever become blocked?

Yes. This may happen as a result of a calculus (stone) or an inflammation of the gland and duct.

How can one tell if a stone is obstructing a salivary duct?

The gland will become hard, swollen, and tender. In some cases the physician will be able to feel the stone by placing his finger in the patient's mouth. X rays sometimes will demonstrate the presence of a salivary stone.

What is the treatment of a stone blocking a salivary duct?

It is removed surgically, usually under local anesthesia.

Do inflammation and abscess formation ever involve the salivary glands in older people?

Yes, particularly inflammation of the parotid gland. This condition, known as parotitis, is sometimes a complication of a debilitating disease in very old people. It also occasionally follows major surgery.

When parotitis affects very old people, recovery is doubtful.

SALIVARY-GLAND TUMORS

Do tumors of the salivary glands occur often in people over sixty?

Yes, especially in the parotid gland at the angle of the jaw. Most of these growths are benign, the so-called mixed tumors of the salivary glands.

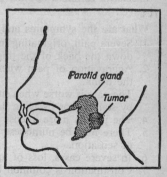

Parotid-gland tumor

What is the treatment of a tumor of the salivary gland in older people?

The tumor and normal surrounding tissue should be surgically removed. Although these operations may take a long time to perform, the results are excellent and older people can withstand them without difficulty.

What are the possible complications of surgery for salivary-gland tumors?

1. The mixed tumors have a tendency to recur locally, if surgery is not extensive.

2. There is considerable danger of cutting or injuring the facial nerve when removing some tumors of the parotid gland. When this happens, paralysis of part of the face will result.

Will there be adequate secretion of saliva after removal of one of the salivary glands?

Yes.

SCIATICA

See Injuries and Accidents; Muscles; Nerves; Rehabilitation and Physical Therapy.

What is sciatica?

A condition in which there is severe pain along the course of the large sciatic nerve. This nerve originates in the spinal cord in the lower back and supplies the muscles of the thighs, legs, and feet.

Is sciatica the same as sciatic neuritis?

Yes.

Is sciatica common in older people?

Yes.

What are the symptoms and signs of sciatica?

1. Severe pain, originating in the lower back and extending down the back of the thighs and into the legs and feet.
2. Aggravation of pain when attempting to move or twist the trunk.
3. The pain is worse when sitting, and is sometimes relieved by standing or by lying flat in bed.
4. The pain is more intense at night.
5. There may be numbness in the feet, with areas of lack of sensation.
6. In severe cases, loss of appetite.
7. Constipation is common because of pain when attempting to move the bowels.
8. Knee and ankle jerk reflexes may disappear in severe cases.
9. Muscle wasting in the thighs and legs develops in cases that last more than a month or two.

What are some of the causes of sciatica?

1. The most frequent cause is pressure on the sciatic nerve from a herniated disk.

2. A severe strain or injury, as occurs in sacroiliac sprain, may trigger sciatica.

3. There may be pressure on the sciatic nerve from a tumor growing in the pelvis or in the region where the nerve exits from the spinal column.

4. Toxins from a distant focus of infection may affect the sciatic nerve, bringing on an attack of sciatica.

What is the treatment of sciatica?

1. If it is found to be caused by a herniated disk, and if symptoms do not subside within 2 to 3 months, surgery should be considered.

2. If the patient is a poor surgical risk, or if the diagnosis of herniated disk is not absolutely certain, sciatica is best treated medically.

What is the usual medical management of sciatica?

1. Absolute bed rest. The patient lies on his back with a pillow under his lower back and under the knees.

2. The mattress should be firm and not bend in the middle. To effect this, boards should be placed between the mattress and the springs.

3. Pain-relieving drugs, such as aspirin, codeine, and some of the newer muscle relaxants, are given.

4. Slow and steady stretching of the sciatic nerve is often accomplished by the attachment of weights to the lower leg. This procedure is called *traction*. The patient may be kept in traction for several days or weeks.

5. Nerve-block injections of such substances as novocaine are often given.

6. Vitamins are given orally and by injection if vitamin deficiency exists.

Are electric pads, hot baths, baking, and diathermy helpful in curing sciatica?

Usually not, although they sometimes bring about temporary relief from pain.

Are there any dangers in hot applications for treatment of sciatica?

Yes; since an older person with this condition often has diminished sensation of heat and cold, severe burns can result.

Does sciatica get well by itself after a period of several weeks or months?

Yes, unless it is secondary to a herniated disk or a tumor pressing on the nerve. However, an older patient should not be left untreated for any length of time, inasmuch as complications may set in.

What are the complications of sciatica in older people?

1. Prolonged bed rest may lead to marked weakness and loss of muscle tone.
2. Prolonged bed rest may lead to pneumonia, owing to insufficient aeration of the lungs.
3. Bedsores may develop.
4. Severe, disabling constipation, with impactions, may develop.
5. Extensive muscle wasting of the legs may take place.

Does sciatica, once cured, have a tendency to recur?

Yes, if it has been caused by a herniated disk or if there is another back injury.

SEX AFTER SIXTY

See CORONARY-ARTERY DISEASE; FEMALE ORGANS; MARRIAGE AFTER SIXTY; PROSTATE GLAND; SEX HORMONES; TESTICLES; WIDOWHOOD.

Do men and women age sexually at different periods in their lives?

Yes, but one must distinguish between aging of the sex organs and strength of sex desire. As we know, the menopause (change of life) causes anatomical changes in the sex organs of women. Generally, this takes place between the ages of 45 and 52. Sexual aging in the male, on the other hand, is a slowly progressive process that starts in the thirties or forties and continues at a rather even pace throughout the remainder of life.

Does the aging process in the sex organs necessarily involve a decrease in the desire for sexual intercourse?

No. The fact that a woman stops menstruating and no longer matures eggs in the ovaries has little to do with decrease in her sexual desires. As for the male, most investigators (including Kinsey) find that his sexual activity reaches it peak during the teens, even before full physical maturity of the sex organs has been attained. He stays at about the same level of sexual activity and desire into his fifties or early sixties.

Rather than an abrupt cessation of sexual desire, there appears to be a gradual decline with each succeeding adult decade. This decline is not closely related to the anatomical changes of aging that occur in the genitals of both the female and the male.

Is a decrease in desire for sexual activity more of a psychological than a physical phenomenon in people past sixty?

A precise answer to this question cannot be given. It is true that most healthy men and women past sixty are physically capable of performing the sex act, although their desire to do so may come at less frequent intervals. Undoubtedly, there is an important physical aspect to decrease in desire, since secretion of sex hormone is diminished in the later years. On the other hand, investigators in this field have discovered that many women past sixty, who produce negligible amounts of ovarian hormone, may have almost as great a desire for sexual activity as they had during their thirties and forties. Similarly, many men in their sixties, although they secrete less testicular hormone, continue to have strong sexual appetites.

What effect does sexual activity have on the general health of people past sixty?

In all probability, sexual activity has little or no effect on the general health of the average female past sixty. It may, however, have a considerable effect on the general health of the male. A man in his late sixties or seventies who engages in strenuous sexual activity, particularly with a much younger woman, can place great strain on his heart and blood vessels. All too often, physicians learn of men in their later years who have suffered coronary thrombosis or cerebral hemorrhage because of sexual overindulgence.

What should people past sixty do about the ordinary physical exertion that accompanies sexual intercourse?

It is not necessary to take special precautions if one is in good health. Nevertheless, the following advice might minimize any strain:

1. Do not have relations when tired or physically exhausted.
2. Do not have relations soon after eating a heavy meal.
3. Do not attempt to hurry.
4. If there is any difficulty in consummating the act, abandon the effort rather than strain for completion.

Is the physical exertion of intercourse greater for the male past sixty than for the female?

Yes.

In general, what effect does normal sex activity have on the heart of an older person?

If the heart is normal to begin with, if there is a minimal amount of coronary arteriosclerosis, if moderation is practiced, then there is little or no harm in sexual intercourse. On the other hand, if angina pectoris is present, if the individual has already suffered an attack of coronary thrombosis, or if the sexual act is repeated too often within a short space of time, then serious strain to the heart muscle and the coronary artery may result.

Does sexual activity tend to raise blood pressure?

Yes, but this is not dangerous to older people who ordinarily have normal blood pressure. It may, however, place a severe strain on the blood vessels of the brain in those who have very high blood pressure.

What restrictions on sexual activity should be placed on healthy men and women past sixty?

None; they will usually govern themselves.

Are homosexual activities common among people past sixty?

If such tendencies exist, they are almost always evident at a much earlier period in life. It is rare to find homosexuality developing in an older person who has been heterosexual throughout earlier years. (It might be mentioned in passing that occasionally a physician will encounter sexual aberration in an older patient who has deteriorated mentally.)

How does the aging process affect sexual desire and activity in men?

Most men retain their sexual desires well into their seventies and eighties. As mentioned previously, the peak of activity is reached early—in the teens or early twenties—and undergoes a slight, gradual decline thereafter.

Is an abrupt loss in sexual desire in a man usually a physical or a psychological phenomenon?

When a man who has been interested in sex throughout his adult life suddenly loses interest, it is most often due to a psychological factor. Proof of this contention is amply provided by men who have been widowed and without sexual desire for several years, who, upon remarrying, regain sexual desire and ability.

What percentage of married couples between the ages of sixty and sixty-five engage in sexual intercourse?

According to Kinsey, approximately 80 to 85 percent.

What percentage of married couples between the ages of sixty-five and seventy engage in sexual intercourse?

Approximately 70 percent.

Do the majority of men retain their potency after seventy years of age?

According to Kinsey, approximately 50 percent will remain potent until seventy-five years of age.

What percentage of men are still potent up to eighty years of age?

About 25 percent.

What is the frequency of marital relations among couples between the ages of sixty and seventy?

According to Kinsey, those couples in which the man is between sixty and sixty-five will have intercourse about once a week; those in which the man is between sixty-five and seventy have intercourse about once a month. Those couples in which the man remains potent and is beyond seventy will probably have relations only two or three times a year.

Are there marked individual variations in the sexual capabilities of men past sixty?

Yes. Many different factors are involved in the retention or loss of virility, and individual variations are great. Experts in this field report that loss of sexual ability in healthy men between the ages of sixty and seventy is usually emotional, rather than physical, in origin.

Are extramarital contacts frequently practiced by men past sixty?

Yes. Here again, the major source of information on this subject comes from the Kinsey investigations. The Kinsey report states, "41% of the outlet in the sixty year age group of men comes from extra-marital relations." It should be noted in interpreting this data that the sampling included a rather limited number of people, and it is doubtful that the statistics would be as high for the entire over-sixty population.

If a man past sixty is potent, does this necessarily mean that he is able to discharge live sperm?

No. Some men are potent but no longer emit live sperm. Conversely, others are impotent but their testicles continue to produce live sperm.

Is male fertility affected by the aging process?

Yes. As one advances into the seventies and eighties the testicles produce fewer live sperm and eventually stop producing them altogether. The majority of men, even though they may be capable of sexual intercourse, stop producing live sperm when they reach the mid-seventies. A very small percentage are capable of manufacturing sperm during their eighties and nineties.

How can a man past sixty discover whether or not he is still fertile?

An examination of the semen for the presence of live sperm can be carried out by a urologist. This test is performed by massaging the prostate gland after inserting a finger into the rectum. The semen thus obtained is placed under a microscope and examined for the presence or absence of live sperm.

Does the presence of live sperm in a man over sixty mean that he is able to impregnate a woman?

Yes. Unless repeated examinations show that no live sperm are present in the ejaculation, a man must be presumed to be capable of causing pregnancy.

Until what age does the average male continue to produce live sperm?

About three out of four males will retain this physiological ability until they reach the age of seventy.

Does the amount of sexual activity during the younger years influence the age at which men lose their desire for sex or their ability to consummate the sex act?

No, unless events earlier in life have caused some disease in the genital tract that restricts sexual desire and competence.

What is the greatest cause of impotence in otherwise healthy men of sixty?

In healthy men, impotence is most often caused by emotional instability or conflicts. Few healthy men of sixty are impotent because of physical factors, inasmuch as the testicles are capable of secreting adequate amounts of the male sex hormone until this age, and the physical mechanism that controls erection of the penis usually remains intact well beyond the sixtieth year.

What is "male menopause"?

This is a very loosely used term, and many physicians doubt the actual existence of a true male menopause. If one means by it that there is a slackening of sex desire and activity in aging men, then, in all probability, the idea has validity. The age at which this occurs, however, varies greatly, and may be anywhere from forty to eighty years of age.

What are some of the symptoms of the so-called male menopause?

To be scientifically accurate, the only specific proof that male menopause has taken place is the finding that the testicles are no longer capable of producing motile, live sperm and that the male is no longer able to have an erection and to consummate the sex act. Stated in more general terms, the symptoms of male menopause are:

1. Mental depression and listlessness.
2. Excessive dryness of the skin.

3. Lower than normal metabolism.
4. Low blood pressure.
5. Loss of interest in one's friends, family, and surroundings.
6. Lack of sexual desire and inability to perform the sex act.

When a male past sixty loses his virility, how can it be determined whether the impotence is psychological or physical in origin?

This is an extremely difficult diagnosis to make. One way to make the differentiation is to administer large doses of the male sex hormone (testosterone). If this brings back virility, it can be presumed that the impotence was physical in origin. If, on the other hand, male-sex-hormone therapy fails to reestablish potency, it can be presumed that the impotence is due largely to psychological factors.

Is it harmful or dangerous to treat impotence with male sex hormones?

In certain cases sex-hormone treatment is inadvisable; in others, it may be pursued for several weeks, but not longer. It has been found that large doses of male sex hormone given over many months may stimulate a quiescent tumor of the prostate to grow. For this reason, male sex hormones should not be given to a man who has an enlarged prostate gland or other evidence of a possible growth of that gland.

It should be emphasized that any beneficial effect from hormone treatment will show up within a few weeks; if the patient fails to show return of potency within that period of time, hormones should be discontinued.

Will giving the male sex hormone relieve symptoms of the so-called male menopause?

If the symptoms are truly due to a diminution in the amount of hormone being secreted, then this form of treatment may be beneficial. Here, too, it should be mentioned that if no improvement is noted within a few weeks, the hormones should be stopped.

What precautions should an older man take when marrying a woman who is many years his junior?

He should seek professional advice before marriage, particularly with reference to performing the sexual act. If moderation is practiced there need be no fears about disparity in age.

Is it natural for men past sixty to take longer to reach climax (orgasm)?

Yes. As a general rule, the older the man, the longer he may take to reach climax.

How does the aging process affect sexual desire in women?
Most studies show that women retain their sexual desires for years after menopause, even though they may not actually participate in marital relations. Moreover, the Kinsey studies indicate that most women undergo very little loss in sexual desire because of aging, even in their seventies or eighties.

Is there a decrease in sexual desire because of menopause?
No. On the contrary, many women show increased interest in sex after change of life. This is thought to be due to relief from the fear of pregnancy.

Is indulgence in strenuous sexual activity dangerous to the heart and blood vessels of healthy older women?
No. For some unknown reason, the heart and the arteries are much less vulnerable in women.

What percentage of healthy women over sixty continue to have sexual intercourse?
Approximately 40 percent of married women, according to Kinsey. (This statistic does not include those who have sexual desires but, for one reason or another, do not have intercourse.)

Do women tend to become frigid as they grow older?
No.

What role do the female sex hormones play in sexual desire?
They seem to play a rather minor role, as shown by the fact that women who have had their ovaries removed retain their usual desires.

Is it harmful physically for older women to overindulge in sexual intercourse?
The term "overindulgence" defies accurate description when applied to sexual intercourse. Perhaps one can say that whatever frequency husband and wife mutually agree upon is the "correct frequency." And the "correct frequency" for a particular couple will rarely cause physical harm. Potential danger exists when the frequency exceeds that of which the wife feels capable.

Is it inadvisable for an older woman to marry a younger man?
It may not be physically harmful, but statistics show that there is a greater incidence of incompatability when older women marry younger men. Furthermore, such women should make certain, prior to marriage, that the underlying motive of the mate is love rather than a desire for economic or social advancement.

Can older women achieve sexual compatability with younger men?

Yes, although it may be a bit more difficult to attain.

Will female sex hormones reestablish sexual desire in an older woman who has lost interest in this phase of living?

No. The loss of sexual desire in women is predominantly a psychological phenomenon.

Is it common for older women who have been sexually dormant for many years to regain interest in sex upon remarrying?

Yes.

Is there usually a change in a woman's ability to reach climax as she ages?

No. Age has relatively little to do with this capacity.

Should women past sixty take any special measures prior to intercourse?

Yes; inasmuch as there is a tendency for the vaginal mucous membranes to secrete less mucus, they should apply a lubricating jelly to the genital area before intercourse.

Does the removal of the uterus and the ovaries influence the sexual desire or capabilities of women?

Not in the least.

Is there any tendency for women past sixty to develop sexual aberrations?

No. On the contrary, the Kinsey investigations indicate that abnormal relations tend to decrease markedly among women who are past the menopause.

SEX HORMONES

See ADRENAL GLANDS; ENDOCRINE GLANDS AND HORMONES; FEMALE ORGANS; OVARIES; PROSTATE GLAND; SEX AFTER SIXTY; TESTICLES.

What are sex hormones?

They are chemical substances produced and secreted by the ovaries in women and by the testicles in men.

Do the testicles continue to secrete male sex hormones throughout life?

Yes, but the quantity is markedly decreased during the later years.

Do the ovaries continue to secrete female sex hormones after the menopause?

Only in minute quantities.

Do glands other than the ovaries or testicles secrete sex hormones?

It is thought that the pituitary gland in the base of the skull and the adrenal glands lying just above the kidneys produce hormones with many of the same actions as those secreted by the ovaries and testicles. When the ovaries and testicles no longer function or when they have been removed, the pituitary and the adrenals take over.

Do the production and secretion of sex hormones have anything to do with the aging process?

Many physicians feel that the sex hormones, particularly the *androgenic* (male) hormone, have much to do with the maintenance of muscle tone and protein metabolism. It is thought that the androgenic hormone (present in slight quantities in the female also) is necessary to the maintenance of normal health among the aged. If it is lacking, people tend to become weak and debilitated.

Will giving sex hormones delay the onset of aging?

No. Although menopause can be delayed by giving female sex hormones, they cannot be used permanently for this purpose. Similarly, although there may appear to be a prolongation of virility in the male as a result of therapy with male sex hormones, the effect cannot be maintained over a period of years.

Are there any harmful effects from giving sex hormones for long periods of time?

Yes. This practice is considered unwise. Large doses of the female sex hormone may stimulate a dormant tumor in the ovaries, breast, or uterus to start growing. By the same token, giving large doses of male sex hormones may stimulate the growth of a dormant tumor in the prostate gland.

Are sex hormones ever used in the treatment of diseases of aging people?

Yes. For some unknown reason, giving male sex hormones to the female often inhibits and arrests the growth of a tumor in the breast or ovary. Conversely, giving female sex hormone to the male may inhibit the growth and spread of a tumor of the prostate gland.

Recent experiments have been carried out in which male sex hormone has been given to both the female and the male in order to stimulate energy and muscle tone. In a certain number of cases this may be effective, but it should not be continued on a long-term basis because of possible harmful effects. Also, in certain cases of osteoporosis in women, female sex hormone will have a beneficial effect.

Will giving large doses of male sex hormone to a female bring on male physical characteristics?

Yes, if it is given over a period of months. Hair may grow on the face and chest, and there may be a deepening of the voice.

Will giving female sex hormones to the male produce female characteristics?

Large doses of female sex hormones, given over a long period of time (as they are in some cases of cancer of the prostate), may cause enlargement of the breasts.

Will the taking of female sex hormones restore a youthful appearance to the skin of an older woman?

No. Millions of dollars have been spent by women who harbor false hopes that the taking of female sex hormones will restore their youthful appearance.

Can large doses of female sex hormone stimulate a woman over sixty to begin to menstruate again?

Yes, occasionally, but it is more likely to happen in a woman in her fifties.

Will large doses of female sex hormone cause an increase in sexual desire in an older woman?

No. For some unexplained reason, sexual desire has relatively little to do with the secretion of sex hormones. Many women continue to have sexual desires long after they have stopped menstruating.

Can itching in the genital region and dryness of the vagina be relieved by using ointments containing female sex hormones?

Some gynecologists believe that relief from these symptoms can be derived from this form of treatment. However, the use of hormone ointments must be carefully supervised. If relief is not obtained within a few weeks, treatment should be discontinued.

Are there any beneficial effects from the so-called youth balms?

No. As stated above, the public has wasted much money on hope that cannot be fulfilled through the use of these "medications."

Is impotence in an aging man always due to a decrease in the amount of hormone secreted by the testicles?

Impotence in a healthy man in his sixties is more likely to be of psychological origin. Impotence in a man in his late seventies or eighties is probably due to a decrease in the amount of male sex hormone.

Will giving male sex hormone correct impotence?

Only if impotency is due to a lack of production of male sex hormone by the testicles. As stated above, in a great many cases impotency in men in their sixties and early seventies is psychological rather than physiological in origin.

Until what age can the average man produce active live sperm?

This varies markedly among different men, races, and climates. There are cases on record of men who have produced live, active sperm when they were in their eighties or nineties.

Is there always a correlation between fertility (the ability to produce live sperm) and potency (the ability to consummate the sex act)?

No. There is relatively little relationship between these two phenomena. A man may be perfectly able to perform the sexual act and yet not produce sperm. On the other hand, a man may be producing live, active sperm in his testicles but may be totally impotent.

Will taking female sex hormone by a man, in order to slow down the growth of a cancer of the prostate, produce changes in his appearance?

Slight to moderate breast enlargement is the only noticeable change.

What role does heredity play in the loss of virility and potency in the male?

Other things being equal, heredity plays an important role in determining the age at which these changes take place.

What can be done to stimulate the secretion of male sex hormone and to restore virility in an aging man?

If it can be determined that psychological factors are not the cause of the loss of virility, giving male sex hormone may help to restore potency. If, after a trial period of several weeks, virility is not restored, the hormones should be discontinued.

Will taking male sex hormones stimulate improved health in an undernourished, debilitated older man?

The male sex hormone *testosterone* is supposed to be a potent anabolic agent. This means that it can aid in building up muscle tissue and help to improve the metabolism of proteins. Therefore, it can be tried for a few weeks, but should be stopped if it is not producing the desired result.

Can the male sex hormone help an undernourished and debilitated older woman?

In some instances. The male hormone has much the same effect on debilitated older women as it has upon men.

Is there such a thing as a male menopause?

Many physicians believe that there is such a period during a man's life, although the changes are not as obvious and abrupt as those that take place in the female. In men, there may be increased irritability, anxiety, and unfounded doubts about his ability to continue to function efficiently. There are also fears over loss of potency and the possibility of a premature death. Most investigators in this field agree that these reactions are psychological rather than physical, yet one cannot completely ignore the physical factors of the aging process.

Should men who show symptoms of "change of life" take hormones to relieve the condition?

It is perhaps best that they let nature take its course rather than attempt to reverse an inevitable trend. Well-integrated men can readily accept the knowledge that they are growing old. Furthermore, there are dangers associated with giving large doses of male hormone. This does not imply, however, that there can be no treatment of the anxiety and emotional stress that affect older men. A visit to the family physician or to a psychiatrist may be helpful.

SHOCK

See ARTIFICIAL RESPIRATION; BLOOD PRESSURE; CIRCULATION; FAINTING; FIRST AID; FRACTURES; INJURIES AND ACCIDENTS; SURGERY.

Do older people tend to go into shock more readily than younger people?

Yes. For this reason it is essential that first aid be given immediately following an accident or injury.

What are the symptoms and signs of shock?

1. In some cases there is loss of consciousness; in others, there is marked apprehension and evidence of fright.

2. If the patient is conscious, he complains of weakness, extreme thirst, and hunger for air.
3. The body is bathed in a cold, clammy perspiration.
4. The pupils of the eyes become dilated.
5. Breathing is rapid and shallow.
6. The skin may take on a gray appearance.
7. The pulse is rapid and weak.
8. Blood pressure is usually very low.

What first aid should be given for shock?

1. The patient should be placed flat on his back. If the shock is profound, some books should be placed under the legs of the bed at the foot, so that the patient's head and chest are lower than the rest of the body.
2. Attempts should be made to relieve pain, since this is one of the precipitating causes of shock.
3. If the cause of the shock is obvious, as when it is secondary to a severe laceration with blood loss, the local condition should be treated immediately. (A tourniquet should be applied to stop the bleeding.) If the shock is secondary to a fracture, the limb should be splinted. In many cases, prompt treatment of the precipitating factor is sufficient to bring the patient out of shock.
4. Blankets should be used to cover the patient, but he should not be too warm.
5. As soon as possible, the patient should be transported on a stretcher to the emergency room of the nearest hospital.

Do people past sixty recover from shock as readily as younger people?

No. Shock of more than a few hours' duration is often fatal to older people, whereas young people may be able to recover even after a day or two in shock.

Should attempts be made to arouse someone who is in shock?

No. If he is unconscious, it will do no good to try to awaken him. If he is sleeping, he should be permitted to do so.

Should whiskey, tea, or coffee be given to someone in shock?

No. It is best to give nothing by mouth until so ordered by a physician.

SKIN

See ALLERGY; BURNS AND FROSTBITE; CLIMATE; CLOTHING; DERMATITIS; FUNGUS INFECTIONS; HAIR; HERPES ZOSTER; HYGIENE; LEUKOPLAKIA; MOLES AND MELANOMAS; PLASTIC SURGERY; PREMATURE AGING; TRICHIASIS; XANTHELASMA.

What are the signs of aging skin?

1. There is a progressive loss of elastic tissue. This can be readily demonstrated by picking up and pinching the skin on the back of the hand and noting the speed with which it resumes its normal shape. In older people, the skin takes much longer to return to normal position.
2. The superficial layers of the skin thin out.
3. Small, patchy areas of skin overgrowth may develop. These look much like flat warts, and are known as hyperkeratoses.
4. The sweat glands tend to become less active, secreting less oil and sweat.
5. Because of the decrease in the number of functioning sweat glands, there is increased dryness of the skin.
6. Pigment changes take place, with loss of pigment in some areas and increased pigmentation in other areas. This results in the "brown spots" of aging, seen so often on exposed surfaces.

If the skin appears old and wrinkled, does this mean that vital organs inside the body are also showing signs of aging?

Not necessarily. Care of the skin during the younger years often determines how soon it will show signs of advancing age. Neglected skin may age prematurely, even though vital organs function normally and show few signs of aging. In other words, an individual may appear old but still have relatively young internal organs.

What can cause skin to age prematurely?

1. Overexposure to sunlight.
2. Constant exposure to wind and frigid climates. (One need only look at the weather-beaten faces of seamen to see how inclement weather can age skin prematurely.)
3. Poor skin hygiene.
4. Constant exposure to irritating substances, such as coal dust, greases, oils, etc.
5. Chronic states of malnutrition.
6. Chronic vitamin deficiency.

Can careful attention to the care of the skin delay the onset of its aging?

Yes. One should note the youthful appearance of aging actors and actresses to see the results of constant care of the skin. Most of these people carefully avoid overexposure to sun, wind, and irritating substances. In addition, they take great pains to see that their skin is clean and well lubricated.

Does itching of the skin occur more frequently as one gets older?

Yes.

Does the skin tend to become "dried out" as one advances in age?

Yes, since the sweat glands secrete less perspiration and oil.

What can be done to prevent dryness and itching of the skin?

1. Since itching is usually worse with low humidity and cold temperatures, homes should be kept comfortably warm and humid.
2. Older people with tendencies toward itching skin should limit bathing to two or three times a week.
3. Strong soaps should be avoided. Some older people may have to abandon soaps entirely because of their irritating effect on the skin. They should substitute superfatted soaps or should cleanse the skin with cold cream or other lubricants.
4. An ounce or two of olive oil or mineral oil placed into the bath water may cut down somewhat on itching.
5. Dry, itching skin feels much better when it is lubricated. Olive oil, mineral oil, or commercial bath oils can be applied for this purpose.
6. Sometimes, dryness and itching of skin are a result of vitamin A deficiency. Replacement of that vitamin may help to alleviate the symptoms considerably.
7. Within the past few years, many women have been using ointments containing the female sex hormone (estrogen). Such ointments have been described as having the ability to rejuvenate the skin and to restore its youthful appearance. In addition, it is claimed that itching and dryness of the skin will be relieved. Although there may be some beneficial effects from using these ointments, they should not be used unless prescribed by a doctor.
8. Much of the itching of the skin in older people can be attributed to nervousness, anxiety, and stress situations. The relief of these states is often followed by cessation of itching.

9. There is a tendency for people to require more drugs as they advance in age. Many drugs, when taken over a number of years, will lead to hypersensitivity reactions manifested by itching of the skin. The itching is often relieved by discontinuing the drug.

10. Itching of the skin in older people may be due to a general disease such as diabetes, kidney disease, or liver disease. A thorough physical examination should be performed to rule out these possibilities. The control or cure of a general condition will often result in cessation of itching.

Does frequent bathing always cause dryness and itching of the skin?

No. This varies from individual to individual, depending on the amount of natural oils in the skin.

How often should healthy older people bathe?

If the skin does not become too dry, and if harsh soaps are avoided, it is perfectly permissible for them to bathe daily or as often as they wish. If, on the other hand, dryness and itching do ensue, they should limit bathing to twice or three times a week. Between baths, they can maintain cleanliness by washing with a cloth and warm water.

It should be mentioned that bathing in a warm, moist climate can be tolerated better than bathing in a cold climate where the humidity is low.

Is there any harm in using commercial bath oils?

No. On the contrary, bath oils lubricate the skin and reduce dryness.

Are older people more susceptible to skin infections and diseases?

Yes, for the following reasons:

1. The blood supply to the skin diminishes as one advances in age. For this reason, it is less resistant to bacterial invasion.

2. Older people's skin cracks more readily, rendering it more susceptible to bacterial and fungus growth.

3. Natural skin oils, which act as a protective mechanism, are secreted in decreasing amounts as one grows older.

4. Older people are more subject to allergies, which often affect the skin.

5. Fungus infections of the skin often follow the prolonged use of antibiotic drugs. Since older people are often forced to take these medications, they will have a greater incidence of fungus infections.

6. Older people are prone to undernourishment and to vita-

min deficiencies, which are conducive to skin afflictions.

7. As a consequence of the aging process, and as a result of long exposure to irritants, skin cancer develops frequently in people past sixty.

What causes wrinkles in the skin?

Degeneration of elastic fibers in the deeper layers of the skin and loss in the amount of fat tissue lying directly beneath the skin.

Is there any way to combat wrinkles?

One of the best ways is to maintain a good level of nutrition. Undernourished, underweight older people will show wrinkles to a much greater extent than those who maintain satisfactory nutrition.

Plastic operations can remove some wrinkles, but the effect of these procedures is usually not permanent. (*See* PLASTIC SURGERY.)

Is it safe to receive injections of paraffin beneath the skin in order to remove wrinkles?

No. This is a dangerous procedure. Paraffin injections are often followed by the formation of paraffin tumors (*paraffinomas*) or even malignant growths.

Are there plastic materials that can be inserted beneath the skin to obliterate wrinkles?

Yes, but many of these materials are not yet fully tested and the ultimate results of their insertion beneath the skin must be further investigated.

Will repeated applications of hormone creams, especially those containing female sex hormones, help to reduce wrinkling?

Most skin specialists agree that their effect on wrinkles is negligible. Moreover, definite harm can result from their indiscriminate use without medical supervision.

Is massage helpful in doing away with wrinkles?

In all probability, it does little permanent good. On the other hand, it may stimulate the blood supply to the massaged area and thus improve skin appearance.

Are face lifting and other kinds of plastic surgery helpful in restoring a more youthful appearance to the face?

Yes. (*See* PLASTIC SURGERY.)

Is there an inherited tendency toward premature wrinkling of the skin?

Yes. Many people inherit this tendency; others retain their youthful appearance until late in life.

How can the onset of wrinkles be delayed?

1. Throughout the early and middle years the skin should be kept clean and free from infections.
2. Overexposure to sunlight, harsh winds, and cold should be avoided.
3. A good nutritional state should be maintained.
4. Excessive use of cheap cosmetics should be avoided.

What is the significance of the brown spots seen so often on the skin of older people?

Senile freckling is a common condition that has no clinical significance other than to denote the fact that one is growing older. Pigment changes are a normal part of the aging process.

Is there any way to prevent freckling and pigment changes?

No, but avoidance of sunburn will make such changes less obvious.

Can local application of ointments do away with pigment changes?

No, although there are cosmetics that may hide skin blemishes.

Does the skin become more sensitive to heat and cold as one grows older?

Yes, especially to intense cold. It is important, therefore, to protect it from prolonged exposure.

Why is it harmful for older people to overexpose themselves to heat and sunlight?

1. Overexposure to sunlight, over the years, predisposes to skin cancer.
2. Intense heat will cause excessive perspiration, with the loss of important body fluids containing such chemicals as sodium and chloride. This loss can lead to heat exhaustion or heat stroke—very serious conditions in older people.
3. Severe sunburn can be a dangerous condition in people in their seventies or eighties.
4. Constant overexposure to the sun will exaggerate the aged appearance of the skin.

Will the skin of healthy older people heal as quickly following surgery or laceration?

Yes, provided the patient is in good general health.

Do older people tend to perspire less?

Yes. The sweat glands, like most other glands, secrete less as time goes on.

What effect does a decreased ability to perspire have on the body?

It will interfere with the heat-regulating mechanism. Also, it will cut down on the elimination of water, carbon dioxide, and other waste materials that usually takes place through the skin.

Does the skin become more sensitive as one gets older?

Yes. It is less able to tolerate medications applied directly to the skin, and it becomes more sensitive to such things as nylon, wool, dyes, cosmetics, and oils from plants. It also may display an increased sensitivity to medications taken internally.

What should be done if someone develops a skin sensitivity?

1. All drugs or medications that are being taken internally should be stopped until it is determined which one is causing the trouble. A substitute drug should then be prescribed.
2. Ointments should be discontinued.
3. New or recently dyed clothing should not be worn.
4. Whenever possible, wool should not be worn.
5. New house plants should be taken out of the house.
6. A doctor may prescribe antihistamine drugs or other desensitizing medications.

Are new undergarments often the cause of allergic reactions of the skin?

Yes.

Where are the most common sites of itching and allergic manifestations?

In the folds and creases, such as the elbow region, the folds of the knee joint, beneath the breasts, in the armpits, in the folds of abdominal fat, and in the creases of the groin.

What special advice should older women follow in the use of cosmetics?

1. Cosmetics may be used so long as they do not produce irritation, itching, puffiness, or swelling of the skin.
2. Cosmetics should be removed before bedtime.
3. If there is any doubt as to a possible harmful reaction to a particular cosmetic, a skin specialist (dermatologist) should be consulted.
4. It should be determined, before a new cosmetic is used, that it does not contain harmful substances, such as arsenic or lead.
5. Cosmetics should not be used to cover up sores or skin growths.

Are there medications that are helpful in controlling fungus infections of the skin?

Yes. *See* FUNGUS INFECTIONS.

SKIN TUMORS

Does the incidence of skin tumors increase as one gets older?

Yes. Perhaps the most common site of a tumor in people over sixty is the skin. The majority are nonmalignant (benign) growths, but skin cancer also occurs more frequently in older people.

What are some of the more common forms of benign skin tumors?

1. *Senile keratoses.* These are localized, brownish thickenings of the skin, usually seen on exposed surfaces. The back of the hands, the face, and the neck are the most frequent sites. It is thought that overexposure to the sun will aggravate and accentuate keratoses.
2. *Seborrheic keratoses.* These are thickened, wartlike, raised, light-brown patches. They represent true warty growths originating from the deep layers of the skin.
3. *Sebaceous adenomas.* These are true benign skin tumors, small in size, originating from the sweat glands or from the deeper layers of the skin.
4. *Papillomas* (or "skin tags") of the skin. These are projected, usually nonpigmented, dumbbell-shaped tumors. They vary in size from that of a pinhead to that of a golf ball.
5. *Angiomas.* These are small, superficial blood-vessel tumors that appear as red spots. Some are the size of a pinhead; others are the size of a pea.

What is the treatment of benign skin tumors?

1. Some can be removed locally with an electric needle (electrical coagulation). This procedure can be carried out in a doctor's office, with or without local anesthesia.
2. Many of the larger benign growths are removed surgically by elliptical incision. Such procedures are carried out in the doctor's office under local anesthesia, or in a hospital.
3. Certain types of benign skin tumors, particularly the blood-vessel angiomas, can be destroyed by the application of carbon dioxide snow. This procedure is carried out in the doctor's office.

4. Certain types of benign tumors, particularly warts, are occasionally treated by X ray rather than by surgery or electrical coagulation.

Are the above methods of treatment effective in curing skin tumors?

Yes, and they are not at all dangerous.

SKIN CANCER

Is skin cancer common in people past sixty?

Yes. It is one of the most common cancers in older people.

Do skin cancers usually spread from their original site to other parts of the body?

No. The great majority remain localized.

Are most skin cancers curable?

Yes, unless they are neglected for a long period of time.

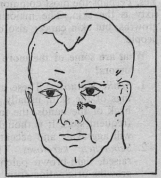

Epithelioma (skin cancer) of face

What are predisposing factors toward development of a skin cancer?

1. Constant or repeated irritation of a benign growth.
2. Repeated injury to a nonmalignant tumor.
3. Overexposure to sunlight throughout life.
4. Neglect of a benign skin condition.

Where do most skin cancers form?

On the exposed surfaces of the body, for example, the nose, the cheeks, the lips, the temples, the scalp, the external ear, the back of the hands. They may also form where skin irritation is most likely to occur, such as the heel, the toes, or the belt region.

What is the treatment of skin cancer?

Most skin cancers are treated in the same way as benign tumors. Surgical excision, electrical coagulation, and X-ray therapy are all good methods of treatment, depending on the specific type of growth. Of course, treatment is more extensive in that the excision of a cancer will be wider, the X-ray dosage will be greater, and the extent of electric-needle application will be deeper and more extensive than for a benign tumor.

Who should treat skin cancers?

A surgeon or a skin specialist. Most general practitioners are not equipped to give this kind of treatment.

How can one tell if he is developing a skin cancer?

Any sore that fails to heal over a period of several weeks or any tumor that shows rapid growth or change in color should be suspected as being a skin cancer. A visit to one's doctor will result in a diagnosis, sometimes obtained by taking a biopsy of the growth.

MOLE, NEVUS, MELANOMA

Are moles very common in older people?

Yes. Although these growths may appear at any age, they tend to increase in number and size as one ages.

Is a mole the same as a nevus?

Yes.

How does the appearance of a mole differ from that of a melanoma?

Often they appear the same. However, a melanoma is a malignant growth and usually undergoes rapid increase in size and changes in color.

Does an ordinary mole ever turn into a melanoma?

Yes. For this reason it is very important to consult a doctor when a mole enlarges, changes color, or is subject to constant irritation.

How often do benign moles turn into malignant melanomas?

Infrequently. However, when they do, the life of the patient is endangered.

Do melanomas occur more often in younger people?

Yes. The incidence in children and young and middle-aged adults is much greater than in those past sixty.

Should an older person have moles removed?

Yes, if they change in color, grow larger, or are subject to repeated irritation.

What are the dangers of a melanoma?

A melanoma is one of the worst kinds of malignant growths. It tends to spread via the bloodstream to distant parts of the body. Eventually, it will invade so many vital structures that the patient will die.

What is the treatment of melanoma?

It should be removed locally with a very wide surgical incision. If there are enlarged glands in the area, they too should be removed.

Within recent years, several chemical agents have been found that are helpful in delaying the growth and spread of melanomas. Perfusion techniques have been devised whereby chemotherapeutic agents are injected into arteries supplying the area of the melanoma, thus bringing a heavy concentration of the drug to the tumor.

Is the surgical removal of a melanoma a serious operation?

Yes, if it is accompanied by a dissection to remove the glands that drain the area of the melanoma. Local removal, by means of a large elliptical excision of the tumor-bearing area, is not a serious operation.

If a melanoma is widely excised locally, can one look forward to a cure?

If the malignancy has not spread to other parts of the body, a cure will result. If cells have already spread to other parts of the body, local excision will not result in a cure.

SLEEP AND REST

See DRUGS AND MEDICINES; LONGEVITY; PHYSICAL ACTIVITY AND EXERCISE; RETIREMENT; SOCIAL BEHAVIOR.

Do people past sixty require more rest and sleep as they grow older?

Yes, although healthy people in their early and mid-sixties may not show evidence of increased need.

Is the need for additional rest a natural phenomenon in older people?

Yes, especially for those who are in their seventies and eighties. An afternoon nap for an hour or an hour of physical inactivity following meals will always have beneficial effects.

Why do people tire more easily as they advance in age?

Fatigue is a chemical and physiological reaction. Waste products are built up in the muscles and other structures of the body as a result of the expenditure of energy; these waste products must be eliminated or reconstituted into chemicals the body can use again for the expenditure of more energy. To effect this process, the body requires rest and sleep. As people age, the accumulation of waste products takes place more rapidly, and it becomes more difficult for the body to eliminate unusable substances and to resynthesize usable ones.

What are the normal sleep requirements for the average individual past sixty?

If he is actively working, he should have eight hours of sleep a night. If he is retired or not working, six hours will usually suffice.

Is bed rest without sleep helpful in restoring a fatigued body?

Yes, although actual sleep is more beneficial.

Is it necessary for active, healthy people in their sixties to take a nap in the afternoon or to rest after meals if they do not feel the need for it?

No, but much benefit can result from this practice.

Is it natural for some elderly people to develop fears about going to sleep?

This sometimes occurs when people have an inordinate fear of death. To their unconscious minds, going to sleep symbolizes dying. Without their awareness of it, such people will fear going to sleep. But most older people do not develop such anxieties.

Is it natural for older people to have periods of dozing and daydreaming?

Yes, especially those in their seventies and eighties. When involuntary dozing or daydreaming develops, it is an indication to begin a routine of daily rest periods.

Do older people dream at night as much as younger people?

Yes. Psychiatrists believe that all people dream continuously. However, young people recall their dreams more readily than older people.

Is there a tendency for older people to have nightmares?

Yes, if they are emotionally disturbed or have unresolved anxieties and fears.

Many older people claim that they regularly sleep for only an hour or two a night. Is this true, or do they imagine it?

There are several levels of unconsciousness during sleep, some of them so deep that the individual is unaware of the passage of time. During other periods, sleep is so light that a semiconscious state is maintained, during which there is an awareness of the passage of time. Although this latter state is actually sleep, it may not be interpreted as such by the older person.

Is there an increased tendency toward sleeplessness (insomnia) as one advances in age?

Yes.

What are some common causes of insomnia?

1. Fear and anxiety, especially fear of death.
2. Excitement, annoyance, or excessive mental stimulation before attempting to sleep.
3. Eating a large meal before going to bed.
4. Drinking coffee or other stimulants before going to bed.
5. Drinking large quantities of fluids before retiring.
6. Sleeping in a room in which the temperature and humidity are not adjusted correctly.
7. Sleeping in a room with a sick person for whom one feels responsible.
8. Sleeping in a noisy atmosphere.

How can one eliminate sleeplessness?

By avoiding or eliminating the stimulating and irritating conditions listed above. Also, a warm bath, a warm glass of milk, and a mild sedative are often helpful in relieving insomnia.

Is it harmful for older people to take sleeping pills, such as the barbiturates?

When these medications are prescribed by a doctor, they are harmless. One should not fear the use of these drugs insofar as addiction is concerned, but they should be taken only when prescribed by a physician.

Is there any harm in sleeping while sitting in a chair?

No, although it is better to sleep in bed so that the blood in the lower extremities can return to the heart more readily. When an older person can only sleep sitting up, he should be permitted to do so.

Does someone with heart or lung trouble who must sleep in a sitting position derive the same rest and restoration from fatigue as one who can sleep lying down?

Yes. The position in which one sleeps is not very important, provided he is able to sleep.

Should old people sleep in the dark, or should a light be left on?

Since most older people get out of bed once or twice during the night, it is perhaps wise to have a night light burning so that they will not stumble in the dark.

Should older people sleep in the same room with children?

Since their sleeping habits usually differ considerably from those of children, it is not a good practice. Not only may it have an adverse effect on a child but also anxiety about a child's welfare may keep the older person awake.

Why should older people refrain from drinking large quantities of fluid before retiring?

Because the need to void may disturb an otherwise comfortable night's sleep.

Is there a tendency in some older people to sleep during the daylight hours and remain awake at night?

This phenomenon does occur sometimes, especially in those who have an inordinate fear of death. If this does take place, medical advice should be sought.

Will a long nap during the day interfere with sleep at night?

Yes. For this reason, the rest period during the day should be limited to one hour.

Does reading just before retiring promote sleep?

For some people it may; for others, it may have the opposite effect. It is important to select the reading material carefully, avoiding subjects that might overstimulate.

Do the decaffeinated drinks actually remove most of the stimulating effects of coffee?

Yes, although some caffein still remains.

Should windows be left open at night?

Yes. Some air circulation should be provided during sleep. This does not mean that a window should be thrown wide open or that a direct flow of air is always essential. There are many good methods of indirect ventilation—and, of course, ventilation nowadays is often supplied by air conditioners.

Should a bedroom be kept dry or humid?

Since the mucous membranes of the respiratory passages of older people may be dry, it is important that the atmosphere contain adequate moisture. Water should be placed in the troughs above the radiators during the winter.

Is it harmful for older people to sleep in the same room with plants or large bouquets of flowers?

No. This is an old misconception with no basis in fact.

Is it safe for older people to go to sleep with a hot-water bottle or electric heating pad?

No. This is an extremely hazardous procedure.

Should older people be permitted to smoke in bed before going to sleep?

No person should smoke in bed at any time.

Is sleepwalking common among older people?

No, but they often wake at night and walk about.

What precautions are necessary for older people who get up from sleep during the night?

1. If they wear eyeglasses, they should put them on before getting out of bed.

2. Furniture, articles of clothing, packages, and other obstructions should be kept out of the passageway from the bed to the bathroom.

3. A light should be put on by an older person before he gets out of bed.

4. It is good practice for older people to sit on the edge of the bed for a minute or two after arising from a deep sleep, since balance and equilibrium may take a little while to be reestablished.

5. If one is getting up in order to take a medication, he should first turn on the light in the bathroom. Many serious accidents have resulted from reaching for a medicine in the dark.

6. If an older person plans to leave his bedroom for any length of time, he should inform his spouse so as not to frighten her.

SMOKING

See ALLERGY; ANESTHESIA; ANGINA PECTORIS; ARTERIOSCLEROSIS; ASTHMA; BLOOD PRESSURE; BRONCHITIS; CANCER AND OTHER MALIGNANT GROWTHS; CIRCULATION; CLAUDICATION; CORONARY-ARTERY DISEASE; COUGHS; HEART; LEUKOPLAKIA; LUNG TUMORS; RESPIRATORY TRACT; TEETH; ULCERS OF STOMACH AND DUODENUM.

Is the use of tobacco harmful to healthy older people?

Most doctors now agree that smoking may have harmful effects on all people, regardless of age. This does not imply that all those over sixty should be advised to discontinue the practice. An important consideration is the fact that a great number of people who have been addicted to smoking for many years will develop serious emotional disturbances if forced to stop.

Of course, it is obvious that those who have illnesses or conditions that might be aggravated by the use of tobacco should stop smoking.

Should healthy older people be advised to stop smoking if they feel capable of discontinuing it?

Yes. This will benefit their respiratory system and circulation, as well as their digestion. But, again, it should be emphasized that if the distress created by abandoning tobacco is too great, they should not do so.

What special rules should older smokers follow?

1. They should *never* smoke in bed. Many an individual has dozed off while smoking and the bed has caught fire. Those who habitually take sleeping pills should be especially careful not to smoke in bed.
2. They should get out of the habit of smoking a cigarette or cigar down to the very end. Often their fingers are less sensitive to heat, thus permitting a burn to occur unnoticed.
3. They should never smoke while driving.
4. They should refrain from smoking while walking in a wind or when exposed to a draft. This may cause clothing to catch fire.
5. They should not smoke before eating, since it may spoil the appetite.
6. They should stop smoking if they have a cold or other respiratory infection.
7. They should abandon smoking if they have chest pain.
8. They should stop smoking if they have a chronic cough or a lung infection.
9. They should give up smoking if they have a circulatory disturbance, such as claudication or numbness and tingling in the hands and feet. (*See* CLAUDICATION.)

What constitutes excessive smoking?

This is a difficult question to answer. What is excessive for one individual may be moderate for another. In general, it can be said that excessive smoking is any amount that induces symptoms. If no symptoms are produced and if physical examination reveals the person to be in good health, then, for him, there is probably no clear-cut dividing line between moderate and excessive use of tobacco. On the other hand, if symptoms do arise, even one cigarette or cigar may be excessive.

Is it better to smoke filtered cigarettes than those without filters?

A filter does remove some of the tars and nicotine from the smoke, but it has not been determined whether or not the amount is great enough to reduce the harmful effects of these substances.

Is it true that those who smoke a cigarette down to the "bitter end" will get more tar and nicotine into their systems?

Yes.

Is cigar smoking less harmful than cigarette smoking?

Yes, probably because cigar smokers inhale less smoke.

Is pipe smoking less harmful than cigarette smoking?

Yes, for the same reason as that given above.

Is there a connection between smoking and the development of leukoplakia of the mouth or tongue?

Yes. There is a definite relationship between the use of tobacco and development of leukoplakia. This does not mean that nonsmokers are immune to leukoplakia, only that heavy smoking is conducive to the development of this condition. (*See* LEUKOPLAKIA.)

Will leukoplakia disappear if one stops smoking?

In some instances it does. In other cases, its progress is retarded considerably. In all cases, leukoplakia is aggravated by continued heavy smoking.

Is the appearance of leukoplakia an indication to stop smoking permanently?

By all means.

Does pipe smoking ever lead to cancer of the lip or tongue?

Infrequently. Modern pipes have good filters that reduce the heat of the smoke. Formerly, pipestems would become intensely hot and would repeatedly irritate and burn the lips or tongue. Such irritation, continued over many years, predisposed toward cancer.

Does a cigarette holder with a filter reduce the effects of the tar and nicotine in tobacco?

Not significantly.

Will the use of "denicotinized" cigarettes cut down on the harmful effects of smoking?

Yes, but only to a limited extent, because much of the tar and nicotine will remain even after the "denicotinizing" process.

How does smoking affect the teeth?

It encourages the deposit of tartar between the gums and the teeth. This may lead to bleeding gums and secondary infection. Moreover, teeth can be permanently stained by the prolonged use of tobacco.

Should those with tuberculosis be permitted to continue smoking?

No, since the smoke may irritate the respiratory passages. It must be stated, however, that tobacco itself has no adverse influence on the progress of the disease.

What is the relationship between smoking and the development of lung cancer?

Most medical investigators are in agreement that the prolonged and heavy use of tobacco, especially cigarettes, is conducive to the development of lung cancer, particularly in men. According to the most recent statistics, lung cancer is several times more prevalent in smokers than in nonsmokers. Nonsmokers are not immune to this disease, however.

Is it the nicotine or the tar in smoke that predisposes to lung cancer?

This cannot be answered with certainty, but most medical men think that the tar is the provoking agent.

If someone has been smoking for many years and is past sixty, should he stop smoking to avoid the possible development of lung cancer?

If he has been smoking for twenty or thirty years and has not developed lung cancer, discontinuing at such a late date will probably have little influence. In other words, the irritating factors that might predispose toward cancer have had plenty of time to produce their effects.

Will smoking filtered cigarettes cut down on the chances of getting lung cancer?

Probably not, but it should be realized that filtered cigarettes have not been in use long enough to reach a definite conclusion. The final answer to this question cannot be given for another fifteen to twenty years.

What effect does smoking have on the circulation?

Nicotine causes blood vessels to contract, and sometimes to go into spasm. Thus, in older people who already have some narrowing of their blood vessels, tobacco will cause further impairment of circulation.

Are there tests that reveal whether or not smoking is causing impaired circulation?

Yes. A lowering of the skin temperature in the hands or feet following the use of tobacco will indicate that there has been contraction or spasm of blood vessels. Also, an oscillometric test may demonstrate decreased pulsations in the extremities.

What effect does smoking have on people with high blood pressure?

Since smoking can cause constriction of blood vessels, it may lead to aggravation of high blood pressure. For this reason, many physicians advise their older patients with high blood pressure to stop smoking.

Is there a test that indicates whether or not someone with high blood pressure should stop smoking?

Yes. Immediately before, during, and after a patient has smoked four or five cigarettes in a row, blood-pressure readings are taken. If there is no elevation of the pressure as a result of smoking, then the practice can, in all probability, be continued. If there is marked elevation of blood pressure, smoking should be discontinued.

What effect does smoking have on the heart?

If the heart is relatively normal, the moderate use of tobacco will in all probability do little harm. If, on the other hand, the individual has angina pectoris (heart pain), or if he has evidence of coronary-artery sclerosis, smoking may cause great damage.

Can heavy smoking cause heart pain in an otherwise healthy individual?

Yes. Anginal attacks can be brought on by the excessive use of tobacco. Such pain is usually caused by the constricting effect of nicotine on the coronary artery.

Should people who are subject to attacks of angina pectoris give up smoking?

Yes.

Should a patient who has recovered from an attack of coronary thrombosis be permitted to resume smoking?

Only if the physician is sure that the smoking will not induce spasms of branches of the coronary artery. If it is resumed at all, smoking should be moderate.

How can one tell if smoking is having a deleterious effect on the heart?

1. By noting the onset of heart pain after heavy smoking.
2. By noting an elevation in the pulse rate.
3. By noting changes in the electrocardiogram after smoking.

Does the use of tobacco ever spoil one's appetite?

Yes, especially in those older people who already have poor appetites.

Does heavy smoking affect digestion adversely?

Yes, especially among those who have a tendency toward indigestion.

Does heavy smoking ever cause the stomach to secrete excessive amounts of acid?

Yes, but this happens more often in young people.

What effect does smoking have on people who have ulcer of the stomach or duodenum?

Since smoking increases acidity, it will aggravate an ulcer.

What is generally considered to be "moderate smoking"?

For pipe smokers 3 pipefuls a day.

For cigar smokers: 2 to 3 cigars a day.

For cigarette smokers: 8 to 10 cigarettes a day.

Can moderate smoking for one person be excessive for another?

Yes. This depends on the state of health of the smoker and his particular sensitivity or lack of sensitivity to the effects of tobacco.

Are people ever allergic to smoking?

Not in the same manner in which they are allergic to pollens, molds, or dusts. However, there is such a thing as hypersensitivity to tobacco.

What are some of the evidences of hypersensitivity to tobacco?

1. Congestion of the mucous membranes of the nose, sinuses, and respiratory passages. This often leads to the excretion of large quantities of mucus.
2. Inflammation of the lining of the eyes (conjunctivitis).
3. Fits of coughing.
4. Loss of appetite, occasionally accompanied by nausea.
5. Pain in the heart region.
6. Dizziness, headache, or loss of equilibrium.
7. Coldness, numbness, or tingling in the hands and feet.
8. Severe cramps in the calves when walking (claudication).
9. Elevation of the blood pressure.
10. Rapid pulse rate.

How does a doctor decide when to advise his patient to stop smoking?

If the symptoms enumerated above appear after smoking, the doctor will probably advise discontinuance of the practice.

SOCIAL BEHAVIOR

See ALCOHOL AND ALCOHOLISM; CLOTHING; FAMILY RE-
LATIONSHIPS; HEARING AND DEAFNESS; HOBBIES; HOTELS,
APARTMENTS, AND COMMUNITIES FOR THE AGING; INSTI-
TUTIONAL CARE; MENTAL CHANGES; PSYCHOTHERAPY;
RETIREMENT.

Does one's social behavior tend to change with advancing age?

This varies so much from one individual to another that no
generalizations can be made. However, it is common knowledge that those who have been socially adjusted during their
earlier years will continue to be so in old age, unless some
illness, such as arteriosclerosis, affects their mental abilities
and attitudes. Conversely, those who have always found it
difficult to adjust to their surroundings will find it increasingly
difficult as they get older.

Are there any special rules to be followed in dealing with the behavior problems of older people?

Yes. One should appreciate that many of the problems originate from irreversible changes. Thus, tolerance and kindness
should be the guiding principles in one's attitude toward them.
The knowledge that they are still important to their family
and friends is the best medicine for older people during
periods of maladjustment.

Is it natural for aging people to become fixed in their habits?

Yes. They are most comfortable doing things they have been
accustomed to doing for years. If they had firmly established
habits during youth and middle age, it is likely that these patterns of behavior will be accentuated during the later years.
If they lived a disorganized existence, it will tend to be even
less organized as they advance in age.

Should those closely associated with older people attempt to alter their patterns of behavior?

Not unless their mode of living makes them or those around
them unhappy.

What can be done about people whose social behavior be-comes unacceptable?

It must first be determined whether physical changes are responsible, or whether the behavioral changes are emotional

in origin. Professional help is necessary in order to make this determination. Treatment will depend on the cause of the disturbance. (*See* INSTITUTIONAL CARE.)

Are specially planned social activities helpful to those who have become socially maladjusted?

Yes. There are many agencies to which one can turn for help in planning social activity for elderly people. Church organizations, social welfare agencies, and city, state, and governmental agencies are alert to the needs of aging people and can be most helpful in advising on activities that will lead to greater social happiness. (*See* ORGANIZATIONS AND AGENCIES.)

When should older people receive guidance about their social life?

Mainly when they themselves feel the need for such help. Most people in their sixties and seventies are able to care for themselves and will resent suggestions that they require special social planning.

Should older people be encouraged to join social clubs for the aging?

Yes, if their social life is barren or if they feel the need for this type of activity. It is a mistake to pressure them if they do not wish to participate.

Is there a tendency for older people to want to be alone more than when they were young?

Some may become more self-sufficient; others may feel a greater need for companionship. The important thing to remember is that if they are content in the way they are living, they should not be disturbed.

Do people often become more active socially as they grow older?

Usually a retiring person will continue his pattern of behavior throughout life. Those who were very active during their younger days may continue the pattern insofar as they are able.

What can be done to help those aging people who lose interest in physical appearance, manners, and observance of the social amenities?

Most older people are unaware that they are acting differently. When it is brought to their attention by someone in whom they have confidence, they will often modify their behavior. Success lies in being kind and in pointing out their omissions in a sympathetic manner. Older people will resent sermons and lectures from younger people.

Should aging people be encouraged to seek the company of people their own age, or should they be encouraged to mix with younger people?

This is a matter of personal preference and varies from individual to individual. Some older people are greatly in demand by younger people and mix with them extremely well. Their greater wisdom and knowledge is often a particular source of pleasure to younger people who seek their company. Other aging people will prefer friends their own age.

When aging people insist on the company of younger people who do not wish to reciprocate, a real problem presents itself. If this occurs, it is important to seek professional advice so that family relationships are not endangered.

What measures should be taken to avoid embarrassing older people who live with their children?

In the great majority of instances no special measures are necessary, but children should avoid making excuses for their parents in front of others. Most people are fully aware that there are changes in social behavior as one ages. They need no special reminder of this obvious fact.

The children of aging parents should avoid situations that might become embarrassing. For instance, if a party is being given and it is known beforehand that there will be drinking or that the conversation might become unacceptable to an older person, arrangements should be made to permit that person to be out of the house.

Do people tend to become less punctual as they age?

Yes, except those who were sticklers for punctuality in their younger days. Much anxiety could be avoided if the children of aging parents would realize that punctuality is less important to those in their seventies or eighties.

Do older people tend to become less modest?

This may occur, but when it does, it is usually a sign of senility.

THE SOCIAL SECURITY MANUAL

See HEALTH INSURANCE AND HOSPITAL INSURANCE; ORGANIZATIONS AND AGENCIES; RETIREMENT.

THE BASIC IDEA

The basic idea of social security is a simple one: During working years employees, their employers, and self-employed people pay social security contributions which are pooled in special trust funds. When earnings stop or are reduced because the worker retires, dies, or becomes disabled, monthly cash benefits are paid to replace part of the earnings the family has lost.

Part of the contributions made go into a separate hospital insurance trust fund so that when workers and their dependents reach 65 they will have help in paying their hospital bills. Voluntary medical insurance, also available to people 65 or over, helps pay doctors' bills and other medical expenses. This program is financed out of premiums shared half-and-half by the older people who sign up and by the Federal Government.

Nine out of ten working people in the United States are now building protection for themselves and their families under the social security program.

YOUR SOCIAL SECURITY

MONTHLY CASH BENEFITS

To get monthly cash payments for yourself and your family, or for your survivors to get payments in case of your death, you must first have credit for a certain amount of work under social security. This credit may have been earned at any time after 1936.

Most employees get credit for ¼ year of work if they are paid $50 or more in covered wages in a 3-month calendar quarter. Four quarters are counted for any full year in which a person has $400 or more in self-employment income. A

575

worker who receives farm wages gets credit for ¼ year of
work for each $100 of covered wages he has in a year up
to $400.

You can be either fully or currently insured, depending
on the total amount of credit you have for work under social
security and the amount you have in the last 3 years. The table
on page 583 shows which kinds of cash benefits may be paid
if you are fully insured and which kinds may be paid if
you are currently insured.

If you stop working under social security before you have
earned enough credit to be insured, the cash benefits will be
payable to you. The earnings already credited to you will remain on your social security record; if you later return to
covered work, regardless of your age, all your covered earnings will be considered.

Fully Insured

Just how much credit you must have to be fully insured
depends upon the year you reach 65 if you are a man, or
62 if you are a woman, or upon the date of your death or
disability.

The amount of credit you will need is measured in quarter-
year units of work called quarters of coverage; but for convenience, the table on this page is given in years. The people
in your social security office will be glad to give you further
details if you have questions.

You are fully insured if you have credit for at least as many
years as shown on the appropriate line of the following chart.

If you reach 65 (62 if a woman) or die or become disabled	You will be fully insured if you have credit for this much work
In 1965	3½ years
In 1967	4
In 1969	4½
In 1971	5
In 1975	6
In 1979	7
In 1983	8
In 1987	9
In 1991 or later	10

If you become disabled or die before reaching 65 (62 for a
woman), you are fully insured if you have credit for ¼ year
of work for each year after 1950 and up to the year of your

disability or death. In counting the number of years after 1950, omit years before you were 22.

No one is fully insured with credit for less than 1½ years of work and no one needs more than 10 years of work to be fully insured. Having a fully insured status, however, means only that certain kinds of cash benefits may be payable—it does not determine the amount. The amount will depend on your average earnings.

Currently Insured

You will be currently insured if you have social security credit for at least 1½ years of work within the 3 years before you die or become entitled to retirement benefits.

AMOUNTS OF MONTHLY PAYMENTS

The amount of your monthly retirement or disability benefit is based on your average earnings under social security over a period of years. The amount of the monthly payments to your dependents or to your survivors in case of your death also depends on the amount of your average earnings.

The exact amount of your benefit cannot be figured until there is an application for benefits. This is because all of your earnings up to the time of the application may be considered in figuring your benefit. The Social Security Administration will, of course, figure your exact benefit at that time.

You can estimate the amount of the worker's benefit, however, by following these steps:
• If you were born before 1930, start with 1956;
1. Count the number of years to be used in figuring your average earnings as follows:
• If you were born after 1929, start with the year you reached 27.
Count your starting year and each year up until (but not including):
• The year you reach 65, if you are a man;
• The year you reach 62, if you are a woman;
• The year the worker becomes disabled or dies, for disability or death benefits.

(Note: At least 5 years of earnings must be used to figure retirement benefits and at least 2 years to figure disability or survivor benefits.)

2. List the amount of the worker's earnings for all years beginning with 1951. (Include earnings in the year of death or the year disability began.) Do not count *more than*

$3,600 for each year 1951 through 1954; $4,200 for each year 1955 through 1958; $4,800 for each year 1959 through 1965; $6,600 for 1966 and 1967; $7,800 for 1968 through 1971; and $9,000 for 1972 and after.

3. Cross off your list the years of lowest earnings until the number remaining is the same as your answer to step 1. (It may be necessary to leave years in which you had no earnings on your list.)

4. Add up the earnings for the years left on your list, and divide by the number of years you used (your answer to step 1).

The result is your average yearly earnings covered by social security over this period.

Look in the table on page 579 and estimate your benefit from the examples given there.

Increasing Payments by Additional Work

If you work after you start getting benefits and your added earnings will result in higher benefits, your benefit will be automatically refigured after the additional earnings are credited to your record.

Special Payments

Special payments of $48.30 a month ($72.50 for a couple) can be made under the social security program to certain people 72 and over who are not eligible for social security benefits. These payments are intended to assure some regular income for older people who had little or no opportunity to earn social security protection during their working years.

People who reached 72 in 1968 or later need credit for some work under social security to be eligible for special payments. Those who reached 72 in 1968 need credit for ¾ year of work under social security. The amount of work credit needed increases gradually each year for people reaching 72 after 1968, until it is the same as that required for retirement benefits. (This will be in 1972 for men and 1970 for women.)

The special payments are not made for any month for which the person receives payments under a Federally-aided public assistance program. The special payments are reduced by the amount of any other governmental pension, retirement benefit, or annuity.

Payments to people who have credit for less than ¾ of a

EXAMPLES OF MONTHLY CASH PAYMENTS

Average yearly earnings after 1950*	$923 or less	$1,800	$3,000	$4,200	$5,400	$6,600	$7,800
Retired worker—65 or older / Disabled worker—under 65	70.40	111.90	145.60	177.70	208.80	240.30	275.80
Wife 65 or older	35.20	56.00	72.80	88.90	104.40	120.20	137.90
Retired worker at 62	56.40	89.60	116.50	142.20	167.10	192.30	220.70
Wife at 62, no child	26.40	42.00	54.60	66.70	78.30	90.20	103.50
Widow at 60	61.10	80.10	104.20	127.20	149.40	171.90	197.30
Widow or widower at 62	70.40	92.40	120.20	146.70	172.30	198.30	227.60
Disabled widow at 50	42.80	56.10	72.90	89.00	104.50	120.30	138.00
Wife under 65 and one child	35.20	56.00	77.10	131.20	181.10	194.90	206.90
Widowed mother and one child	105.60	167.90	218.40	266.60	313.20	360.60	413.80
Widowed mother and two children	105.60	167.90	222.70	308.90	389.90	435.20	482.70
One child of retired or disabled worker	35.20	56.00	72.80	88.90	104.40	120.20	137.90
One surviving child	70.40	84.00	109.20	133.30	156.60	180.30	206.90
Maximum family payment	105.60	167.90	222.70	308.90	389.90	435.20	482.70

* Generally, average earnings are figured over the period from 1951 until the worker reaches retirement age, becomes disabled, or dies. Up to 5 years of low earnings or no earnings can be excluded. The maximum earnings creditable for social security are $3,600 for 1951-1954; $4,200 for 1955-1958; $4,800 for 1959-1965; and $6,600 for 1966-1967. The maximum creditable for 1968-1971 is $7,800, and beginning in 1972, $9,000; but average earnings usually cannot reach these amounts until later. Because of this, the benefits shown in the last column on the right generally will not be payable until later. When a person is entitled to more than one benefit, the amount actually payable is limited to the larger of the benefits.

year of work covered by social security are made from general revenues, not from social security trust funds.

DISABILITY PAYMENTS

If you become disabled before 65, you and certain members of your family may be eligible for benefits.

Do not wait too long after you are disabled to apply for benefits; if you wait more than a year, you may lose benefits. Payments may begin with the 7th full month of disability.

If you are found eligible for disability insurance benefits, you will remain eligible as long as you are disabled. When you reach 65, your benefit will be changed to retirement payments at the same rate.

Who Is Considered Disabled?

A person is considered disabled only if he has a severe physical or mental condition which—

- Prevents him from working, and
- Is expected to last (or has lasted) for at least 12 months or is expected to result in death.

A person with a severe medical condition could be eligible even if he manages to do a little work.

How Much Work Credit Is Required for a Disabled Worker?

If you become disabled before you are 24, you need credit for 1½ years of work in the 3 years before you became disabled.

If you become disabled between 24 and 31, you need social security credits for half the time after you are 21 and before you become disabled.

To get disability benefits if you become disabled at 31 or later, you must be fully insured and have credit for 5 years of work in the 10 years just before you become disabled.

The Amount of Your Disability Benefit

The amount of your monthly disability payment is generally the same as the retirement benefit you would get if you were 65. Figure your average earnings as if you reached 65 (62 for a woman) at the time you become disabled. If you are a disabled widow, surviving divorced wife, or dependent widower, the amount of your benefit is figured from what your spouse would have received. (See page 579.)

Vocational Rehabilitation

Everyone who applies for social security disability benefits is referred for possible services to his State rehabilitation agency. These services help many people to return to productive employment. Social security often helps pay the cost of services provided to applicants by rehabilitation agencies.

For more information about the disability benefits for blind people and disabled widows, disabled surviving divorced wives, and disabled dependent widowers, get in touch with your social security office.

FAMILY PAYMENTS

Monthly payments can be made to certain dependents:
- When the worker gets retirement or disability benefits;
- When the worker dies.

These dependents are—
- Unmarried children under 18, or between 18 and 22 if they are full-time students;
- Unmarried children 18 or over who were severely disabled before they reached 18 and who continue to be disabled;
- A wife or widow, regardless of her age, if she is caring for a child under 18 or disabled and the child gets payments based on the worker's record;
- A wife 62 or widow 60 or older, even if there are no children entitled to payments;
- A widow 50 or older (or dependent widower 50 or older) who becomes disabled not later than 7 years after the death of the worker or, in the case of a widow, not later than 7 years after the end of her entitlement to benefits as a widow with a child in her care;
- A dependent husband or widower 62 or over;
- Dependent parents 62 or over after a worker dies.

In addition to monthly benefits, a lump-sum payment may be made after the worker's death.

Under the law in effect before February 1968, there were circumstances in which benefits could be paid to children of a woman worker only if she had worked 1½ out the the last 3 years before she retired, became disabled, or died, or if she had actually provided most of the child's support. This provision, which prevented payment of benefits in some cases, has been removed. Now children are considered dependent on both their mothers and their fathers, and they may become eligible for benefits when either parent becomes entitled to retirement or disability benefits or dies.

Payments may also be made under certain conditions to a divorced wife at 62 or a surviving divorced wife at 60 (or a disabled surviving divorced wife 50 or older). To qualify for benefits, a divorced wife must have been married to the worker for 20 years and also meet certain support requirements. Benefits also can be paid a dependent surviving divorced wife at any age if she is caring for her deceased former husband's child under 18 or disabled who is entitled to benefits. For more information about this provision, get in touch with your social security office.

Monthly payments to the wife or dependent husband of a person entitled to retirement or disability payments generally cannot be made until the marriage has been in effect at least 1 year unless the couple are parents of a child. Payments can be made to the widow, stepchild, or dependent widower of a deceased worker if the marriage lasted 9 months or longer; or in the case of death in line of duty in the uniformed services, and in the case of accidental death if the marriage lasted for 3 months, under special circumstances.

Amount of Your Family's Benefits

Cash benefits to your dependents, and to your survivors in case of your death, are figured from the amount of your retirement or disability benefit.

Permanently reduced benefits are received by:

- Workers and their wives who choose to start receiving retirement benefits while they are between 62 and 65;
- Widows who choose to start receiving benefits between 60 and 62; and
- Disabled widows and disabled dependent widowers 50 or older who receive benefits before they reach 62.

The amount of the reduction depends on the number of months they receive benefits before they reach 65 (62 for widows and disabled dependent widowers). On the average, people who choose to get benefits early will collect about the same value in total benefits over the years, but in smaller installments to take account of the longer period during which they will be paid.

If a person could be entitled to monthly benefits based on the social security records of two or more workers, he will receive no more than the largest of the benefits.

TYPES OF CASH BENEFITS

This table shows the principal types of payments and the insured status needed for each.

Retirement

Monthly payment to—	If you are—
* You as a retired worker and your wife and child	Fully insured.
Your dependent husband 62 or over	Fully insured.

Survivors

Monthly payments to your—	If at death you are—
* Widow 60 or over or disabled widow 50-59	Fully insured.
* Widow (regardless of age) if caring for your child who is under 18 or disabled and is entitled to benefits	Either fully or currently insured.
Dependent child	Either fully or currently insured.
Dependent widower 62 or over and disabled dependent widower 50-61	Fully insured.
Dependent parent at 62	Fully insured.
Lump-sum death payment	Either fully or currently insured.

Disability

Monthly payments to—	If you are—
You and your dependents if you are disabled	Fully insured and if you meet work requirements explained on page 580.

* Under certain conditions, payments can also be made to your divorced wife or surviving divorced wife.

The lump-sum payment at a worker's death is ordinarily three times the amount of his monthly retirement benefit at 65, or $255, whichever is less.

Benefits Not Taxable

Social security benefits you receive are not subject to Federal income tax.

AN APPLICATION IS NECESSARY

Before payments can start, an application must be filed.

When you are nearing 65 or if you become disabled, get in touch with your social security office.

It is important for you to inquire at your local social security office 2 or 3 months before you reach 65, not only for the possibility of retirement benefits, but also for Medicare benefits, which are available whether or not you retire. If you wait until the month you reach 65 to apply for the medical insurance part of Medicare, you will lose at least one month of protection. It is always to your advantage to apply before you reach 65, even if you do not plan to retire. If you have high earnings which would increase the amount of your benefit in the year you are 65 or later, your benefit amount will be refigured. You will always be sure of receiving benefits at the highest possible rate.

When a person who has worked under the social security law dies, some member of his family should get in touch with the social security office.

If you cannot come to the social security office—perhaps because you are housebound or hospitalized—write or telephone. A social security representative can arrange to visit you.

Long delay in filing an application can cause loss of some benefits, since back payments for monthly cash benefits can be made for no more than 12 months.

An application for a lump-sum death payment must usually be made within 2 years of the worker's death.

Proofs Needed

When you apply for social security benefits, take your own social security card or a record of your number; and if your claim is based on the earnings of another person, his card or a record of the number.

You will need proof of your age. If you have a birth certificate or a baptismal certificate made at or shortly after your birth, take it with you when you apply. If you are applying for wife's or widow's benefits, take your marriage certificate; if your children are eligible, their birth certificates.

Take your Form W-2, Wage and Tax Statement, for the previous year; if you are self-employed, a copy of your last Federal income tax return.

Proof that the applicant was being supported by the insured person is required before benefits can be paid to a parent after the death of a working son or daughter, or to a husband or widower whose working wife has retired, become disabled, or died. Generally, this proof must be furnished within 2 years after the worker dies, or, in the case of husband's benefits, within 2 years after his wife applies for cash benefits.

Do not delay applying because you do not have all of these proofs. When you apply, the people in your social security office can tell you about other proofs that may be used.

If you apply for retirement or survivor payments and supply all of the necessary information and then 4 to 6 weeks go by after the time you thought your benefits should start and you do not hear about your claim, get in touch with your social security office. There are special procedures for speeding payments in these cases and your social security office will be glad to do everything possible to prevent delays in your payments.

Information Is Confidential

Under the law and regulations, social security records are confidential. Information from your record may not be disclosed without proper authorization.

If You Work After Payments Start

When you apply for retirement or survivors insurance benefits, your social security office will explain how any future earnings you may have will affect your payments and when and how to report your later earnings to the Social Security Administration. The explanation that follows is intended to give a general idea of the conditions under which benefits are paid to people who are still working.

For taxable years ending after 1967, the following rules apply:

If you earn $1,680 or less in a year, you get all the benefits.

If you earn more than $1,680 in a year while you are under 72, the general rule is that $1 in benefits to you (and your family) will be withheld for each $2 you earn from $1,680 to $2,880. In addition, $1 in benefits will be withheld for each $1 of earnings over $2,880.

Exception to the general rule: Regardless of total earnings

in a year, benefits are payable for any month in which you
neither earn wages of more than $140 nor perform substan-
tial services in self-employment.

*The decision as to whether you are performing substantial
services in self-employment depends on the time you devote
to your business, the kind of services you perform, how your
services compare with those you performed in past years, and
other circumstances of your particular case.*

Benefits are also payable for all months in which you are
72 or older, regardless of the amount of your earnings in
months after you reach 72.

Your earnings as a retired worker may affect your own
and your dependents' right to benefits. If you get payments as
a dependent or survivor, your earnings will affect only your
benefit and not those of other members of the family.

Earnings which must be counted—

Earnings from work of any kind must be counted, whether
or not the work is covered by social security. (There is one
exception: tips amounting to less than $20 a month with any
one employer are not counted.) Total wages (not just take-
home pay) and all net earnings from self-employment must
be added together in figuring your earnings for the year. However, income from savings, investments, pensions, insurance,
or royalties you receive after 65 because of copyrights or
patents you obtained before 65, does not affect your benefits
and should not be counted in your earnings for this purpose.

In the year in which your benefits start and the year your
benefits end, your earnings for the entire year are counted in
determining the amount of benefits that can be paid.

Earnings after you reach 72 will not cause any deductions
from your benefits for months in which you are 72 or over.
However, earnings for the entire year in which you reach 72
count in figuring what benefits are due you for months before
you are 72.

For more information about how working after you apply
for benefits will affect your retirement or survivors payments,
inquire at your social security office.

Beneficiaries Outside the United States

Special rules affect the payment of benefits to people outside the United States. If you intend to go outside the United
States for 30 days or more while you are receiving benefits,
ask your social security office for Leaflet No. SSA-609.

If you are not a citizen or national of the United States,
your absence from this country may affect your right to bene-

fits. The people in your social security office will be glad to explain these provisions to you.

Reasons Why Payments Stop

When monthly payments are started, they continue until they must be stopped for one of the reasons given below. If any of these occurs, it must always be promptly reported to the Social Security Administration.

Marriage—Benefits for a child, an aged dependent parent, a disabled dependent widower, a divorced wife, a disabled widow, or widow receiving mother's benefits generally stop when the beneficiary marries a person who is not also getting social security dependent's or survivor's benefits.

There is an exception for the widow who remarries after reaching age 60. If she could have qualified for benefits on her deceased husband's record, she may still get benefits on that record. She would qualify for ½ of her deceased husband's retirement benefit, or (at 62) for the amount of the wife's benefit on her later husband's record, whichever is larger. A similar provision applies to widowers who remarry after 62.

Divorce—Payments to a wife or a dependent husband generally end if a divorce is granted. However, if a wife 62 or older and her husband are divorced, benefits to the wife may continue if the marriage lasted at least 20 continuous years before the divorce. (If a wife under 65 and her husband are divorced after 20 continuous years of marriage, she may receive benefits at 62 or later provided certain conditions are met. For more information, get in touch with any social security office.)

No child "in her care"—Payment to a wife under 62 or to a widow or surviving divorced wife under 60 will generally stop when she no longer has in her care a child under 18 or disabled. A widow or surviving divorced wife who is 50 or over and is severely disabled should get in touch with her social security office for information about any benefits that may be payable.

Child reaches 18—When a child reaches age 18, his payments stop unless he is—

- Disabled (if so, he and his mother may be eligible for benefits for as long as he is disabled), or
- A full-time, unmarried student (if so, he may be eligible for benefits until he reaches 22).

Adoption—When a child is adopted, his payments end unless he is adopted by his stepparent, grandparent, aunt, uncle, brother, or sister after the death of the person on whose record he is receiving benefits.

Death—When any person receiving monthly benefits dies, his or her payments end.

Disability benefits—When the benefits payable to a person stop because he is no longer disabled, the benefits payable to his dependents also stop.

If payments end because of any of these reasons, the last check due is the one for the month before the event.

FINANCING THE PROGRAMS

Federal retirement, survivors, and disability benefits, and hospital insurance benefits are paid for by contributions based on earnings covered under social security.

If you are employed, you and your employer share the responsibility of paying contributions. If you are self-employed, you pay contributions for retirement, survivors, and disability insurance at a slightly lower rate than the combined rate for an employee and his employer. However, the hospital insurance contribution rate is the same for the employer, the employee, and the self-employed person.

As long as you have earnings that are covered by the law, you continue to pay contributions regardless of your age and even if you are receiving social security benefits.

How Contributions Are Paid

If you are employed, your contribution is deducted from your wages each payday. Your employer sends it, with an equal amount as his own share of the contribution, to the Internal Revenue Service.

If you are self-employed and your net earnings are $400 or more in a year, you must report your earnings and pay your self-employment contribution each year when you file your individual income tax return. This is true even if you owe no income tax.

Your wages and self-employment income are entered on your individual record by the Social Security Administration. This record of your earnings will be used to determine your eligibility for benefits and the amount of cash benefits you will receive.

The maximum amount of earnings that can count for social security and on which you pay social security contributions is shown in the following table:

Year	Amount
1937-50	$3,000
1951-54	3,600
1955-58	4,200
1959-65	4,800
1966-67	6,600
1968-71	7,800
1972 and after	9,000

Earnings over the maximums may have been reported to your social security record and may appear on your earnings statement, but cannot be used to figure your benefit rate.

When you work for more than one employer in a year and pay social security contributions on wages over $7,800 for 1968 through 1971 or on wages over $9,000 in 1972 or later, you may claim a refund of the excess contributions on your income tax return for that year. If you work for only one employer and he deducts too much in contributions, you should apply to the employer for a refund.

A refund is made only when more than the required amount of contributions has been paid.

Questions about contributions or refunds should be directed to the Internal Revenue Service.

This table shows the schedule of contribution rates now in the law:

CONTRIBUTION RATE SCHEDULE FOR EMPLOYEES AND EMPLOYERS (EACH)

Years	Percent of Covered Earnings		
	For Retirement, Survivors, and Disability Insurance	For Hospital Insurance	TOTAL
1969-70	4.2	0.6	4.8
1971-72	4.6	.6	5.2
1973-75	5.0	.65	5.65
1976-79	5.15	.7	5.85
1980-86	5.15	.8	5.95
1987 and after	5.15	.9	6.05

CONTRIBUTION RATE SCHEDULE FOR SELF-EMPLOYED PEOPLE

Years	Percent of Covered Earnings		
	For Retirement, Survivors, and Disability Insurance	For Hospital Insurance	TOTAL
1969-70	6.3	0.6	6.9
1971-72	6.9	.6	7.5
1973-75	7.0	.65	7.65
1976-79	7.0	.7	7.7
1980-86	7.0	.8	7.8
1987 and after	7.0	.9	7.9

THE TRUST FUNDS

Social security contributions for retirement, survivors, and disability insurance go into the Federal Old-Age and Survivors Insurance Trust Fund and the Federal Disability Insurance Trust Fund. They are used to pay the benefits and administrative expenses of these programs and may be used for no other purpose.

There are two other trust funds—a Federal Hospital Insurance Trust Fund, into which hospital insurance contributions are placed, and out of which hospital insurance benefits and administrative expenses are paid; and a Federal Supplementary Medical Insurance Trust Fund, into which the enrollees' premiums, along with the Government's matching contributions, are placed, and out of which the benefits and administrative costs of the medical insurance program are paid.

Funds not required for current benefit payments and expenses are invested in interest-bearing U.S. Government securities.

Certain costs, however, are financed from general funds of the U.S. Treasury, including the cost of hospital insurance benefits for people who are uninsured for cash social security benefits; the Government's share of the cost for supplementary medical insurance; and cash payments for certain uninsured people 72 and over.

KINDS OF WORK COVERED

Almost every kind of employment and self-employment is covered by social security. Some occupations, however, are covered only if certain conditions are met.

Farming

You receive social security credit as a farm operator or rancher if your net earnings from self-employment are $400 or more in a year. You must report your net earnings from self-employment as a part of your income tax return.

If your gross earnings from farming in a year are between $600 and $2,400, you may report two-thirds of your gross earnings, instead of your net earnings, for social security purposes. If your gross earnings from farming are more than $2,400 and your net earnings are less than $1,600, you may report $1,600 for social security purposes.

If you rent your farm land to someone else, you receive social security credits for your rental income if you "materially participate" in the actual production of the farm commodities or the management of production.

Ministers and Members of Religious Orders

Before 1968 income from the ministry received by a clergyman (ordained, commissioned, or licensed ministers, Christian Science practitioners, and members of religious orders who have not taken a vow of poverty) was not covered by social security unless the clergyman signed a form stating that he wanted it to be covered.

For taxable years ending after December 1967, earnings from services as a clergyman will automatically be covered unless the clergyman files an application to have it excluded, stating that he is conscientiously opposed, or opposed by reason of religious principles, to receiving social security benefits based on services as a clergyman.

A clergyman who qualifies to be excluded from coverage may complete Form 4361 and file it with the Internal Revenue Service. This form may be secured at any social security office or at any Internal Revenue Service office. Once this form is filed it cannot be withdrawn.

Clergymen who elected coverage for any year before 1968 will not be affected by the new provisions. They will continue to be covered.

A clergyman reports his income and makes his tax contributions as if he were self-employed, even though he may be working as an employee.

Members of religious orders who have taken a vow of poverty are not covered by social security.

For more information about social security coverage for clergymen, ask for a copy of Leaflet No. 9 at your social security office.

Family Employment

Work done by a parent as an employee of his son or daughter in the course of the son's or daughter's trade or business is covered by the law. Domestic work in the household of a son or daughter is not covered unless special conditions are met.

Work for a parent by a daughter or son (also a stepchild, adopted, or foster child) under 21 is not covered.

Also not covered is any work performed by a wife for her husband or by a husband for his wife.

Household Workers

A domestic worker's cash wages (including transportation expenses if paid in cash) for work in a private household are covered by the law if they amount to $50 or more from one employer in a calendar quarter.

If you employ a household worker who will come under the law and you are not receiving the forms for making the earnings reports, ask your social security office or your Internal Revenue Service office for a copy of Leaflet No. 21. This leaflet explains how to get the forms and make the reports.

Employees Who Receive Tips

Cash tips amounting to $20 or more in a month with one employer are covered by social security.

You must give your employer a written report of the amount of your tips within 10 days after the month in which you receive them. Your employer will collect your contributions due on these tips from other wages he owes you or from funds you turn over to him for that purpose. Otherwise, your contribution must be paid by you to the Internal Revenue Service.

If your report is late or incomplete, you will be liable for your social security contribution on tips not reported, and you may also be subject to a penalty in an amount equal to ½ of that contribution.

Your employer includes your tips reported to him along with your other wages in his social security wage reports and on Form W-2, but he does not have to match your social security contribution on the tips.

If you receive tips, you can get further information at your social security office.

Employees of Non-profit Organizations

Employees of non-profit organizations operated exclusively for religious, charitable, scientific, literary, educational, or humane purposes, or for testing for public safety, may be covered by the social security law if—
- The organization waives its exemption from the payment of social security contributions by filing a certificate (Form SS-15) with the Internal Revenue Service, and
- Those employees who wish to be covered indicate their desire to participate by signing the Form SS-15a that goes with the certificate.

Employees who sign the form and employees who are hired or rehired after the calendar quarter in which the waiver certificate is filed are covered. If any employee of a non-profit organization earns wages of less than $50 in a quarter, his wages for that quarter are not covered.

Employees of State and Local Governments

State and local government employees may be covered by social security under voluntary agreements between the individual State and the Federal Government.

Farm Employees

When you work for a farmer, a ranch operator, or a farm labor crew leader, you earn social security credits:
- If the employer pays you $150 or more in cash during the year for farm work, or
- If you do farm work for the employer on 20 or more days during a year for cash wages figured on a time basis (rather than on a piece-rate basis).

For more information about farm labor crews and the conditions under which the farmer or the crew leader is the employer, get Leaflet No. 15 from your local security office.

Household workers employed on a farm or ranch operated for profit are covered under the same rules as other farm employees.

Federal Employment

Most employees of the Federal Government not covered by their own staff retirement system are covered by social security.

Military Service

Active duty or active duty for training you perform as a member of the uniformed services of the United States after 1956 counts toward social security protection for you and your family. From 1957 through 1967 your basic pay was credited to your social security record.

For active duty after 1967, your credits for each month of active duty will generally amount to your basic pay plus $100. No additional deductions will be made from your pay for the extra $100 credits. You cannot, however, get social security credit for more than $7,800 in any year ($9,000 starting in 1972), including the extra credits.

For Active Duty After September 15, 1940, and Before 1957—

Social security credits of $160 a month are given to most veterans who served during this period. When credits are given, they count the same as wages in civilian employment. These credits are not actually listed on your record, but if they would affect your benefit, the people in the social security office will ask for proof of your military service when an application is filed on your record.

Railroad Employment

Earnings from railroad work are reported to the Railroad Retirement Board and not to the Social Security Administration. Your social security record will not include any work you may have done for a railroad.

Benefits based on work for a railroad are ordinarily paid by the Railroad Retirement Board. However, if you have less than 120 months (10 years) of railroad service when you retire or become disabled, your earnings for railroad work after 1936 are considered in figuring your disability or retirement payments under the social security law.

A retired worker who has at least 120 months of railroad service and who has also done enough work under social security to qualify for social security benefits may receive retirement benefits under both railroad retirement and social security.

Survivors of a worker can be entitled under one system only, either railroad retirement or social security, even though the worker may have been entitled during his lifetime under both. Regardless of which program will pay the benefits, records of the deceased worker's railroad earnings after 1936 and his earnings under social security will be combined to determine payments to survivors.

Railroad workers or their survivors can get further information from any social security or railroad retirement office, or they may write to the Railroad Retirement Board, 844 Rush Street, Chicago, Illinois 60611.

American Citizens Working Abroad

U.S. citizens employed by American employers in foreign countries or aboard vessels or aircraft of foreign registry are covered by social security. Seamen and airmen employed on American vessels or aircraft are usually covered regardless of citizenship.

U.S. citizens working abroad for a foreign subsidiary of an American corporation may be covered if the parent firm makes an agreement with the Secretary of the Treasury to see that social security contributions are paid for all U.S. citizens employed abroad by the foreign subsidiary.

Foreign Agricultural Workers

Agricultural work performed by foreign workers admitted to the United States on a temporary basis to do agricultural work is not covered.

Foreign Exchange Visitors

Work performed by foreign nationals temporarily in the United States to study, teach, conduct research, etc., under a foreign exchange program is not covered under social security if it is performed to carry out the purpose for which they were admitted to the country.

SOCIAL SECURITY CARDS

You must have a social security number if your work is covered by the social security law or if you receive certain kinds of taxable income. Your social security number is also used for income tax purposes. Show your card to each of your employers when you start to work. Upon request, show it to anyone who pays you income that must be reported.

You can get a social security card at any social security office. The number on your card is used to keep a record of your earnings and of any benefits to which you and your dependents become entitled.

You need only one social security number during your lifetime. Notify your social security office if you ever get more than one number.

If you change your name, or if you lose your social security card, go to a social security office to get a card showing your new name or a duplicate of the card you lost.

CHECKING YOUR RECORD

Each employer is required to give you receipts for the social security contributions he deducts from your pay. He does this at the end of each year and also when you stop working for him. These receipts, such as Form W-2, will help you check on your social security record. They show the amount of your wages that counts for social security. For most kinds of work, your wages paid in forms other than cash—for instance, the value of meals or living quarters—must be included. For domestic work in a private household or for farm work, only cash wages count.

You should keep a record of the amount of self-employment income you have reported.

You should check your record from time to time to make sure your earnings have been correctly reported. This is especially important if you have frequently changed jobs. Simply ask your social security office for a postcard form to use in requesting a copy of your record, complete, sign, and mail it.

If Your Records Do Not Agree

If your records of your earnings do not agree with the amounts shown on the statement you get from the Social Security Administration, get in touch with your social security office promptly. If you write, give your social security number, the periods of work in question, your pay in each period, and your employer's name and address. If the earnings in question were from self-employment, include the date your tax return was filed and the address of the Internal Revenue Service office to which the return was sent.

RIGHT OF APPEAL

If you feel that a decision made on your claim is not correct, you may ask the Social Security Administration to reconsider it. If, after this reconsideration, you are not satisfied the decision is correct, you may ask for a hearing by a hearing examiner of the Bureau of Hearings and Appeals. And, if you are not satisfied that the decision of the hearing examiner is correct, you may request a review by the Appeals Council. The Social Security Administration makes no charge for any of these appeals. You may, however, choose to be represented by a person of your own choice, and he may charge you a fee. The amount of such a fee is limited and must be approved by the Social Security Administration.

Someone in your social security office will explain how you may appeal and will help you get your claim reconsidered, or request a hearing.

If you are still not satisfied, you may take your case to the Federal courts.

SOCIAL SECURITY OFFICES

The Social Security Administration has over 850 offices conveniently located throughout the country. These offices have representatives who regularly visit neighboring communities.

If any of your questions about monthly social security benefits or Medicare are not answered in this book, call, write, or visit your social security office. The people who work there will be glad to answer questions and to explain your rights. They will also assist groups and organizations in informing their members about social security through talks, films, and other planned activities.

For the address of your social security office, look in the telephone directory under Social Security Administration, or ask at the post office.

YOUR MEDICARE HANDBOOK

HEALTH INSURANCE UNDER SOCIAL SECURITY

Dear Beneficiary:

This is Your Medicare Handbook. It explains the benefits you are entitled to under Medicare and tells how the program works. I believe this handbook will answer most of your questions about Medicare, but some details have necessarily been omitted.

Should you ever have a question about the amount of a bill Medicare helped pay, get in touch with the organization that handled the payment.

If you need further information or want help concerning your Medicare protection or any other social security matters, please get in touch with your social security office. The people there are always glad to help you.

Sincerely yours,

ROBERT M. BALL
Commissioner of Social Security

P.S.: The cost of health care has been rising faster than other costs of living. When health care costs go up, Medicare costs more too.

You can help slow down the rise in health care costs in two ways:

1. If you know you are going to have to see a doctor about some ailment, don't put it off too long. If you wait too long, the ailment may be much harder to cure, or even impossible. And it could cost much more.

2. Don't ask your doctor to prescribe more medicine or more treatments or a longer stay in a hospital or extended care facility than he thinks you really need.

LIKE MEDICARE, YOUR HANDBOOK HAS TWO PARTS . . .

PART A

• The *first* section describes *hospital insurance,* often called *Part A* of Medicare. This is the part that helps pay for your care when you are in the hospital and for related health services, when you need them, after you leave the hospital.

PART B

• The *second* section describes *medical insurance,* often called *Part B* of Medicare. This is the part that helps pay your doctor bills and bills for other medical services you need.

YOUR MEDICARE HEALTH INSURANCE CARD SHOWS THE PROTECTION YOU HAVE

The people at the hospital, doctor's office, or wherever you get services, can tell from your health insurance card that you have both hospital and medical insurance and when each started. This is why you should always have your card with you when you receive services.

When a husband and wife both have Medicare, they receive separate cards and claim numbers.

If you ever lose your health insurance card, the people in your social security office will get you a new one.

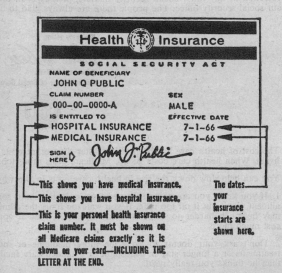

Health (⚕) Insurance

SOCIAL SECURITY ACT

NAME OF BENEFICIARY
JOHN Q PUBLIC

CLAIM NUMBER   SEX
000–00–0000–A   MALE

IS ENTITLED TO   EFFECTIVE DATE
HOSPITAL INSURANCE   7–1–66
MEDICAL INSURANCE   7–1–66

SIGN HERE ⊳ *John J. Public*

This shows you have medical insurance.

This shows you have hospital insurance.

This is your personal health insurance claim number. It must be shown on all Medicare claims exactly as it is shown on your card—INCLUDING THE LETTER AT THE END.

The dates your insurance starts are shown here.

HOSPITAL INSURANCE—PART A OF MEDICARE

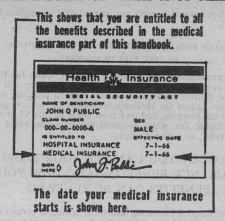

This shows that you are entitled to all the benefits described in the medical insurance part of this handbook.

Health 🔥 Insurance

SOCIAL SECURITY ACT

NAME OF BENEFICIARY
JOHN Q PUBLIC

CLAIM NUMBER   SEX
000-00-0000-A   MALE

IS ENTITLED TO   EFFECTIVE DATE
HOSPITAL INSURANCE   7-1-66
MEDICAL INSURANCE   7-1-66

SIGN HERE ◊ *John J. Public*

The date your medical insurance starts is shown here.

How Hospital Insurance Works

Your hospital insurance helps pay for medically necessary covered services provided by health facilities participating in Medicare when you are:

- ### A Bed Patient in a Hospital

And . . . if you need further care *after* a hospital stay, when you are:

- ### A Bed Patient in an Extended Care Facility, or

- ### A Patient at Home Receiving Services From A Home Health Agency.

The services hospital insurance helps pay for are called *covered services*. When you meet the conditions described on the following pages, your hospital insurance *covers almost all of the services* you would ordinarily receive as a bed patient in a participating hospital or extended care facility or as a patient at home receiving services from a participating home health agency. Your hospital insurance will also, in some cases, help pay for care in certain hospitals that do not participate in Medicare (see page 606).

When you receive covered services from a participating hospital, extended care facility, or home health agency, you do not need to make any claim for your hospital insurance benefits. These institutions or agencies make the claims and receive the Medicare payment. They have agreed to charge you only for services which are not covered by Medicare.

You will always receive a notice from the Social Security Administration when a payment has been made on your behalf.

All outpatient hospital services are covered only by medical insurance. See page 611.

HEALTH FACILITIES MUST MEET CERTAIN CONDITIONS TO TAKE PART IN MEDICARE

To participate in the Medicare program, health facilities must meet standards which help assure that they will be able to provide high quality health care. In addition, they must not charge the Medicare beneficiary for services paid for by the program, and they must abide by title VI of the Civil Rights Act, which prohibits discrimination based on race, color, or national origin.

HOW OFTEN YOU CAN USE YOUR HOSPITAL INSURANCE BENEFITS—AND HOW YOUR BENEFITS CAN BE RENEWED

Your use of hospital insurance benefits is limited to certain *maximum* amounts for certain periods of time—but there is a way for your hospital insurance benefits to *start over again* (except the "lifetime reserve" described on page 602). You can figure out yourself how this works:

HOW THE USE OF HOSPITAL INSURANCE BENEFITS IS COUNTED

WHEN YOU RECEIVE COVERED SERVICES AS—	YOUR PART A BENEFITS ARE—
• A bedpatient in a hospital.	• Up to 90 "hospital days" for *each* "benefit period."
• A bed patient in an extended care facility.	• Up to 100 "extended care days" for each "benefit period."
• A patient at home receiving home health services.	• Up to 100 "home health visits" for *each* "benefit period." (Page 605 describes the 1-year time limit on these visits.)

These three kinds of benefits and how you qualify for them are described in more detail on the following pages. But, as you can see, you can get covered services for up to these total numbers of "days" and "visits" for *each* "benefit period." So you need to know what a "benefit period" is to know how often you can use your hospital insurance benefits.

WHAT IS A "BENEFIT PERIOD"?

A "benefit period" is simply a period of time for measuring your use of hospital insurance benefits. (In the first Medicare Handbook and in some other Medicare publications, we called this period of time a "spell of illness," which is the term used in the law. But because many people thought this term had something to do with a single illness or a particular "spell" of sickness, we are now calling it a "benefit period.") This is how it works.

The first time you enter a hospital after your hospital insurance starts will be the beginning of your *first* benefit period. Your first benefit period *ends* as soon as you have not been a bed patient in any hospital (or any facility that mainly provides skilled nursing care) for *60 days in a row*. After that, a *new* benefit period begins the next time you enter a hospital—and *that* benefit period ends as soon as you have *another* 60 days in a row when you are not a bed patient in any hospital (or any facility that mainly provides skilled nursing care). Then *another* benefit period can begin the *next* time you enter a hospital—and so on.

There is no limit to the number of benefit periods you may have. There is an easy way to remember the rule. Just keep in mind that *any time* you are not in any hospital or other facility mainly providing skilled nursing care for *60* days in a row a *new* benefit period will begin the next time you go into a hospital. And, of course, for each new benefit period, your full hospital insurance benefits are available again to use as you need them.

YOU GET A PERSONAL RECORD OF BENEFITS USED

You don't have to bother about trying to keep track of how many "days" or "visits" you use in each benefit period. The notice you receive from the Social Security Administration after you have used any hospital insurance benefits will tell you how many benefit "days" and "visits" you have left in that benefit period. But, very few people who enter a hospital or extended care facility, or use home health services, need these services long enough to use all the benefits they have for a benefit period. So most people will never run out of "days" or "visits," because a new benefit period will almost always start with full benefits available again the next time they are needed.

EXAMPLE: Mr. L was in the hospital for 14 days and then went home.

After being at home for 80 days, Mr. L needs to return to the hospital. When Mr. L is admitted this time, he is in a new benefit period. That means he is again eligible for up to 90 hospital days because more than 60 days have gone by since he was last in a hospital (or other facility that mainly provides skilled nursing care). The benefit days Mr. L used the time before do not matter because he is in a new benefit period.

However, because Mr. L had been in the hospital only 14 days, he still had 76 hospital benefit days left in the original benefit period. If he had had to go back to the hospital within 60 days, instead of 80, he could have used any of these remaining days that he needed during this second stay.

HOW HOSPITAL INSURANCE BENEFITS ARE FINANCED

The hospital insurance program is financed by special contributions from employees and self-employed persons, with employers paying an equal amount. These contributions are collected along with regular social security contributions from the wages and self-employment income earned during a person's working years.

The contribution rate for the hospital insurance program is six-tenths of one percent of the first $7,800 of earnings. It will increase gradually until 1987 when it will reach the final rate of nine-tenths of one percent.

These contributions are put into the Hospital Insurance Trust Fund from which the program's benefits and administrative expenses are paid. Funds from general tax revenues are used to finance hospital insurance benefits for people who are covered under the program but are not entitled to monthly social security or railroad retirement benefits.

In addition, the law provides that the various dollar amounts for which the patient is responsible be reviewed annually. These dollar amounts include the first $60 of hospital charges in each benefit period and different per-day amounts after certain periods of benefit use in hospitals and extended care facilities. These are described on the following pages. The law also provides that if this annual review shows that hospital costs have changed significantly these amounts must be adjusted for the following year.

WHAT HOSPITAL INSURANCE CAN PAY
WHEN YOU ARE A HOSPITAL BED PATIENT

In *each* benefit period, your hospital insurance can help pay for *up to* 90 days of bed patient care in any participating general care, tuberculosis, or psychiatric hospital.

- For the first 60 days—hospital insurance pays for all covered services, *except for the first $60.*
- For the 61st through the 90th day—hospital insurance pays for all covered services, *except for $15 a day.*

IMPORTANT!

Once you have taken care of the **first $60** of hospital expenses in each benefit period, **you do not have to pay it again,** even if you have to go back in a hospital more than once in that same benefit period.

ALSO, YOU HAVE A "LIFETIME RESERVE"
OF 60 ADDITIONAL HOSPITAL DAYS

This is like a "bank account" of extra days to draw from if you need them. You can use them if you ever need more than 90 days of hospital care in the same benefit period. For each "lifetime reserve" day used, hospital insurance pays for all covered services, *except for $30 a day.*

Each lifetime reserve day you use permanently reduces the total you have left.

Usually you will want to use your lifetime reserve days if you need hospital care after you have used all your 90 days in a benefit period. *Unless* you decide *not* to use them, the extra days of hospital care that you use are automatically taken from your lifetime reserve.

If for any reason you do not wish to use your reserve days, the hospital will ask you to say so in writing. In making your decision, you should consider any private insurance you have which may pay for some or all of your additional hospital care. And, of course, you may wish to talk to your doctor or the people at the hospital about whether in your particular situation you should draw on your lifetime reserve.

EXAMPLE: Mrs. S had to go to the hospital a number of times in the same benefit period and used up all her 90 days. Before a new benefit period could start, she again needed to go to a hospital. She can draw from her "lifetime reserve" days to help her pay for the hospital care.

SPECIAL RULES FOR BENEFITS IN PSYCHIATRIC HOSPITALS

For care in a psychiatric hospital, there is a lifetime limit of 190 hospital benefit days. Also, for a beneficiary who is a patient in a psychiatric hospital on the day his hospital insurance starts, there is a special limitation which is described in Question 5 on page 607.

YOUR BENEFITS WHEN YOU ARE A BED PATIENT IN A PARTICIPATING HOSPITAL

PART A HELPS PAY FOR:

The list below describes the kinds of benefits that hospital insurance will help pay for when you are a bed patient in a hospital and some of the services that it cannot pay for.

- Bed in a semiprivate room (2-4 beds in a room) and all meals, including special diets.
- Operating room charges.
- Regular nursing services (including intensive care nursing).
- Drugs furnished by the hospital.
- Laboratory tests.
- X-ray and other radiology services.
- Medical supplies such as splints and casts.
- Use of appliances and equipment furnished by the hospital such as a wheelchair, crutches, and braces.
- Medical social services.

PART A DOES NOT PAY FOR:

- Personal comfort or convenience items (such as charges for telephone, radio, or television furnished at your request).
- Private duty nurses.
- Any extra charge for use of a private room, unless you need it for medical reasons.
- Noncovered levels of care.
- Doctors' services (medical insurance helps pay for these).

AN EXAMPLE OF HOW HOSPITAL INSURANCE HELPS PAY FOR HOSPITAL CARE

Mrs. C was in the hospital for 14 days.

During her stay in the hospital, Mrs. C had an operation. Her bill included the hospital charges for semiprivate room and all meals, including special diet; use of the operating room; X-rays, laboratory tests; oxygen; and drugs furnished by the hospital. There was also a charge of $9.25 for television and telephone services.

Of the total hospital bill of $798.25, Mrs. C paid $69.25. (This was the first $60 for that benefit period plus the charges for the television and telephone.) Her hospital insurance took care of the remaining $729. (And, of course, Mrs. C's medical insurance helped pay her doctor bills.)

EXTENDED CARE BENEFITS AFTER YOU LEAVE THE HOSPITAL

Sometimes a patient no longer needs all the care which hospitals provide, but still needs full-time skilled nursing care and other health services which cannot be furnished in his home. In these cases, the doctor may transfer the patient from the hospital to an extended care facility. This is a specially qualified facility which is staffed and equipped to furnish full-time skilled nursing care and many important related health services.

Hospital insurance pays for all covered services in a participating extended care facility for the first 20 days you receive such services in each benefit period and all but $7.50 a day for up to 80 more days in that same benefit period, *but only if all the following are true:*

1. Your medical needs require continuing skilled nursing care;
2. A doctor determines that you need extended care and orders such care for you;
3. You have been in a participating (or otherwise qualified) hospital for at least 3 days in a row before your admission;
4. You are admitted within 14 days after you leave the hospital; and
5. You are admitted for further treatment of a condition for which you were treated in the hospital.

If you leave an extended care facility and are readmitted to one within 14 days, you can continue to use your additional extended care benefit days for that benefit period without a new 3-day stay in a hospital.

The following list describes some of the kinds of extended care services hospital insurance will help pay for and some of the services that it cannot pay for.

PART A HELPS PAY FOR:

- Bed in a semiprivate room (2-4 beds in a room) and all meals, including special diets.
- Regular nursing services.
- Drugs furnished by the extended care facility.
- Physical, occupational, and speech therapy.
- Medical supplies such as splints and casts.
- Use of appliances and equipment furnished by the facility such as a wheelchair, crutches, and braces.
- Medical social services.

Part A Does NOT Pay For:

- Personal comfort or convenience items (such as charges for telephone, radio, or television furnished at your request).
- Private duty nurses.
- Any extra charge for use of a private room, unless you need it for medical reasons.
- Noncovered levels of care.
- Doctors' services (your medical insurance helps pay for these).

HOME HEALTH BENEFITS AFTER YOU LEAVE THE HOSPITAL

After you have been in a hospital (or in an extended care facility *after* a hospital stay), your doctor may decide that the continued care you need can best be given in your own home through a home health agency. If the continuing care you need in your home includes part-time skilled nursing care or physical or speech therapy, Medicare can pay for this care and also for certain additional health care services you may need.

Hospital insurance pays for all covered services—for as many as 100 home health visits after the start of one benefit period and before the start of another.

The visits must be medically necessary and be furnished by a participating home health agency. Benefits can be paid for up to a year after your most recent discharge from a hospital or participating extended care facility *but only if all the following are true:*

1. You were in a participating (or otherwise qualified) hospital for at least 3 days in a row;
2. The continuing care you need includes part-time skilled nursing care or physical or speech therapy;
3. You are confined to your home;
4. A doctor determines that you need home health care and sets up a home health plan for you within 14 days after your discharge from the hospital or a participating extended care facility; and
5. The home health care is for further treatment of a condition for which you received services as a bed patient in the hospital or extended care facility.

For an explanation of how "visits" are counted, see Question 8 on page 607.

The following list describes the kinds of home health services that hospital insurance will help pay for and some of the services that it cannot pay for.

Part A Helps Pay For:

- Part-time nursing care, physical therapy, or speech therapy.

  And if you need any of the above services, the following services are also covered:

  - Occupational therapy.
  - Part-time services of home health aides.
  - Medical social services.
  - Medical supplies and appliances furnished by the agency.

PART A DOES NOT PAY FOR:

- Full-time nursing care.
- Drugs and biologicals.
- Personal comfort or convenience items.
- Noncovered levels of care.
- Meals delivered to your home.

BENEFITS FOR CARE IN HOSPITALS THAT DO NOT TAKE PART IN MEDICARE

Nearly all hospitals in the country take part in Medicare. But if you are admitted for emergency care to a hospital that does not take part in Medicare, hospital insurance may still be able to help pay some of the bills.

Your hospital insurance can help pay for emergency care if the hospital: (1) meets certain conditions listed in the law; (2) is the closest or the quickest one to get to that has a bed available; and (3) is equipped to handle the emergency.

If you receive emergency care in such a hospital, the benefit payment will usually be made to the hospital. If the hospital decides to bill you instead of Medicare, the benefit payment will be made to you. The people at your social security office will help you make your claim.

UTILIZATION REVIEW

Each hospital and extended care facility has a Utilization Review Committee. The purpose of this committee is to help assure the most effective utilization of hospital or extended care facility services. The committee, which includes at least two physicians, reviews admissions on a sample basis and reviews ALL long-stay cases.

In some cases, the review will show that a patient's stay in the hospital or the extended care facility is no longer medically necessary. For a hospital inpatient, the review could indicate that a different kind of care would be more appropriate, for example, care in an extended care facility which Medicare could help pay for. For the patient in the extended care facility, the review might show that the patient was no longer receiving the kind of care for which Medicare could pay extended care benefits.

When this happens, the committee talks the matter over with the patient's doctor and then makes a decision. If the decision is that the patient can receive the kind of care he needs elsewhere, the patient, his doctor, and the hospital or extended care facility are advised in writing.

Three days after this notice, Medicare, by law, has to stop paying inpatient benefits even if the patient stays in the facility.

QUESTIONS AND ANSWERS ABOUT HOSPITAL INSURANCE

1. **Where can I find out if a hospital, extended care facility, or home health agency is participating in Medicare?**

   Your doctor, or someone at the institution or agency, can tell you. Or you can ask the people in any social security office.

2. If I am injured while at work and my medical expenses are (or could be) covered by the workmen's compensation law, will my hospital insurance also pay?

No.

3. Does hospital insurance pay for services in a foreign hospital?

No, but there is one exception: if (1) you are in the United States when an emergency arises and (2) the foreign hospital is closer than the nearest hospital in the United States which could provide the emergency care you need. Then hospital insurance will help pay for the emergency care.

4. Can hospital insurance pay anything toward the cost of my care in a Christian Science sanatorium?

Yes. Your hospital insurance can cover certain hospital and extended care services furnished to inpatients of a sanatorium operated, or listed and certified, by the First Church of Christ, Scientist, in Boston. For more information, ask at any social security office.

5. Is there a special rule for beneficiaries who are in a psychiatric hospital when their hospital insurance protection starts?

Yes. When a person is a patient in a psychiatric hospital *at the time* his hospital insurance starts, the days in the mental hospital during the 150-day period just before his hospital insurance starts count against the total number of benefit days he can use in a psychiatric hospital in his first benefit period.

These days, however, do not count against his lifetime maximum of 190 days of payment for care as a patient in a psychiatric hospital. Nor do they count against his benefit days in his first benefit period if he goes to a *general hospital* for treatment of a condition other than mental illness. (For more information, get in touch with your social security office.)

6. What can I do if I think a mistake has been made in the amount of my hospital insurance benefits?

The first thing to do is to ask someone at the hospital, extended care facility, or home health agency that provided the services. Usually they can answer your questions. Sometimes, however, they may need to refer you to the organization that handles their Medicare payments. If you are still not satisfied, get in touch with your social security office for information about your right to formal appeal.

7. What if I cannot pay the amounts that hospital insurance does not pay?

You may want to ask at your local public assistance office about help under a State program such as old-age assistance or medical assistance (sometimes called "medicaid").

8. What is a home health "visit"?

One "visit" is counted *each* time you receive a covered health care service from a home health agency. If you receive two *different* services on the same day (for example, both a nurse and a physical therapist call on you), that would be *two* "visits". It would also be two "visits" if you received the *same* service twice in a day (such as two calls by a nurse).

MEDICAL INSURANCE—
PART B OF MEDICARE

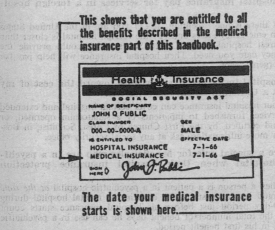

This shows that you are entitled to all the benefits described in the medical insurance part of this handbook.

The date your medical insurance starts is shown here.

YOU PAY HALF THE COST OF YOUR
MEDICAL INSURANCE PROTECTION

The basic medical insurance premium for each person is $5.30 a month through June 1971. It will be increased to $5.60 for the 12-month period starting in July 1971. Those who delayed signing up for a long period of time after their first chance or who signed up again after canceling this insurance in the past are required by law to pay an additional 10 percent for each full year they were eligible but not enrolled. Starting in July 1971, the premium will be $6.20 a month for those who did not enroll for a year or longer after they were eligible, $6.70 a month for those who delayed 2 years or longer, and $7.30 for those who delayed 3 years or longer.

Your premium covers half the cost of your medical insurance protection. The Federal Government pays the other half for you.

The medical insurance premium rate must be reviewed annually. If necessary, the rate is changed to make sure that the total amounts collected in premiums and the equal amounts provided by the Government will continue to meet the full costs of the program. The results of the annual review are announced in December of each year. The change in the premium, if any, is effective for the 12-month period beginning the following July.

Medical insurance premiums are automatically deducted from monthly checks for those who receive social security benefits, railroad retirement benefits, or a civil service annuity. Those who do not receive any of these monthly checks pay their premiums directly to the Social Security Administration (or, in some cases, have premiums paid on their behalf under a State assistance program).

IF YOU EVER DECIDE TO CANCEL

You can cancel your medical insurance at any time. Your protection and your premiums will stop at the end of the calendar quarter after the quarter your notice is received. (A calendar quarter is any of the 3-month periods beginning with January 1, April 1, July 1, or October 1.)

If you do cancel your medical insurance, you have only one chance to get it back. You may sign up again in one of the "general enrollment" periods which begin within 3 years after you cancel your medical insurance. There is a general enrollment period *every* year—from January 1 through March 31.

If you should ever think of canceling your medical insurance protection, remember that you may not be able to get equal protection from other sources. Many Blue Cross-Blue Shield plans and commercial insurance companies do not offer broad coverage policies for people 65 and over, but only *extra* insurance for those who already have medical insurance under Medicare.

HOW MEDICAL INSURANCE WORKS

Your medical insurance helps pay for—
    Doctor's Services
    Outpatient Hospital Services
    Medical Services and Supplies
    Home Health Services
    Outpatient Physical Therapy
    —and other health care services.

To understand the way medical insurance works, it will help to know the following terms.

COVERED SERVICES:

These are the kinds of services medical insurance can help pay for.

$50 DEDUCTIBLE:

For each calendar year, medical insurance does not pay any of the first $50 of reasonable charges for covered services.

REASONABLE CHARGES:

Reasonable charges are determined by the Medicare carriers—the organizations selected in each State by the Social Security Administration to handle medical insurance claims—and take into consideration the customary charges of your doctor (or supplier) as well as the charges made by other doctors and suppliers in your locality for similar services.

After Medicare records show that your bills for covered services are over $50 for a calendar year, medical insurance will pay 80 percent of the reasonable charges for covered services for the rest of that year. (There are two exceptions to this rule. One is the special rule on page 611, and the other is described in Question 2 on page 629.) Be sure to send in a claim as soon as your bills reach $50 so the Medicare records will show the first $50 as well as the rest of your bills.

Important: There is only *one* $50 medical insurance deductible each year—not a separate $50 deductible for each kind of covered service. Also, medical expenses in the last 3 months of one year can sometimes count toward the $50 deductible for the next year. This carry-over rule is described on page 617.

EXPLANATION OF BENEFITS NOTICE

Whenever a medical insurance claim is sent in, you will receive a statement showing your use of medical insurance benefits. This statement will show you how much of your expenses have been credited to your $50 deductible and the amount of the benefit payment if any. The explanation of benefits statements are important because you can use the latest one to show your doctor and others when they want to know how much of the $50 deductible you have met.

WHEN A DOCTOR TREATS YOU

Medical insurance will help pay your doctor bills for all covered services you receive in the United States. Payment can be made no matter where a doctor treats you—in a hospital, his office, an extended care facility, your home, or at a group practice or other clinic.

You select your own doctor. He does not have to "sign up" or make any other special arrangements with Medicare.

For covered services you receive from your doctor, the medical insurance payment can be made either to you or to your doctor. See page 615 for the two ways payment can be made.

The following list shows the kinds of doctors' services that medical insurance will help pay for and some of the services it cannot pay for.

PART B HELPS PAY FOR:

- Medical and surgical services by a doctor of medicine or osteopathy.
- Certain medical and surgical services by a doctor of dental medicine or a doctor of dental surgery.
- Services by podiatrists which they are legally authorized to perform by the State in which they practice.
- Other services which are ordinarily furnished in the doctor's office and included in his bill such as:
    Diagnostic tests and procedures
    Medical supplies
    Services of his office nurse
    Drugs and biologicals which cannot be self-administered.

PART B DOES NOT PAY FOR:

- Routine physical checkups.
- Routine foot care and treatment of flat feet and partial dislocations of the feet.
- Eye refractions and examinations for prescribing, fitting, or changing eyeglasses.
- Hearing examinations for prescribing, fitting, or changing hearing aids.
- Immunizations (unless directly related to an injury or immediate risk of infection such as a tetanus shot given after an injury).
- Services of certain practitioners, for example:
    Christian Science practitioners
    Chiropractors
    Naturopaths

COVERAGE OF DENTAL SERVICES

Medical insurance covers the services of dentists only when the services involve surgery of the jaw or related structures or setting of fractures of the jaw or facial bones.

Medical insurance does *not* pay for dental services such as the care, filling, removal, or replacement of teeth, or treatment of the gum areas nor for surgery or other services related to these kinds of dental care.

RADIOLOGY AND PATHOLOGY SERVICES BY DOCTORS WHEN YOU ARE A BED PATIENT IN A HOSPITAL

Medical insurance pays *all* (100 percent) of the reasonable charges by doctors for radiology services such as X-rays, and pathology services such as blood and urine tests you receive as an inpatient in a participating or otherwise qualified hospital.

You may not receive any doctor bills for these services because many hospitals and the doctors who perform these services have agreed that the hospital will collect the payments due from your medical insurance. If you do receive doctor bills for these services, send them in as described on page 615 for full payment of the reasonable charges even though you have not met the full deductible.

Medical insurance pays 80 percent of the reasonable charges by doctors for all other covered services you receive. Full payment can be made only for radiology and pathology services.

SPECIAL RULE: Because the full reasonable charges are taken care of when you receive radiology and pathology services as a hospital inpatient, these charges do not count toward the $50 deductible.

AMBULANCE SERVICES

Medical insurance will help pay for ambulance transportation by an approved ambulance service to a hospital or skilled nursing home only when (1) the ambulance, its equipment, and personnel meet Medicare requirements, (2) transportation by other means could endanger the patient's health, and (3) the patient is taken to a facility serving the locality, or the *nearest* facility that is equipped to take care of him.

Under similar restrictions, medical insurance can help pay for ambulance services from one hospital to another, from a hospital to a skilled nursing home, or from a hospital or skilled nursing home to the patient's home if his home is in the same locality as the hospital or skilled nursing home.

OUTPATIENT HOSPITAL BENEFITS

When people go to the hospital for diagnosis or treatment and are not admitted as bed patients, the services they receive are called *outpatient hospital services.*

Covered outpatient services whether for diagnosis or treatment are paid by medical insurance.

After the $50 deductible has been met, Medicare takes care of 80 percent of the reasonable charges for all covered outpatient hospital services you receive.

The hospital will apply for the Medicare payment and will charge you for any part of the $50 deductible you have not met plus 20 percent of the remaining reasonable charges for the outpatient services.

If the charge is $50 or less and the hospital cannot determine how much of the $50 deductible you have met, then the hospital may ask you to pay the entire bill. If you pay the bill, any Medicare payments that are due will be paid directly to you. Except in unusual circumstances, the hospital will prepare the Medicare claim for you. If you ever need help with your claim, get in touch with your social security office.

When you pay an outpatient bill of $50 or less, here is what happens:

- *If you have already met the $50 deductible*—Medicare will pay you 80 percent of the amount you paid the hospital.

- *If you have not met the $50 deductible*—Medicare will credit the amount you paid toward your $50 deductible. If that amount plus any part of the deductible you have previously met for the year adds up to more than $50, medical insurance will pay you 80 percent of the amount above the $50 deductible.

EXAMPLE: During the year, Mrs. J had bills of $45 for covered services *before* she received treatment in the hospital outpatient department. The hospital charged her $10 and she paid the bill at their request. When her claim is received, $5 of the outpatient bill is used to make up her $50 deductible and Mrs. J receives 80 percent of the remaining $5, which would be $4.

IMPORTANT!

When you go to a hospital for outpatient services, be sure to show the people there your most recent explanation of benefits statement (see page 610). From this form, they can tell how much of the $50 deductible you have met and how much of the deductible, if any, they may charge you.

The following list describes the kinds of outpatient hospital services that medical insurance will help pay for and some of the services that it cannot pay for:

PART B HELPS PAY FOR:

- Laboratory services.
- X-ray and other radiology services.
- Emergency room services.
- Medical supplies such as splints and casts.
- Other diagnostic services.

PART B DOES NOT PAY FOR:

- Tests given as part of a routine checkup.
- Eye refractions and examinations for prescribing, fitting, or changing eyeglasses.

- Immunizations (unless directly related to an injury or immediate risk of infection such as a tetanus shot given after an injury).
- Hearing examinations for prescribing, fitting, or changing hearing aids.

OUTPATIENT PHYSICAL THERAPY SERVICES

Outpatient physical therapy services are covered by medical insurance when they are furnished under the direct and personal supervision of a doctor or when they are furnished as part of covered home health services.

Also, physical therapy services you receive as an outpatient are covered when they are furnished by a qualified hospital, extended care facility, home health agency, clinic, rehabilitation agency, or public health agency, and they are furnished under a plan established and periodically reviewed by a doctor.

EMERGENCY OUTPATIENT CARE FROM CERTAIN NONPARTICIPATING HOSPITALS CAN ALSO BE COVERED

If you receive emergency outpatient care from a nonparticipating hospital which meets certain conditions, the hospital will usually bill Medicare for its share of the charges. It will then bill you for any part of the $50 deductible you have not met plus 20 percent of the remaining reasonable charges.

The hospital may choose instead to bill you for the entire amount. In this case, your medical insurance will pay you 80 percent of the reasonable charges (after the $50 deductible has been met).

For help in making your claim, get in touch with your social security office.

HOME HEALTH BENEFITS

Your medical insurance will help pay for up to 100 home health visits each calendar year *but only if all the following are true:*

1. You need part-time skilled nursing care, or physical or speech therapy services;
2. You are confined to your home;
3. A doctor determines you need home health care;
4. A doctor sets up and periodically reviews the plan for home health care; and
5. The home health agency is participating in Medicare.

For an explanation of how home health "visits" are counted, see Question 8 on page 607.

The home health agency always makes the claim for the benefit payment, so you do not submit a *Request for Medicare Payment* form when you receive home health services. Since medical insurance takes care of 80 percent of the reasonable charges, the agency will bill you for any part of the $50 deductible you have not met plus 20 percent of the remaining reasonable charges.

The following list describes the kinds of home health services that medical insurance will help pay for and some of the services that it cannot pay for.

PART B HELPS PAY FOR:

- Part-time nursing care, physical therapy, or speech therapy.
  And if you need any of the above services, the following services are
  also covered:

  - Occupational therapy.
  - Part-time services of home health aides.
  - Medical social services.
  - Medical supplies and appliances furnished by the agency.

PART B DOES NOT PAY FOR:

- Full-time nursing care.
- Drugs and biologicals.
- Personal comfort or convenience items.
- Noncovered levels of care.
- Meals delivered to your home.

OTHER MEDICAL SERVICES AND SUPPLIES

This benefit helps you pay for a number of different medical services
and supplies which may be necessary in the treatment of an illness or
injury. They may be furnished in connection with treatment by your
doctor, a medical clinic, or other health facility.

When a participating hospital, extended care facility, or home health
agency provides covered services and supplies, it will make the claim
for the Medicare payment and will bill you for any of the $50 deductible
you have not met and 20 percent of the remaining reasonable charges.
Otherwise you or the supplier of services will make the claim, as described on page 615.

The following list shows the kinds of medical services and supplies
that medical insurance can help pay for when they are medically necessary and ordered by your doctor and some that it cannot pay for.

PART B HELPS PAY FOR:

- Diagnostic laboratory tests furnished by approved independent laboratories.*
- Radiation therapy and diagnostic X-ray services.*
- Portable diagnostic X-ray services furnished in your home under a
  doctor's supervision.
- Surgical dressings, splints, casts, and similar devices.*
- Rental or purchase of durable medical equipment prescribed by a
  doctor to be used in your home: for example, a wheelchair, crutches,
  or oxygen equipment.
- Devices (other than dental) to replace all or part of an internal body
  organ. This includes corrective lenses after a cataract operation.
- Certain ambulance services (see page 611).

* If you are a patient in a hospital or extended care facility and, for
some reason, your hospital insurance cannot pay for these services (for
example, because you have used up your benefit days), medical insurance can help pay for them.

PART B DOES NOT PAY FOR:

- Prescription drugs and drugs you can administer yourself. For example, insulin injections for a diabetic condition.
- Hearing aids.
- Eyeglasses.
- False teeth.
- Orthopedic shoes or other supportive devices for the feet—except when shoes are a part of leg braces.

HOW TO CLAIM MEDICAL INSURANCE BENEFITS

1. PAYMENT TO YOUR DOCTOR OR SUPPLIER

If you and your doctor (or supplier) agree that he will apply for the medical insurance payment, it will be made directly to him. This is called "assignment" of the benefit.

A. Complete and sign Part I of the *Request for Medicare Payment* (Form SSA-1490). (A copy of this form is on page 618.) Often your doctor's office or the supplier will complete Part I as a convenience to you.

B. Your doctor or supplier completes Part II of the form.

C. Your doctor or supplier sends in the *Request for Medicare Payment* form.

When your doctor or supplier accepts assignment, he agrees that his total charge will not exceed the reasonable charge (see page 609). This means that you are responsible only for any of the $50 deductible not yet met, plus 20 percent of the balance of the "reasonable charges."

2. PAYMENT TO YOU

If either you or the doctor (or supplier) do not want to use the assignment method, the medical insurance payment can be made directly to you. **You can make a claim whether or not the bill has been paid.**

A. Complete and sign Part I of the *Request for Medicare Payment* form. Often your doctor's office or the supplier will complete Part I as a convenience to you.

B. Your doctor or supplier will either complete Part II or give you an itemized bill. An itemized bill shows the date, place, and description of each service, and the charge for each service. (Be sure your name and claim number are on each bill exactly as they are shown on your health insurance card.)

C. You send in the *Request for Medicare Payment*, with either Part II completed or with itemized bills, to the organization which handles claims for the *area where you received services*. These organizations are listed on pages 622 to 628.

NOTE:

You may send in a number of bills from the *same* doctor or supplier (or from different doctors or suppliers) with a single *Request for Medicare Payment* form.

Also, whichever method you use, if you have health insurance in addition to Medicare or you are covered under a State program which pays all or part of your health care, be sure to fill in Item 5 of your *Request for Medicare Payment* form. (See page 618.)

WHEN TO SEND IN YOUR FIRST CLAIM EACH YEAR

Medical insurance does not pay any part of the first $50 of covered medical expenses in each year. After the first $50, medical insurance pays 80 percent of the reasonable charges.

Before *any* payment can be made, your record must show that you have met your deductible. So, as soon as your bills come to $50, send them to the office that will be handling your medical insurance claims (see page 622). If the charges for covered services are $50 or more, an entry will be made in your record to show that you have met the deductible for the year, and any payment due at the time will be made.

In some cases, of course, you may want to send them in before you have a total of $50. For example, you may already have $40 in small medical bills when you receive services from a doctor for $25 and he agrees to take your assignment. In that case, you would send in your $40 in prior bills, so that when the assignment is processed for payment the record will show that you have met $40 of the $50 deductible.

Your social security office will always be glad to answer your questions about when to send in your first claim.

IF YOU BELONG TO A GROUP PRACTICE PREPAYMENT PLAN

Group practice prepayment plans represent a special way of making health services available to their members. Generally, each member pays regular premiums to the plan in advance and this entitles him to receive any of the health services the plan provides, whenever he needs them, without paying a separate fee for each health service he receives. Congress took steps to assure that these plans could participate in the Medicare program while continuing their established method of operation.

Almost all group practice prepayment plans have made special arrangements with the Social Security Administration to receive direct payment for covered services they furnish their members who are medical insurance beneficiaries.

If you are a member of a plan which has made these special arrangements:

You **DO NOT** need to make a claim for any covered services which are provided through your group practice prepayment plan.

You **DO** need to make a claim for any covered services you receive which are not provided by your plan. In making your claim, you use one of the two methods described on page 615.

In addition, each plan has developed special methods to credit your membership premium payments or your use of plan services to the $50 deductible. Your plan will, of course, advise you of its method.

If you need more information, get in touch with your group practice prepayment plan.

WHEN THE CARRY OVER HELPS YOU

To help the beneficiary who might otherwise need to meet the $50 annual deductible twice in a short period, there is a special carry-over rule.

If you have expenses in the last 3 months of a year which can be counted toward your $50 deductible for that year, they can also be counted toward the $50 annual deductible for the next year. This is called the carry over. So, even if you have not met the $50 deductible before October, be sure to send in all the bills for covered services you receive in October, November, or December. The carry over will be credited to your deductible for both years.

TIME LIMITS FOR PAYMENT OF CLAIMS

Under the law, there are some time limits for making payment on claims you send in. These limits are as follows:

WHEN SERVICES WERE RECEIVED	WHEN CLAIMS MUST BE FILED
October 1, 1969—September 30, 1970	By December 31, 1971
October 1, 1970—September 30, 1971	By December 31, 1972
October 1, 1971—September 30, 1972	By December 31, 1973

NOTE: These time limits for sending claims in are very important. *Medicare can pay your claim only if it is sent in within the time limits shown above.* Don't lose money by waiting too long to send in your claim.

THE REQUEST FOR PAYMENT FORM

Pages 618–619 shows the *Request for Medicare Payment* form. If you do not have a claim form, you can use the form on pages 618–619. Just cut it out along the line.

REQUEST FOR MEDICARE PAYMENT

MEDICAL INSURANCE BENEFITS—SOCIAL SECURITY ACT (See Instructions on Back—Type or Print Information)

Form Approved
Budget Bureau No.
72–R0730

NOTICE—Anyone who misrepresents or falsifies essential information requested by this form may upon conviction be subject to fine and imprisonment under Federal Law.

PART I—PATIENT TO FILL IN ITEMS 1 THROUGH 6 ONLY

A Copy from your **HEALTH INSURANCE CARD** (See example on back)

1 Name of patient

□ Male □ Female

2 Health insurance claim number Letter

Telephone Number

3 Patient's mailing address

City, State, ZIP code

4 Describe the illness or injury for which you received treatment (Always fill in this item if your doctor does not complete Part II below)

Was your illness or injury connected with your employment?
□ Yes □ No

5 If you have other health insurance or if your State medical assistance agency will pay part of your medical expenses and you want information about this claim released to the insurance company or State agency upon its request, give the following information.

Insuring organization or State agency name and address

Policy or Medical Assistance Number

6 I authorize any holder of medical or other information about me to release to the Social Security Administration or its intermediaries or carriers any information needed for this or a related Medicare claim. I permit a copy of this authorization to be used in place of the original, and request payment of medical insurance benefits either to myself or to the party who accepts assignment below.

Signature of patient (See instructions on reverse where patient is unable to sign)

Date signed

SIGN HERE ▶

PART II—PHYSICIAN OR SUPPLIER TO FILL IN 7 THROUGH 14

7

A. Date of service	B. Place of service (*See Codes below)	C. Fully describe surgical or medical procedures and other services or supplies furnished for each date given	D. Nature of illness or Injury requiring services or supplies	E. Charges (If related to unusual circumstances explain in 7C)	Leave Blank
				$	
			9 Total charges	$	
			10 Amount paid	$	
			11 Any unpaid balance due	$	

8 Name and address of physician or supplier (Number and street, city, State, ZIP code)

Telephone No.

Physician or supplier code

13 Show name and address of facility where services were performed (If other than home or office visits)

12 Assignment of patient's bill (See reverse)

☐ I accept assignment ☐ I do not accept assignment

☐ MD ☐ DO ☐ DDS

Other degree _____

14 Signature of physician or supplier (A physician's signature certifies that physician's services were personally rendered by him or under his personal direction)

Date signed

*O—Doctor's Office
IL—Independent Laboratory

H—Patient's Home (If portable X-ray services, identify the supplier)
IH—Inpatient Hospital

ECF—Extended Care Facility
OH—Outpatient Hospital

OL—Other Locations
NH—Nursing Home

FORM SSA-1490 (10-69)

Department of Health, Education, and Welfare
Social Security Administration

HOW TO FILL OUT YOUR MEDICARE FORM

There are two ways that Medicare can help pay your doctor bills

One way is for Medicare to pay your doctor.—If you and your doctor agree, Medicare will pay him directly. This is the assignment method. You do not submit any claim; the doctor does. All you do is fill out Part I of this form and leave it with your doctor. Under this method the doctor agrees to accept the charge determination of the Medicare carrier as the full charge; you are responsible for the deductible and coinsurance. Please read Your Medicare Handbook to help you understand about the deductible and coinsurance. (Because Medicare has special payment arrangements with group practice prepayment plans these plans handle all claims for covered services they furnish to their members.)

The other way is for Medicare to pay you.—Medicare can also pay you directly—before or after you have paid your doctor. If you submit the claim yourself, fill out Part I and ask your doctor to fill out Part II. If you have an itemized bill from him, you may submit it rather than have him complete Part II. (This form, with Part I completed by you, may be used to send in several itemized bills from different doctors and suppliers.) Bills should show who furnished the services, **the patient's name and number,** dates of services, where the services were furnished, a description of the services, and charges for each separate service. It is helpful if the diagnosis is also shown. Then mail itemized bills and this form to the address shown in the upper left-hand corner, Block A. If no address is shown there, use the address listed in Your Medicare Handbook—or get advice from your nearest social security district office.

SOME THINGS TO NOTE IN FILLING OUT PART I
(Your doctor will fill out Part II).

1 & 2 Copy the name and number and indicate your sex exactly as shown on your health insurance card. Include the letters at the end of the number.

3 Enter your mailing address and telephone number, if any.

4 Describe your illness or injury. Be sure to check one of the two boxes.

5 If you have other health insurance or expect a welfare agency to pay part of the expenses, complete item 5.

6 Be sure to sign your name. If you cannot write your name, sign by mark (X), and have a witness sign his name and enter his address on this line.

If the claim is filed for the patient by another person he should enter the patient's name and write "By," sign his own name and address in this space, show his relationship to the patient, and why the patient cannot sign. (If the patient has died the survivor should contact the nearest social security office for information on what to do.)

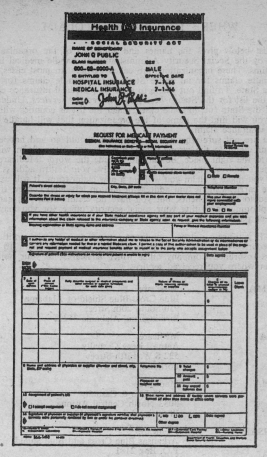

IMPORTANT NOTES FOR PHYSICIANS AND SUPPLIERS

Item 12: Acceptance of an assignment requires the physician (or supplier), to accept the charge determination of the Medicare carrier as his full charge for the service.

This form may also be used by a supplier, or by the patient to claim reimbursement for charges by a supplier for services such as the use of an ambulance or medical appliances.

If the physician or supplier does not want Part II information released to the organization named in item 5, he should write "No further release" in item 7C following the description of services.

WHERE TO SEND YOUR CLAIM

The list below gives the names and addresses of the organizations selected by the Social Security Administration to handle medical insurance claims. These organizations are called carriers. In most cases, carriers handle claims for an entire State; a few handle claims for only part of a State. To find out where to send your medical insurance claim, look in the list for the State *where you received the services.* Under the name of the State (or, in some cases, under the list of counties within a State), you will find the name of the organization that will handle your medical insurance claim.

If you are not sure where your first claim should go and happen to send your claim to the wrong office, don't worry. Your claim will be sent on to the right place. Be sure to include the word "Medicare" in the carrier's address on the envelope, and give *your* return address.

After you make a claim you will get a new claim form. It will usually show the carrier's name and address in the top left-hand corner. If you ever need to claim benefits, but you have no claim form, you can get one by phoning or writing your social security office (or you may use the one on pages 618–619 of this handbook).

NOTE: If you are a railroad annuitant (even if you are also entitled to social security benefits), send your medical insurance claim to The Travelers Insurance Company office which is nearest to your home— no matter where you received services.

ALABAMA	Medicare Blue Cross-Blue Shield of Alabama 930 South 20th Street Birmingham, Alabama 35205
ALASKA	Medicare Aetna Life & Casualty 522 S.W. Fifth Street Portland, Oregon 97204
ARIZONA	Medicare Aetna Life & Casualty 3033 North Central Avenue Phoenix, Arizona 85012
ARKANSAS	Medicare Arkansas Blue Cross and Blue Shield P.O. Box 2181 Little Rock, Arkansas 72203
CALIFORNIA Counties of Los Angeles, Orange, San Diego, Ventura, San Bernardino, Imperial, San Luis Obispo, Riverside, Santa Barbara	Medicare Occidental Life Insurance Co. of California Box 54905 Los Angeles, California 90054
Rest of State:	Medicare California Blue Shield P.O. Box 7968, Rincon Annex San Francisco, California 94119

COLORADO

Medicare
Colorado Medical Service, Inc.
P.O. Box 6410
Denver, Colorado 80206

CONNECTICUT

Medicare
Connecticut General Life Insurance Co.
71 Catlin St.
Meriden, Connecticut 06450

DELAWARE

Medicare
Blue Cross and Blue Shield of Delaware
201 West 14th Street
Wilmington, Delaware 19899

DISTRICT OF
COLUMBIA

Medicare
Medical Service of D.C.
550—12th St., S.W.
Washington, D.C. 20024

FLORIDA

Medicare
Blue Shield of Florida, Inc.
P.O. Box 2525
Jacksonville, Florida 32201

GEORGIA

The Prudential Insurance Co. of America
Medicare Part B
P.O. Box 7340, Station C
1175 Peachtree St., N.E.
Atlanta, Georgia 30309

HAWAII

Medicare
Aetna Life & Casualty
P.O. Box 3947
Honolulu, Hawaii 96812

IDAHO

Medicare
The Equitable Life Assurance Society
P.O. Box 8048
Boise, Idaho 83707

ILLINOIS
Counties of Cook,
DuPage, Kane, Lake, Will

Medicare
Illinois Medical Service
222 N. Dearborn
Chicago, Illinois 60601

Rest of State:

Medicare
Continental Casualty Co.
P.O. Box 910
Chicago, Illinois 60690

INDIANA

Medicare
Mutual Medical Insurance, Inc.
110 North Illinois Street
Indianapolis, Indiana 46204

IOWA   Medicare
                              Iowa Medical Service
                              Liberty Building
                              Des Moines, Iowa 50307

KANSAS   Medicare
Counties of Johnson,   Blue Shield of Kansas City
Wyandotte   P.O. Box 169
                              Kansas City, Missouri 64141

Rest of State: Medicare
                              Kansas Physicians' Service
                              P.O. Box 953
                              Topeka, Kansas 66601

KENTUCKY   Medicare
                              Metropolitan Life Insurance Co.
                              1218 Harrodsburg Road
                              Lexington, Kentucky 40504

LOUISIANA   Medicare
                              Pan-American Life Insurance Co.
                              P.O. Box 60450
                              New Orleans, Louisiana 70160

MAINE   Medicare
                              Union Mutual Life Insurance Co.
                              P.O. Box 4629
                              Portland, Maine 04112

MARYLAND   Medicare
Counties of Montgomery,   Medical Service of D.C.
Prince Georges   550—12th St., S.W.
                              Washington, D.C. 20024

Rest of State: Medicare
                              Maryland Blue Shield, Inc.
                              Box 202
                              Baltimore, Maryland 21203

MASSACHUSETTS   Medicare
                              Massachusetts Medical Service
                              P.O. Box 2194
                              Boston, Massachusetts 02106

MICHIGAN   Medicare
                              Michigan Medical Service
                              P.O. Box 2201
                              Detroit, Michigan 48231

MINNESOTA   Medicare
Counties of Anoka,   The Travelers Insurance Co.
Dakota, Hennepin,   515 Marquette Avenue, South
Ramsey, Washington   Minneapolis, Minnesota 55402

Counties of Filmore, Goodhue, Houston, Olmstead, Wabasha, Winona	Medicare The Travelers Insurance Co. 201 First Avenue, S.W. Rochester, Minnesota 55902
Rest of State:	Medicare Blue Shield of Minnesota P.O. Box 7899 Minneapolis, Minnesota 55404
MISSISSIPPI	Medicare The Travelers Insurance Co. P.O. Box 22545 Jackson, Mississippi 39201
MISSOURI Counties of Andrew, Atchison, Bates, Benton, Buchanan, Caldwell, Carroll, Cass, Clay, Clinton, Daviess, DeKalb, Gentry, Grundy, Harrison, Henry, Holt, Jackson, Johnson, Lafayette, Livingston, Mercer, Nodaway, Pettis, Platte, Ray, St. Clair, Saline, Vernon, Worth	Medicare Blue Shield of Kansas City P.O. Box 169 Kansas City, Missouri 64141
Rest of State:	Medicare General American Life Insurance Co. P.O. Box 505 St. Louis, Missouri 63166
MONTANA	Medicare Montana Physicians' Service P.O. Box 2510 Helena, Montana 59601
NEBRASKA	Medicare Mutual of Omaha Insurance Co. P.O. Box 456, Downtown Station Omaha, Nebraska 68101
NEVADA	Medicare Aetna Life & Casualty P.O. Box 3077 Reno, Nevada 89502
NEW HAMPSHIRE	Medicare New Hampshire-Vermont Physician Service Two Pillsbury Street Concord, New Hampshire 03301
NEW JERSEY	Medicare The Prudential Insurance Co. of America P.O. Box 6500 Millville, New Jersey 08332

NEW MEXICO

Medicare
The Equitable Life Assurance Society
P.O. Box 3070, Station D
Albuquerque, New Mexico 87110

NEW YORK
Counties of Bronx,
Columbia, Delaware,
Dutchess, Greene, Kings,
Nassau, New York,
Orange, Putnam,
Richmond, Rockland,
Suffolk, Sullivan, Ulster,
Westchester

Medicare
United Medical Service, Inc.
Two Park Avenue
New York, New York 10016

County of Queens

Medicare
Group Health Insurance, Inc.
227 West 40th Street
New York, New York 10018

Counties of Livingston,
Monroe, Ontario, Seneca,
Wayne, Yates

Medicare
Genesee Valley Medical Care, Inc.
41 Chestnut Street
Rochester, New York 14604

Counties of Allegany,
Cattaraugus, Erie,
Genesee, Niagara,
Orleans, Wyoming

Medicare
Blue Shield of Western New York, Inc.
298 Main Street
Buffalo, New York 14202

Counties of Albany,
Broome, Cayuga,
Chautauqua, Cheming,
Chenango, Clinton,
Cortland, Essex, Franklin,
Fulton, Hamilton,
Herkimer, Jefferson,
Lewis, Madison,
Montgomery, Oneida,
Onondaga, Oswego,
Otsego, Rensselaer,
Saratoga, Schenectady,
Schoharie, Schuyler,
Steuben, St. Lawrence,
Tioga, Tompkins,
Warren, Washington

Medicare
Metropolitan Life Insurance Co.
258 Genesee Street
Utica, New York 13502

NORTH CAROLINA

The Prudential Insurance Co. of America
Medicare B Division
P.O. Box 1482
High Point, North Carolina 27261

NORTH DAKOTA

Medicare
North Dakota Physicians Service
301 Eighth Street, South
Fargo, North Dakota 58102

OHIO
Counties of Ashtabula,
Cuyahoga, Geauga, Lake,
Loraine

Medicare
Medical Mutual of Cleveland, Inc.
2060 East Ninth Street
Cleveland, Ohio 44115

Rest of State:

Medicare
Nationwide Mutual Insurance Co.
P.O. Box 57
Columbus, Ohio 43216

OKLAHOMA

Medicare
Aetna Life & Casualty
7 South Harvey
Oklahoma City, Oklahoma 73102

OREGON

Medicare
Aetna Life & Casualty
522 S.W. Fifth Street
Portland, Oregon 97204

PENNSYLVANIA

Medicare
Pennsylvania Blue Shield
Box 65
Camp Hill, Pennsylvania 17011

RHODE ISLAND

Medicare
Physicians' Service
444 Westminster Mall
Providence, Rhode Island 02901

SOUTH CAROLINA

Medicare
Blue Shield of South Carolina
Drawer F, Forest Acres Branch
Columbia, South Carolina 29206

SOUTH DAKOTA

Medicare
South Dakota Medical Service, Inc.
711 North Lake Avenue
Sioux Falls, South Dakota 57102

TENNESSEE

Medicare
The Equitable Life Assurance Society
P.O. Box 1465
Nashville, Tennessee 37202

TEXAS

Medicare
Group Medical and Surgical Service
P.O. Box 22147
Dallas, Texas 75222

UTAH

Medicare
Blue Shield of Utah
2455 Parley's Way,
Salt Lake City, Utah 84110

VERMONT

Medicare
New Hampshire-Vermont Physician Service
Two Pillsbury Street
Concord, New Hampshire 03301

VIRGINIA
Counties of Arlington,
Fairfax
City of Alexandria

Medicare
Medical Service of D.C.
550—12th St., S.W.
Washington, D.C. 20024

Rest of State:

Medicare
The Travelers Insurance Co.
P.O. Box 10166
Richmond, Virginia 23230

WASHINGTON

Medicare
Washington Physicians' Service
Mail to your local Medical Service Bureau

WEST VIRGINIA

Medicare
Nationwide Mutual Insurance Co.
P.O. Box 3183
Charleston, West Virginia 25332

WISCONSIN
County of Milwaukee

Medicare
Surgical Care
P.O. Box 2049
Milwaukee, Wisconsin 53201

Rest of State:

Medicare
Wisconsin Physicians Service
Box 1787
Madison, Wisconsin 53701

WYOMING

Medicare
The Equitable Life Assurance Society
P.O. Box 628
Cheyenne, Wyoming 82001

PUERTO RICO

Medicare
Seguros De Servicio De Salud De Puerto Rico
G.P.O. Box 3628
Hato Rey, Puerto Rico 00936

VIRGIN ISLANDS

Medicare
Mutual of Omaha Insurance Co.
P.O. Box 456, Downtown Station
Omaha, Nebraska 68101

AMERICAN SAMOA

Medicare
Aetna Life & Casualty
P.O. Box 3947
Honolulu, Hawaii 96812

GUAM

Medicare
Aetna Life & Casualty
P.O. Box 3947
Honolulu, Hawaii 96812

QUESTIONS AND ANSWERS ABOUT
MEDICAL INSURANCE

1. **Where can I get more copies of the Request for Medicare Payment form?**

   Generally when you send a claim to the carrier, you will get back a new *Request for Medicare Payment* form to use for your next claim. Also, most doctors' offices have a supply of the forms. And you can always get extra copies from your social security office.

2. **Is there a limit on what medical insurance will pay for doctors' services when the services are mainly for the treatment of mental illness?**

   Yes. When such services are furnished outside a hospital, the payment is limited to a maximum of $250 a year.

3. **Who makes the decision whether to rent or purchase durable medical equipment my doctor has prescribed for use in my home?**

   You do. When considering purchase, particularly of expensive equipment, you should keep in mind that the Medicare payments are made over a period of time, based on the reasonable rental rate for the equipment, and that these payments stop when your need for the equipment ends. So in deciding whether to purchase equipment, you may wish to talk to your doctor about how long you may need it. Your social security office can also help when you have any questions.

4. **What happens if I want to assign the payment to a doctor, but he doesn't want to accept an assignment?**

   That is his right. He does not have to take an assignment of your benefits. If your doctor doesn't agree to take your assignment, the payment will be made directly to you, whether or not the bill has been paid.

5. **If I assign the benefit to my doctor or supplier, does this mean all my future benefit claims must also be handled on an assignment basis?**

   No. The payment can be made directly to your doctor or supplier one time and the next time it can be made to you.

6. **I understand that the medical insurance benefits are paid on a "reasonable charge" basis. Who decides what the reasonable charge is, and how does this affect payment?**

   The carrier determines "reasonable charge" for covered services. If there is an assignment, the doctor or supplier agrees that the reasonable charge will be his total charge and that he will charge *you* only for any of the $50 deductible not yet met and 20 percent of the balance of the "reasonable charge." If there is no assignment, medical insurance can pay *you* only 80 percent of the reasonable charge (after the $50 deductible is met), even if the bill exceeds the "reasonable charge." (See page 609.)

7. **What can I do if I disagree with the amount paid on my claim?**

   Write to the carrier which handled the claim and tell why you disagree with the amount allowed. If you are still not satisfied with the reply, you can request a hearing from the carrier.

8. Medicare does not pay all the doctor's bills. What can I do if I can't pay the rest?

If you do not have any other insurance or other resources with which you can pay the amounts due, you may want to ask at your public assistance office about help. The people there can give you information about a State program such as old-age assistance or medical assistance for the aged (sometimes called "medicaid").

SOME HEALTH SERVICES AND ITEMS THAT NEITHER HOSPITAL INSURANCE NOR MEDICAL INSURANCE WILL PAY FOR

Under each kind of benefit described under hospital insurance, there is a list of items and services hospital insurance will not pay for. The medical insurance part of the book also has a list of items and services that medical insurance will not pay for. But there are some other items or services that are not covered under either part of Medicare. These are shown in the following list:

- Services that are not reasonable and necessary for the diagnosis or treatment of an illness or injury.
- Cosmetic surgery—*except when furnished in connection with prompt repair of accidental injury or for the improvement of the functioning of a malformed body member.*
- Services for which neither the patient nor another party on his behalf has a legal obligation to pay—*such as free chest X-ray.*
- Certain services payable under other Federal, State, or local government programs.
- Services furnished by immediate relatives or members of the patient's household.

THE FIRST 3 PINTS OF BLOOD

Medicare cannot pay for the first 3 pints of whole blood (or units of packed red blood cells) that you receive either under hospital or medical insurance.

- Hospital insurance cannot pay for the first 3 pints of blood you receive in a *benefit period*. Usually, when you receive blood under hospital insurance it will be as a bed patient in a hospital.
- Medical insurance cannot pay for the first 3 pints of blood you receive in a *calendar year*. Usually, when you receive blood under medical insurance it will be in a doctor's office, a clinic, or the outpatient or emergency department of a hospital.

These are *separate* rules and they operate independently of each other. For example, if you receive blood under both hospital insurance and medical insurance, Medicare could not pay for the first 3 pints of blood under *either* program. But the blood you get under hospital insurance is fully paid for starting with the fourth pint during a benefit period; medical insurance will help pay for the blood you get starting with the fourth pint during a calendar year.

How to Get Help to Replace Blood

Some people are able to arrange for the replacement of these first 3 pints of blood—that way they don't have to pay for them. There are two ways this can be done. First, you may arrange for replacement from a friend or relative or you may be a member of a blood donor group that will replace these first 3 pints of blood for you. Second—and this is often overlooked—your children (or your son-in-law or daughter-in-law) may belong to a blood replacement plan that includes you as a beneficiary. In that case, you would be eligible for blood on the basis of *their* membership.

You might want to check with your children and children-in-law about this so you'll have the information handy if you ever need it.

In almost all blood donor plans, blood replacement credit can be arranged anywhere in the United States.

SPEECH

See APOPLEXY, OR STROKE; HEARING AND DEAFNESS; MENTAL CHANGES; PARKINSON'S DISEASE AND PALSY; REHABILITATION AND PHYSICAL THERAPY; TEETH.

Do speech changes often take place after sixty?

Healthy people in their sixties rarely show changes in their manner of speaking, although those in their seventies and eighties may.

What changes in speech normally take place as people age?

1. Speech becomes slower.
2. Older people tend to articulate less clearly.
3. There is often hesitation in finding the right word, especially if it is one that is used infrequently.
4. Words may be slurred.
5. The voice may drop in volume toward the end of a sentence.
6. There may be stammering or, less often, stuttering.
7. Older people who spoke another language in their youth tend to revert to their native tongue. This peculiar phenomenon takes place mainly among those in their late seventies or eighties who are showing signs of cerebral arteriosclerosis.

Does the amount of speaking that one has done in earlier life affect the age at which speech changes take place?

Definitely. Those who have done a great deal of public speaking or who have been accustomed to addressing large groups of people will retain their speaking abilities far longer and better than those who have not been so trained. As a matter of fact, some people perform best in their sixties and seventies because they are so familiar with the methods of effective communication. As we know, some of the world's greatest orators have been men in their sixties and seventies.

Is there a natural tendency for aging people to forget names and places?

Yes, especially for those names and places they have known for only a short time, but they can often remember the names of people and places they knew fifty or sixty years earlier.

Do poorly fitting dentures interfere with speech?

Yes. Older people should have their dentures checked regularly.

What routine should be followed by older people who have difficulty with speech?

1. They should write down the essential things they want to say before they are confronted with the need to say them.
2. If they are to give a speech, they should read it rather than speak extemporaneously.
3. If there is impairment of vision, the speech should be written in capital letters or should be printed in large block letters on cards.
4. Companions of older people should explain to others that there is need for particular attention lest the speaker be upset or confused by inattentiveness.

Can an older person who stammers or searches for words be aided by those to whom he is speaking?

Yes. Those who have contact with older people should be exceptionally tolerant and should permit them plenty of time in which to make themselves understood. It is also helpful to supply the missing word when it can be anticipated. Further help can be given by asking others within earshot of the speaker to be quiet.

Should those who are in the company of people with speech difficulties take over for them, or should they be permitted to "go it alone"?

It hurts the pride of an older person to have someone speak for him. It is much better to aid him, as outlined above, rather than to take over completely.

What are other methods for aiding older people in speech communication?

1. Listen carefully, so that it is unnecessary for them to repeat.

2. Urge those who are in the same room not to talk at the same time.

3. Look directly at the speaker. Often it will be possible to read his lips and thus obviate the necessity for repetition.

4. Supply the missing word or thought if the speaker is groping too long.

5. Do not walk out of the room while an older person is speaking.

6. Do not permit others to interrupt while he is speaking.

7. If he is speaking too softly, tell him so at the beginning of the conversation.

8. If the speaker has a hearing loss, suggest that he wear a hearing aid. This device will help him speak better.

Why is it that some people lose their power of speech as a result of a stroke, whereas others retain normal speech?

This will depend on which area of the brain was affected by the hemorrhage or blood clot. If the stroke is in the area of the patient's speech center, the power of speech is usually lost; if not, speech is retained. (The speech center in a right-handed person is on the left side of the brain. In a left-handed person, the speech center is located on the right side of the brain.)

Can people who have lost their power of speech as a result of a stroke ever be retrained to speak?

Yes. Speech rehabilitation can sometimes accomplish startling results. If the afflicted individual is exceptionally intelligent, his chances for regaining power of speech are greater. Furthermore, if the damage to the speech center is only slight or moderate, the chances of recovery are greater.

If regaining speech is not possible, can rehabilitation still be helpful?

Yes. There are experts in this field who can train the patient to make his needs easily understood by those around him. Also, one who has lost the power of speech may retain the power of writing and so be able to communicate in that manner.

SPLEEN

See ANEMIA; BLOOD; LEUKEMIA; LYMPH GLANDS.

What is the spleen?

It is a solid, reddish-purple gland located near the stomach toward the back of the abdominal cavity on the upper left-hand side beneath the ribs. It measures approximately five inches in length, three inches in width, and two inches in thickness.

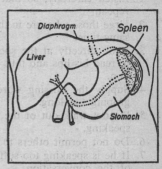

The spleen and organs to which it is attached

What are the functions of the spleen?

It is a blood-lymph gland concerned with blood-cell storage, manufacture and destruction of red blood cells, and iron metabolism. During development of the embryo, the spleen produces both red and white blood cells. After birth, this function is taken over by the bone marrow, and the spleen normally confines its activities to the production of certain white blood cells and to red-blood-cell storage, iron metabolism, and disposition of worn-out red blood cells. It has the additional function of destroying bacteria that reach it through the bloodstream.

Does the spleen usually function normally throughout life?

Yes. The changes of age may lead to some replacement of its functioning tissue by fibrous tissue, but, by and large, most older people have normal splenic function.

Does disease or disturbance in function of the spleen ever affect older people?

Occasionally. It has been found that upset in function of this organ may lead to anemia, to impaired function of the bone marrow, or to failure of the blood-clotting mechanism.

What does "hypersplenism" mean?

It is a vague term used to denote excessive function of the spleen. In hypersplenism, the ability of the bone marrow to produce red blood cells may be impaired and a disturbance in the blood-clotting mechanism may result. Severe anemia may follow.

What is the treatment of hypersplenism?

If the spleen functions so abnormally that an uncontrollable anemia results, it should be removed. This operation, although of major proportions, can be performed safely on older people.

Is the spleen essential to normal living?

No.

Is the spleen often the primary site of a tumor?

No. Although cancer that is primary elsewhere in the body will often spread to the spleen, rarely does a tumor originate in this organ.

STOMACH AND DUODENUM

See DIET; ESOPHAGUS; GASTRITIS; HERNIA; INTESTINES; ULCERS OF STOMACH AND DUODENUM.

How much of the digestive process takes place in the stomach?

Contrary to common belief, the stomach plays a small role in the digestion and absorption of food. Its main functions are to churn food and to break it down into smaller particles. Digestion is initiated in the stomach with the action of hydrochloric acid, but only water, alcohol, and a small quantity of proteins are absorbed through the stomach

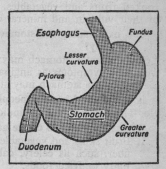

Stomach

wall. The major part of the digestive process takes place farther on in the small intestines.

Is the stomach an essential part of the intestinal tract?

Life can be sustained even after the entire stomach has been removed. However, the stomach is important in maintaining general nutrition. People who have undergone total stomach removal become markedly anemic and underweight. Those who have had two-thirds or even three-quarters of their stomachs removed can maintain fairly normal nutrition and weight.

Does stomach capacity tend to decrease as one grows older?

Yes.

Should people eat less food as they grow older?

Yes, since caloric requirements will lessen with decreased physical activity. Moreover, older people find it more difficult to digest large meals.

Is it good practice for older people to cut down on the amount of spices and condiments they eat?

Yes. A bland diet is much more digestible.

Should older people cut down on the amount of fried and fatty foods they eat?

Yes, because bile secretion tends to slow down during the later years, which makes the digestion of fats and greases more difficult.

Should older people cut down on the amount of raw fruits and vegetables they eat?

Only if they cause indigestion. Despite the fact that raw fruits and vegetables may be more difficult to digest than cooked fruits and vegetables, they should be eaten because of their vitamin and mineral content.

Can overloading the stomach do harm to other organs of the body?

Yes, a distended stomach may cause pressure upon the heart, with such symptoms as angina pectoris. Also, repeated over-loading of the stomach may strain the liver and pancreas.

Is it natural for older people to belch or have heartburn?

No. These symptoms are indicative of disturbed digestion.

What foods tend to create gas, belching, and heartburn?

1. Fruit skins and vegetables containing a large amount of fiber, such as celery, cabbage, and lettuce.
2. Fatty or fried foods.
3. Highly seasoned foods.
4. Rich foods, such as custard, and foods containing large quantities of cream.
5. Any food taken in large amounts.

How much do the emotions affect stomach function?

Emotional upsets almost invariably upset digestion. The upper or lower end of the stomach may go into spasm as the result of an emotional disturbance. The most frequent symptoms are loss of appetite, pain in the upper abdomen, nausea, and vomiting.

Does smoking affect digestion?

In all probability, moderate smoking does not disturb digestion. However, heavy smoking (a package or more of cigarettes a day) will cause excessive secretion of acid and gastric juices.

Can healthy older people drink alcoholic beverages without hurting digestion?

Yes, if they drink in moderation. A small amount of alcohol will actually aid digestion.

How can an older person find out whether or not there is anything wrong with his stomach?

By having stomach X rays taken each year, even if he has no symptoms.

What symptoms should alert one to possible stomach trouble?

1. Loss of appetite for more than a few days.
2. Frequent episodes of nausea or vomiting.
3. Heartburn, belching, and flatulence.
4. The onset of anemia.
5. Pain in the upper part of the abdomen.
6. Jet-black, tarry stools.
7. Loss of weight.

Are loss of appetite and loss in weight early symptoms of stomach trouble?

Not necessarily. Serious stomach disorders may be present for several weeks or even months with little effect on appetite or weight.

Does the stomach secrete less acid as one grows older?

Yes. It is estimated that approximately one out of four people over sixty-five years of age secrete no hydrochloric acid at all.

Can one live normally without the secretion of hydrochloric acid?

Yes. The great majority of those who secrete no acid have normal digestion. If indigestion does develop, it can usually be relieved by taking dilute hydrochloric acid drops in milk or fruit juice. Some people whose stomachs do not secrete hydrochloric acid will become anemic.

Will diminished acid secretion lower the chances of developing an ulcer of the stomach or duodenum?

Yes. (*See* ULCERS OF STOMACH AND DUODENUM.)

What is pylorospasm?

The pylorus is the outlet of the stomach. At this site there is a thick muscle sphincter that opens and closes, allowing small quantities of food to pass from the stomach into the duodenum (the beginning of the small intestine). The pyloric sphincter, when irritated, may go into such spasm that it will not emit any food for a period of several minutes or even hours.

What are the symptoms of pylorospasm?
When the pylorus goes into severe spasm, a sharp pain in the upper midabdomen, beneath the breastbone, may ensue. This is sometimes followed by nausea and vomiting.

What causes pylorospasm?
1. Stress, tension, excitement, annoyance, etc.
2. Eating too large a meal.
3. Eating very spicy, highly seasoned foods.
4. Drinking too much alcohol.
5. Eating greasy foods.
6. Eating too quickly and failing to chew food sufficiently.

What is the treatment of pylorospasm?
Most of the time the spasm will subside spontaneously within a few minutes or an hour or two. When it doesn't, a doctor should be called. He will, in all probability, give an injection of an antispasmodic drug and prescribe antispasmodics to be taken by mouth.

TUMORS OF THE STOMACH

How common is cancer of the stomach in people past sixty?
The greatest incidence of cancer of the stomach is between the ages of fifty and sixty. The next most common age is from sixty and after.

Are all tumors of the stomach cancerous?

No. Benign tumors, such as lipomas (fatty tumors), myomas (muscle tumors), or polyps of the mucous membrane, do occur.

What are the early symptoms of cancer of the stomach?

Unfortunately, most stomach cancers grow stealthily, without symptoms, for a period of several months. For this reason it is important that older people have their stomachs X-rayed each year.

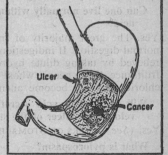
Diagram of stomach ulcer and stomach cancer

What are some of the late symptoms of cancer of the stomach?
1. Loss of appetite.

2. Nausea and vomiting.
3. Anemia.
4. Loss of weight.
5. Pain in the upper abdomen.

How can a tumor of the stomach be diagnosed?
1. By stomach X rays.
2. By examining stomach contents for tumor cells.
3. By performing a gastroscopy.
4. By surgical examination.

What is gastroscopy?
It is the passing of a long, metal, hollow tube through the mouth and down the esophagus into the stomach. The examining physician can sometimes see the tumor directly through the gastroscope.

What is the treatment of cancer of the stomach?
Surgical removal of the cancer-bearing portion of the stomach, leaving behind only the uninvolved stump. The remaining stump of the stomach is then stitched to the small intestine, allowing food to pass through into the small intestine. This procedure is called a gastrectomy.

Is cancer of the stomach ever curable?
Yes, if it is operated on before it has spread to distant structures. With earlier diagnosis, an even greater number of people are being saved, although this type of cancer is still one of the most lethal of all malignancies.

Is there any way to prevent cancer of the stomach?
No.

What is the treatment of a benign tumor of the stomach?
It should be removed surgically. Most stomach tumors can be removed locally, leaving the stomach behind. In some cases in which the tumor involves a large portion of the stomach, a subtotal gastrectomy is performed. This will mean the removal of two-thirds to three-quarters of the stomach.

SURGERY

See ANESTHESIA; APPENDICITIS; CANCER AND OTHER MALIGNANT DISEASES; HERNIA; PLASTIC SURGERY.

Is there increasing need for surgery as one advances in age?
Yes. As one ages, more organs require repair, removal, or replacement. Modern surgical techniques have been developed

for repair of such organs as the heart, some major blood vessels, the intestines, the kidneys, and other major structures. Just as there is no need to move out of a house because it has become old and requires repairs, so there is no need to consign an older patient to invalidism when he shows a defect in one of his important structures.

Is advanced age in itself a contraindication to surgery?

No. Within the past twenty to thirty years, physicians and surgeons have learned a great deal about supporting the aging individual so that he can withstand surgery.

Does the expression "too old to be operated on" hold true in most cases today?

No. Many years ago, surgeons would often refrain from surgery on older people because of the fear of anesthetic difficulties, lung complications, heart or kidney failure, and other problems. Today, most of these dangers can be eliminated or controlled.

How much greater is the risk of surgery for older patients than for younger ones?

If they are in satisfactory general health, there is very little added risk. On the other hand, if major degenerative changes have taken place, the risk is considerably greater.

What are the most important contraindications to surgery on older people?

Heart failure or inadequate heart function; extensive coronary-artery disease; marked arteriosclerosis; extremely high blood pressure; cirrhosis or other liver disease; extensive kidney damage; unusual resistance to the idea of being operated on.

What special precautions will a surgeon take before operating on a patient who is in his seventies, eighties, or nineties?

1. He will ascertain to the best of his ability the cardiac condition of the patient. This will be done by taking an electrocardiogram and by having an internist in consultation. If necessary, the heart will be treated with digitalis, and the patient will be given diuretics (medications to get rid of excess body fluids).

2. The adequacy of kidney, liver, adrenal, and pancreatic function will be determined through chemical analysis of the blood. In particular, the levels of blood sugar, urea, uric acid, proteins, sodium, chloride, and potassium will be noted. If major impairment of these organs is

discovered, and if the contemplated surgery is elective rather than essential, postponement or cancellation will probably be recommended.

3. A blood count will be taken to ascertain whether anemia is present and whether the patient has a blood disease. Tests to note the adequacy of the blood-clotting mechanism will be carried out.

   If anemia or impaired blood clotting is found, transfusions, chemicals, and vitamins will be prescribed preoperatively.

4. An X ray of the lungs will be taken. If impairment, such as emphysema, bronchitis, or bronchiectasis is noted, appropriate preoperative medication will be given.

5. The physician and surgeon will always attempt to evaluate the mental attitude of the older patient toward the surgery that is about to be performed. If he has great resistance to being operated on or inordinate fear of death, the surgeon will think twice before operating, unless it is absolutely necessary. A "will to live" is an essential component of smooth recovery after surgery.

6. Finally, the surgeon must judge the overall ability of his patient to withstand the surgery. Fortunately, because of greater knowledge in prevention of postoperative complications, advances in anesthetic methods, availability of blood for transfusion, increased knowledge of chemical requirements, and the advent of the antibiotic drugs, most surgery can now be performed safely, regardless of the age of the patient.

Are such elective operations as repair of hernia or removal of hemorrhoids or gallstones safe to perform on most older patients?

Yes. These operations have extremely low mortality rates, provided the patient is in a satisfactory state of health.

Should the surgeon explain the exact nature of the operation to the patient before performing it?

Yes, and it is perhaps more important to do this with older patients than with younger ones. The former are usually better able to adjust to the realities of the situation. Moreover, if information is unnecessarily withheld from older people, they are more likely to come to erroneous conclusions concerning the ultimate outcome.

Should older patients engage the services of an internist before surgery?

Yes. Since older people are more susceptible to postoperative complications involving organs such as the heart, lungs, liver, and kidneys, it is important that they have an expert to care for them before and after the operation.

Is an adequate oxygen supply during surgery important for older patients?

Yes. The brain, the heart, and other organs will suffer inordinately in older people if there is the slightest oxygen shortage during the operation. Extra oxygen may be needed because of diminished respiratory function in this group of patients.

How is extra oxygen administered to patients after surgery?

1. By placing in the nose a rubber tube that is attached to an oxygen tank.
2. By placing an oxygen mask over the face.
3. By placing the patient in an oxygen tent.

Do older people tend to react differently from younger ones to pre- and postoperative medications?

Yes. The dosage of morphine, scopolamine, phenobarbital and other barbiturates, atropine, etc., must be modified for older patients. Their age and weight must be given careful consideration in calculating dosages.

Is anemia a deterrent to surgery on older patients?

Since the tissues of older people are more sensitive to lack of oxygen, anemia assumes a role of great importance. Insufficient red blood cells will lead to inadequate oxygen supply to the tissues. It is therefore important that anemic patients be given blood transfusions to tide them over the operative period. After the patient has recovered from surgery, the anemia can be attacked more vigorously.

Are blood transfusions safe for older people?

Yes.

Is high blood pressure (hypertension) a contraindication to surgery in older people?

If people in their seventies or eighties have blood-pressure readings above 200, elective operations may be postponed until the pressure can be brought down to a more normal level. However, if surgery is necessary, the high pressure should not act as a deterrent. Special measures will be taken by the internist and the anesthetist so that the operation can proceed with relative safety.

Does high blood pressure increase the risks of surgery?

Yes.

Is there a greater tendency for older patients to go into surgical shock?

Naturally, they do not withstand extensive procedures as well as younger people do, and therefore have a higher incidence of shock. However, the overall incidence of shock is not great because of improved pre- and postoperative care. Control of blood loss, maintenance of chemical and mineral balance, adequate oxygen supply, and more refined operative techniques have cut down tremendously on the incidence of this grave complication.

How is the condition of the heart checked during surgery?

By observing a continuous tracing of the heart action with a cardioscope. This instrument, which is similar to an electrocardiogram, projects a tracing of the heart's action on a screen. Deviations from normal can be seen immediately, and appropriate measures to correct them will be taken instantly.

What measures are taken to support the heart and blood vessels both before and after major surgery?

1. An electrocardiogram is taken and studied.
2. If there is evidence of inadequate heart function, digitalis or a similar drug may be prescribed.
3. If the body contains extra fluid, diuretics are given to increase fluid output.
4. If the blood pressure is extremely high, several days of preoperative bed rest may be prescribed. (Medications to lower high blood pressure preoperatively are no longer being prescribed; the artificially lowered pressure creates a false picture during surgery and may lead to cardiac failure.)
5. Marked anemia is treated by giving transfusions preoperatively.
6. If there is marked hardening of the arteries, drugs to cause blood-vessel dilatation are sometimes given.
7. Ample supplies of oxygen will always be maintained.

Is liver function of particular importance in operations on older patients?

Yes. Impaired liver function is one of the most frequent causes of death from surgery.

The liver can best be supported preoperatively by giving large amounts of protein and sugar, both orally and intravenously. At the same time there should be a very low intake of fat. If the flow of bile is obstructed, as in cases of jaundice, vitamin K is given to prevent excessive operative or postoperative bleeding.

What measures are taken to aid liver function during the postoperative period?

Large quantities of sugar in the form of glucose are given. Also, proteins and vitamins B, C, and K may be prescribed.

What special measures are taken to aid kidney function after surgery?

The major consideration is that the patient's output of urine is adequate. Also, the chemical balance of the patient must be maintained. This will involve a constant survey of the amounts of sodium, chlorides, potassium, phosphorus, calcium, albumin, globulin, and urea that circulate in the blood or appear in the urine. Specific measures may have to be taken from time to time to increase the amount of certain chemicals or to decrease the amount of others that are present in too great concentration.

Failure of kidney function is one of the most common causes of surgical mortality in older patients.

What special preoperative measures can be taken to prevent lung complications?

1. If the patient is a heavy smoker, he should stop smoking for several days prior to admission to the hospital.
2. If a respiratory infection is present and the surgery is elective, it should be postponed until the infection has been brought under control.
3. If there is a tendency toward repeated lung infections, antibiotics should be given before, during, and after surgery.
4. The patient should be instructed that it will be necessary for him to breathe deeply and to cough up all mucus, even if these measures cause pain.

Is it common practice to keep older patients in recovery rooms after surgery?

Yes. All facilities for treating postoperative patients are concentrated in the recovery room. Such rooms have a constant supply of oxygen, drugs for postoperative patients, suction apparatus to keep the breathing passages open, and—most important of all—a staff of specially trained nurses and doctors in constant attendance.

How long are patients kept in recovery rooms?

Those with minor conditions may be kept for only an hour or two. Those who have had extensive surgery may be kept for an entire day or even for several days. Families should know of this practice in advance, so that they do not worry unnecessarily.

What can the patient do postoperatively to aid his own recovery?

1. He should breathe deeply, to expand his lungs fully.
2. He should cough up mucus, even if it causes pain in the incision.
3. He should move about in bed and get out of bed as soon as permitted. This will aid his circulation and help to prevent blood clots from forming in veins.
4. He should inform his surgeon or nurse if he has any unusual symptoms or discomfort.
5. He should force himself to eat whatever is permitted to him, even if he has no appetite.

Do older surgical patients require longer periods of postoperative bed rest?

On the contrary. It is more important that older patients get out of bed early in order to prevent complications such as pneumonia and phlebitis. The latter conditions occur more often in the older age groups.

Will physical activity after surgery delay wound healing?

No. It has been shown that wounds will heal more quickly if the patient is active after surgery.

What is early ambulation?

It means getting out of bed and walking soon after surgery. In most instances, this will be within a day or two after the operation has been performed. Such early ambulation stimulates circulation and tends to lead to better aeration of the lungs.

What preoperative precautions are necessary concerning the patient's teeth?

1. The surgeon and anesthetist should be notified if there are any loose teeth. All too often a loose tooth will be knocked out during anesthesia, and it may be swallowed or aspirated into the windpipe. Such teeth should be removed prior to surgery.
2. Patients should inform the anesthetist about all dentures. All removable dentures should be taken out before the patient undergoes anesthesia.
3. If the surgery is elective, all decayed or abscessed teeth should be removed before the patient enters the hospital. They are frequently the source of postoperative infections.

Are any special anesthetic procedures designed for older surgical patients?

Yes. (*See* ANESTHESIA.)

Are special measures necessary to promote wound healing in older surgical patients?

Not if the patient is in good general health. However, if he is debilitated or undernourished, supplementary proteins and vitamins B and C may be given during the postoperative period. Also, it is well known that anemic patients tend to heal more slowly. In such cases, blood transfusions are often given pre- and postoperatively.

Is it important to know that the body contains an adequate vitamin supply prior to surgery?

Yes. Vitamin deficiencies may lead to poor wound healing and, in some instances, to uncontrollable hemorrhage. It is therefore common practice to give large doses of supplementary vitamins to older surgical patients.

How can one determine whether or not a preoperative patient has an adequate supply of body proteins?

By analyzing the blood for the amount of circulating albumin and globulin. If these substances are deficient, blood will be given.

Is it important to regulate fluid intake and output when operating on an older patient?

Yes. Too much fluid may place a strain on the heart and lungs. Too little fluid may endanger kidney function. Maintaining the delicate balance between fluid intake and output is one of the most difficult problems of surgery on older people.

Do older patients find it more difficult to void after surgery?

Yes, especially while remaining in bed. Men, in particular, may find it more difficult because of enlargement of the prostate gland.

To encourage spontaneous urination, patients should be gotten out of bed as soon as possible after surgery. If they still cannot void, a rubber catheter is passed into the bladder.

Are older patients more susceptible to postoperative infections?

Not if they are in good general health. However, if they are anemic, underweight, or suffer from a vitamin deficiency, they are more susceptible.

What can be done to overcome postoperative infections in older patients?

As stated elsewhere, older people respond well to the antibiotic drugs. These are often given prophylactically to those in whom one expects a possible postoperative infection.

Is it necessary for older patients to remain in the hospital longer after surgery?

Their rate of recovery might be slightly slower than that of younger patients, but this is usually a matter of a few days. Of course, if they are exceptionally debilitated and aged, the time needed for recovery will be much longer.

How soon after major surgery can most patients bathe?

When the surgical wound has healed completely. If there is an opening, or drain, in the wound, showers and baths cannot be taken.

How soon after major surgery can patients go out of the house?

By the time most patients are discharged from the hospital, they have been walking about the hospital corridors for several days. If the weather is pleasant, there is no reason why they should not go for a walk or sit out of doors when they go home.

Can older patients climb stairs after coming home from the hospital?

Yes, provided they climb only a flight or two.

How soon after surgery can the average surgical patient drive his car?

It is perhaps best for older patients to wait six to seven weeks, even though driving modern automobiles demands very little physical effort. The necessity to stop or swerve suddenly may place too great a strain on a recent surgical wound.

Is it good practice for older patients to take extra vitamins after surgery?

Yes, since appetite and food intake are often decreased after major surgery.

Is it advisable for older patients to wear a support after an abdominal operation?

This question can be answered only by the attending surgeon. It will depend on the type of operation that has been performed and on how satisfactorily the wound has healed. In many instances, an abdominal support gives the sensation of added protection even though it is not actually doing much good. When a support is worn, it is best to use an ordinary two-way elastic support. Trusses and complicated surgical belts are rarely indicated after abdominal surgery.

Is it natural to have some pain, tingling, a sensation of numbness, and a feeling of tightness in a wound area?

Yes. Such sensations may persist for weeks or even months

after an operation. Nerves and muscles are severed in surgery, and these structures may take a long time to grow together again. If wound pain becomes severe, the surgeon should be notified.

SYPHILIS

See ANEURYSMS; GONORRHEA; MENTAL CHANGES; NERVES; OPTIC-NERVE ATROPHY; TESTS.

Can older people contract syphilis as readily as younger people?

Yes, if they are exposed to it. There is no natural or acquired immunity to venereal disease. Naturally, people in their sixties, seventies, and eighties are less likely to be exposed to a syphilitic contact.

What is the most common form of syphilis seen in older people?

Tertiary syphilis. This is the late stage of syphilis, seen in those who failed to receive adequate treatment during the early stages of the disease.

What are some of the organs affected by tertiary syphilis?

Any organ may be affected, but the following are most likely to be involved:

1. The brain. This will result in extreme mental disorder and paralysis (paresis).
2. The spinal cord. This will cause a condition known as locomotor ataxia or tabes dorsalis.
3. The blood vessels. One of the most frequent sites of involvement is the aorta, the large blood vessel leading away from the heart. It may lead to aneurysm of the aorta. (*See* ANEURYSMS.)
4. The liver. The most common effect on this organ is formation of a gumma, or syphilitic abscess.
5. The skin. Syphilitic lesions (nonhealing ulcers and rashes) may appear.

Does tertiary syphilis respond well to treatment?

No. Primary and secondary syphilis respond very well to the newer antibiotic medications, but tertiary syphilis is much less responsive to treatment. For this reason it is very important to treat syphilis vigorously during its early stages.

Can older people transmit syphilis to others?

If it is tertiary syphilis, it is not usually contagious. However, if an older person contracts a primary syphilitic lesion, it is just as contagious as when it is contracted by a younger individual.

Does tertiary syphilis ever cause blindness?

Yes, since it may produce inflammation of the optic nerves.

How can one tell if he has syphilis?

By any of several accurate blood tests.

How does tertiary syphilis affect the heart?

Long-standing, untreated syphilis damages the aortic valve, which often leads to heart failure.

Does syphilis often attack the nervous system?

Yes, but this is not nearly so common today as it was thirty or forty years ago. In the days when syphilis went untreated and when treatment was less effective, involvement of the nervous system was extensive.

How does syphilis affecting the nervous system evidence itself?

1. *Paresis.* This is a form of psychosis due to syphilis affecting the brain. It is usually associated with delusions of grandeur and lack of contact with reality.
2. *Locomotor ataxia* or *tabes dorsalis.* This is syphilis affecting the spinal cord, which results in loss of the sense of position in the lower extremities. It leads to a peculiar gait on walking, occasioned by the necessity of watching where the feet are being placed.

Is there any satisfactory treatment of paresis?

Yes, in a sizable number of cases the condition can be brought under control either by the administration of large doses of penicillin or by the "malaria" treatment. This latter method consists of giving the patient malaria in order to produce the accompanying chills and high fever. The high fever will often kill the syphilitic germs. Similar results have also been obtained by placing the patient in heat cabinets to raise body temperature.

Is there a cure for locomotor ataxia?

No, since the condition is associated with destruction of nerve cells. Once a nerve cell is destroyed, it cannot regenerate. Nevertheless, treatment of locomotor ataxia is important in preventing further spread of the syphilis.

TEETH

See DIET; LEUKOPLAKIA; MOUTH, LIPS, AND TONGUE; SMOKING; SPEECH; VITAMINS.

If one's general health remains good, and if the teeth have been well cared for during the early years, are the chances good that they will stay healthy when one gets older?

Yes. Teeth can remain in good condition throughout the lifespan if they are properly cared for. But most people neglect their teeth and so there is dental deterioration earlier than necessary. Furthermore, most people at one time or another during their lives develop generalized diseases that influence the health of the teeth.

Is it natural for teeth to fall out as people enter their sixties or seventies?

Actually, this is not a natural phenomenon. As mentioned above, loss of teeth is due either to neglect or to some underlying disease or disturbance in body function.

Do older people have a greater tendency to develop dental caries?

Yes, because calcium deficiency in the aging is quite common.

Is an increase in the number of caries an indication that there is something wrong with the general health?

It may or may not be, but one should undergo a complete physical examination to rule out a systemic disease. Blood-chemistry analysis and bone X rays will usually uncover any calcium deficiency.

Is it natural for teeth to show evidences of wear from prolonged use?

Yes. They will wear down along the edges and the gums may recede. With loss of strength in the jawbone, teeth may loosen in their sockets. If the contour of the jawbone changes, teeth may get out of alignment and the bite will suffer.

How often should older people have their teeth examined?

At least twice a year, and, of course, whenever they develop symptoms.

Does disease of the gums often indicate that there is something wrong with the general state of health?

Yes. Vitamin deficiency and blood diseases may first evidence themselves by gum inflammation, swelling, and bleeding.

Upper

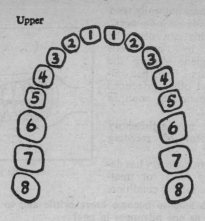

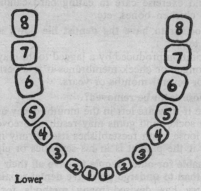

Lower

Full set of adult teeth

1. Middle incisor teeth
2. Lateral incisors
3. Canine teeth
4. Premolar teeth
5. Bicuspid teeth
6. Molar teeth
7. Molar teeth
8. Wisdom teeth

Do the gums naturally tend to recede as one ages?

Yes, but this can often be overcome by continuous mouth hygiene during the earlier years. Pyorrhea alveolaris and other infections must be treated as soon as they appear.

Is there any satisfactory treatment of receding gums?

Yes. Modern dentistry has devised many forms of treatment to control this condition.

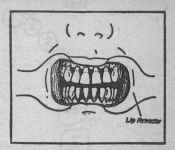

Receding gums

Do teeth tend to become more brittle and to break more easily as one advances in age?

Yes, much in the same manner as bones tend to lose strength and become more susceptible to fracture. For this reason, older people should exercise care in eating hard candies, chewing on meat or chicken bones, etc.

Is it important to have the dentist file down a broken or jagged tooth?

Yes. The irritation produced by a jagged tooth may cause cancer of the tongue or cheek membranes if it is permitted to go untreated for several months or years.

Should loose teeth be removed?

Yes, because if they are left in the mouth, decay and infection of the tooth socket and gums may result. Moreover, it is rare that a very loose tooth reestablishes itself firmly in its socket, particularly if the patient is in his seventies or eighties.

Is it advisable for older people to have all their teeth pulled rather than to undergo extensive dental repair?

No. Dentistry has devised many methods for preserving teeth. Every attempt should be made to save the tooth before extracting it. Artificial teeth, although satisfactory in many instances, are not a complete substitute for one's own teeth.

What are some of the adverse results of loss of teeth in older people?

1. Loss of teeth is often associated with disturbance in chewing. Marked disturbances of this nature may eventually lead to malnutrition.
2. It may be associated with improper alignment of the jawbone and faulty occlusion of the teeth.

3. Pain in the joint connecting the lower jaw to the temple region may result.
4. The appearance of the face is often altered markedly by the loss of several teeth. This, in turn, may cause considerable emotional upset to an older individual.
5. Speech is frequently altered and impeded by loss of teeth.
6. The mere knowledge that there has been tooth loss can produce depression in aging people, since it indicates so clearly that they are showing the effects of age.

Do teeth tend to get out of alignment as people grow older?

Yes. If teeth wear down unevenly, they will get out of alignment. Also, there is a tendency for the shape of the jawbone to change with age, and this will contribute to faulty alignment.

Will the loss of molar teeth ever lead to pain in the joint connecting the lower jaw to the face (temperomandibular joint)?

Yes, since it often causes malocclusion of the teeth, with subsequent strain on the muscles of mastication (chewing).

What can be done to remedy pain in the temperomandibular joint?

Dentures may replace the lost teeth, or extensive dental rehabilitation of all the remaining teeth may be necessary in order to reestablish proper alignment.

Is loss of teeth a common cause of malnutrition in older people?

Yes. People shy away from foods that require much chewing. They thereby omit many essential food elements from their diets. When chewing is impaired, older patients should get a list of essential and nourishing foods that require no mastication. Also, during this period, they should take supplementary vitamins and minerals.

Do teeth usually become discolored as people age?

Yes, particularly if they are heavy smokers. The condition should be treated by frequent visits to the dentist for removal of stains and tartar.

Can the teeth become discolored as a result of taking medications?

Yes. Certain drugs will eventually lead to discoloration of the teeth and gums. Any medication taken over a period of years should be suspected if tooth discoloration develops.

Is it dangerous to have the teeth X-rayed?

No. Recently the dangers of diagnostic X rays have been grossly exaggerated.

What special precautions should be taken by older patients before they visit a dentist?

1. Do not eat for several hours before visiting a dentist, for nausea and vomiting sometimes accompany extensive dental work or the giving of a local or general anesthetic. Moreover, it is dangerous to receive a general anesthetic shortly after eating.
2. If the patient knows himself to be sensitive to any drug or medication, he should so inform his dentist. This is particularly important if one is sensitive to novocaine or adrenalin.
3. If one is especially sensitive to pain, he should take a sedative before leaving for the dentist's office.
4. If the patient has a heart condition or any other major debility, the dentist should be informed before he begins work on the teeth. Also, it is perhaps best to get permission from one's doctor before receiving major dental treatment.
5. Preferably, dental work on older people should be performed in the dentist's office only if it can be accomplished with no anesthesia or with only local anesthesia. It is much safer to hospitalize an older patient who requires general anesthesia.

What is the significance of bleeding gums?

It may indicate the presence of a local infection in the mouth, or it may be part of a generalized disorder. Some of the common causes of bleeding gums are:

1. Pyorrhea alveolaris.
2. A Vincent's infection of the gums.
3. A loose tooth.
4. Injury secondary to strenuous brushing of the teeth.
5. Deposits of tartar between the gums and the teeth.
6. Vitamin deficiencies, especially of vitamins C and K.
7. Scurvy.
8. Hemophilia (inherited condition characterized by excessive bleeding).
9. Prolonged jaundice.
10. Blood diseases, with impairment of the blood-clotting mechanism.

Is it wise for people whose gums bleed to consult their dentist and physician?

Yes. *Both* should be consulted.

Does pyorrhea alveolaris occur often in older people?

Yes, especially when oral hygiene has been neglected.

What is pyorrhea alveolaris?

It is a general term used to describe any infection of the gums and the roots and sockets of the teeth.

What causes pyorrhea alveolaris?

Bacteria. Many varieties can and do grow in the mouth. Most pyorrheic infections are caused by a combination of several different bacteria.

What is the treatment of pyorrhea alveolaris?

1. Regular brushing and cleansing (by a dentist) of the teeth.
2. Regular removal of collected food particles and tartar from the area between the teeth and between the gums and the teeth.
3. Removal of decayed or loose teeth.
4. Filling of all dental caries (cavities).
5. Removal of abscessed teeth.
6. Application of medications locally. These may include sodium perborate and various antibiotic medications.
7. Treatment of the general condition of the patient with special attention to nutritional deficiencies, vitamin deficiencies, and anemic states.

Does infection of the teeth, gums, or mouth ever lead to infection elsewhere in the body?

Yes. Infected teeth are frequently the source of distant infection, including infections of the valves of the heart, kidney infections, and joint infections. It should be remembered that the tooth socket has small blood vessels at its base, and these vessels drain into the general circulation.

Does smoking affect the teeth?

The use of tobacco does not directly damage a tooth, but it does cause the deposit of tartar between the tooth and the surrounding gum. If tartar is permitted to collect, it can lead to infection and bleeding of the gums. Also, heavy smokers often develop discolored teeth.

Is it important for older people to be in good general health in order for dentures to be fitted accurately?

Yes. Poor general health may be accompanied by a condition in which there is swelling or retraction of the gums and mucous membranes in the mouth. If artificial teeth are fitted at such a time, they will not fit when the general state of health has improved.

What is the usual treatment of a root abscess or an infected tooth?

Rarely can the involved tooth be saved. It is common practice to remove teeth so afflicted.

Will drinking large quantities of milk help to prevent tooth decay and prolong the life of teeth?

Although it is essential that there be an adequate intake of calcium for the maintenance of healthy teeth, it is doubtful that drinking extra amounts of milk will do very much to prevent decay or to prolong the life of the teeth.

Will taking extra vitamins help to preserve the teeth?

Extra vitamins are of little value when intake is adequate. It should be stressed, however, that vitamin deficiency will often lead to infections and formation of dental caries.

What is the most common cause of acute toothache in older people?

An abscess at the base of a tooth or in the gum surrounding a tooth.

Should older patients with infections of the teeth or gums be given antibiotics?

Yes, if they are cardiac patients or if their general health is poor. This will protect against spread of the infection from the mouth to vital structures, such as the heart, kidneys, and liver. On the other hand, if they are healthy, robust people, they will usually not require antibiotics for a tooth or gum infection.

When in doubt in cases of this kind, the dentist will undoubtedly consult with the patient's doctor.

Does bad breath often originate from the teeth?

Yes. The following dental conditions may contribute toward bad breath:

1. Failure to remove and cleanse dentures regularly.
2. Infection of the gums.
3. Failure to brush teeth regularly and to remove food particles.
4. Failure to have decayed teeth removed.

If bad breath persists, even though none of the conditions above is present, then it most likely is caused by some condition unrelated to the teeth.

What special care of the teeth should older people take?

1. Teeth should be brushed gently after each meal. Strenuous brushing may cause injury to the gums.
2. Broken or jagged edges of teeth should be filed down by the dentist.

3. A dentist *and* physician should be consulted for repeated bleeding from the gums.

4. All removable dentures should be taken out and cleansed regularly.

5. The dentist should be visited at least twice a year, even if there is no apparent trouble with the teeth or gums.

DENTURES

Is it true that dentures tend to lose their accurate fit if they are not worn steadily?

Yes.

How often should removable dentures be cleaned?

If possible, after each meal, and certainly before retiring at night.

Should any special materials be used to cleanse or soak dentures?

Yes. The dentist should supply the names of products he prefers.

What special precautions concerning dentures should be taken by those who are to undergo surgery?

All removable dentures must be taken out of the mouth prior to surgery. If this is not done, small dentures may be swallowed or aspirated into the lungs during the administration of anesthesia or during the immediate postoperative period. Large dentures, if inadvertently left in place, may break, causing smaller parts to be swallowed or aspirated.

Is it safe for older people to have their teeth capped?

Yes, provided they are in good general health and the remaining portion of the tooth underlying the cap is healthy.

TESTICLES

See ADRENAL GLANDS; ENDOCRINE GLANDS AND HORMONES; MARRIAGE AFTER SIXTY; PROSTATE GLAND; SEX AFTER SIXTY; SEX HORMONES.

What are the usual changes that take place in the testicles as men grow older?

There is a gradual decline in the amount of male sex hormone secreted into the bloodstream and a decreasing ability to produce sperm cells. Ultimately, both of these functions come to a halt. The female has a rather abrupt cessation in ovarian function. The male's testicular changes take place slowly over a period of many years. Regardless of these physical evidences of aging, sexual desire and potency may persist long after sperm production has ceased.

What symptoms can result from lack of circulating male sex hormones?

In some men there are no symptoms. In others, the following may result:

1. Listlessness and fatigue.
2. Diminished muscle tone and muscle weakness.
3. Calcium withdrawal from the bones with resultant brittleness (osteoporosis).
4. Mental depression with loss of zest for living.

Do the above symptoms constitute a "male menopause"?

If there is such a thing, the above symptoms do constitute it. It must be stated, however, that these symptoms may never occur in some men, whereas *all* women sooner or later go through the menopause.

How can a man tell if he is continuing to produce live sperm?

By having a specimen of semen obtained through prostatic massage. The semen is then examined under a microscope for the presence or absence of live sperm.

Will giving male sex hormone restore the ability of the aging testicle to produce live sperm?

Once a testicle has stopped producing live sperm, giving hormones does relatively little good.

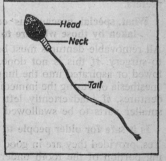
Sperm

What is the average age at which a man ceases to produce live sperm?

Generally, the testicles usually continue to produce live sperm until the age of seventy. There are many exceptions to this, and cases have been recorded in which the testicles have continued to produce live sperm well into the eighties and nineties.

Will the administration of male sex hormone prolong the period of potency?

Only when the loss of potency is due to insufficient secretion of the male sex hormone. (As stated elsewhere, the most frequent cause of loss of potency is psychological rather than physical.)

Is it dangerous to give male sex hormones over a prolonged period of time?

Yes, for it may stimulate a dormant tumor of the prostate gland to grow or to become cancerous.

Is it ever advisable to remove the testicles of an older man?

Yes, when there is a cancer of the prostate gland. Removal will slow down the growth and spread of the malignancy. Also, if a man past sixty develops a tumor in one testicle, it is usually advisable to remove both glands.

Will surgical removal of the testicles shorten the life-span?

No.

Does the surgical removal of the testicles always lead to the development of symptoms ascribed to deficient male-hormone secretion?

No. The cortex of the adrenal glands usually takes over the secretory and hormonal functions of the testicles. The chemicals so secreted are called testoids and their action is quite similar to that of the male sex hormone.

Is it possible for a man to have intercourse after his testicles are removed?

In the majority of cases, the testicles are removed only in aged men who have already become impotent. However, there are a few cases on record in which the ability to have intercourse has continued.

Will the removal of the testicles in an elderly man cause him to lose male characteristics, such as beard growth and masculine voice and appearance?

There are no resulting changes in appearance.

What is the significance of an enlarged testicle in a man past sixty?

It may be due to one of the following:

1. A tumor, either malignant or benign.
2. A hydrocele, a collection of fluid in the sac surrounding the testicle.
3. An inflammation (orchiditis or epididymitis).
4. A hernia that has extended down into the scrotum will give the appearance of an enlarged testicle, even though the gland is not actually enlarged.

What is the treatment of a tumor of the testicle?

Surgical removal of the gland and its attached cord. If the

tumor is malignant, it is advisable to remove the other testicle as well. This is done because the secretion of male hormone by the normal testicle may stimulate and further the growth of cancer cells that may have spread to other parts of the body. Moreover, there is a tendency for the remaining testicle to develop a tumor.

How common are tumors of the testicle in older men?

Tumors are uncommon in this age group. Young adults are much more likely to develop testicular growths.

Is surgical removal of a testicle a serious operation?

No, but the dissection of the lymph glands in the groin and lower abdomen that accompanies an operation for cancer of the testicle is serious. Nevertheless, recovery after surgery takes place in almost all cases.

Why are the testicles sometimes removed when a man has cancer of the prostate gland?

It has been discovered that the continued secretion of the male sex hormone will stimulate the further growth of cancer cells. By removal of the testicles, this stimulation is removed.

TESTS

What diagnostic tests are performed most often on older patients?

acid phosphatase A blood test that sometimes indicates the presence of a cancer of the prostate gland and its spread to other parts of the body.

after image An eye test demonstrating the degree of strabismus (crossed eyes).

agglutination A test to demonstrate the presence of antibodies in the blood.

albumin The presence of albumin in the urine may indicate kidney disease.

alkaline phosphatase A blood test that, when elevated, indicates obstruction of the flow of bile into the intestine. A valuable test in cases of jaundice.

allergy Any test used to demonstrate the presence of an allergy.

amylase A blood test for the enzyme amylase. When there is an abnormally high level of amylase, it may indicate an inflammation of the pancreas (pancreatitis).

amyloid A blood test for the substance amyloid. When there is an abnormally high level of amyloid, it indicates the presence of degeneration (amyloidosis) in certain organs, such as the liver, kidney, or spleen.

aptitude A psychological test to determine the potential ability of someone in a special field of endeavor.

association A psychological test in which the patient is given a series of words and is asked to state what other words they make him think of.

auditory The use of the audiometer to determine ability to hear.

Bachman A test to determine the presence of trichinosis (an infection caused by eating diseased pork or ham).

Bárány's A test to determine the presence of disease in the inner ear (labyrinth).

basal metabolism A breathing test that measures the amount of energy expended when the body is at rest.

Bence Jones protein A urine test that, when positive, indicates the presence of a tumor known as myeloma.

Benedict's A urine test for the presence of sugar.

benzidine A test for the presence of blood. It can be performed on urine, stool, sputum, or other body substances.

benzodioxane The intravenous injection of this substance brings about a lowering of the blood pressure in people who have a tumor (pheochromocytoma) of the adrenal gland.

bilirubin A blood test for the presence of bile pigment. Increased bilirubin indicates the presence of jaundice.

bilirubin clearance The ability of the liver to remove injected bilirubin from the bloodstream is a test of adequacy of liver function.

biopsy The surgical removal of tissue in order to determine the exact diagnosis.

bleeding time Puncturing the finger and noting how long it takes for the bleeding to stop.

blind A *blind test* is one in which both the observer and the one being tested are unaware of the end result.

bone conduction A hearing test in which a vibrating tuning fork is placed against the mastoid bone behind the ear. Failure to hear the vibrations indicates bone-conduction deafness.

Bromsulphalein Failure of the liver to eliminate injected Bromsulphalein from the blood is an indication of impaired liver function.

capillary resistance A test for the resistance of small blood vessels (capillaries) to stress. A tourniquet is applied to an arm; if capillaries break, it shows lowered resistance.

cephalin flocculation A liver-function test based on its ability to flocculate (clot) cholesterol.

cholesterol A blood test to determine the quantity of cholesterol in circulating blood.

circulation time A test to determine how rapidly blood circulates throughout the body. Circulation is impaired in certain types of heart disease.

clearance A test of the efficiency of the kidney in clearing certain substances that come to it in the circulating blood.

coagulase A test for the virulence (strength) of staphylococcal germs. A positive coagulase test shows these germs to be more dangerous and resistant to destruction.

coccidioidin A skin-sensitivity test to determine the presence of a coccidioidomycosis infection. This fungus infection is also called *San Joaquin Valley fever.*

coin Striking coins against one another on the chest wall while the physician listens with a stethoscope on the opposite chest wall. A clear bell tone indicates pneumothorax, or air in the space between the lung and the chest cage. (The normal sound is dull and muffled.)

cold agglutination A test for blood antibodies that are present in certain peculiar types of pneumonia (atypical pneumonia).

cold pressor People with a tendency to high blood pressure will show a marked rise in blood pressure when a hand is immersed in ice-cold water for one minute.

colloidal gold A test for syphilis affecting the brain or spinal cord.

color vision The viewing of multicolored cards with numbers on them; given to determine if a man is color-blind.

concentration-dilution A test for adequacy of kidney function based on its ability to concentrate and dilute urine.

Congo red A test to detect amyloid degeneration of organs or tissues.

conjunctival An allergic test in which the substance suspected of being the cause of the allergy is dropped into the eye. Inflammation and redness are positive reactions.

Coombs A blood test to detect Rh antibodies.

cross-matching A test to determine whether the donor's and recipient's blood will mix without clotting; performed before giving a blood transfusion.

Davidsohn differential A test to determine the presence of infectious mononucleosis; a heterophile test.

exercise tolerance A test for heart function, angina pectoris, etc. A patient steps up and down two stairs in the physician's office. It is noted how much exercise he can do before developing chest pain.

Fehling's A urine test for the presence of sugar.

ferric chloride A urine test for the presence of diacetic acid, an indication of acidosis.

finger to finger A test of cerebellar function in which the patient, from an outstretched-arm position, must bring his two index fingers together. Normally, this is easy to do.

finger to nose A test of cerebellar function in which the patient, from an outstretched-arm position, must bring his index finger smoothly to the tip of his nose.

Fishberg's A test for kidney function in which the concentration (specific gravity) of the urine is calculated twelve hours after he has not had any fluid. Normally, the kidneys concentrate urine without difficulty.

Folin-Wu A blood chemical test for the amount of urea. Excess amounts of urea in the blood may lead to uremic poisoning.

fragility A test to note the strength of red blood cells by putting them in salt solutions of varying strengths.

Frei A skin-sensitivity test to determine whether the patient has lymphogranuloma venereum.

galactose tolerance A test for liver function to see if it can utilize galactose (milk sugar). Failure to do so indicates poor liver function.

glucose tolerance A blood test to determine the presence of diabetes or a tendency toward its development. It also is used to determine the presence of hypoglycemia.

Gmelin's A test to detect the presence of bile in the urine.

Gofman A blood test to determine tendencies toward development of hardening of the arteries (arteriosclerosis).

Graham-Cole A test for gallbladder function and to see if it contains stones. A dye is swallowed or injected, following which, X rays are taken.

guaiac A test for the presence of blood in the stool, urine, sputum, etc. A positive guaiac test result denotes the presence of blood.

heterophile A test to detect the presence of infectious mononucleosis.

hippuric acid A chemical test to determine adequacy of liver function.

histamine The injection of histamine normally causes secretion of hydrochloric acid in the stomach.

icterus index A test for the presence of bile pigments in the blood. The index is elevated in cases of jaundice.

indigo carmine This chemical dye is injected intravenously. If the kidneys are functioning normally, the dye should appear in the urine within seven minutes.

iodine tolerance A test for overactivity of the thyroid gland.

Kahn A blood test for the presence of syphilis.

kidney function Any one of many tests to determine adequacy of kidney function.

Kline A blood test for syphilis. A positive test indicates the presence of the disease.

L.E. A test for the presence of lupus erythematosus, an inflammation of the skin.

liver function Any one of the many tests to determine the adequacy of the numerous liver functions.

manometric A test performed on the spinal fluid, after spinal puncture, to note the pressure of the fluid within the cerebrospinal space.

Mantoux A skin-sensitivity test for tuberculosis.

Mazzini A test for syphilis. (A positive result indicates the presence of syphilis.)

methylene blue This dye is injected and should appear in the urine within thirty minutes if kidney function is adequate.

Mosenthal A kidney-function test in which the various levels of concentration of the urine are determined over a twenty-four-hour period.

Naffziger's Pressing the jugular veins in the neck will cause increased pain in the back in a patient with a herniated disk.

pancreatic function Any one of several tests to determine the adequacy of pancreatic function.

Papanicolaou A vaginal smear test for cancer.

parallax An eye test to detect cataracts or opaque areas in other parts of the eyeball.

patch An allergy test in which the substance suspected of causing the allergy is applied to the skin and held in place for a day or two with an adhesive patch.

penicillin sensitivity A test to discover how sensitive a particular germ is to the action of penicillin.

Perthes A test performed to discover whether the deep veins in the legs are open or clotted. (This test is sometimes performed before operating for varicose veins.)

phenolsulfonphthalein (P.S.P. test) This dye is injected intravenously and its presence is noted in the urine. Failure to find it in the urine indicates kidney disease.

plasma L.E. A test for the presence of lupus erythematosus.

potassium tolerance A potassium salt is swallowed. If the patient has inadequate adrenal-gland function, the potassium blood quantity is markedly increased.

pronation-supination A test of cerebellum (part of the brain) function determined by having the patient rapidly rotate his hands up and down.

prothrombin time A blood test to determine adequacy of the blood-clotting mechanism. A prolonged *prothrombin time* indicates impairment of this mechanism.

Queckenstedt-Stookey Pressing the jugular veins in the neck normally causes a rise in the pressure of the cerebrospinal fluid surrounding the brain and spinal cord. Failure of this to take place indicates disease within the skull (intracranially).

reduction Any test demonstrating the presence of sugar, as in the urine.

Rh A blood test for the presence of the Rh factor.

Rorschach A psychological test for the presence of neurotic tendencies.

rose bengal A liver-function test based on its ability to remove this dye from the circulating blood.

scratch An allergy test in which the skin is scratched and the substance suspected of causing the allergy is applied to the scratched area.

sedimentation The time it takes blood cells placed in a glass tube to settle out and separate from the serum. (It happens more rapidly in people harboring infections.)

serologic Test performed on the serum of the blood.

Takata-Ara A liver-function test.

tannic acid A test for the presence of carbon monoxide in the blood.

therapeutic Any test in which the response to treatment is used as an aid to diagnosis, such as giving iodine to a suspected case of overactivity of the thyroid gland. If the patient improves, it indicates that the diagnosis was correct.

thymol turbidity A liver-function test, often used to determine whether the outlet of the bile duct is obstructed.

Töpfer's A test to determine the presence of hydrochloric acid in the gastric (stomach) juice.

Trendelenburg's A test to note the extent of varicosities of the veins in the legs.

tuberculin A skin test to determine the presence of the germ causing tuberculosis in the system. A positive response does not necessarily indicate that an active tuberculosis infection exists, but rather that the person has at one time or another harbored the tuberculosis germ in his body.

two-step An exercise test performed to note the response of the heart to exertion. In angina pectoris, this test may bring on heart pain.

urea clearance A test of kidney function depending on the amount of urea (a waste product) the kidneys can remove (clear) from the blood in one minute.

van der Bergh's A blood test to determine whether jaundice is caused primarily by liver disease or by obstruction of the bile ducts leading to the intestines.

vestibular Tests to determine the adequacy of function in the inner ear. Disturbance of such function may indicate the presence of a brain tumor.

vital capacity Tests to determine the adequacy of lung function.

von Pirquet A skin test for the presence of the tuberculosis germ in the body.

Wassermann A blood test for the presence of syphilis. A positive Wassermann result usually indicates the presence of syphilis.

water A test of adrenal-gland function. People with diseased adrenal glands do not urinate in large quantities after drinking large quantities of water.

Weber's A tuning fork hearing test carried out by placing the vibrating tuning fork on the forehead.

Weill-Felix A test for the presence of one of the rickettsial infections.

Widal A test for the presence of typhoid fever.

THROMBUS AND THROMBOSIS

See APOPLEXY, OR STROKE; ARTERIOSCLEROSIS; CIRCULATION; CORONARY-ARTERY DISEASE; EMBOLUS AND EMBOLISM; POLYCYTHEMIA; RETINAL THROMBOSIS; SMOKING; VEINS AND VARICOSE VEINS.

What is a thrombus?

A clot of blood that has formed or lodged in an artery or vein.

What causes thrombosis (the formation of a thrombus)?

There are many causes. When a thrombus forms in the passageway of an artery, it is most often secondary to advanced arteriosclerosis. When it occurs in a vein, it may be due to a breakdown of the valves, as occurs in varicose veins, or to inflammation of the wall of the vein, as occurs in phlebitis.

Injuries to blood vessels, stagnation of blood, interference with free flow of blood by an enlarging infection or tumor, or upset in the blood-coagulation mechanism can also cause a thrombus to form.

What is an embolus?

It is a piece of clotted blood that has broken off from a thrombus in a vein or on the inner wall of the heart. An embolus travels through the bloodstream from one part of the body to another, where it lodges and forms a thrombus, a condition called thrombosis.

Does thrombosis occur very frequently in people past sixty?

Yes. As one might expect, the aging process produces those conditions that predispose to thrombosis—arteriosclerosis, varicose veins, impaired heart function, etc.

What are common types of thrombosis in elderly patients?

1. Coronary thrombosis.
2. Cerebral thrombosis.
3. Carotid-artery thrombosis (in the neck).
4. Mesenteric thrombosis (in the abdomen).
5. Thrombosed hemorrhoids.
6. Phlebitis.
7. Thrombosed varicose veins.

What is the treatment of a thrombosed artery?

1. All measures should be taken to dilate those arteries that are uninvolved. In other words, attempts should be made to develop collateral circulation. (*See* CIRCULATION.)
2. If a major artery is clotted and no longer functioning,

immediate investigations should be undertaken to see if an arterial graft can be performed.

3. If an embolus has lodged in an artery, causing a thrombosis, immediate surgery should be carried out to remove the clot.

What is the treatment of a thrombus or a thrombosis of a vein in the leg?

If it is caused by an inflammation (thrombophlebitis), the following measures should be taken:

1. The patient should stay in bed, with the limb at body level.
2. Anticoagulants, such as heparin or dicoumarol, may be given to reduce the possibility of a piece of blood clot breaking away and causing embolism.
3. Antibiotics should be given to control any infectious element in thrombophlebitis.
4. Medications should be given to cut down on the swelling, pain, and inflammatory reaction.
5. If emboli are repeatedly breaking off and traveling to other parts of the body, the vena cava (the large vein in the abdomen) will probably be tied off surgically. This drastic procedure is seldom necessary.

Is there any way to prevent thrombosis from taking place?

Yes, by prophylactic measures during middle age. If one has a tendency toward high blood pressure, which ultimately damages the blood vessels, he should be treated continuously during his early years. If his blood-cholesterol content is high, he should go on a low-cholesterol diet in order to delay the onset of arteriosclerosis.

If there are extensive varicose veins, they should be ligated and stripped. Finally, if one has a tendency toward phlebitis or clot formation, he should be given anticoagulants.

THYROID GLAND

See ADRENAL GLANDS; ENDOCRINE GLANDS AND HORMONES; HEART; PARATHYROID GLANDS; TESTS; WEIGHT.

What is the thyroid gland and where is it located?

It is a U-shaped endocrine gland lying in the front of the lower portion of the neck, surrounding the trachea (windpipe). It is made up of three portions: a large lobe on either side and a small connecting isthmus.

The thyroid gland is one of the most important glands in the body, since it regulates the rate and manner in which we turn food into energy and expend that energy. In other words, it regulates metabolism.

How does the thyroid gland regulate metabolism?

It produces a hormone, thyroxine, which enters the bloodstream and affects tissue function throughout the entire body. Thyroxine governs

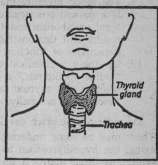

Thyroid gland

body growth and development, the production of muscular energy and body heat, and the regulation of salt and water storage.

Is thyroid function usually slower in people past sixty?

To a certain extent. However, older people tend to need less energy and are less active physically. The gland does continue to produce sufficient hormones throughout the life-span.

What is a goiter?

Any enlargement of the thyroid gland. It may be a uniform or an irregular enlargement. It may be associated with normal, overactive, or deficient gland function.

How can one tell if the thyroid is underactive?

This condition, called hypothyroidism, evidences itself in the following manner:

1. There may be a uniform swelling in the neck, due to thyroid enlargement.
2. There is a tendency to gain weight, even though the appetite may not increase noticeably.
3. The tissues tend to become waterlogged, particularly the tissues directly beneath the skin. When the skin over the legs or arms is pressed down, the tissues fail to rebound to the surface and "pitting" (depression) appears.
4. The patient is constantly fatigued, lacks energy, and feels cold even in warm weather.
5. The skin becomes dry and scaly, and perspiration is slight, even in hot weather.
6. If the patient is female, there may be cessation of menstruation and inability to conceive.
7. The pulse rate slows to 40 to 50 beats per minute.

8. The blood pressure may drop below normal.
9. If a patient is suspected of having hypothyroidism, a basal metabolism test (BMR) may be performed. The results will demonstrate whether or not there is underactivity of function and to what degree.
10. By doing a chemical test of the blood known as an "iodine-uptake test," a doctor can tell rather accurately whether the thyroid is underactive, overactive, or is functioning normally.

Do older people often develop hypothyroidism?

There may be some underactivity of thyroid function due to aging, but hypothyroidism to a degree sufficient to cause the symptoms listed above is uncommon.

How does one make a diagnosis of overactivity of the thyroid gland (hyperthyroidism)?

1. A swelling in the neck, either uniform or irregular, may develop as a result of enlargement of the thyroid.
2. The pulse rate becomes rapid, from 100 to 140 beats per minute.
3. Blood pressure tends to rise.
4. Appetite increases markedly, but weight loss takes place despite the greater food intake.
5. The skin becomes moist, perspiration is excessive, and the eyes may begin to bulge.
6. The patient becomes irritable and nervous, cries easily, and develops a tremor of the hands.
7. A basal metabolism test (BMR) will reveal overactivity of the gland.
8. The iodine-uptake test will reveal thyroid overactivity.

Do people past sixty frequently develop overactivity of the thyroid gland?

No. Hyperthyroidism is uncommon, although older people do occasionally develop goiters with overactivity of gland function. This condition is seen more often in young adults, however.

What is an apathetic goiter?

This is an unusual condition in which older people are apathetic and appear to have underactivity of the thyroid but, in actuality, have overactivity of the gland. The diagnosis may be difficult to make because the gland swelling is often negligible and the symptoms are not characteristic of an overactive thyroid. A BMR or an iodine-uptake test will confirm the diagnosis.

Does the thyroid often form a goiter in people past sixty?
It is not as common as in younger adults, but it does occur.

What is the main treatment of underactivity of the thyroid gland?
People of all ages respond quite well to administration of thyroid hormone. This can be given in the form of a tablet. Although this type of replacement therapy does not cure the condition, the symptoms will disappear, so long as the patient continues to take the thyroid medication.

What is the treatment of overactivity of the thyroid gland?
1. If the overactivity is due to a goiter with irregular swelling of the gland, surgery should be performed. During this procedure, the major portion of the involved lobe of the thyroid is removed. The operation can be carried out safely and with excellent results, even on patients in their sixties or seventies.
2. If the overactivity is due to a uniform swelling of the entire gland, and a diagnosis of exophthalmic goiter (Graves' disease or hyperthyroidism) has been made, then medical treatment rather than surgery is indicated. This condition is exceedingly rare in people over sixty; but, should it occur, antithyroid drugs, such as Tapazole, or radioactive iodine will overcome the overactivity of the gland and restore the patient to normal.

Is it dangerous for older people to take thyroid-hormone tablets without the advice of a physician?
Yes. This is a most powerful hormone and should never be taken unless a doctor has prescribed it. Thyroid tablets can cause overactivity of gland function and may cause considerable damage to the heart. It is especially dangerous for older people whose heart muscle is already weakened by arteriosclerosis.

Will the removal of the thyroid (thyroidectomy) shorten the life-span?
No. If the operation is carried out successfully—as almost all operations on the thyroid are—there will be no undesirable aftereffects.

Does the thyroid gland ever become cancerous?
Yes. It is estimated that one out of every ten goiters that have been present for more than fifteen to twenty years will develop cancer.

What is the treatment of cancer of the thyroid?
Certain types of cancer will not respond to any form of treat-

ment. But the great majority of cancers of the thyroid can be treated successfully by surgical removal of the gland or, in an occasional case, by the administration of radioactive iodine.

What are the indications for surgery on a goiter in a patient who is past sixty?

1. When the thyroid is markedly overactive and is causing damage to the heart.
2. If the patient has not responded to the administration of radioactive iodine or to the antithyroid drugs.
3. If a goiter has grown to such size that it compresses the windpipe and interferes with normal breathing.
4. If a quiescent nodule that has been present in the gland for years begins to grow.
5. In any case in which the surgeon suspects that cancerous changes may be developing.

Does treatment of the thyroid gland ever benefit older people who have heart disease?

Yes. If the heart disease is associated with overactivity of the thyroid, the administration of radioactive iodine may result in great improvement. Even if the heart condition is not accompanied by an overactive thyroid, radioactive-iodine therapy may prove beneficial. It will cause the thyroid to become underactive, thus lowering metabolism and creating a situation in which fewer demands will be made on the heart muscle. This form of treatment is especially helpful to some older people who suffer from angina pectoris or coronary arteriosclerosis.

When performing a thyroidectomy, does the surgeon usually remove the entire gland?

No. He will usually leave behind about 10 percent of each lobe, which can produce sufficient hormone to maintain normal metabolism. Exceptions to this are when the thyroid is removed in an attempt to aid a failing heart or when cancer is present. In such cases, the entire gland is removed.

TIC DOULOUREUX

See CONJUNCTIVITIS; EYES; NERVES.

What is tic douloureux (trigeminal neuralgia)?

It is a recurrent condition in which there are sudden paroxysms of excruciating pain along the course of one or more branches of the trigeminal nerve in the face. The spasms of pain come on abruptly, often triggered by touching the side of the face or by exposing it to a draft. At other times an attack will come on from drinking a cold liquid, sudden exposure to cold, or for no apparent reason.

What parts of the face are most frequently involved in the attacks?

The eye, the cheek, and the side of the mouth and chin.

Is tic douloureux seen very often in older people?

Yes. It occurs most often after sixty.

What causes tic douloureux?

The cause is unknown.

What is a trigger point?

These are areas on the face that, when touched or irritated, can precipitate an attack.

Does tic douloureux occur on both sides of the face in the same patient?

No. It is confined to one side of the face.

What is the usual frequency of attacks?

In mild cases, an attack may occur only once every few weeks or months. In severe cases—and these are quite numerous—there may be several attacks a day. In this latter group, it is not unusual for drug addiction to result, as the need for relief of pain becomes imperative. Also, there are cases on record of suicide committed in order to be rid of the awful attacks.

What is the treatment of tic douloureux?

1. In the very mild case in which the attacks come on only once or twice a year, treatment may be limited to giving of pain-relieving medications for the isolated paroxysm.
2. In those cases in which the attacks are spaced more closely, alcohol injection directly into the involved branch of the nerve may be carried out. This will cause a certain degree of paralysis and degeneration of the nerve, thus freeing the patient from attacks for periods of several months. When the attacks recur, an injection can be given again.
3. In the most severe cases, neurosurgery will be carried out. This entails a brain operation in which the particular branch or branches that are subject to the attacks are cut.

Is surgery for tic douloureux safe and effective?

Yes. Almost all older people who are otherwise in a satisfactory state of health can undergo this type of surgery. In the great majority of instances, complete relief ensues.

Will cutting the trigeminal nerve cause facial paralysis?

No, but if the branch of the nerve going to the eye region is cut, special postoperative care will be necessary. In such cases, there may be loss of sensation on the surface of the eyeball, causing the patient to be unaware of dirt or dust that might enter. To safeguard against this, the patient must wear goggles when out of doors or when exposed to wind or dust.

Will tic douloureux recur after surgery?

Not if the involved branch of the nerve has been cut. Rarely does another branch of the same nerve subsequently become afflicted.

TRANSPLANTATION OF ORGANS

See ANATOMICAL CHANGES IN ORGANS; ARTERIOSCLEROSIS;
DEGENERATIVE CHANGES OF AGING; LONGEVITY.

Can diseased or worn-out tissues or organs be replaced?

Yes. Tissues and organs can be grafted, but at the present time the end results are successful in only a few cases. Most tissues transplanted from one individual to another, or from an animal to a human, will degenerate and die within a few days or weeks.

Can tissues be successfully transplanted from one part of a patient's body to another?

Yes, this can often be accomplished successfully. The most commonly transplanted tissue, of course, is skin, but bone, cartilage, and blood vessels can frequently be transplanted from one part of the body to another.

What is an autotransplant?

Tissue transplanted from one part of the same body to another.

What is a homotransplant?

Tissue transplanted from one human to another.

Why do transplants from another individual (homotransplants) degenerate and die?

All humans have immune bodies and antibodies circulating in their blood. It is the function of these substances and the cells to which they are attached to protect the individual against foreign bodies. Bacteria, viruses, inert particles such as dirt or debris, and tissue cells from others are all considered "foreign material" by the host. Transplanted tissue, acting as a foreign body, stimulates the host's antibodies and protective cells, resulting in the ultimate destruction of the graft. This reaction is called *transplantation immunity*.

Is it ever possible to transplant an entire organ successfully?
Yes, if identical twins are involved. In several cases on record a kidney has been removed from a healthy twin and transplanted successfully into the body of a twin suffering from diseased kidneys.

Are there instances of successful transplantation of pieces of tissue from one individual to another?
Yes. The cornea (the clear, thin membrane covering the pupil of the eye) can often be transplanted successfully.

Are there instances of successful transplants of animal tissue to humans?
Yes. Animal cartilage has often been used successfully in plastic surgery to build up a receding chin or a saddle nose.

Are there instances of successful transplants of nonliving substances?
Yes. Dacron, nylon, and other plastics are often used successfully as replacements for segments of blood vessels.

Are attempts being made to overcome transplantation immunity?
Yes, a great deal of intensive research is going on in this field. It is widely recognized that once transplantation immunity has been overcome, it will be feasible to replace diseased and worn-out structures with healthy, younger tissues from the bodies of other individuals. The solution to this problem revolves around immobilization of the antibodies of the recipient of the transplant. So far, no one has been able to overcome this resistance.

What might be the medical and social significance of overcoming transplantation immunity?
It would open the door to widespread use of homotransplantation. A time may come, in the not-too-distant future, when it will be commonplace to replace a diseased or worn-out heart, major blood vessel, lung, kidney, pancreas, thyroid, or other diseased organ with a healthy organ taken from the body of a young person. This will result in tremendous changes both in attitudes toward and in treatment of the aging process.

Is it surgically feasible to transplant major organs?
Yes, and refinements of present-day surgical techniques will undoubtedly permit such operations in an ever increasing number of cases. Even now, techniques have been elaborated

to permit the successful transplantation of a heart, an aorta, a kidney, a lung, and other organs from one animal to another.

Does a successfully transplanted organ always react normally in its new environment?

No, and this is one of the factors that might conceivably limit the usefulness of organ transplantation. It has been found in animal experiments that a healthy transplanted organ sometimes develops the same disease as the structure it has replaced.

Is it logical to look forward to a prolongation of the life-span of an individual through organ transplant?

Yes, provided his life-span is endangered as the result of disease within one or two organs. In other words, if someone is in relatively good health except for a diseased kidney or a diseased heart, then a successful transplant may afford him many extra years of life. On the other hand, one who shows the generalized effects of aging in all his organs will be helped little by replacement of one or two diseased structures.

TRAVEL

See DIET; DRIVING; FIRST AID; INJURIES AND ACCIDENTS; PHYSICAL ACTIVITY AND EXERCISE; RETIREMENT.

What precautions should older people take before taking a long trip?

1. If an older person has a medical problem that might need attention, he should find out beforehand what medical care will be available along the route. It is especially important to check on medical facilities before one takes an automobile trip across long stretches of uninhabited country.

2. Before departure, an older person should write to the Information Bureau of the American Medical Association for the names of hospitals and reputable physicians in the areas in which he will remain during his trip. (*See* ORGANIZATION AND AGENCIES.)

3. The possibilities of physical strain should be carefully evaluated. Certainly, airplane and boat travel will be accompanied by less physical effort than automobile travel. On the other hand, an automobile trip can usually be interrupted at frequent intervals for needed rest periods.

4. The altitude at which one will travel should be checked beforehand. Many older people, especially those with heart conditions, cannot withstand high altitudes.

5. The climate of the places to be visited should be checked. Extremes of temperature for long periods should be avoided.

6. The availability of personnel to handle heavy baggage should be known beforehand.

7. Medications that might be needed, as well as a first-aid kit, should be taken along. Also, prescriptions that might have to be refilled during the trip should be taken along.

8. An extra pair of eyeglasses and the eyeglass prescription should be brought along by the traveler.

9. Appropriate immunization and vaccinations should be obtained well in advance of an extended trip, especially if travel to a foreign land is anticipated. Certificates of proof of immunization must be carried by the traveler.

10. If special foods will be required, information as to their availability should be obtained before setting out on a trip.

What are some additional items to be checked before an older person goes on a long automobile trip?

1. Availability of toilet facilities along the route. An ample supply of toilet tissue should be taken along.

2. The conditions of the roads over which one will travel. Older people often tolerate rough roads poorly.

3. The availability and quality of the restaurants along the way.

4. The spacing of stopping-off places should be planned in advance.

What should be the limit of automobile travel for older people?

Much will depend on the condition of the roads and on who is doing the driving. Approximately 250 to 300 miles per day is usually a comfortable distance.

Is it safe for older people to travel to high altitudes in automobiles?

Yes, provided they are in good health and will not exert themselves while at altitudes over a few thousand feet. Walking and sightseeing at heights above 5,000 feet may bring on symptoms of oxygen deprivation. If at any time there is shortness of breath or chest pain, the trip should be interrupted and the person should promptly return to a lower altitude.

Should eating be restricted at high altitudes?

Yes. A heavy meal may precipitate great discomfort—and even heart symptoms.

Should older people be restricted in the length of time they spend in high altitudes?

Only if there are adverse symptoms, such as those mentioned above.

Are high-altitude precautions also necessary for air travel?

No. Practically all modern airplanes are pressurized, so that the pressure in the cabin is no higher than that at a few thousand feet. Moreover, passengers rest quietly in their seats, thus eliminating the factor of exertion. In addition, oxygen is carried in planes and can be given if symptoms of oxygen deficiency do develop.

If older people find it necessary to stay in very hot climates, what precautions should they take?

1. They should stay out of the sun, except for very brief periods.
2. They should dress lightly.
3. They should drink large quantities of water.
4. If they perspire profusely, they should take a 10-grain salt tablet two or three times a day. (This procedure may have to be modified for those who are on salt-restricted diets.)
5. They should not engage in strenuous physical activities.
6. Frequent cool showers or baths should be taken.
7. Food intake should be limited to light meals, perhaps only two a day.
8. They should not drink alcoholic beverages.

If older people find it necessary to stay in very cold climates, what precautions should they take?

1. They should, of course, take along plenty of warm clothing. Heavy woolen socks, earmuffs, and fur-lined gloves are particularly important.
2. They should avoid overexposure to strong winds and should stay indoors as much as possible.
3. They should remain indoors and should avoid walking for at least one hour after eating a heavy meal.
4. They should drink plenty of hot liquids.

Do older people have difficulty adjusting to very humid climates?

Yes. Such places should be avoided whenever possible, because excessive perspiring may lead to serious upset in the heat-regulating mechanism.

What special accessories should older people take on extended trips, if possible?

1. A small pillow to be placed behind the back or under an arm.
2. A favorite sleeping pillow. Many older people get so attached to a particular pillow that they will sleep poorly if deprived of it.
3. Favorite soaps and other toilet articles.
4. An enema bag, especially for those who have a tendency toward constipation.
5. An electric blanket, if they are traveling to cold climates.
6. Favorite items of clothing, even if they appear beforehand not to be suitable for the place to be visited. Considerable discomfort may be felt by leaving behind an article of clothing to which one has become attached.

Is it especially important for older people to travel with light baggage?

Yes. They should not lift luggage weighing more than 20 to 30 pounds. If an extended trip is planned, trunks should be sent ahead.

Is it wise for older people to be met upon arrival at a destination?

Yes. This is extremely important to arrange in advance.

What special precautions should be taken before going on a boat trip?

1. Information should be gathered concerning the available medical facilities. Inquiry should be made concerning the qualifications of the ship's doctor. Older people should not go on extended cruises unless there is a competent physician on board.
2. If the boat will travel through rough seas, adequate supplies of motion-sickness pills should be taken along.
3. Information should be obtained concerning the medical and hospital facilities at ports to be visited. Older people in poor health should not take cruises that stay at sea for more than a few days at a time.
4. They should learn about the excursions that will be taken while in port. Some of the side trips may be too strenuous for older people to take.
5. They should be certain of the climates they will encounter.
6. They should know about the diseases that exist in the areas to which they intend to travel.
7. They should find out what foods should be avoided in the ports of call.

Should older people observe strict precautions about eating strange foods and drinking unbottled water when traveling to foreign lands?

Yes. Age brings with it no immunity to diseases acquired from eating or drinking infected foods and liquids. The safe procedure is to eat only cooked foods and to drink only bottled water.

What items should go into a medical kit to be taken on an extended trip?

The same items one keeps in a medicine cabinet at home. (*See* FIRST AID.) Also, one's family doctor should be consulted concerning specific antibiotic drugs and antidiarrheal medications that should be taken along.

How does one know what immunizations and vaccinations are necessary when traveling to foreign countries?

The tourist agent will know the answer to this question. If the agent does not know, a letter should be written to the consulate of the country to which one intends to travel.

Here is a list of vaccinations and immunizations that should be obtained before one goes to a foreign country:

1. Smallpox vaccination (for travel anywhere).
2. Typhoid vaccination—three injections or one booster shot at yearly intervals (for travel outside continental United States).
3. Influenza vaccination—two or three injections (for older people traveling during the winter).
4. Typhus fever vaccination—two injections (for travel to certain East European countries and the Orient).
5. Cholera vaccination—two injections (for travel to India and the Orient).
6. Plague vaccination—two injections (for travel to the Orient and India).
7. Yellow fever vaccination—one injection (for travel to the Orient and certain parts of Central and South America).

How soon before departure on a trip should the above injections be taken?

Since many of them may cause older people to develop a fever and feel quite sick, it is good practice to space them out for 2 to 3 months before departure. Longer periods than 6 months are not advisable, since some of the immunizations are effective for only a few months.

TREATMENT

See CANCER AND OTHER MALIGNANT GROWTHS; CONTAGION AND CONTAGIOUS DISEASES; DIAGNOSIS OF DISEASE; DRUGS AND MEDICINES; FIRST AID; GAS AND SMOKE POISONING; INJURIES AND ACCIDENTS; REHABILITATION AND PHYSICAL THERAPY; SURGERY.

How effective is treatment of people in their sixties, seventies, or eighties?

Many conditions that afflict older people are degenerative in nature. These diseases are part of the aging process and response to treatment is, therefore, not very effective.

Modern medicine has been reluctant to concede that nothing can be done about the problems brought on by old age. As a consequence, many conditions that were previously thought to be irreversible are today responding to new methods and techniques of treatment. The recent development of surgery for repair or replacement of arteriosclerotic blood vessels is one example of medicine's response to the challenge of the problems of aging. Ten or fifteen years ago, an attitude of defeatism invariably followed a diagnosis of impaired circulation. If the impairment was in the leg, amputation was the sole method of treatment. Today, surgical restoration of blood supply to a limb has already proved successful in thousands of cases. Arterial grafts have also benefited patients suffering from cerebral arteriosclerosis. The day may not be far off when we may be able to save kidneys that have been damaged by the passage of time.

Is prophylactic treatment especially important during the middle years of life?

Yes. The degenerative changes that are likely to occur as one advances into the later years can often be anticipated, and early preventive measures, if pursued vigorously, may delay their onset. For instance, it is well known that obesity predisposes to diabetes, high blood pressure, and liver disease. If treatment is directed against obesity and weight is restored to normal levels, the aforementioned diseases may be prevented. Similarly, if a patient shows a progressive increase in blood pressure with advancing age, he should avoid strenuous pursuits and emotional excitement.

Are there any major differences in the reactions of older people to treatment?

Yes. A wise physician keeps in mind the fact that as people grow older they adjust less readily to marked change in their pattern of living. Thus, a course of treatment that creates a great upheaval in their mode of existence may be an unwise form of therapy, even though it may be effective from a medical point of view. If major changes do become necessary, they should be carried out as gradually as possible. For example, the overweight older person should reduce slowly, and should never be placed on a "crash" diet. The patient with high blood pressure should have it lowered slowly over a period of weeks or months.

Do medications produce the same reactions in older patients as they do in younger ones?

Reactions to most medications are the same throughout life, but they often become intensified as one grows older. For instance, a sleeping pill that will cause only slight drowsiness in a man of thirty-five may produce ten or twelve hours of complete unconsciousness in a man of seventy-five.

Are drugs as readily absorbed into the body by older people?

Yes, but the *rate* of absorption may be slightly less rapid than that of younger people.

Do older patients require smaller doses of narcotics than younger patients?

Yes.

Do older people eliminate drugs from the body as quickly as younger people?

No. Most drugs are eliminated from the body through the lungs, the kidneys, and the liver. Since these organs function more slowly as one ages, medications tend to remain in the body for longer periods of time. Thus, the effects of a sleeping pill may last well into the next day.

Is there a tendency for older people to develop resistance to various medications?

Yes. Perhaps the best-known example of this resistance is the loss of effectiveness of laxatives that have been taken over a long period of time. The same applies to sedatives, tranquilizers, and some of the antibiotics. Other drugs such as the pain-relieving salicylates and the antacids usually retain the same degree of effectiveness.

Do older patients respond as well to antibiotics as younger patients?

Usually they do, but some antibiotics, such as penicillin, may cause an allergic reaction if they have been given on several occasions previously. Fortunately, if a patient fails to respond to one antibiotic, another can be found to which he will respond.

Is there such a thing as being too old to take a certain medication?

Most drugs and forms of treatment can be given to people of all ages, but the physician who treats large numbers of people in their seventies or eighties is alert to variations in their response to medications. As a consequence, he will often vary dosages considerably.

What are some good general rules for older people to follow in regard to medications and treatments?

1. They should not indulge in self-treatment. No matter what their economic status, medical care can be obtained, even if it is at the clinic level.

2. They should not take a medication or follow a course of treatment merely because a friend or acquaintance advocates it.

3. They should always carry with them, in a wallet or purse, information concerning the drugs they are taking and the telephone number of their physician. This will help anyone who might aid them in an emergency. For example, if an individual is subject to insulin shock or to convulsions, he should always have specific instructions on his person for those who might wish to help him.

4. When in doubt as to whether or not a medication should be taken, they should always check with the physician by telephone. Medications prescribed several months previously may no longer be indicated.

5. When in doubt as to dosage, call the physician or pharmacist.

6. Patients should never withhold information from their doctor. There is a great tendency among older patients to hold back information for fear they will learn that their condition is serious.

7. If there has once been a sensitivity or allergic reaction to a drug, the physician must be informed.

8. Patients should not hesitate to tell their physician of a poor response to a medication he has prescribed.

9. Patients should discontinue any medication that causes nausea, vomiting, conjuctivitis (inflammation of the eyes), hives, or a skin rash.

10. Older patients should discontinue any course of treatment that is too strenuous or that leads to exhaustion.

TRICHIASIS

See BLEPHARITIS; CONJUNCTIVITIS; ECTROPION AND ENTROPION; EYES; HAIR.

What is trichiasis?

It is a condition in which the eyelashes tend to grow in different directions. Some point inward and scratch the surface of the eyeball.

Do older people often develop trichiasis?

It is not a very common condition. When it does occur, it is very likely to affect people in their seventies who have had a chronic inflammation of the eyelids.

What is the treatment of trichiasis?

The eyelashes must be plucked regularly by an ophthalmologist. In severe cases it may be necessary to perform an operation on the lid in an attempt to reshape it so that the margins point away from the surface of the eyeball.

What is trichiasis of the anus?

It is a condition in which there is an overgrowth of hair about the anal orifice. Some of the hairs get into the opening and cause irritation and itching. It is rare in people past sixty.

TUBERCULOSIS

See RESPIRATORY TRACT; X RAY.

How common is tuberculosis in people past sixty?

According to most statistics, the mortality rate from tuberculosis in the United States is higher after fifty than at any other age. It is a common misconception that older people develop immunity to tuberculosis.

Is tuberculosis more common in older men than women?

Yes. It occurs four times more often in men.

When tuberculosis affects older people, can it be transmitted by them to younger people who live with them?

Yes. At any stage in life, tuberculosis is contagious. Unprotected coughing and poor hygiene spread the disease.

How is tuberculosis diagnosed?

1. By taking an X ray of the chest.

2. By noting symptoms such as chronic cough, coughing up of blood, loss of appetite and weight, anemia, and malaise.
3. By finding the tuberculosis bacillus in the sputum.

Does treatment of tuberculosis in older people differ markedly from that for younger people?

No.

Is isolation of the older patient just as important as isolation of a younger one?

Yes.

Does coughing spread tuberculosis?

Yes. This is by far the most frequent mode of transmission.

What is the treatment of tuberculosis?

The answer to this question would take a great deal more space than is available here. It is therefore possible only to outline briefly some of the methods of treatment.

1. Rest in bed.
2. Isolation, so that the disease will not be transmitted to others.
3. High-calorie diet, including adequate amounts of vitamins and minerals.
4. The giving of specific antituberculosis drugs, such as isoniazid, streptomycin, or para-aminosalicylic acid.
5. Surgical removal of the infected portion of the lung, if the disease is limited to one lung or one segment of a lung. Surgery is advocated most often in those cases in which damage to the lung is extensive.
6. Collapse of the involved lung by injecting air into the chest cavity surrounding it.
7. Thoracoplasty, an operation in which several ribs are removed in order to bring about collapse of a tuberculous cavity.

Can older people with tuberculosis be treated at home, or is it necessary to hospitalize them?

This will depend largely on the extent of the disease and the living conditions at home. If there are small children in the household, it is best to institutionalize the tubercular patient. Contagion is too great a risk. If, on the other hand, the patient lives alone with his or her spouse, and if adequate nursing care is available, he may be treated adequately at home.

Of course, if surgery is contemplated, or if the disease is progressing rapidly, hospitalization is essential.

What is the outlook for older people who have tuberculosis?

Today, the chances of arresting the disease are much greater than ever before. The antituberculosis drugs, the advent of safe chest surgery, and improved medical management have raised the recovery rates tremendously.

ULCERS OF THE STOMACH AND DUODENUM

See Diet; Esophagus; Gastritis; Intestines; Stomach and Duodenum.

How common are ulcers of the stomach or duodenum in people past sixty?

They occur, but less often than in younger people. In the majority of cases, the patient has had a history of stomach trouble. An exception is the ulcer found in association with marked arteriosclerosis. In these cases, the blood supply to the mucous membrane lining the stomach or duodenum may diminish to such an extent that a localized area of ulceration takes place.

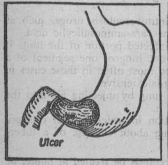

Peptic ulcer

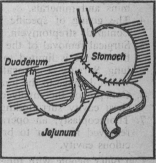

End result of partial stomach removal for ulcer

Should ulcer patients avoid aspirin and other salicylate medications?

Recent investigations indicate that ulcer patients should not use aspirin or other salicylates. It is thought that their use might stimulate the ulcer to bleed.

Are older patients with ulcer more likely to hemorrhage?

Yes. This is because their blood vessels are apt to be arteriosclerotic and therefore possess less elastic tissue. When the blood vessel is eroded, it is less able to contract and to stop the bleeding. Massive hemorrhage is one of the commonest and most serious complications of ulcers in older people.

What is the significance of the vomiting of blood?

1. The most common cause is an ulcer of the stomach or duodenum.
2. Varicose veins of the esophagus, associated with cirrhosis of the liver, may cause vomiting of blood.
3. Acute or chronic gastritis (inflammation of the stomach) may be accompanied by the vomiting of blood. (*See* GASTRITIS.)
4. An acute intestinal upset (gastroenteritis), in which the patient has had several episodes of violent vomiting, may cause bleeding to occur.
5. A benign or malignant tumor of the stomach is often associated with the vomiting of blood.

What is tarry stool?

A jet-black stool caused by bleeding from the stomach, duodenum, or intestinal tract. The bright red blood is oxidized during its passage through the intestinal tract and emerges from the rectum jet black.

Can cortisone or any of the other steroids cause ulceration of the stomach or duodenum?

Yes. It is thought that in some instances, particularly in those people who have been taking large doses of cortisone or similar substances for many months, ulcerations can be produced.

How does a doctor diagnose ulcer of the stomach or duodenum?

1. By taking a careful history and noting the characteristic abdominal pain, usually occurring between meals, when the stomach is empty.
2. By noting that there is relief of pain on taking milk or antacid medications.
3. By noting the presence of tarry stool or the vomiting of blood.
4. The most accurate method of diagnosing an ulcer is to take an X ray after the patient has swallowed barium.

Is it dangerous for people to medicate themselves with antacids?

No. However, it is unwise to continue this practice if the stomach symptoms continue. A serious stomach ailment can be masked by the temporary relief obtained by taking antacids.

Do ulcers ever cause obstruction of the outlet of the stomach?

Yes. This is a common complication of chronic ulcer in an older person. In some cases, the scar tissue that forms around the ulcer completely closes off the outlet of the stomach.

What can be done to relieve an obstruction of the outlet of the stomach?

In all probability, surgery will be necessary.

What is the standard medical treatment of an ulcer of the stomach or duodenum?

The methods used are essentially the same for older people as for younger ulcer patients. They consist of the following:

1. Frequent taking of small meals, usually no more than three hours apart.
2. Drinking large quantities of milk, especially between meals.
3. Avoiding spicy, greasy, and fried foods.
4. Avoiding alcoholic beverages.
5. Taking antacid medications.
6. Taking medications such as Banthine, which cuts down on the amount of acid secreted by the stomach.
7. Avoiding undue stress.
8. Avoiding the use of tobacco.

What are the indications for surgery for an ulcer?

1. Repeated, severe hemorrhages that require transfusions and endanger life.
2. Obstruction of the outlet of the stomach (pyloric obstruction).
3. Perforation of an ulcer and resultant peritonitis.
4. A suspicion that the ulcer has become cancerous.
5. Persistence of severe pain and indigestion despite medical treatment.

Can people in their sixties or seventies successfully withstand surgery for an ulcer of the stomach or duodenum?

Yes, if their general health is satisfactory.

What operations are now being performed for ulcer of the stomach or duodenum?

The surgery for older people differs very little from that for younger people. Some surgeons advocate a subtotal gastrectomy, the removal of approximately three-quarters of the stomach. When this is done, the remaining quarter of the stomach is stitched to the small intestine. This procedure removes the acid-secreting portion of the stomach and excludes from the stream of food the site where the ulcer had existed. In other cases, the surgeon may recommend a vagotomy, the cutting of the main nerve to the acid-secreting cells of the stomach. Along with vagotomy, the surgeon will remove half the stomach or will cut the pyloric sphincter (pyloroplasty). This will allow the alkaline juices of the small intestine to back up into the stomach and neutralize any acid that may still be secreted by the stomach.

There are at present about ten to twelve effective operations for curing an ulcer.

Can people who have had part of the stomach removed eat normally?

Yes. Even if three-quarters of the stomach has been removed, the remaining portion will dilate sufficiently within a period of a few months to permit the patient to eat full-sized meals.

Is it necessary for people who have undergone surgery for ulcer to maintain a strict diet?

No. They can be much more liberal than they were prior to surgery. However, it is imprudent for them to drink large quantities of alcohol or to eat highly spiced and seasoned foods.

Is there any way for older people to prevent ulcer formation?

1. Avoiding unnecessary emotional strain will undoubtedly reduce the chances of getting an ulcer. It has been shown that emotional stress is a primary factor in the development of ulcers.
2. People should eat a sensible diet and not overload their stomachs if they wish to avoid an ulcer.
3. There is an exceptionally high incidence of ulcers in alcoholics. Alcoholic beverages in moderation are all right, but if one has a tendency toward excessive acid secretion, alcohol should be avoided.
4. Those people who do secrete large quantities of acid should be particularly careful to avoid spicy and highly seasoned foods.
5. Those people who secrete large quantities of acid should neutralize it by taking milk between meals and by taking antacid medications.

How can one tell if he has excessive acid secretion?

In the best test, the doctor passes a rubber tube through the patient's nose into his stomach and analyzes the stomach contents. This will show quite accurately whether or not the stomach is secreting too much acid. Recently, tests on the urine have been developed to show the level of acid secretion.

URINARY BLADDER AND URETHRA

See Bed-Wetting; Cystitis and Interstitial Cystitis; Cystocele and Rectocele; Gonorrhea; Kidneys; Prostate Gland.

Does the holding capacity of the urinary bladder tend to decrease during the later years?

Not in the normal bladder. However, if chronic cystitis is present, there will be irritability and spasm, thus decreasing the bladder's capacity to hold urine. In older women, a condition known as interstitial cystitis (a chronic inflammation and thickening of the bladder wall) may be present; this will lead to contraction and consequent lessened bladder capacity.

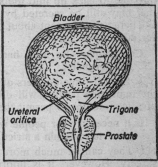

Normal male bladder and outlet

Do older people tend to void more frequently?

Yes, because the male usually has a certain amount of enlargement of the prostate and the female often develops weakness of the muscles and ligaments that control the bladder and its outlet (the urethra). It is not uncommon for older people, even when they are perfectly healthy, to get up at least once during the night to void.

What can be done to cut down on frequency of urination during the night?

Of course, the primary cause must be treated and eliminated. However, the following measures are helpful:

1. No fluids should be taken after the regular evening meal.
2. Evening meals should be eaten at least 3 to 4 hours before retiring.
3. Alcohol and coffee, since they stimulate voiding, should be avoided in the evenings.
4. Diuretic medications, which increase voiding, should be taken in the mornings or early afternoons.
5. Medications in the belladonna group can be given before retiring. They will cut down on bladder irritability and will tend to cut down on the desire to void.

6. Sedatives and sleeping pills should not be taken if one can sleep without them. They tend to make one sleep more deeply and thus be less conscious of the need to void.

7. Medications can also be given that will act directly to reduce bladder irritability.

What are some of the more frequent causes of irritability and spasm of the urinary bladder?

In the male:

1. Enlargement of the prostate gland, with partial obstruction of the bladder outlet.

2. Infection of the urine left behind in the bladder because of incomplete emptying.

3. An infection in the kidney or the outlet of the kidney, resulting in the passage of infected urine down to the bladder.

4. Pus in the urine secondary to a diverticulum of the bladder. (A diverticulum is an outpouching through the wall of the bladder, which may contain stagnant, infected urine.)

5. Infection of the urine due to gonorrhea, or to a staphylococcus, streptococcus, or colon bacillus entering the bladder from the outside.

6. Infection of the bladder secondary to infection in the prostate gland.

In the female:

1. Constriction of the outlet (neck) of the bladder as the result of a long-standing chronic inflammation of the urethra. (The urethra is the tube leading from the bladder to the outside.) Since the urethra in the female is short, infection may occur from bacteria in the vagina.

2. Development of interstitial cystitis, a condition of unknown origin, with thickening of the muscle wall of the bladder.

3. Infection of the urine of the bladder due to stagnation of urine secondary to cystocele and incomplete emptying.

4. Cystitis due to infected urine coming down from the kidneys.

5. Cystitis secondary to infection reaching the bladder from the outside.

What can be done to prevent the development of bladder irritation as one gets older?

Men should seek treatment from a urologist whenever there is difficulty in voiding. If there is bladder obstruction due to an enlarged prostate, and if this is relieved early, irritability of the bladder will not develop later on. Also, all urinary infections should be treated vigorously as soon as they appear. In women, most cystoceles develop during the childbearing age or during menopause (change of life). If surgical repair is carried out early, bladder irritability will be avoided in later life. Also, if there is a chronic urinary infection, it should be brought under control by vigorous treatment.

Does eating sharp, salty, or spicy foods cause one to void more frequently?

Yes, because greater liquid intake is needed to dilute the spices and salt. This added fluid intake will necessitate frequent voiding.

Is it natural for the urinary stream to be less forceful in men past sixty?

Yes. There is loss in the force of the urinary stream as the muscles that control urination lose some of their tone.

Why do some older women lose their urine when coughing, sneezing, or laughing?

This condition usually indicates loss in muscle tone at the outlet of the bladder. It is caused most often by a cystocele (*see* CYSTOCELE AND RECTOCELE) or by weakening of the muscle controlling the urethra.

What can be done to overcome loss of urine when coughing, sneezing, or laughing?

Surgical correction is necessary in most cases. Operations for repair of cystocele (hernia of the bladder) or loss of sphincteric control at the bladder outlet are not serious, and healthy women in their seventies and eighties can safely undergo them.

If an older person wets the bed, what can be done?
See BED-WETTING.

What is residual urine?
The urine left behind in the bladder after urination.

What are causes of residual urine in the female?
1. A cystocele (a hernia of the bladder into the vaginal canal).
2. A stricture (contracture) of the bladder outlet.
3. A diverticulum (outpouching of the wall) of the bladder secondary to a stricture of the outlet of the bladder.
4. A tumor of the bladder.

What are causes of residual urine in the male?
1. Enlargement of the prostate gland, with obstruction of the outlet of the bladder.

2. The development of a diverticulum of the bladder, which will contain stagnant urine.

3. A stricture of the urethra (the tube leading from the bladder to the outside) secondary to an old infection.

Is it common for healthy older men to dribble urine after voiding?

Yes. Small drops of urine may continue for several seconds after the main stream has been passed. This phenomenon occurs in many older men and is not significant. It merely means that urination will take a little longer.

Dribbling *is* indicative of bladder obstruction if it continues for several minutes after the main stream has been passed.

What should be done about dribbling of urine?

If the prostate is not so enlarged that it requires treatment, men should not discontinue voiding until all the drops have emerged. If, on the other hand, dribbling is associated with a markedly enlarged prostate, it can be helped only through surgery. (*See* PROSTATE GLAND.)

Dribbling in the female, if associated with cystocele or urethrocele, will require surgical repair.

Does it take longer to empty the bladder as one grows older?

Yes. The bladder tends to contract less forcefully and the stream tends to flow at a slower pace. This is particularly true of men.

What is cystoscopy?

An examination in which a long, hollow, metal tube is inserted through the urethra (the passageway from the bladder to the outside) into the bladder. Cystoscopes are equipped with lights and lenses, which permit an excellent view of the interior of the bladder. In addition, the outlet of the ureters from the kidneys can be studied through the cystoscope and catheters can be passed up the ureters to the kidneys.

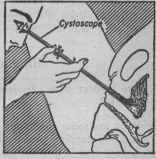

Cystoscope

Is cystoscopy very painful?

In the female it is almost painless. In the male, there is some discomfort, but this can be minimized by giving narcotics and local anesthetic agents. In children, cystoscopy is performed under general anesthesia.

Where can a cystoscopic examination be performed?
In a urologist's office or in a hospital.

Is a cystoscopic examination dangerous for someone past sixty?
No.

Of what value is a cystoscopic examination?
It is often of great value. Some of the major uses are:

1. To make a diagnosis of an inflammation of the bladder.
2. To treat with medications and to wash out an infected bladder.
3. To view a tumor of the bladder wall and to take a specimen for biopsy examination.
4. To destroy and remove small bladder tumors by means of an electric needle inserted through the cystoscope.
5. To crush large stones in the bladder and to wash them out through the cystoscope.
6. To diagnose a diverticulum of the bladder.
7. To dilate the urethra or a stricture of the outlet of the bladder.
8. To diagnose enlargement of the prostate gland.
9. To remove an enlarged portion of the prostate gland, thus relieving obstruction of the bladder. This is a common procedure, and is called transurethral resection.
10. To pass special catheters up the ureters toward the kidneys. This procedure permits diagnostic X-ray examination for kidney disease and for abnormalities or obstruction in the ureters. Frequently, it results in dislodging a stone caught in the ureter.

BLADDER STONES

Are bladder stones frequently encountered in people past sixty?
Yes.

What are some conditions that cause bladder stones?

1. Long-standing obstruction to the outlet of the bladder may lead to the formation of stones. This is considerably more common in men than in women, since obstruction to urinary outflow occurs more frequently in men.
2. Chronic cystitis, with inflammation of the bladder wall, may also lead to the formation of stones.
3. Stones often develop within a diverticulum (outpouching of the wall) of the bladder.
4. Many bladder stones originate in the kidneys and reach the bladder through the ureters.

What are the symptoms of bladder stone?
Painful, frequent, bloody urination. Small bladder stones may pass out with the urine, but larger ones may cause an abrupt, sudden blockage of the urinary outlet.

How is the diagnosis of a bladder stone made?
By X-ray examination, which will show the presence of the stone, or by direct observation through a cystoscope.

What is the treatment of bladder stones?
1. Small stones can be left alone; they may eventually pass out of the body spontaneously.
2. Larger stones can sometimes be crushed with a specially designed instrument passed through a cystoscope. This procedure is called lithopaxy.
3. Stones that cannot be passed or crushed are removed surgically by making an incision into the bladder.

What is the best way to prevent formation of bladder stones?
Vigorous treatment to eradicate such conditions as the following:
1. Chronic cystitis.
2. Enlargement of the prostate gland.
3. Contracture of the neck of the bladder.
4. Diverticulum of the bladder wall.
5. Kidney or ureter stones.

In addition, one should maintain an adequate fluid intake and have regular checkups, with particular attention to blood-chemistry findings.

DIVERTICULUM OF THE BLADDER

What is a diverticulum of the bladder?
It is a pouch originating from the bladder wall; it usually contains stagnant urine.

What causes a diverticulum?
Long-standing infection and obstruction of the outlet to the bladder. As one strains in an attempt to pass urine the muscle wall of the bladder is weakened. Eventually it gives way in a weak spot and a diverticulum results.

Are diverticula of the bladder wall very common?
Yes, especially in men with chronic cystitis and enlargement of the prostate.

How does a physician diagnose diverticulum of the bladder?
In the majority of cases, a diverticulum does not cause

symptoms. However, in people with chronic cystitis and pus in the urine, the diagnosis is made by cystoscopic examination or by taking X rays of the bladder.

What is the treatment of diverticulum of the bladder?

If it causes no symptoms, is small in size, and contains only small quantities of urine, no treatment is necessary. However, if it is large and contains large amounts of infected urine, it should be removed surgically.

Is an operation for the removal of a diverticulum dangerous?

No, but it is a major operation.

What is the operative procedure for diverticulum?

An abdominal incision is made just above the pubic bone, the bladder is exposed, and the diverticulum is removed. The bladder wall is sutured, a drain is inserted, and the abdominal wall is closed. Recovery takes place in almost all cases without complications.

What is the significance of markedly concentrated, dark-yellow urine?

In most instances, this is due to insufficient fluid intake. Older people whose fluid intake is restricted will pass this type of urine. In some instances, the urine is deep yellow because of jaundice. However, that condition also has other symptoms; the whites of the eyes turn yellow and the stool often becomes clay-colored.

How can one overcome markedly concentrated urine?

If there are no restrictions on fluid intake, more fluids should be taken. Healthy people should drink eight to ten glasses of liquid daily.

How often should older people have their urine examined?

Older people should have two physical checkups each year, including a urine examination.

What is a neurogenic bladder?

A bladder that fails to function properly because of a nerve disease or disorder.

Do older people often develop a neurogenic bladder?

Not if they are in good health. It is almost always associated with a nerve disease, such as multiple sclerosis; paralysis, such as that produced by a stroke; a spinal-cord tumor; or an injury to the spine affecting the nerves to the bladder. (*See* NERVES.)

BLADDER TUMORS

Are bladder tumors common in older people?
Yes. Bladder tumors occur frequently in people past sixty.

Are bladder tumors more common in men?
Yes, but women may also develop them.

What are the most common bladder tumors?
1. *Benign papillomas.* These are cauliflower-shaped growths arising from the lining membrane of the bladder wall. They vary in size from that of a pea to that of a plum.
2. *Malignant or cancerous tumors* originating from the cells lining the bladder. These are called transitional-cell cancers.

What is the most characteristic symptom of a bladder tumor?
The painless passage of blood in the urine. Frequency of urination and pain come late in the course of the disease.

How is diagnosis of a bladder tumor made?
By a cystoscopic examination. A piece of the tumor is cut off, removed through the cystoscope, and microscopically examined.

Are the majority of bladder tumors malignant?
Yes, but they generally grow very slowly over a period of years and are usually amenable to cure if discovered early.

What is the treatment of a bladder tumor?
1. If the tumor is small, it can usually be completely destroyed through the cystoscope. A cystoscope is passed into the bladder, and the growth is burned away from the bladder wall by an electric needle.
2. Large growths confined to one area can be removed surgically by excision of that portion of the bladder wall.
3. In some instances, the tumor grows to such proportions that the entire bladder must be removed—an operation of great magnitude. Today, however, it is being carried out successfully in an ever-increasing number of cases. When the entire bladder is removed, as in cases of cancer, the ureters (the tubes leading down from the kidneys) are implanted into an isolated segment of the small intestine (ileum), which is prepared to receive them. This loop of intestine is thus used as a substitute for the bladder. The open end of the intestine, which contains the ureters, is stitched onto the abdominal wall; a bag, to catch the urine, is worn at all times.

What are the chances for recovery after surgery for a malignant bladder tumor?

1. If the growth is small and has been burned away through a cystoscope, recovery will take place. There may be a recurrence several months or years later, but, in most instances, it too can be controlled in a similar manner.

2. If the cancer is limited to one section of the bladder, the removal of that segment of the bladder results in a cure in the majority of cases.

3. When the tumor has grown to such proportions that the entire bladder must be removed, cure is not easy to effect. In all probability, the cancer cells have already spread to other structures. However, many people who have this operation survive for several years after surgery.

Do tumors of the bladder tend to grow and spread quickly to other organs?

Not nearly as quickly as most other tumors. It is not unusual for someone to have cancer of the bladder for eight or nine years.

THE URETHRA

What is the urethra?
It is the tube leading from the urinary bladder to the outside. Its sole function is to convey urine.

Does the male urethra differ from that of the female?
Yes. The male urethra is much longer, extending from the outlet of the bladder through the penis. The female urethra is very short, extending from the bladder to the urinary opening in the vagina.

What are some of the conditions affecting the urethra in older people?

1. *Strictures.* These can result from long-standing inflammation, with the eventual formation of fibrous scar tissue. Inflammation of the female urethra is common, as it is so close to the vagina, where bacteria often grow. One of the most frequent causes of stricture of the male urethra is gonorrhea.

2. *Infections of the urethra.* These are most frequently caused by nonspecific germs, such as the staphylococcus, streptococcus, and colon bacillus. Cases of acute gonorrhea in people past sixty are infrequent.

3. *Caruncles of the urethra in the female.* These are

small pieces of over-grown tissue located at the opening of the urethra in the vaginal orifice. The condition is caused by chronic irritation and localized infection.

4. *Diverticulum of the urethra.* This is an out-pouching, or bulge, through the wall of the urethra, usually occurring in women as the end result of a chronic infection.

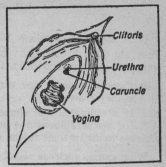

Caruncle of the urethra

What is the treatment of the various conditions affecting the urethra?

1. If a stricture of the urethra interferes with passage of urine, or if it results in retention of urine in the bladder or attacks of cystitis, it should be treated by repeated dilatation. This is accomplished by the passage of special instruments called "atsounds." If dilatation does not relieve the stricture, it should be cut surgically. In some cases it is necessary to do a plastic repair of the passageway.

2. A caruncle of the urethra may become very painful, particularly when one is passing urine. It may also lead to frequency of urination and stress. If a caruncle causes such symptoms, it should be destroyed with an electric needle or should be removed surgically. Very small caruncles can sometimes be controlled by application of silver nitrate.

3. A diverticulum of the urethra may be associated with recurrent attacks of cystitis or with obstruction to passage of urine. In some cases, there is pain during intercourse. When symptoms are severe, the diverticulum should be excised by surgery.

4. Infections of the urethra, whether caused by nonspecific organisms or by the gonorrheal germ, must be treated vigorously in order to prevent spread of the infection to the bladder and kidneys. The patient should drink large quantities of fluid, local antiseptics are applied, and antibiotic drugs are administered until all signs of infection have disappeared.

VEINS AND VARICOSE VEINS

See CIRCULATION; EMBOLUS AND EMBOLISM; THROMBUS AND THROMBOSIS.

What are varicose veins?

They are dilated, enlarged veins with damaged valves. Blood stagnates in them and often forms blood clots.

Is there a tendency for varicose veins to form in people as they grow older?

Yes. It is estimated that almost half of the women over fifty years of age and about one out of four men over fifty have varicose veins in their thighs or legs.

What causes varicose veins?

It is thought that constant back pressure on veins, over a period of years, will eventually cause their valves to break down. This condition is especially prevalent in people who, because of the nature of their work, must stand for many hours at a time.

What are the symptoms produced by varicose veins?

When they are large and contain a great deal of stagnant blood, there is a heavy, dragging sensation in the legs. This is often accompanied by a general feeling of tiredness and lack of energy. Occasionally—particularly in older people, varicose veins may so impair circulation that heart symptoms will develop. Also, untreated varicose veins may lead to phlebitis (inflammation in a vein), thrombosis (a clot in a vein), skin ulcerations, hemorrhage from a ruptured vein, or eczema.

How does one know if he has varicose veins?

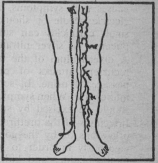

Most varicosities are plainly visible, appearing as large bluish swellings and irregularities beneath the skin of the thighs and legs.

What is the treatment of varicose veins?

In most instances, the best treatment is surgical. This will involve tying off the main veins and removing all those that lend themselves to this

Varicose veins and method of stripping

procedure (called stripping). The stripping of the main saphenous vein in the thigh and legs often leads to obliteration of many other varicosities of veins leading into the main vein. Those varicosities that remain after surgery can be injected with a substance to cause clotting.

Surgical treatment gives excellent results in the great majority of cases.

Can surgery for varicose veins be performed safely on people who are past sixty?

Yes. However, it must first be ascertained that the *deep* vein circulation is adequate. If the superficial veins are tied off or removed when the deep veins are unable to transport blood, the results will be poor.

Can varicose veins be treated by means other than surgery?

Yes. The wearing of compression bandages or elastic stockings will frequently give substantial relief to those who, for one reason or another, cannot safely undergo surgery.

How effective is the injection treatment of varicose veins?

If the varicosities are large, injection therapy is not very satisfactory. It is particularly ineffectual for varicose veins located above knee level.

This form of treatment will clot some of the varicosities, thus causing the blood to travel through the deeper, more normal, veins. Today, the injection treatment is reserved for small varicosities or for those patients who can not safely undergo surgery.

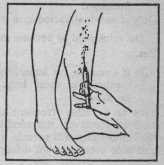

Injection treatment of varicose veins

What is the injection treatment?

A "sclerosing" solution is injected with a small needle directly into a varicosed vein. This will cause a clot to form, thus obliterating the passageway and forcing the blood to travel through a more normal vessel.

Does the blood clot formed by injection of a varicose vein ever break loose and enter the general circulation?

Almost never.

Is varicose-vein ligation and stripping a dangerous operation?

No. The operation is not risky, and successful results can be anticipated in the vast majority of cases, even if the patient is in his eighties or nineties.

What are varicose ulcers?

Skin ulcerations that develop as a result of stagnation of blood in varicosities. They usually form on the inner side of the leg above the ankle after years of neglect or inadequate treatment of the varicosities.

What is the treatment of varicose ulcers?

1. Bed rest for a period varying from a week to a month.
2. Warm, moist soaks for any infection of the ulceration.
3. Application of antibiotic solutions or ointments.
4. Surgical ligation and stripping of the varicosities responsible for the ulceration.

Should people who have been operated on for varicose veins continue to wear compression bandages or elastic stockings?

Only if residual varicosities continue to cause discomfort.

Do veins tend to become more fragile as people age?

Yes.

Is it common for superficial veins in the thighs or legs to rupture and cause large black-and-blue marks beneath the skin?

This is a rather frequent occurrence, especially in older women. However, the condition requires no treatment and the hemorrhage will subside spontaneously, although the black and blue area may not disappear for several weeks.

Is a rupture of a vein beneath the skin a warning that the same thing might happen to a vein located in a vital area of the body?

No. The superficial veins are especially fragile in older people and are apt to rupture with even slight injury. Important, deep veins are much better protected and therefore do not rupture easily.

PHLEBITIS

What is phlebitis?

An inflammation of a vein.

Do older people often develop phlebitis?

Yes, because the walls of the veins become more fragile and because the aging process makes them more susceptible to inflammation. Moreover, in the later years, circulation slows and blood tends to stagnate and clot.

What are the symptoms of phlebitis?

1. A cordlike, firm swelling along the course of the vein.
2. Pain, redness, and tenderness along the course of the vein.
3. The entire limb may feel hot and may become swollen.
4. Body temperature may be elevated by one or two degrees.
5. The pulse rate may become more rapid.
6. Pain on attempting to walk or exercise the limb.

Is phlebitis ever serious when it affects older people?

Yes, particularly when it involves the deep veins of the legs or the veins in the pelvis or the abdomen.

What is the main danger of phlebitis?

A piece of clotted blood from the passageway of the vein may break off and travel to other parts of the body. This is called an embolism. (*See* EMBOLUS AND EMBOLISM.)

What is the treatment of phlebitis?

1. Bed rest, with the affected limb kept at body level.
2. If pain is marked, luke-warm, wet compresses may be applied.
3. Medications to ease the pain and reduce the inflammatory process—aspirin or some other analgesic, butazolidin, or similar medications.
4. Antibiotics to overcome any infection in the area.
5. The administration of anticoagulant drugs, such as heparin or dicoumarol, to prevent the spread of clotting and to reduce the chances of an embolus taking place.
6. Surgery to tie off the main saphenous vein in the groin or, if embolus has already occurred, to tie off the vena cava in the abdomen. The latter is done very rarely, when life is endangered by the possibility of repeated embolization.

How can older people guard against the development of phlebitis?

1. By exercising regularly, even when confined to bed by an illness. This will aid normal circulation through the veins.
2. Regular walking, if the general health permits.
3. By treatment of varicose veins, even if they cause no symptoms, so that phlebitis does not eventually set in.

4. Wearing of elastic stockings or compression bandages by those who have small varicosities and by those who are not able to undergo surgery.

5. By eliminating constricting garters.

6. By undergoing surgery for the removal of any growth that causes back pressure on the veins in the thighs or legs.

7. If possible, by giving up a job that requires standing in one position for long periods of time.

8. By seeking early treatment for any infection of the legs or feet, especially a fungus infection of the toes.

VERTIGO AND DIZZINESS

See BLOOD PRESSURE; CIRCULATION; FAINTING; HEADACHE; HYPERTENSION; NERVES.

What is vertigo?

It is the loss of the sense of balance, equilibrium, and position. In vertigo, the patient complains that the room seems to be spinning or that the whole world seems to be whirling around.

Do staggering, nausea, vomiting, and a faint feeling often accompany vertigo?

Yes.

Do people lose consciousness during an attack of vertigo?

No.

What are some of the most common causes of vertigo in older people?

1. Disturbance in the inner ear (the cochlea), where the sense of balance is controlled.

2. Ear infections involving the middle and inner ear.

3. Deafness caused by inner-ear disturbance.

4. Blockage of the eustachian tube, which leads from the throat to the ear.

5. Taking large doses of certain drugs, for example, quinine.

6. Excessive use of alcohol.

7. Excessive use of tobacco.

8. Abrupt changes of body positions, such as getting up quickly from a lying-down position.

9. Abrupt changes in blood pressure, especially a sudden drop in pressure.

10. Sudden spasm of a blood vessel in the brain, with temporary deprivation of sufficient oxygen supply.

11. Arteriosclerosis of the blood vessels to the brain.
12. Hemorrhage in the brain (stroke, cerebral hemorrhage).
13. Inadequate heart function, with irregular heartbeats.
14. Otosclerosis (*see* HEARING AND DEAFNESS).
15. Encephalitis or meningitis (inflammation of the brain or of the meninges, the tissues covering the brain).
16. Syphilis affecting the brain.
17. A tumor of the nerve of hearing (acoustic-nerve tumor).

What is the treatment of vertigo?

Naturally the treatment will depend entirely on which of the above-mentioned factors is found to be responsible for the symptoms. Such drugs as Dramamine and Bonamine are very helpful in relieving vertigo and dizziness temporarily, but they should not be taken until the cause of the condition has been determined.

What measures can older people take to minimize vertigo or dizziness?

1. They should receive treatment as soon as they discover that the symptom is recurrent.
2. Any nose, throat, or ear infection should be treated promptly and vigorously.
3. If deafness accompanies the dizziness, an ear specialist should be consulted.
4. Any medication or drug that causes vertigo or dizziness should be discontinued.
5. Excessive use of alcohol and tobacco should be stopped.
6. Treatment of heart conditions, high blood pressure, and arteriosclerosis should be undertaken.
7. Body positions should be changed slowly, especially standing up from a lying-down position.

VITAMINS

See ANEMIA; DIET; HEPATITIS; SURGERY; WEIGHT.

What are vitamins?

They are chemical compounds contained in various foods. Vitamin D is also present in sunlight.

Are vitamins essential to health?

Yes. Vitamin deficiencies can lead to many diseases, some of which may seriously endanger life.

Do older people usually require supplementary vitamins, or do they obtain a sufficient quantity from their ordinary diet?

Most physicians who treat large numbers of patients over sixty feel that supplementary vitamins are of considerable help to the patient in maintaining a good state of health. Despite a well-rounded diet, the intestinal tract in older people may fail to absorb the necessary amounts of vitamins from the ingested food. For this reason, it is common practice to advise those in their seventies or eighties to take vitamin pills.

Will extra vitamins help those who are already in good health?

Although the body utilizes only as much of each vitamin as it needs, a doctor cannot always be sure when a minor deficiency exists. Therefore, doctors often prescribe extra vitamins to insure that there will be no deficiency. Furthermore, the onset of a relatively minor illness in an older individual may cause a major vitamin deficiency.

What happens if an excess amount of vitamins is taken?

The body eliminates it. It would take a huge amount to produce harmful results.

Are vitamins beneficial to people who are undernourished and debilitated?

Yes. Such people usually have an insufficient vitamin intake or their intestinal tract fails to absorb those vitamins that are taken.

How does a physician make a diagnosis of vitamin deficiency when the patient has no overt symptoms of a vitamin-deficiency disease?

1. If the patient is undernourished or debilitated, it can be assumed that a vitamin deficiency exists.
2. If there is marked anemia, there is, in all probability, a coexisting vitamin deficiency.
3. If food intake is restricted to a limited number of substances because of an underlying disease, such as an ulcer or gallstones, it can be assumed that a deficiency of certain vitamins will occur.

What are some of the more common vitamin-deficiency states and what symptoms do they cause?

1. Vitamin A deficiency will produce:
   a. Dryness of the skin and tissues about the eyes.
   b. Decreased acuteness of night vision.
2. Vitamin B_1 (thiamine) deficiency will cause:

    a. Weight loss, poor appetite, loss of strength, and neuritis.

    b. In rare instances, older people may develop beriberi—with characteristic loss of muscle tone and strength —neuritis, mental confusion, and impaired heart action.

3. Vitamin B_2 (riboflavin) deficiency will result in cracking of the skin at the corners of the mouth, scaliness in the skin folds—especially about the face—redness and inflammation of the inside of the mouth and tongue, and photophobia (fear of light).

4. Nicotinic acid deficiency will cause the development of pellagra, with its characteristic rash on exposed body surfaces, intestinal upset, and emotional instability.

5. Folic acid deficiency will cause marked anemia, often of the pernicious type. (*See* ANEMIA.)

6. Vitamin B_6 deficiency can lead to:

    a. Marked general weakness.

    b. Irritability and nervousness.

    c. Intestinal upset.

7. Vitamin B_{12} deficiency can cause:

    a. Pernicious anemia.

    b. Nerve-tissue damage and neuritis.

8. Vitamin C (ascorbic acid) deficiency can result in:

    a. Scurvy, with bleeding, especially from the gums and in the intestinal tract. Hemorrhage into the joints may also occur. Extreme weakness often ensues.

    b. Large black-and-blue areas beneath the skin, evidence of subcutaneous hemorrhage.

9. Vitamin D deficiency causes:

    a. An upset in calcium metabolism, with bowing and thinning out of the bones. This condition is called rickets. (Not seen among older people.)

    b. Marked anemia.

10. Vitamin E deficiency in advanced states may cause:

    a. Weakening of heart muscle, with impaired function.

    b. Inflammation of nerve and muscle tissues.

11. Vitamin K deficiency causes upset in the blood-clotting mechanism, with increased tendency to hemorrhage.

12. Vitamin F deficiency often leads to an upset in function of connective tissues and capillaries (the tiny blood vessels that transport blood cells to the areas surrounding the body cells).

Will a vitamin deficiency always produce the symptoms listed above?

No. A minor deficiency will result in no obvious symptoms.

Nevertheless, with even a minor vitamin deficiency, the level of general health may drop insidiously.

Do people develop a deficiency of just one vitamin, or do they develop a simultaneous deficiency of several vitamins?

Vitamin deficiencies are usually multiple.

How long must a patient take vitamins before their beneficial effects are apparent?

If vitamins are taken by mouth, several weeks may pass before maximum benefits are seen. If they are given by intramuscular or intravenous injection, results may be seen within several days to a week or two.

What foods should older people eat in order to ensure high vitamin intake?

Vitamin A: milk, eggs, fish, liver, green vegetables.

Vitamin B_1 (thiamine): vegetables, liver, eggs, whole grains, meat.

Vitamin B_2 (riboflavin): meat, eggs, dairy products.

Vitamin B_6 (pyroxidane): meat, fish, liver, yeast, grains, vegetables.

Nicotinic acid: wheat germ, peanuts, yeast.

Vitamin B_{12}: meat, liver, eggs, dairy products.

Vitamin C: grapefruits, lemons, oranges, other citrus fruits, cabbages, tomatoes, potatoes.

Vitamin D: fish-liver oils, eggs, dairy products, milk.

Folic acid: green vegetables, liver, kidney, yeast.

Vitamin K: meat and vegetable fats.

Vitamin E: wheat germ, whole grains.

Can older people take supplementary vitamins on their own, or should vitamins be prescribed by a physician?

Vitamins are potent chemicals, and although they cannot do much harm, they should nevertheless be prescribed by a doctor. People usually cannot diagnose which vitamin is lacking, and it is wasteful to take vitamins that are already present in ample quantities. Furthermore, stomach upset may follow the taking of certain vitamins in capsule or pill form. Another factor that argues against self-medication is that a patient rarely knows the proper dosage. He may lack one vitamin in particular but will receive an inadequate amount of that vitamin in an ordinary multivitamin capsule. Hence, even though he is taking a pill containing all the essential vitamins, his symptoms will not be relieved.

Is there a natural decrease in the ability to absorb vitamins as one grows older?

Healthy older people can absorb normal amounts of vitamins

from the intestinal tract. However, when they are ill, anemic, or convalescing from a serious disease, ability to absorb swallowed vitamins may be markedly decreased. For this reason, it is frequently necessary to give vitamins by injection.

Are vitamins helpful in cases of anemia?

Yes, but vitamins alone will not relieve the anemia. Many doctors think that a high vitamin intake will aid the absorption and utilization of iron, thus helping to overcome the anemia. Liver extract, iron, folic acid, and other chemicals are usually required to cure many types of anemia.

Will taking supplementary vitamins cut down on the incidence of colds and respiratory infections?

Yes, provided there is an existent vitamin deficiency.

Will taking extra vitamins cause the average older person to gain weight?

No. However, if someone is undernourished and has a vitamin lack, vitamins will help to improve appetite and thus lead to gaining weight.

Is there a tendency for diabetics in particular to develop vitamin deficiencies?

Yes, mainly because of their restrictions in diet. Also, vitamin metabolism is erratic in certain cases of long-standing diabetes.

Is it important for an older person who contemplates surgery to make sure that he has no vitamin deficiency?

Yes. In order to ensure good wound healing, the levels of vitamins B and C in the blood must be adequate. Also, vitamin K must be present in adequate amounts to ensure proper blood clotting.

How can postoperative patients who are not permitted to eat maintain an adequate supply of vitamins?

For the first few days after surgery it may be necessary to administer vitamins intravenously or intramuscularly. As soon as eating is resumed, a diet rich in vitamins is given.

Is vitamin A ever helpful in improving eyesight?

Yes, in an occasional case where there is a vitamin A deficiency.

Is vitamin A ever helpful in treating leukoplakia of the mouth or tongue?

Yes. (*See* LEUKOPLAKIA.)

Is vitamin B ever helpful in relieving pain or a burning sensation on the tongue?

Yes. Large doses sometimes will alleviate this condition.

Is vitamin B$_{12}$ ever helpful in relieving the neuritis seen in some cases of diabetes?

Yes.

Will taking large doses of antibiotics ever interfere with the absorption of vitamins from the intestinal tract?

Yes. In cases where it is essential to give the antibiotics, supplementary doses of vitamins B, C, and K should be administered.

Will vitamins ever benefit older people with arteriosclerosis?

Yes. Their general condition will improve after prolonged use of large doses of vitamins.

Do people with cirrhosis of the liver require extra vitamins?

Yes. Such patients should receive vitamins by injection, as there is frequently malabsorption from the intestines.

Will excessive vitamin D intake increase the chances of developing kidney stones?

This has happened in a very few cases. Most kidney stones are caused by infection plus an upset in uric acid, calcium, or phosphorus metabolism.

Is it important for older people who have chronic diarrhea to take supplementary vitamins?

Yes, because diarrhea may cause vitamins to be eliminated before they have had time to be absorbed.

Is it important for older people with ulcers or other stomach disorders to take supplementary vitamins?

Yes, because ulcer diets omit certain vitamin-rich foods.

Is it important to give vitamin K to someone who will undergo surgery on the gallbladder or intestines?

Yes, especially in cases of jaundice. Vitamin K will help combat the usual bleeding tendency in these cases.

Should people with hepatitis take supplementary vitamins?

Yes. Large doses of vitamins B, C, and K should be given for the duration of the illness.

Should people with tuberculosis take extra vitamins?

Yes.

Is it important for older people who are on reducing diets to take extra vitamins?

Yes, since their limited food intake may deprive them of many essential vitamins.

WEIGHT

See ANEMIA; DIABETES MELLITUS; DIET; HEART; LONGEVITY; PHYSICAL ACTIVITY AND EXERCISE; RETIREMENT; TEETH; THYROID GLAND; VITAMINS.

Does the appetite normally increase or decrease as one enters the later years?

As a general rule, the appetite tends to slacken as one grows older. The main reason for this is that the caloric requirements decrease as one expends less physical energy.

It is estimated that the average person over sixty requires only 75 percent of the food that someone in his twenties or thirties requires.

Is there a constitutional tendency toward being fat or thin?

There is considerable difference of opinion among medical men as to whether or not one inherits a weight tendency. If it were true, it would imply that there were two different types of endocrine-gland systems—one that caused an individual to become fat and another that caused him to remain thin. This theory has never been substantiated.

Almost all investigators do agree, however, that food habits develop along specific lines almost from the time of birth. Thus, in certain families, the parents overfeed their children and thereby set a pattern of eating that may last throughout life. All the members of such a family may be fat. Conversely, in families in which everyone is thin, the family custom may be to eat small amounts of food at each meal.

What should the normal caloric intake be for an average healthy male past sixty years of age?

According to the National Research Council, the average healthy American male past sixty weighs 154 pounds; he is five feet nine inches tall; and he requires approximately 2,500 calories a day, of which 70 grams should be protein.

What should the normal caloric intake be for an average healthy woman past sixty years of age?

According to the National Research Council, the average American woman past sixty weighs 128 pounds; she is five feet four inches tall; and she requires a minimum of 1,800 calories a day, of which 59 grams should be protein.

Does the average person who is thin tend to live longer than one who is fat?

All longevity statistics tend to show that the average thin person in good health will live longer than the average fat person. (*See* LONGEVITY.)

What types of foods should older people eat to maintain a normal weight?

Although healthy people in their sixties and seventies usually require no special diet, it is better that their food be bland and not spicy. Rich sauces, stuffings, fats, gravies, and greases should be omitted from the diet. Fried foods and rich desserts should be eaten sparingly. The diet should include adequate protein and vitamins. (*See* DIET.)

What are good weights for people over sixty to maintain?

Below is a chart of average weights for men and women between sixty and seventy years of age:

MEN		WOMEN	
Height	Average Weight (lbs.)	Height	Average Weight (lbs.)
5'0"	133	4'10"	127
5'2"	139	5'0"	131
5'4"	146	5'2"	137
5'6"	154	5'4"	145
5'8"	163	5'6"	153
5'10"	173	5'8"	161
6'0"	183		
6'2"	193		
6'4"	204		

ABNORMAL WEIGHT

Is there a natural tendency for people to become fat after sixty?

Not unless they have lived very active physical lives in the forties and fifties and then abruptly retire to a life of inactivity.

What is the main cause of obesity in older people?

The same as that for younger people; that is, eating more calories than are required to maintain normal body weight.

Is obesity in older people often caused by glandular imbalance?

No. Obesity is seldom caused by upset gland function. It can usually be traced to the intake of more food than is needed by the body.

Is lowered metabolism often the cause of obesity in older people?

No. Although his metabolism may slow down, an older person will not put on weight if he maintains a caloric intake no greater than his own specific requirements. Of course, this does not apply to the sick older person who retains excessive fluids in his body. Such people, usually those suffering from heart conditions, may put on weight because of the accumulation of excessive body fluids. This kind of extra weight is lost when the patient is dehydrated with specific diuretics.

What are some of the dangers of becoming overweight after sixty?

1. It has been found that overweight people tend to have a shorter life-span.
2. Obesity predisposes toward the development of certain diseases, such as diabetes, high blood pressure (hypertension), heart failure, arteriosclerosis, gallbladder disease, varicose veins, and hernia.
3. Obesity increases the surgical risk if an operation becomes necessary.
4. Stout people tend to lose their balance more easily and therefore have a greater incidence of fracture and other injuries.
5. Obesity leads to shortness of breath and makes walking, climbing stairs, and sleeping more difficult.
6. Fat people have a much greater incidence of pneumonia.
7. Obese people have more complaints of the intestinal tract, for example, pain in the abdomen, indigestion, belching, flatulence, and constipation.
8. Headache, lassitude, and irritability are seen more frequently in obese people.

Is there much truth to the statement, made by many older people, that they eat less but still gain weight?

No. Most people who have put on weight tend unconsciously to fabricate about how much they eat. They convince themselves that their intake is low, whereas, in reality, it may be far in excess of their requirements.

Are strenuous "crash" diets safe for people over sixty?

No. Moreover, *all* dieting by older people should be done under medical supervision. Obesity should be considered a problem requiring expert medical care and advice.

Are some of the "reducing" drugs harmful to older people?

Yes. Some may raise the blood pressure to a dangerous level; others may adversely affect heart function. They should never be taken unless prescribed by a physician.

What are some important general instructions for the older individual who wants to lose weight?

1. Eat only those foods listed on the diet that the physician has prescribed.

2. Do not eat between meals.
3. Avoid the use of sugar, cream, and butter.
4. Limit the fluid intake each day.
5. Limit the quantity of salt taken each day.
6. Avoid the use of highly seasoned foods, which may increase the intake of fluid.
7. The bowels should be moved daily. If necessary, a lubricant or mild laxative should be prescribed.
8. The quantities of food eaten daily should be carefully measured and the calories calculated.
9. A daily weight record should be kept. Weigh-in should be at the same time each day.
10. If there is a question about an item on the diet, the doctor should be asked about it.

What is an adequate caloric intake per day for a reducing diet?

Approximately 1,200 calories per day, or about half of the normal requirement.

Are psychological factors important in getting an overweight person to reduce?

Yes. If the person is hostile to the idea of weight loss, no diet will be very effective.

What are some complications of surgery to which overweight people are susceptible?

1. Bronchitis and pneumonia.
2. Heart irregularities and heart failure.
3. Thromboses and clots in blood vessels.
4. Slow wound healing.
5. Tendency toward wound rupture and subsequent hernia through the incision.
6. Increased incidence of wound infection.

Should people be placed on reducing diets before undergoing elective surgery?

Yes.

Is obesity harmful to older people who have heart disease or high blood pressure?

Definitely. One of the first things a doctor does when he treats obese patients with these conditions is to place them on a reducing diet. Elimination of unnecessary fat will ease the load on an ailing heart and on sclerotic blood vessels.

Should older people who have a tendency to become obese stop eating cholesterol-containing foods?

Yes, since these foods are fattening. However, it should be understood that the tendency to deposit cholesterol in the blood vessels begins in childhood and early youth, and very little can be done to reverse the process once a person has passed sixty years of age.

Does obesity during the earlier years of life tend to cause premature hardening of the arteries?

Yes. Most physicians today believe that the intake of large quantities of fat does lead to premature hardening of the arteries.

Is obesity especially harmful to the older diabetic?

Yes. Obese diabetics should be placed on reducing diets.

Does obesity affect those who have joint pains or arthritis?

Yes. It has been shown that overweight people usually suffer much greater discomfort from their arthritis than thin people.

Does physical exercise help greatly in losing weight?

No. Normal physical exercise is all that is required. It has been proved quite definitely that weight loss is difficult to accomplish solely through physical exercise.

Does cancer develop more often in fat people than thin people?

Yes. Statistics show this to be true, although the reason is not known.

Is there a tendency for older overweight people to develop angina pectoris, coronary thrombosis, and other heart conditions more frequently than thin people?

Yes. This is a well-known fact. Weight reduction *prior to the development of heart symptoms* is a sound course of action.

Is it advisable for people past sixty who are on reducing diets to take supplementary vitamins and minerals?

Yes, because most reducing diets contain insufficient quantities of vitamins and minerals.

What is a good reducing diet for an older person?

See DIET.

What are the special dangers for people over sixty of being underweight and undernourished?

1. Failure to maintain an adequate protein intake will result in the wasting away of essential muscle and organ tissue.
2. Those who are underweight and undernourished usually take in an insufficient quantity of amino acids (protein components), which are essential for tissue metabolism.

3. Underweight, undernourished people usually fail to take in a sufficient quantity of essential vitamins and thus may develop deficiency diseases. (*See* VITAMINS.)

4. Undernourished people usually have an inadequate intake of minerals, such as iron, calcium, phosphorus, potassium, sodium, and chlorides. These are essential to maintenance of normal organic function.

5. Malnutrition is associated with an increased incidence of infection. Although healthy, thin people exhibit a greater resistance to infections, those who are undernourished have a decreased resistance to infections and have more trouble overcoming those that are present.

Do undernourished people have an inordinate number of complications after surgery?

Yes. Wound healing is inhibited greatly if body proteins, vitamins, and minerals are inadequate. However, it should be emphasized that the *healthy* thin person does better in surgery than the healthy fat person.

Should undernourished older people receive special preoperative care?

Yes. Their lack of proteins, vitamins, and minerals should be overcome, insofar as possible, by giving them blood transfusions, a high-protein diet, and large doses of vitamins and minerals.

Does being underweight, even though one has an adequate caloric intake, indicate that some underlying disease might be preventing a gain in weight?

Yes. It is not normal to be underweight when an adequate diet is being eaten. If this happens, a thorough physical examination is called for.

What are some common causes of an underweight condition in people who maintain a normal caloric intake?

1. Episodes of vomiting, in which the ingested food is ejected before it has been absorbed.

2. Diarrhea, causing the food to pass through the intestinal tract before it can be properly absorbed.

3. Upset in the function of the pancreas and in bile secretion. This condition may result in inadequate digestion of food and in incomplete absorption from the intestinal tract.

4. Disease in the liver or kidneys.

5. Malignant growths, in which the cancer cells use up so many of the food elements that there is weight loss.

6. Overactivity of the thyroid gland.

When a healthy person past sixty begins to lose weight, is an underlying disease always the cause?

Not by any means. Emotional upset, unattractively prepared food, inadequate teeth or dentures, and other factors may cause loss of appetite and, therefore, of weight.

Many older people are diverted from eating because of the presence of noisy children, the blaring of loud radios or television sets, or the nagging by members of the family who urge them to eat more than they want.

A change in food fare, a more attractive setting, the solution of some petty emotional problem—any of these may bring about marked changes in an older person's eating habits.

Can extra vitamins and minerals help undernourished people regain normal weight?

Yes. It is not enough merely to eat more calories, since absorption and utilization of food by the body may not be possible if the intake of essential vitamins and minerals is inadequate.

What are special hazards in operations on elderly people who are undernourished?

1. Tissues that have an inadequate supply of protein, vitamins, and minerals tend to heal very poorly.
2. Liver and kidney function may be disturbed by inadequate intake of proteins and vitamins, especially of vitamins K and C.
3. Markedly undernourished people are usually anemic, and this condition will interfere with wound healing and postoperative recovery.

Does the average older individual require as much protein in his diet as the younger person?

No. Younger people need protein to build new tissues and for growth. Obviously, this is not as essential in those past sixty. It is estimated that the average healthy older person requires about 75 percent of the protein intake of the younger individual.

Should older underweight people be given high-fat diets?

No. It is much better to increase the quantity of protein and sugars.

What measures can be taken to stimulate the appetites of older people?

1. See to it that their surroundings at mealtime are pleasant and quiet.
2. Make sure that they are not having trouble with their teeth or dentures.

3. Discuss with them the foods they like and dislike. Cater to their whims and prejudices.

4. Do not attempt to force them to eat. This may cause rebellion, as it does with children.

5. Discuss food seasoning. Many older people will reject foods that are too highly seasoned or are not seasoned sufficiently.

6. Do not discuss important family problems at mealtime.

7. If they prefer to eat alone, permit them to do so.

8. Often, appetite is stimulated by a small quantity of alcohol. Permission to serve this should be obtained from the family doctor.

9. Appetite is often stimulated by moderate physical exercise. If the doctor permits it, older people should be encouraged to take a walk out of doors before sitting down to a meal.

What is a good high-calorie diet for older underweight people?

See DIET.

WIDOWHOOD

See FAMILY RELATIONSHIPS; LONGEVITY; MARRIAGE AFTER SIXTY.

What is the expectancy of widowhood for the average American woman?

According to reliable life-expectancy statistics, the average American male will live four to five years less than the average American female. Also, the average American marries a woman four years his junior. Thus, the average American woman must anticipate about eight years of widowhood.

If these statistics are related to people in older age groups, one notes that the average American man of sixty will live 15.7 years after that age. His wife—who is fifty-six years of age—can look forward to 22.4 more years. Therefore, she will be widowed for 6.7 years.*

Should married couples prepare for the possibility of widowhood?

Yes. It is wise to attempt to prepare and plan for the time when one of them—most often, the wife—will be on her own.

*Courtesy of the Metropolitan Life Insurance Co.

Older couples, instead of becoming more dependent on each other, should consciously try to attain greater independence. Society, too, should assume a greater role in this area and should make plans that allow aging widows or widowers to lead more productive and better-adjusted lives.

Older husbands have the responsibility of instructing their wives on economic and financial matters so that they can more easily manage their affairs when they are alone. If husbands have, in the past, withheld intimate financial information, they should, when they enter their later years, confide in their wives and familiarize them with specific details of importance.

What advice should be given to persons who have recently lost a spouse?

Perhaps the most important thing for them to know is that there is *no one pattern* of acceptable behavior. Men and women who have been loyal, devoted, and loving spouses may, within a few months after being widowed, lead an active social life and remarry. This is not necessarily an indication of lack of love for the deceased. For emotional health during widowhood, it is often wise for couples to discuss with each other how they expect the survivor to act. Thus, a husband may specifically urge his wife to remarry after he is gone. Such advice will often relieve the sense of guilt that overwhelms a widow who is attempting to reestablish herself in life.

Periods of mourning, too, very greatly among different peoples, races, and religions. Joint decision on this subject will dispel the survivor's guilt feelings later on. Modern Western society no longer holds to rigid standards concerning mourning attire or the length of time mourning must be observed. And it should never be forgotten that, often, the best adjustment to widowhood is attained by those who were happiest during their marriage. Excessive mourning is no longer considered to be a compliment to the deceased. Rather, it may indicate the deceased's inability to properly prepare the survivor for a life alone.

Are remarriages often successful for people past sixty?

Yes. However, as might be expected, statistics show that the incidence of incompatibility is much greater in this age group. Patterns of behavior and habits become more set as people age, and their ability to make adjustments to others diminishes markedly.

Are the chances for a happy remarriage greater when people past sixty marry into their own age group?

Yes. The greatest incidence of unsuccessful remarriage is

when a woman past sixty marries a younger man or when a
man past sixty marries a very young woman.

XANTHELASMA

See EYES; SKIN.

What is xanthelasma?

It is a harmless condition in which yellow plaques form on
the eyelids, most often on the upper lids. They range in size
from that of a pinhead to that of a lima bean.

Do older people get xanthelasma?

Yes. It is most common in people past sixty, and is more
prevalent in women.

What causes xanthelasma?

The cause is unknown, but it appears to be part of the general
aging process. The chemical composition of the plaques is
quite similar to that of the cholesterol deposited in the walls
of arteriosclerotic blood vessels.

What is the treatment of xanthelasma?

The plaques are not harmful if left alone. However, since they
are unsightly, many people want them removed. This is done
either by surgical removal with a scalpel or with an electric
needle. Local anesthesia can be used to eliminate pain.

X RAY

See ANATOMICAL CHANGES IN ORGANS; BONES AND JOINTS;
CANCER AND OTHER MALIGNANT GROWTHS; DIAGNOSIS OF
DISEASE; PAGET'S DISEASE.

Are there any valid reasons why older people should not be subjected to diagnostic X rays?

No. Much misinformation has been disseminated concerning
the dangers of diagnostic X rays. Whatever the merit of this
position, it does *not* apply to people past sixty.

What are the supposed dangers of X rays?

In recent years, the danger of diagnostic X rays has been
greatly exaggerated. The theory is that excessive X rays may

damage the reproductive organs and thereby be reflected in deformities in offspring. Since very few men and no women past sixty will become parents, the matter is quite unimportant. Another theory is that multiple X-ray examinations may stimulate malignancy, especially leukemia. This has not been definitely established as yet.

What evidences of aging can be seen on X ray?

1. The bones appear thinner and show less calcium.
2. Cartilage may show calcium deposits, especially in the ribs.
3. Spaces occupied by cartilage (which does not show up on X ray) have become narrower.
4. The stomach may have dropped to a lower position in the abdomen.
5. The various sphincters of the intestinal tract may show loss of tone.
6. The large bowel may have developed pouches, or diverticula.
7. The lungs may show more fibrous tissue, and the air spaces may be enlarged.
8. The contour of the heart and aorta may have changed in a characteristic manner.
9. Blood vessels may show calcium deposits as a result of arteriosclerosis.
10. Innumerable other changes in organs and structures of the body will have occurred as a result of aging.

Are X rays helpful in diagnosing the stage of the aging process?

Yes. X ray is one of the best methods of finding out how far the aging process has advanced. In this form of examination, special attention is paid to the appearance of the bones (especially the skull), the blood vessels, the contour of the heart, and other important structures.

Is it safe to fluoroscope older patients?

Yes, but since more X rays are absorbed during fluoroscopy than during the taking of an X-ray picture, overexposure should be avoided.

Are special precautions necessary before one undergoes a barium X-ray examination of the intestinal tract?

Yes. Older people often are constipated, and it is necessary to make sure that the lower intestinal tract is empty before the barium is swallowed. Also, since they have a tendency toward constipation, it is important that the barium be evacuated from the bowel after the X rays have been completed.

Are special precautions advisable when X-raying the kidneys of older people?

Yes. Tests should be carried out to make sure that the patient is not sensitive (that is, allergic) to the material to be injected into the veins. (As explained elsewhere, dye must be injected into the bloodstream for the kidneys to show up on X ray.)

What is an arteriogram?

It is an X ray of an artery, and is taken after the injection of a dye directly into the arterial system. It will outline the contour of the artery, thus showing whether the passageway is normal, narrowed, or closed. It will also demonstrate the extent of arteriosclerosis.

Are arteriograms particularly helpful in diagnosing disease in older people?

Yes, since older people are likely to develop arteriosclerosis.

What is an aortogram?

It is an X ray of the aorta, the large blood vessel leading from the heart down through the chest and into the abdomen. A dye is injected through a needle, directly into the aorta. The needle is inserted through the muscles of the lower back. Then an X ray is taken.

What will an aortogram show?

It will show the extent of arteriosclerosis in the aorta, the arteries to the kidneys, and the arteries going to the thighs and legs. It will also demonstrate the presence of an obstruction or aneurysm. A lumbar aortogram is essential before an arterial graft or other operation on the aorta is performed.

What is a phlebogram?

It is an X ray of a vein, performed by injecting an opaque dye into the veins prior to X ray.

Can defects in the blood vessels of the brain be demonstrated by X-ray examination?

In many instances. Recently, valuable information has been obtained from arteriograms of the blood vessels of the brain. A needle is placed into one of the main arteries of the neck and a dye is injected. An X ray is then taken. A clot, as well as an aneurysm, in a blood vessel of the brain can be demonstrated. Such tests are essential prior to undertaking surgery for a cerebral-blood-vessel defect.

Can X rays help diagnose a stroke?

Yes, especially if there has been a thrombosis.

Do X rays of the gallbladder and bile ducts give as much information about older people?

Yes. These tests can be performed safely and with the same results on people of all ages.

Can older people withstand the effects of X-ray treatments, cobalt radiation, etc., as well as younger people?

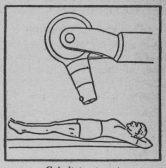

Cobalt treatment

Yes. The dosage may have to be modified in terms of the weight of the individual, but in general, older people tolerate these treatments satisfactorily.

Does the skin demand special attention when X-ray or cobalt treatments are given to older people?

Yes, because their skin is usually thinner and more fragile. Dosages of X ray may have to be reduced somewhat.

Can the radioactive isotopes be given safely to older people?

Yes.

What are some of the diseases affecting older people that may be relieved by treatment with radioactive isotopes?

1. Angina pectoris, the heart pain due to coronary artery insufficiency, can often be relieved by the administration of radioactive iodine.
2. Radioactive iodine will also help in cases of overactivity of the thyroid gland and in a small percentage of cases of cancer of the thyroid.
3. Radioactive phosphorus is sometimes helpful in the treatment of certain blood diseases, such as leukemia and polycythemia.
4. Radioactive gold, when implanted into the abdominal cavity, has been found to be helpful in delaying the progress of cancer of the ovaries.
5. Radioactive cobalt has been found to be helpful in delaying the progress of cancer of the urinary bladder.

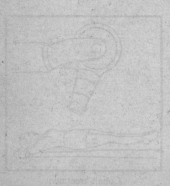

INDEX